D1287771

luisa y. Gan, MD
Dallas, TX
4-21-86

# DIAGNOSIS AND THERAPY OF CORONARY ARTERY DISEASE

# DIAGNOSIS
# AND THERAPY OF
# CORONARY ARTERY DISEASE
## Second Edition

*Edited by*

## PETER F. COHN, M.D.

Professor of Medicine and Chief, Cardiology Division
State University of New York Health Sciences Center
Stony Brook

Martinus Nijhoff Publishing

BOSTON   DORDRECHT   LANCASTER

**Library of Congress Cataloging in Publication Data**
Main entry under title:

Diagnosis and therapy of coronary artery disease.

Includes bibliographies and index.
1. Coronary heart disease. I. Cohn, Peter F.,
1939–     [DNLM: 1. Coronary Disease—diagnosis.
2. Coronary Disease—therapy. WG 300 D536]
RC685.C6D52 1985     616.1'23     84-22685
ISBN 0-89838-693-4

DISTRIBUTORS:

for North America

Kluwer Academic Publishers
190 Old Derby Street
Hingham, MA 02043

for all other countries

Kluwer Academic Publishers Group
Distribution Centre
P.O. Box 322
3300 AH Dordrecht
The Netherlands

*In memory of my parents, Archie and Clare*
*To my sons, Alan and Clifford*
*But most of all, to my wife, Joan, for whose*
*love and understanding my appreciation can*
*never be adequately expressed*

# CONTENTS

# CONTRIBUTING AUTHORS

Joseph S. Alpert, M.D.
Professor of Medicine
Chief, Division of Cardiovascular Medicine
University of Massachusetts Medical School
55 Lake Avenue North
Worcester, Massachusetts 01605, USA

J. Thomas Bigger, Jr., M.D.
Professor of Medicine and Pharmacology
Columbia University
College of Physicians and Surgeons
Department of Medicine
Cardiology Division
630 West 168th Street
New York, New York 10032, USA

Eugene Braunwald, M.D.
Hersey Professor of the
Theory and Practice of Physic (Medicine)
Hermann Ludwig Blumgart Professor of Medicine
Harvard Medical School
Chairman, Joint Department of Medicine
Physician-in-Chief
Brigham and Beth Israel Hospitals
75 Francis Street
Boston, Massachusetts 02115, USA

Robert A. Bruce, M.D.
Professor of Medicine
Department of Medicine
Division of Cardiology
University of Washington School of Medicine,
RG-22
Seattle, Washington 98195, USA

Kanu Chatterjee, M.B., F.R.C.P.
Lucie Stern Professor of Cardiology
Associate Chief, Cardiovascular Division
Department of Medicine, Room 1186
University of California at San Francisco
School of Medicine
San Francisco, California 94143, USA

Joan Kirschenbaum Cohn, M.S.W.
Instructor in Pediatrics
State University of New York
Health Sciences Center
Stony Brook, New York 11794, USA

Lawrence H. Cohn, M.D.
Professor of Surgery
Harvard Medical School

Surgeon
Brigham & Women's Hospital
75 Francis Street
Boston, Massachusetts 02115, USA

Peter F. Cohn, M.D.
Professor of Medicine
Chief, Cardiology Division
State University of New York
Health Sciences Center, T-17-020
Stony Brook, New York 11794, USA

John J. Collins, Jr., M.D.
Professor of Surgery
Harvard Medical School
Chief, Division of Thoracic and Cardiac Surgery
Brigham & Women's Hospital
75 Francis Street
Boston, Massachusetts 02115, USA

David A. Cox, M.D.
Fellow, Cardiology Division
Harvard Medical School
Brigham & Women's Hospital
75 Francis Street
Boston, Massachusetts 02115, USA

R. Curtis Ellison, M.D.
Professor of Medicine and Pediatrics
University of Massachusetts Medical School
55 Lake Avenue North
Worcester, Massachusetts 01605, USA

Sheldon Goldberg, M.D.
Professor of Medicine
Director, Cardiac Catheterization Laboratory
Thomas Jefferson University Hospital
Fifth Floor, Room 5611-D
New Hospital Building
Philadelphia, Pennsylvania 19107, USA

Thomas B. Graboys, M.D.
Assistant Professor of Medicine
Havard Medical School
Brigham & Women's Hospital
Director, Clinical Services, Lown Cardiovascular Laboratory
Richardson Fuller Building Harvard University
School of Public Health
221 Longwood Avenue
Boston, Massachusetts 02115, USA

Herman K. Hellerstein, M.D.
Professor of Medicine
Case Western Reserve University School of Medicine
Head, Cardiology Outpatient Department
Physician, University Hospitals of Cleveland
Cleveland, Ohio 44106, USA

L. David Hillis, M.D.
Associate Professor of Internal Medicine
Director, Cardiac Catheterization Laboratory
University of Texas
Health Science Center at Dallas
5323 Harry Hines Boulevard
Dallas, Texas 75235, USA

William B. Kannel, M.D.
Professor of Medicine
Chief, Section of Preventive Medicine and Epidemiology
Department of Medicine and
Evans Memorial Department of Clinical Research
Boston University School of Medicine
720 Harrison Avenue
Suite 1105
Boston, Massachusetts 02118, USA

William E. Lawson, M.D.
Instructor in Medicine
Director, Echocardiographic Laboratories
State University of New York
Health Sciences Center, T-17-020
Stony Brook, New York 11794, USA

Edward B. Leahey Jr. M.D. (deceased)
Instructor in Medicine
Columbia University College of Physicians & Surgeons
630 West 168th St.
New York, New York 10032 USA

William W. Parmley, M.D.
Professor of Medicine
Chief, Cardiovascular Division
University of California at San Francisco
School of Medicine
San Francisco, California 94143, USA

Claire E. Proctor, R.D.M.S.
Senior Echocardiographic Technician
Echocardiographic Laboratories
State University of New York
Health Sciences Center, T-17-020
Stony Brook, New York 11794, USA

James A. Reiffel, M.D.
Associate Professor of Clinical Medicine
Department of Medicine
Cardiology Division
Columbia University
College of Physicians and Surgeons
630 West 168th Street
New York, New York 10032, USA

Richard J. Shemin, M.D.
Assistant Professor of Surgery
Harvard Medical School
Brigham & Women's Hospital
75 Francis Street
Boston, Massachusetts 02115, USA

Robert Soufer, M.D.
Fellow, Cardiology Section
Yale University School of Medicine
333 Cedar Street, 87 LMP
Post Office Box 3333
New Haven, Connecticut 06510, USA

Joseph Stokes, III, M.D.
Professor of Medicine
Section of Preventive Medicine and Epidemiology
Department of Medicine and
Evans Memorial Department of Clinical Research
Boston University School of Medicine
720 Harrison Avenue
Suite 1105
Boston, Massachusetts 02118, USA

Stephen F. Vatner, M.D.
Associate Professor of Medicine
Harvard Medical School
Brigham & Women's Hospital
Director
New England Regional Primate Center
One Pine Hill Drive
Southboro, Massachusetts 01772, USA

Pantel S. Vokonas, M.D.
Associate Professor of Medicine and Public Health
Boston University School of Medicine
720 Harrison Avenue
Boston, Massachusetts 02118, USA

Barry L. Zaret, M.D.
Professor of Medicine and Diagnostic Radiology
Chief, Cardiology Section
Yale University School of Medicine
333 Cedar Street, 87 LMP
Post Office Box 3333
New Haven, Connecticut 06510, USA

# PREFACE TO THE FIRST EDITION

Because the increasing complexities of diagnosing and treating coronary artery disease are at times overwhelming for many physicians, the purpose of this book is to bring together in one comprehensive yet reasonably concise text a scholarly but clinically oriented analysis of the major aspects of coronary artery disease.

The book is mainly intended for internists and clinical cardiologists as well as for those in training for these respective disciplines, but it should also be of interest to primary care physicians responsible for the management of patients with coronary artery disease. Each of the contributors—whether cardiologist, radiologist, or surgeon—has been selected for his special interest or experience in the respective topic. Since some prefer the terms coronary heart disease or atherosclerotic heart disease, they are considered synonymous with coronary artery disease for purposes of this text.

Current controversies in coronary artery disease are noted in an introductory section, and the book is then organized into two parts. Part I deals with diagnosis and evaluation and part II with prevention and therapy of coronary artery disease. Obviously, these areas cannot be—nor should they be—totally divorced from one another. Furthermore, several subjects (exercise testing and training, for example) are of necessity discussed in more than one chapter with appropriate cross referencing. Special attention has been directed at making the references as current as possible. Since the aim of the book is to do more than just update the concepts, the reader is also informed of the pertinent controversies in the field. The word controversy is used in its most liberal form, so as to include areas of disagreement or of uncertainty as well as changes in traditional views. Each of the contributors has been asked to identify specifically the most important of the controversies in his particular area of interest and to address himself to these issues in the course of the chapter.

This book grew out of clinical and research experiences shared with many staff members and trainees of the Cardiovascular Division, Department of Medicine, Peter Bent Brigham Hospital. For their inspiration and assistance I am especially grateful. I would also like to acknowledge the superb administrative and secretarial help provided by Adele Slatko and the editorial skills of Lin Richter and her staff at Little, Brown and Company. A special word of thanks to members of my family and my wife's family for their continuing encouragement in the preparation of this book.

# PREFACE TO THE SECOND EDITION

The main goal of this book remains the same as it did in the first edition in 1979: to provide a comprehensive yet reasonably concise monograph on coronary artery disease with as many current (1980-84) references as possible. To allow new information to be added while keeping the book at the same size as the first edition, several changes in the format of the book have been made. There are now three parts, rather than two, and several chapters have been merged. Thus, there is now one chapter on management of angina, rather than two, and one chapter on therapy of acute myocardial infarction and its complications (including the use of hemodynamic monitoring), rather than three.

Two totally new chapters have been added, one dealing with effects of ischemia in the experimental animal (by physiologists) and one dealing with the psychosocial aspects of coronary artery disease (by a clinical social worker). These chapters emphasize the important contributions that other disciplines can bring to the modern physician dealing with coronary artery disease.

I wish to thank Jeffrey Smith and his staff at Martinus Nijhoff for their editorial assistance in the preparation of this edition. Marlene Landesman was also particularly helpful in the preparation of this edition, and her secretarial assistance is gratefully acknowledged.

# INTRODUCTION: CONTROVERSIES IN CORONARY ARTERY DISEASE

Eugene Braunwald

Coronary artery disease is now the great scourge of the human population in industrial nations. Indeed, in 1969 the Executive Board of the World Health Organization pointed out that "coronary heart disease has reached enormous proportions . . . [and] will result in coming years in the greatest epidemic mankind has faced unless we are able to reverse the trend by concentrated research into its cause and prevention." Not unlike some of the earlier great scourges—bubonic plague, yellow fever, and smallpox—coronary artery disease suddenly strikes down a significant percentage of the population. It also causes prolonged suffering, disability, and eventually, death in an even larger number. Consider, for a moment, the enormity of the problem. In the United States alone coronary artery disease is responsible for almost 700,000 deaths per year, more than one-third of all deaths; and more than 1.2 million persons with coronary artery disease are hospitalized annually. The costs of this disease in human suffering are incalculable. The direct annual costs are approximately $20 billion; the indirect annual costs have been estimated at $10 billion. The value of future earnings, if death had not occurred, is difficult to estimate but amounts conservatively to another $30 billion!

The principal clinical manifestations of coronary artery disease are sudden death, myocardial infarction, angina pectoris, and chronic congestive heart failure. Although the association between angina pectoris and narrowing of the coronary arteries has been accepted for two hundred years, it is curious that the causes of the two more dramatic manifestations—acute myocardial infarction and sudden death—have become appreciated only during this century.

## Risk Factors

It is now well established that the appearance of any of the clinical manifestations of coronary artery disease signifies that the disease is already far advanced, yet the condition must be *prevented,* as well as treated, if we are to exert a favorable impact from the public health point of view. The risk of developing coronary artery disease is not identical in all individuals, and it is possible to identify a series of traits, conditions, and habits characteristic of individuals at particularly high risk. On the other hand, there is considerable controversy about whether a concerted reduction in the three most important risk factors—hypertension, cigarette smoking, and hypercholesterolemia—will, in fact, materially reduce the incidence of coronary artery disease. Even if it does, a key question remains. If the given risk factor has been present for a long period of time—say, 30 years—can a much shorter period, during which the factor has been reduced or even eliminated, be expected to counteract the longer, earlier period? This question is of enormous importance. Indeed, the National Heart, Lung and Blood Institute has carried out a major study to settle this issue by means of the Multiple Risk Factors Intervention Trial, but unfortunately without a conclusive result.

To examine a narrower issue—the lipid theory of the etiology of atherosclerosis—it is possible to recognize individuals whose concentrations of both serum cholesterol and low-density lipoprotein cholesterol are distinctly elevated and whose risk for developing coronary artery disease is greatly increased. It is also possible to show that experimentally produced atherosclerotic lesions in animals fed high levels of cholesterol can regress following dietary manipulations. However, it is important to remember that human atherosclerotic lesions develop differently from those in experimentally induced atherosclerosis in animals and that there is controversy concerning the extent to which the findings of regression in animals can be transferred to man. Also, while it now seems clear that high-density lipoprotein cholesterol may exert a protective effect on the development of atherosclerosis, we do not know how to intervene and increase the concentration of this important serum fraction.

It is generally agreed that the risk factors can be identified early in life and that many individuals have pathologic evidence of coronary artery disease by the age of 25. Yet the desirability of screening all infants and children for coronary risk factors and attempts to reverse these risk factors early in life remain controversial. In addition to the three well-established risk factors mentioned above, associations have also been demonstrated among the incidence of coronary artery disease and physical inactivity, obesity, hyperuricemia, excessive intake of coffee, high consumption of sucrose and glucose, absence of fiber in the diet, "softness" of drinking water, as well as the so-called coronary-prone behavior patterns: social mobility and status incongruity.

## The Atherosclerotic Plaque

The structure and composition of the atherosclerotic plaque are well defined, but there is considerable debate concerning the genesis of the lesion. Specifically, is the fatty streak commonly found at autopsy in young adults the precursor of the more complex atherosclerotic plaque? What are the roles of adhesion and aggregation of platelets to the endothelium in the genesis of atherosclerosis? How valid is the monoclonal hypothesis, which suggests that atherosclerosis results from the proliferation of a single clone of smooth muscle cells? The answers to these questions obviously have far-reaching implications concerning the prevention of coronary artery disease.

## Acute Myocardial Infarction

Thrombi are frequently found at postmortem in persons with coronary artery disease who died of acute transmural myocardial infarction. Generally the larger the infarction, the worse the prognosis; and it is becoming widely accepted that a variety of therapeutic approaches can reduce extensive myocardial ischemic injury in experimental animals. How this information should be applied to clinical practice remains an issue. First of all, we need to demonstrate unambiguously that the interventions useful in reducing infarct size in experimental animals exert the same effect in humans and that they do improve ventricular function or prognosis, or both. Although debate also persists concerning the many other aspects of the care of patients with acute myocardial infarction, that is, the use of anticoagulants, cardiac glycosides, and other inotropic agents, it appears that patients with uncomplicated infarcts can be discharged from the hospital relatively early—7 to 10 days after infarction—and some question whether these patients really benefit from care in a coronary care unit or even require hospitalization at all.

While the Swan-Ganz catheter can be used readily for measuring cardiac dynamics in acute myocardial infarction and while there is agreement that this technique is essential for the management of patients with complicated infarcts, there is considerable controversy concerning the indications for its use among patients with uncomplicated infarcts or those receiving standard pharmacologic therapy. It is widely accepted that intra-aortic balloon counterpulsation can improve the hemodynamics of patients with acute myocardial infarction with pump failure, and while it may be particularly helpful in patients who need to undergo left heart catheterization and coronary arteriography, there is no agreement concerning the ability of this mode of therapy to improve the long-term prognosis. In addition, while it is feasible to carry out coronary artery bypass grafting in patients with acute myocardial infarction and left ventricular pump failure, there is serious controversy as to the effect this radical form of therapy has on prognosis. By contrast, the advent of intracoronary thrombolysis has proved to be an exciting new form of therapy for acute myocardial infarction.

The majority of patients who survive acute myocardial infarction can be rehabilitated to reasonable functional status in society. However, the value, if any, of complex psychotherapeutic and physical exercise training programs remains controversial. And though active participation in a comprehensive rehabilitation program may improve patient motivation and perhaps the quality of life, what is the mechanism responsible for this improvement? Is it largely a placebo effect? Or are there truly beneficial changes in cardiac function, coronary collateral flow, and severity of atherosclerotic lesions?

## Arrhythmias

The enormous importance of a variety of arrhythmias in acute myocardial infarction is widely appreciated, and there is agreement that these arrhythmias can be treated effectively. However, there is controversy concerning the value of prophylactic use of antiarrhythmic drugs and, in particular, what type of prophylactic antiarrhythmic therapy is indicated in the prehospital phase of acute myocardial infarction. There is agreement that myocardial ischemia may cause ventricular tachyarrhythmias, but there is controversy concerning the mechanism of these tachyarrhythmias. Are they caused by reentry, by enhanced automaticity, or by both? The role of invasive electrophysiologic testing is still controversial, though its advocates now probably outnumber its opponents.

While it is now widely recognized that frequent and complex ventricular premature contractions in patients who have recently suffered a myocardial infarction signal the increased risk of sudden death, and while a variety of antiarrhythmic agents that can reduce the frequency of these premature contractions are available, the protective value of a reduction in premature contractions is not known. Some $\beta$-adrenergic blocking agents improve the prognosis of patients who have recovered from the acute phase of myocardial infarction, but the application of this knowledge remains controversial. Which patients will benefit most? How long will the reported benefits persist?

## Noninvasive Testing

It is now possible to recognize areas of diminished myocardial perfusion and acute myocardial infarction by means of a variety of radionuclide imaging techniques, but the specific indications for "hot spot" and "cold spot" imaging and analysis of ventricular wall motion by radionuclide angiography have not been resolved. These techniques provide fascinating new information, but their clinical value in coronary artery disease has not been clearly established. Can these procedures be applied widely as screening tests in patients with suspected coronary disease and in the follow-up of patients with known disease? Though we have learned how to standardize exercise electrocardiographic tests, to perform them safely and rapidly, and to compare the results obtained with the findings in normal persons, we do not know the precise indications for exercise testing. In whom should these tests be carried out? How should the results be interpreted? For example, there is considerable difference of opinion as to the desirability of carrying out exercise tests in asymptomatic individuals with known risk factors for coronary artery disease and whether these individuals should be followed up by coronary arteriography if the results are positive.

While M-mode echocardiography is a simple (for the patient) noninvasive method for recording abnormalities of motion of the left ventricular wall secondary to coronary artery disease, there still is debate about the sensitivity and specificity of the method. It is appreciated that M-mode echocardiography samples and records the thickness and motion of only a selected segment of the left ventricle and that cross-sectional echocardiographic techniques examine a much larger portion of the ventricle; because of this, the role of two-dimensional or cross-sectional echocardiography in clinical practice is increasing.

## Coronary Arteriography and Hemodynamics

By means of coronary arteriography we know how to evaluate the anatomy of the coronary arterial bed with precision and at a low risk, thereby detecting coronary artery disease and determining its effect on left ventricular function by means of catheterization and left ventriculography. And there is agreement that these procedures should be carried out in most patients with severe angina pectoris, unstable angina, and recurrent angina following coronary bypass surgery. However, still at issue is whether or not coronary arteriography is indicated in patients with mild angina pectoris, in asymptomatic or mildly symptomatic patients who have suffered a myocardial infarction, in patients who have unexplained ventricular failure and ventricular arrhythmias, and in those with clearly atypical chest pain.

Though we recognize that angina pectoris can occur in patients with normal coronary arteriograms and that the prognosis in these patients if often quite favorable, we do not know the etiology of the syndrome or how to recognize it without coronary arteriography; nor do we know how to treat it. And while we know that coronary spasm can occur in the course of coronary arteriography and in patients with variant angina, we now know that the role of a spasm in the usual forms of stable and unstable angina pectoris and perhaps even myocardial infarction is more important than previously realized.

We have learned to recognize angina pectoris in most patients in whom the condition occurs and we know that asymptomatic myocardial ischemia occurs in large numbers of patients with coronary artery disease. However, we do not know why myocardial ischemia is so frequently silent, we have not developed a strategy for its detection, and we do not apreciate the clinical significance of asymptomatic myocardial ischemia.

In coronary artery disease, ventricular end-diastolic pressure and, hence, left atrial and pulmonary capillary pressure rise during ischemia, but what is the mechanism of these pressure elevations? Are they due to transient left ventricular failure, reduced ventricular compliance, or both? We agree that the contractile reserve of the ischemic ventricle can be evaluated by means of the newer techniques of intervention ventriculography, but the value of these studies in patient care remains controversial.

## Coronary Artery Surgery

Probably no aspect of coronary artery disease is now more intensely controversial than the treatment of angina pectoris, both stable and unstable. There is agreement that coronary artery bypass grafting can result in striking symptomatic benefit in a large majority of patients, but the mechanism by which it accomplishes this benefit is not completely clear. There is evidence that at least in some patients it is related to more than simply improving the perfusion of the previously ischemic myocardium. But the real area of controversy concerns the effects of surgical treatment on longevity. Because of several multicenter studies, there is little argument that coronary artery bypass grafting will improve the prognosis in patients with obstructive disease of the left main coronary artery, but there is a great deal of debate concerning the effects of this operation on longevity in patients with other anatomic forms of coronary artery disease. The manner in which age, a history of previous myocardial infarction, left ventricular size and function, and the specific distribution of coronary obstructive lesions modifies the effect of myocardial revascularization on survival is not clear. Nor is it clear how much impact coronary angioplasty will have in reducing the number of patients referred for surgical revascularization.

## Summary

It will be evident to the reader of this book that as a result of considerable effort, and despite major gaps in our knowledge, we have learned a great deal about the etiology, pathogenesis, clinical manifestations, diagnosis, and treatment of coronary artery disease. What do we now have to show for this increased information? Almost miraculously, the frightening and previously inexorable rise in the mortality consequent to this disease has been stopped and has been reversed. Thus, mortality secondary to coronary artery disease has declined by approximately 20 percent in the United States during the past decade. However, the mechanism responsible for this welcome change is not clear. Is it related to (1) an alteration in diet? (2) the reduction in the number of cigarettes smoked by individuals in high-risk groups? (3) the effective control of hypertension? (4) the present national emphasis on physical fitness? (5) improvements in the treatment of acute myocardial infarction, congestive heart failure, and other manifestations and complications of coronary artery disease? (6) a combination of some or all of these factors? or to (7) an as yet unrecognized influence?

Dr. Cohn and his contributors have rendered conspicuous service to patients with coronary artery disease and to the physicians who treat them by effectively summarizing our current knowledge, by pointing out areas of controversy, and by identifying areas of ignorance concerning the most serious life-threatening illness in the industrialized world.

# I. PATHOGENESIS AND PATHOPHYSIOLOGY OF CORONARY ARTERY DISEASE

# 1. EFFECTS OF MYOCARDIAL ISCHEMIA ON REGIONAL MYOCARDIAL FUNCTION IN THE EXPERIMENTAL ANIMAL

David A. Cox

Stephen F. Vatner

The most important aspect of myocardial ischemia is its effect on myocardial mechanical function. For centuries there has been an interest in the effects of coronary artery occlusion on the heart [1]. By the late nineteenth century, it was appreciated that coronary artery occlusion induced a fall in arterial pressure [2], but quantitative measurements of the effects of ischemia on contraction were first described in 1935 by Tennant and Wiggers [3]. One of the goals of this chapter is to review the merits and limitations of various experimental techniques for measurement of regional myocardial function in ischemia. Another is to discuss the effects of ischemia on myocardial contraction immediately after the onset of ischemia, during the steady-state and with chronic ischemia and infarction. Finally, we will examine the reversibility of derangements in myocardial function with reperfusion after brief coronary artery occlusions insufficient to induce infarction and after occlusions of up to several hours duration.

## Experimental Techniques

In 1935 Tennant and Wiggers [3] first documented, in anesthetized, open-chest dogs, systolic expansion of myocardium in the ischemic region of the left ventricle in a quantitative man-

ner by means of an optical myograph with the myograph arms sutured to the epicardial surface. Since the early work of Tennant and Wiggers, investigators have employed a number of techniques to measure various indices of regional function in ischemic and normally perfused myocardium. Some of these techniques, including motion pictures of the beating heart [4, 5] and high-speed cineradiography of metal clips attached across the wall with a flexible band to measure epicardial segment length and wall thickness, have been applied only to anesthetized, open-chest animals [6]. Regional function has also been measured in open-chest animals with isometric force gauges [7–9], epicardial dimension gauges [9–11], and wall thickness gauges [12, 13], all of which result in some distortion of wall motion because of varying degrees of tethering of the myocardium and the measuring device.

The development of miniature ultrasonic transducers has allowed the measurement of regional segment length and wall thickness in anesthetized, open-chest animals [14–17] and conscious animals [18–21]. These devices are imbedded in the left ventricular wall, where they are able to move freely with the surrounding myocardium without exerting tension, providing a more physiological measurement of regional function. Arrays of crystal pairs can be used to measure myocardial function over a sizable region of the left ventricle [18, 20, 22] (figure 1–1). Echocardiography has been used for measurement of regional function in anes-

The work in this chapter is supported in part by USPHS grants HL33065 and HL26215.

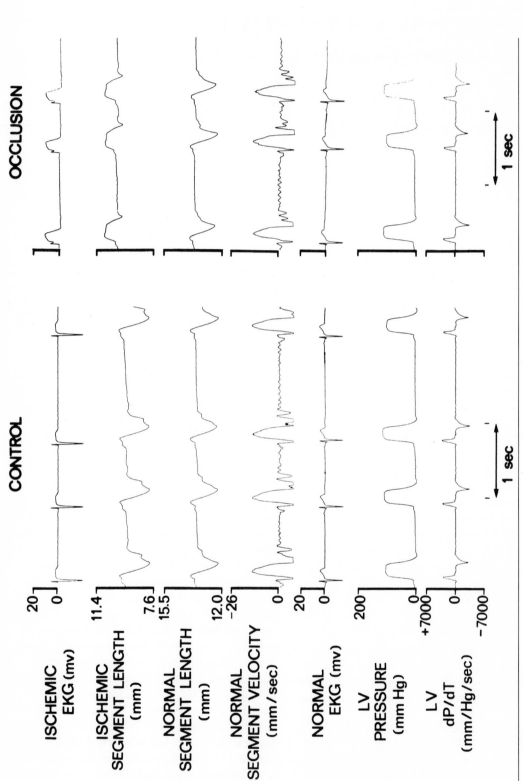

FIGURE 1–1. The effects of an occlusion of the left anterior descending coronary artery are shown on regional segment length and electrograms in the normal and ischemic zones along with LV pressure, dP/dt, and velocity of segment length shortening in the normal zone. During occlusion paradoxical bulging developed in the ischemic zone along with substantial ST segment elevation, while regional function in the normal zone remained essentially constant and no ST segment elevation was observed. (From Heyndrickx, G.R. et al. *The Journal of Clinical Investigation* 56:978, 1975. Reprinted with permission.)

thetized, open-chest [23–25] and closed-chest [26, 27] animals. This offers the potential advantage of noninvasive measurement, but M-mode echocardiography is limited to measurement of wall motion of the posterior wall and septum. Two-dimensional echocardiography allows analysis of larger regions of the left ventricle and can measure wall thickening or radial wall motion at the endocardial surface, but identification of the endocardial surface can be difficult [28]. Cardiac rotation can present difficulties with M-mode and two-dimensional echocardiography, though epicardial markers have been employed as reference points in some experimental studies to minimize this problem [27].

An important concern in any measurement of regional myocardial function is the precise location and orientation of the measuring device in the ventricular wall. One factor is the relationship of the measurement site to the lateral ischemic border. Several studies have provided evidence for an abrupt transition between ischemic and nonischemic tissue [29–31]. In a study of conscious dogs [32], our laboratory implanted pairs of ultrasonic transducers subendocardially such that they subtended adjacent zones of intense ischemia and relatively normal perfusion. These segments of myocardium behaved, in functional terms, almost identically to homogeneously ischemic segments, exhibiting severe reductions in systolic shortening. Thus, inadvertent placement of transducers in zones of heterogeneous perfusion could lead to erroneous interpretation of depressed or absent myocardial function.

Streeter et al. [33] studied fiber orientation in the canine left ventricle and found that fiber angles varied from about 60 degrees from the circumferential at the endocardial surface to about −60 degrees at the epicardial surface, with the midwall fibers oriented approximately circumferentially. Two studies [17, 34] have examined the subepicardial response to subendocardial ischemia using circumferentially oriented pairs of ultrasonic crystals in the epicardium. Under conditions with subendocardial ischemia and maintained subepicardial blood flow, subepicardial segment shortening was severely impaired, correlating with subendocardial blood flow. Under these same condi-

tions, however, Gallagher et al. [17] found that subepicardial segment shortening was maintained in segments, with the crystal pairs parallel to the epicardial surface fibers (approximately, 50 degrees from the circumferential axis) as long as flow remained normal in the outer wall. Thus, measurements of epicardial shortening depend critically on the orientation of the transducers. Whether measurement of shortening in endocardial layers depends strongly on transducer orientation remains an open question.

## Early Adjustments to Regional Ischemia

Brief periods of acute myocardial ischemia induce complex dynamic changes in regional myocardial performance (figure 1–2). Following abrupt occlusion of a coronary artery, the earliest observed change in severely ischemic segments is a small late systolic lengthening, beginning within a few beats after the onset of ischemia [15, 35–39], presumably as the result of a diminished duration of contraction with hypoxia [37, 40]. A progressive reduction in the duration and extent of shortening occurs until there is a paradoxical holosystolic lengthening of the ischemic segment by 30 to 60 seconds after occlusion [15, 35, 38, 39], which persists as long as the occlusion is maintained. These changes are associated with an increase in end-diastolic length of the ischemic segment (15, 35, 38, 39). The decline in the velocity of segment shortening lags several seconds behind the decline in shortening, not being manifested up to 10 to 15 seconds after the onset of ischemia, when shortening is already reduced [38]. This is consistent with experiments in isolated isometric papillary muscle, which showed that the rate of force generated was less sensitive to hypoxia than the amount of force generated [41].

Pressure-length loops instantaneously plotting left ventricular pressure and epicardial [36, 37] or subendocardial [35, 38] segment length have been used to provide an index of regional myocardial work. As a first approximation, left ventricular pressure varies with stress except late in the ejection period [42], and the changes in length and strain are proportional. Therefore, the integral of pressure with respect to length is approximately proportional to the integral of

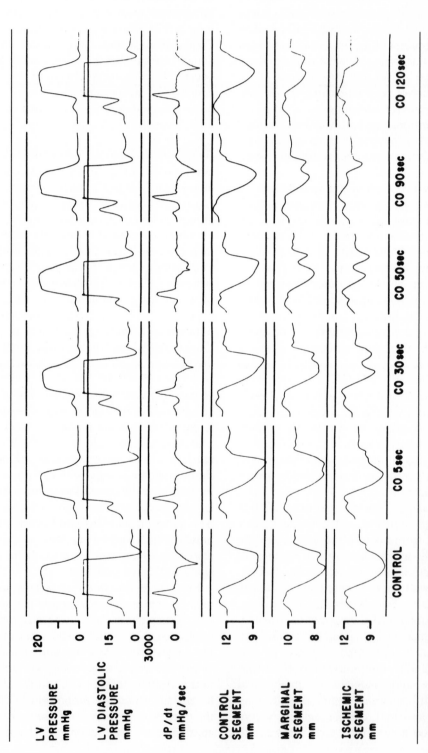

FIGURE 1-2. The progression of changes during acute coronary occlusion (CO) are illustrated by selected beats displayed at rapid paper speed. The control segment shows an initial increase in the extent of shortening, which was no longer evident at 120 seconds. In the ischemic segment there is an early abbreviation of the extent and duration of active shortening at 5 seconds and complete loss of systolic shortening at 90 seconds. (From Theroux, P. et al. Regional myocardial function in the conscious dog during acute coronary occlusion and responses to morphine, propranolol, nitroglycerin, and lidocaine. *Circulation* 53:302, 1976. Reproduced by permission of the American Heart Association, Inc.)

stress with respect to strain, and the area enclosed by this loop over one cardiac cycle thus reflects work during that cycle [36]. Within seconds after the onset of regional ischemia, the area of the pressure—length loop of the ischemic segment is reduced as a result of the late systolic lengthening [35–38], and the area can be markedly reduced even before overall systolic shortening is significantly reduced [38]. With the further reduction in shortening during the ejection phase, the loop assumes a crescent shape with an area approaching zero, a reduction significantly greater than expected from the reduction in shortening [38] (figure 1–3). Within 30 seconds of the onset of profound ischemia the segment exhibits holosystolic lengthening with the development of a clockwise pressure-length loop [35–37] (as opposed to the normal counterclockwise loop), implying that mechanical energy is being dissipated into the ischemic segment.

The effects of acute myocardial ischemia on measurements of regional segment shortening and systolic wall thickening have been compared [19, 38]. Changes in systolic wall thickening paralleled changes in segment shortening; as the extent and velocity of systolic shortening diminished, the degree and velocity of wall thickening decreased proportionally. By 30 to 60 seconds after coronary artery occlusion, when systolic shortening was replaced by holosystolic bulging, systolic wall thinning was observed.

Early changes in systolic function have been examined in the "border zone" of intermediate dysfunction surrounding the severely ischemic zone [15, 35], though it has been acknowledged that a heterogeneous mixture of ischemic and nonischemic cells may be subtended by the transducers in this region [35]. In these marginal segments, within seconds of the onset of ischemia, shortening during ventricular ejection decreased and the segments lengthened during late systole as ventricular pressure fell [15, 35]. After 2 minutes of ischemia the contraction pattern stabilized with intermediate (40 to 50 percent) reductions in shortening, velocity of shortening, and segment work (derived from pressure-length loops).

In nonischemic myocardial segments remote from the ischemic segments in anesthetized,

open-chest [15] and conscious dogs [35, 39], within a few seconds of the onset of regional ischemia a significant increase in shortening (up to 35 percent) occurred without a significant change in end-diastolic length in these segments. It is felt that the late systolic bulging of the ischemic zone seen at this time may serve to reduce the net afterload on the nonischemic myocardium and facilitate its shortening. Beyond the first few seconds the effects of ischemia on the normal myocardium are controversial. Theroux et al. [15] showed in anesthetized, open-chest dogs that the end-diastolic dimensions and contractility in the normal zones increased after the first 15 seconds, and the increased contractility was attributed to the Frank-Starling mechanism. Other studies of conscious dogs by the same group [35] found much smaller increases in contractility. In contrast, Wyatt et al. [43] noted a deterioration in function in the normal zone. Data from our laboratory [18] indicated that the behavior of the nonischemic zone varied but that increases in shortening were generally completely offset by the effects of heart rate, which reduces the extent of shortening. Thus, in situations where heart rate does not increase in response to acute myocardial ischemia, i.e., in the anesthetized, open-chest animal, larger increases in the extent of shortening in the nonischemic zone would be predicted. Another situation in which heart rate does not rise as much with myocardial ischemia occurs in the presence of cardiac denervation. Under these conditions acute myocardial ischemia utilized the Frank-Starling mechanism to a greater extent in the nonischemic zone [44].

In addition to the changes in systolic function induced by ischemia, significant changes occur in diastolic function. Changes in left ventricular relaxation are seen within seconds of the onset of ischemia in conscious dogs [39]. By 5 seconds after occlusion, ischemic segments exhibited late systolic lengthening, as mentioned earlier, and early diastolic shortening. Late systolic shortening was observed in nonischemic segments. These dysynchronous systolic and early diastolic events interrupted the fall of left ventricular pressure during isovolumic relaxation, causing a decrease in the absolute magnitude of peak negative left ventricular dP/dt of the first derivative

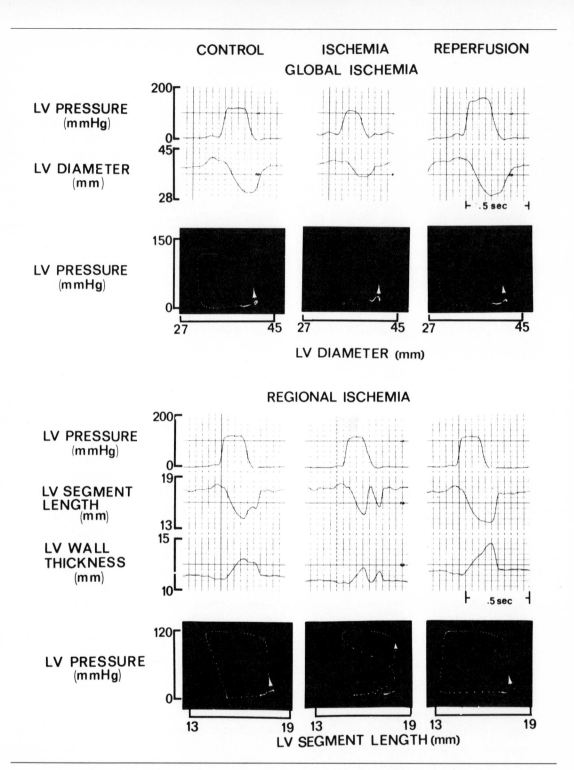

FIGURE 1–3. The effects of ischemia (middle panels) and reperfusion (right panels) are shown on LV pressure, dimensions, and pressure-length loops in an experiment of global ischemia induced by constriction of the left main coronary artery (top) and regional ischemia induced by complete occlusion of the left circumflex coronary artery (bottom). In both cases, ischemia reduced work substantially and was followed by an overshoot during reperfusion. Note that the shape of pressure-dimension loop was altered strikingly in regional but not in global ischemia. (From Pagani, M. et al. Initial myocardial adjustments to brief periods of ischemia and reperfusion in the conscious dog. *Circulation Research* 43:83, 1978. Reproduced by permission of the American Heart Association, Inc.)

of left ventricular pressure with respect to time. By 30 to 60 seconds after occlusion, ischemic segments showed holosystolic bulging, and late systolic shortening was no longer seen in nonischemic segments, at which time peak negative left ventricular dP/dt returned to control. However, the time constant of left ventricular pressure fall remained prolonged, suggesting persistent impairment of relaxation [39].

## Steady-State Adjustments to Regional Ischemia

Within several minutes of the onset of regional myocardial ischemia in experimental animals, a steady-state is achieved in which there is little change in various indices of regional myocardial function for periods of 1 hour or more unless preexisting collateral vessels are available to perfuse the ischemic zone. While recovery of regional function secondary to opening of preformed collaterals is occasionally observed in the canine heart, it is not observed in the primate, where functional collateral vessels are not present.

A number of studies have examined the relationship between reductions of blood flow and function that are induced by coronary artery stenosis. One such study was carried out in our laboratory in conscious dogs with acute, graded levels of coronary stenosis [21]. Regional endocardial segment shortening was measured by the ultrasonic dimension technique and correlated with endocardial blood flow measured by the radioactive microsphere technique. The endocardium was chosen as the site for these measurements because myocardial ischemia tends to be most severe in subendocardial regions [45–47]. An excellent correlation between segment shortening and regional blood flow was obtained using an exponential function [figure 1–4]. Significant impairment in function was found with only 10 to 20 percent reductions in blood flow. Severe reduction in blood flow was required to reduce function completely. In segments exhibiting paradoxical systolic lengthening, blood flow fell by 95 percent from control levels, a significantly greater reduction than the 82 percent reduction in blood flow to akinetic segments. These data indicate that small reduc-

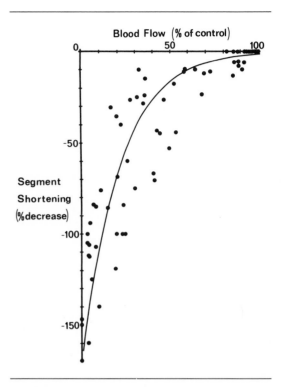

FIGURE 1–4. The curvilinear relationship between percentage of decreases in regional segment length (SL) shortening (ordinate) are plotted against decreases in regional myocardial blood flow (BF) as percentage of control. (From Vatner, S.F. Correlation between acute reductions in myocardial blood flow and function in conscious dogs. *Circulation Research* 47:201, 1980. Reproduced by permission of the American Heart Association, Inc.)

tions in blood flow can significantly impair function, but severe reductions in flow are required to eliminate shortening, indicating sensitive coupling between blood flow and endocardial segment shortening. Earlier studies in open-chest preparations used either less sensitive measures of regional myocardial function [48–50] or a less sensitive indicator of regional myocardial blood flow [48–51]. These latter studies measured coronary artery blood flow, which does not indicate only the change in blood flow to the endocardium of the central ischemic zone. Weintraub et al. [52] observed in anesthetized, open-chest dogs a sigmoidal relationship between regional blood flow measured with radioactive microspheres and endocardial segment length shortening, such that large reductions in blood flow were required to give significant reductions in shortening. In that study, however, heterogeneously perfused segments were not specifically excluded, thus potentially biasing the observed relationship between flow and function [32].

Measurements of epicardial segment shortening in anesthetized, open-chest dogs have been found to correlate poorly with epicardial blood flow measured by the radioactive microsphere technique [34, 52], but correlated rather closely with endocardial blood flow such that severe dysfunction was measured in epicardial layers with endocardial ischemia and normal epicardial blood flow, as often occurs with nonuniform transmural blood flow. Gallagher et al. [17] found that epicardial flow and function do not correlate when the epicardial dimension gauges are aligned circumferentially, in which case epicardial function correlates with endocardial blood flow, but do correlate when the epicardial dimension gauges are parallel to the epicardial surface fibers (approximately 50 degrees from the circumferential axis). Thus, measurements of epicardial shortening are highly dependent on transducer orientation.

The relationship of regional myocardial blood flow and function has also been studied with function expressed in terms of wall thickening measured with ultrasonic dimension crystals [16, 18, 51, 53] or by echocardiography [24]. Gallagher et al. [16], using open-chest dogs, related changes in blood flow induced by coronary stenosis in each of four myocardial layers to changes in wall thickening. They observed that a 77 percent reduction in systolic thickening occurred without significant decreases in the transmural blood flow, although blood flow in the inner half of the ventricular wall was reduced. Akinesis was observed with normal perfusion in the subepicardial quarter of the wall, but systolic thinning occurred only with transmural ischemia. Thus, subendocardial blood flow correlated significantly with wall thickening and better than did transmural blood flow.

In the above studies, regional myocardial blood flow and function were measured in the central ischemic zone with graded reductions in coronary blood flow. In other studies, myocar-

dial blood flow and function were measured in different regions of the left ventricle in the steady-state with severe regional ischemia after complete coronary artery occlusion. Function was measured in terms of endocardial segment shortening [45] and wall thickening [54], and measurements were made in regions with normal function in addition to hypokinetic and dyskinetic (or akinetic) areas of the left ventricle. In less than 5 minutes from the onset of ischemia, myocardial function in these regions had achieved a steady-state, which persisted for 1 to 4 hours. Regions with normal function had insignificant changes in endocardial blood flow with graded levels of depression of blood flow to hypokinetic and dyskinetic segments [45, 54]. As expected, ischemia was most severe in the subendocardial layers. It must be recognized that blood flow measured in hypokinetic regions at the border of the ischemic zone may represent the average of flow to a mixture of severely ischemic and nonischemic myocardium as opposed to tissue with homogeneously intermediate reductions in blood flow. Considerable controversy surrounds the question of the existence of a significant zone of intermediate ischemia surrounding the central ischemic zone. A number of studies have supported the concept of a zone of intermediate ischemia based on analysis of myocardial blood flow [55, 57]. However, analysis of tissue containing an admixture of ischemic and nonischemic myocardium would yield intermediate reductions in blood flow. Other studies, in which efforts were made to minimize or account for admixture of ischemic and nonischemic tissue, showed a sharp interface between ischemic and nonischemic tissue without a significant zone of intermediate ischemia [29–31]. Thus, it appears that under many conditions after acute coronary artery occlusion, normally perfused myocardium can exist adjacent to severely ischemic tissue. In a study of conscious dogs [32] our laboratory measured endocardial segment shortening in segments subtending severely ischemic and adjacent, normally perfused myocardium (figure 1–5). Surprisingly, rather than exhibiting a magnitude of segment shortening intermediate between that observed in ischemic and remote nonischemic myocardium, these segments exhibited severe

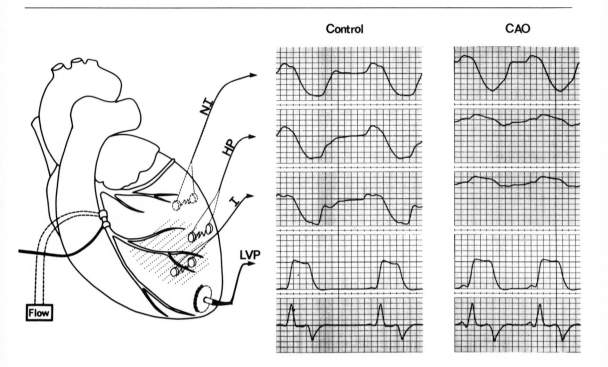

FIGURE 1-5. Techniques: A miniature pressure gauge was implanted in the left ventricle to measure pressure and dP/dt. A hydraulic occluder and flow probe were implanted on the left anterior descending or left circumflex coronary artery to occlude the vessel and to confirm the occlusion. Pairs of miniature ultrasonic crystals were implanted in the potentially ischemic (I) and nonischemic (NI) zones and subtending the border between the two zones to measure endocardial segment shortening. The tracings at the right show the effects of coronary artery occlusion (CAO) on segment shortening in nonischemic, heterogeneously perfused (HP), and ischemic segments and on measurements of left ventricular pressure (LVP) and LV dP/dt. Coronary artery occlusion eliminated active systolic shortening in ischemic segments and in heterogeneously perfused segments, while shortening in nonischemic segments did not change appreciably. (From Cox, D.A. and Vatner, S.F. Myocardial function in the areas of heterogeneous perfusion after coronary artery occlusion in conscious dogs. *Circulation* 66:1154, 1982. Reproduced by permission of the American Heart Association, Inc.)

dysfunction indistinguishable from that in homogeneously ischemic segments in the central ischemic zone. In homogeneously nonischemic segments adjacent to the ischemic zone, shortening was reduced by approximately 50 percent, supporting the concept that myocardial dysfunction extends beyond the ischemic zone. That is, there is a divergence in the expected close correlation between blood flow and function that occurs at the ischemic "border," with greater reductions in function than would be expected from measurement of myocardial blood flow. Abnormalities in function in zones adjacent to acutely ischemic or infarcted regions have been demonstrated in experimental animals by measurement of epicardial shortening

[58]; wall thickening by ultrasonic transducers [59], M-mode echocardiography [24] and two-dimensional echocardiography [25]; and radial wall motion by two-dimensional echocardiography [26, 25]. Though the reason for dysfunction extending beyond the ischemic zone is not known, several possibilities exist. One is that myocytes in these adjacent regions have biochemical derangements despite normal perfusion [60]. Persistent dysfunction after transient, early ischemia is possible as with the "stunned" myocardium [18, 61], but such transient ischemia has not been demonstrated experimentally. The most likely possibility is that "tethering" to adjacent dyskinetic myocardium or mechanical parallel resistance depresses the con-

tractile performance of the adjacent nonischemic tissue [24, 58, 62].

Utilizing two-dimensional echocardiographic techniques in anesthetized, closed-chest dogs, Weyman et al. [27] have shown that with acute myocardial ischemia the majority of dyskinetic radial segments exhibit their maximal systolic bulging in the first half of systole rather than at end-systole. In Weyman's study most of the segments that were dyskinetic in early systole were no longer dyskinetic at end-systole, though there were no data concerning the severity of ischemia in these different segments. They concluded that analyses of regional myocardial systolic function based solely on end-diastolic and end-systolic dimensions may underestimate the extent of myocardial dysfunction with ischemia. However, the question remains whether measurements of maximal systolic bulging correlate better with the degree of reduction in myocardial blood flow in a given ischemic segment than do the differences of end-diastolic and end-systolic dimensions.

Diastolic abnormalities are associated with acute myocardial ischemia and infarction in patients in terms of relaxation abnormalities [63–65], the dynamics of rapid filling [66, 67], and diminished ventricular compliance [63, 68–70]. A number of investigators have examined the regional myocardial diastolic properties contributing to these global changes. Hess and coworkers [71] examined the diastolic properties of the left ventricle during ischemia in the conscious dog. They found that with both partial and complete coronary occlusions the relaxation rate fell in ischemic segments but increased in nonischemic segments, indicating that global relaxation during ischemia represents a composite of varied regional patterns. In patients paced to angina, Bourdillon et al. [72] used M-mode echocardiography to demonstrate a slowed relaxation rate in ischemic myocardium. In patients with coronary artery disease examined angiographically [73], infarcted areas exhibited a relaxation rate paralleling the rate of decrease in pressure, but noninfarcted "ischemic" areas supplied by stenosed coronary arteries had a relaxation rate much slower than the rate of decrease in pressure. Pouleur et al. [73] concluded that the "ischemic" regions were responsible for the slower left ventriclar pressure fall. Hess et al. [71] also showed that with a partial coronary artery stenosis sufficient to decrease but not eliminate systolic wall thickening, myocardial wall stiffness remained normal. However, with complete coronary artery occlusion inducing systolic wall thinning, wall stiffness increased, leading them to conclude that systolic overstretch of the ischemic segments might account for the increased stiffness seen only with severe ischemia. Bourdillon et al. [72] demonstrated increased myocardial stiffness in ischemic myocardium, but this occurred in the absence of systolic wall thinning, arguing against systolic overstretch as the mechanism of increased wall stiffness. Whether the decreased rate of relaxation in ischemia contributes to impaired diastolic filling and decreased compliance is a subject of great controversy. Glantz and Parmley [74] have argued that the prolongations in the time constants for relaxation are small in comparison to the time to end-diastole and should result in negligible increases in diastolic wall stress. However, in anesthetized dogs, Mitchell et al. [75] and Weisfeldt et al. [76] demonstrated incomplete ventricular relaxation with ischemia, potentially retarding ventricular filling at high heart rates, and in one study in patients with ischemia during exercise, impaired relaxation persisted into the left ventricular filling phase [77]. Grossman and Barry [78] have proposed that there may be a persistence of cross-bridges in the ischemic myocardium throughout diastole, contributing to the resistance to filling and the upward shift in the left ventricular pressure-volume relationship. Pouleur et al. [73] argued that because the rate of decrease in local wall stress is slower than the rate of decline in pressure, any analysis based on rate of decline of pressure would underestimate the importance of relaxation abnormalities in later diastolic abnormalities.

## Chronic Adjustments to Regional Ischemia

Several studies have examined regional myocardial function over periods up to 4 weeks in conscious dogs with permanent coronary occlusion. Function has been measured in terms of endocardial segment shortening over a 4-week period [45, 79] and in terms of wall thickening over a 1-week period [20]. In those segments in the central ischemic zone, with the onset of ischemia, end-diastolic length increased significantly [45, 79] but by 4 weeks fell below the preocclusion length, presumably due to the retraction of tissue that occurs with scar formation as evidenced by the observed correlation between the decrease in end-diastolic segment length and the percentage of scar found on histological examination [79]. With coronary artery occlusion, segment length shortening in the central ischemic zone changed to paradoxical systolic bulging [45, 79] and systolic wall thickening changed to paradoxical thinning [20]. With time the systolic bulging and wall thinning in these segments became less pronounced. The paradoxical bulging was gradually replaced by akinesis after 4 weeks [45, 79], though no significant systolic shortening returned over this period. In "hypokinetic" or "marginal" segments located near the perimeter of the ischemic zone, with coronary artery occlusion end-diastolic length increased [45, 79] and end-diastolic wall thickness decreased [20]. This change persisted for several days, then began to diminish such that the end-diastolic length was significantly less than the preocclusion value by 3 to 4 weeks [45, 79]. Shortening [45, 79] and wall thickening [20] were, by definition, reduced to an intermediate degree after occlusion. Though Roan et al. [20] noted no significant change in systolic wall thickening in this region over the first week, with deterioration in some segments and improvement in others, other studies showed slight improvement in shortening over 3 to 4 weeks [45, 79], perhaps due to scarring of infarcted myocardium or hypertrophy of residual viable myocardium.

Shortly after occlusion, nonischemic segments exhibited an increase in end-diastolic length [45, 79] and a decrease in end-diastolic wall thickness [20], which persisted for 3 to 4 weeks [79]. In one study, shortening in this zone was enhanced and remained so for 3 to 4 weeks [79], but in others [20, 45] function did not significantly increase in the nonischemic zone.

In contrast to the acute changes in compliance of ischemic myocardium, Forrester et al. [80] found an increase in left ventricular compliance in the dog heart by 1 hour after myocardial infarction. As cellular infiltration and tissue edema occur over time, the infarcted segment progressively stiffens [81, 82] as soon as hours after the infarction. Within the first few weeks, the infarct can become virtually nondistensible as fibrosis develops. The physical model of Bogen et al. [62] predicts increases in left ventricular systolic function with increases in infarct stiffness up to a point, beyond which further increases in stiffness may retard diastolic filling so much as to counterbalance any further improvements in systolic function.

## Effects of Reperfusion

Coronary artery reperfusion during acute myocardial infarction has become an important clinical tool. Reperfusion is accomplished surgically by emergency coronary artery bypass grafting [83] and nonsurgically by angioplasty [84] and most commonly utilizing either intracoronary or intravenous thrombolytic therapy (see chapter 9). With this in mind, an important component of this discussion concerns the reversibility of the functional changes observed in ischemic myocardium. Coronary artery occlusions of less than 20 minutes duration in canine preparations do not result in myocardial necrosis [85, 86], but this does not necessarily mean that function in the ischemic region returns to normal levels after reperfusion. Studies by Banka et al. [9] and Puri [87] in anesthetized animals reported that epicardial shortening returned rapidly after release of occlusions up to 45 minutes in duration. Subsequent studies have generally shown that the time required for functional recovery of ischemic segments is directly proportional to the duration of the occlusion [18, 88–91]. In a study of conscious dogs by Heyndrickx et al. [18], in ischemic segments exhibiting paradoxical or absent motion during occlusion, reperfusion after 5 minutes of occlusion induced a gradual return of regional endocardial function over the next 6 hours (figure 1–6). End-diastolic segment length remained elevated and segment shortening and velocity of shortening were depressed at 2 hours and did not return to preocclusion levels until 6 hours after reperfusion. A 15-minute occlusion

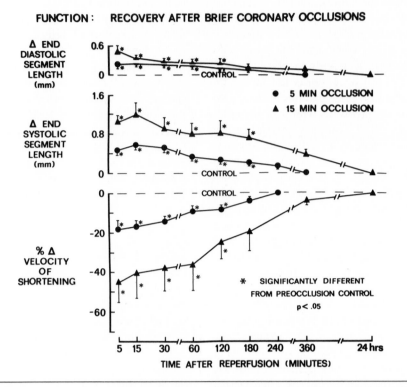

FIGURE 1–6. The prolonged recovery times for end-diastolic and end-systolic segment length and velocity of shortening after 5-minute (circles) and 15-minute (triangles) occlusions are compared. Recovery times from 5 minutes to 24 hours after reperfusion are shown. Values that were significantly different from control are shown by the asterisk (P < 0.01) and cross (P < 0.05). (From Heyndrickx, G.R. et al. *The Journal of Clinical Investigation* 56:978, 1975. Reprinted with permission.)

resulted in derangement of function measured in terms of segment shortening [18] and wall thickening [89], which was even greater and more prolonged, in some dogs returning to control levels only after 24 hours of reperfusion. Evidence exists for several potential mechanisms for this prolonged dysfunction after brief periods of ischemia, termed the "stunned myocardium" [61]. In one study, endocardial blood flow remained significantly depressed 3 hours after reperfusion, following a 15-minute occlusion in conscious dogs [89]. Another potential mechanism is impaired purine metabolism for prolonged periods of time after brief coronary artery occlusion [92–94].

Of interest is that with brief coronary artery occlusions a transient overshoot of regional function above preocclusion levels has been observed after reperfusion in anesthetized [7, 95] and in conscious animals [38]. With release of a 100-second occlusion this transient overshoot was characterized by increases in regional stroke work as reflected by the area of the pressure-length loop, as well as the extent and velocity of shortening [38]. The overshoot was not dependent on adrenergic mechanisms, but was prevented by inhibiting reactive hyperemia. When this restriction to reperfusion was released, the delayed reactive hyperemia was accompanied by a delayed overshoot in function (figure 1–7). With longer occlusions such an overshoot in regional function above preocclusion levels is not observed. During the first few minutes of reperfusion after a 15-minute occlusion, systolic segment shortening and wall thickening have been shown to be higher than that measured over the next few hours, paralleling the reactive hyperemic response [89, 96], but still slightly lower than preocclusion control.

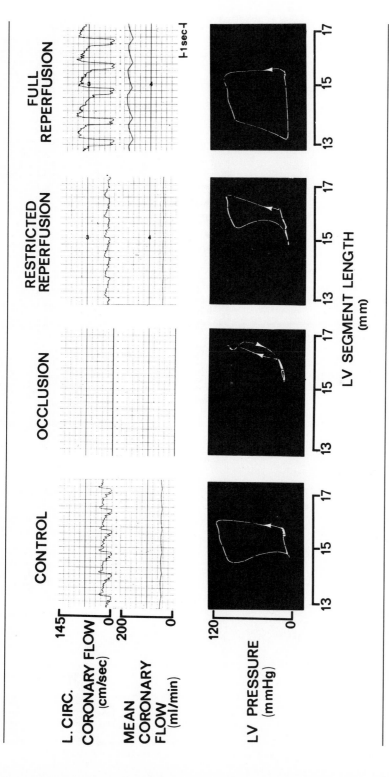

FIGURE 1–7. The effects of regional ischemia (second panel), restricted perfusion (third panel), and full reperfusion (fourth panel) are shown for left circumflex coronary flow (top) and left ventricular pressure-segment length (LVP-SL) (bottom). After 90 seconds of occlusion (second panel), regional function is completely lost (note the clockwise rotation of the LVP-SL loop, showing negative work). Flow was then returned to the control level for 3 minutes by partial release of the cuff occluder and function recovered almost completely (third panel). Finally, after complete release of the coronary occluder, reactive hyperemia and an increase in the area of the loop were observed (fourth panel). (From Pagani, M. et al. Initial myocardial adjustments to brief periods of ischemia and perfusion in the conscious dog. *Circulation Research* 43:83, 1978. Reproduced by permission of the American Heart Association, Inc.)

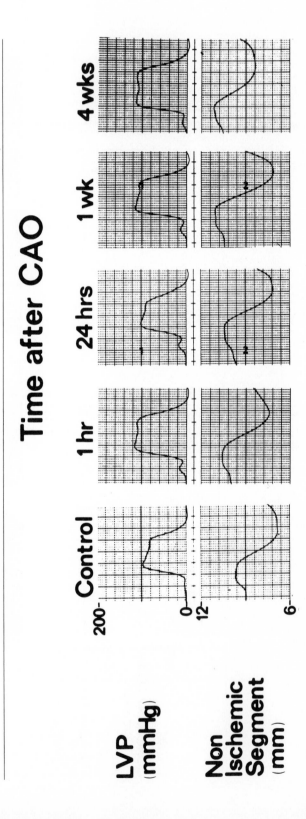

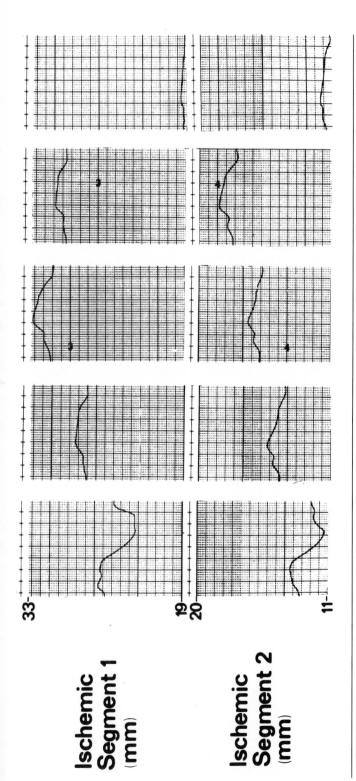

FIGURE 1-8. Phasic recordings of left ventricular (LV) pressure and segmental shortening in one nonischemic and two ischemic segments before coronary artery occlusion (CAO), at 1 hour during CAO and 24 hours, 1 week, and 4 weeks after permanent occlusion. Note that improvement of shortening was not observed in the ischemic segments with permanent CAO. (From Lavallee, M., et al. *European Journal of Cardiology* (in press). Reprinted with permission.)

Examining the effects of reperfusion on regional diastolic properties of the ischemic left ventricle, Hess et al. [71] found that wall stiffness decreased significantly by 1 to 2 minutes after a 2-minute partial or complete occlusion. Interestingly, after a 2- to 3-minute complete occlusion in conscious dogs, Theroux et al. [35] observed recovery of systolic function in ischemic segments within 2 minutes, but abnormal late shortening occurred during isovolumic relaxation in these segments for up to 45 minutes after release of the occlusion. Forrester et al. [37] found a similar pattern after occlusions of varying durations.

As previously mentioned, coronary artery occlusions of less than 20 minutes do not induce myocardial necrosis [85, 97], but occlusions of longer duration are associated with progressive extension of infarction [85, 98]. Studies have shown that reperfusion within 3 hours can reduce myocardial infarct size [99–101], but the extent to which reperfusion salvages regional myocardial function has been elucidated more recently. Lavallee et al. [45] examined the effects of reperfusion for 4 weeks on regional segment shortening in conscious dogs undergoing 1-, 2- and 3-hour coronary artery occlusions and contrasted the results to those in dogs with permanent occlusions (figure 1–8). At 1 hour after coronary artery occlusion, three classes of ischemia-induced dysfunction were observed in the four groups of dogs: dyskinetic or akinetic, severely hypokinetic (systolic shortening depressed by 65 to 95 percent), and moderately hypokinetic (systolic shortening depressed by 40 to 65 percent). In dogs with permanent coronary artery occlusion, little improvement was found in segment shortening in any of the classes of ischemic segments over the 4-week period. In contrast, reperfusion carried out 1 hour after occlusion resulted in recovery of 64 percent of systolic shortening in the dyskinetic segments and almost complete return of contractile function in hypokinetic segments (figure 1–9). In the 2-hour group, systolic shortening returned in the moderately and severely hypokinetic segments, but was slight and not significant in the dyskinetic segments (figure 1–10), compatible with the findings of Theroux et al. [102] for reperfusion for 4 weeks after a 2-hour occlusion in conscious

dogs and of Ellis et al. [103] for reperfusion for 2 weeks after a 2-hour occlusion in anesthetized dogs. In the 3-hour group, significant improvement in systolic shortening occurred only in the moderately hypokinetic segments. However, when analyzing the severely hypokinetic and dyskinetic segments in one group, a small but significant return of function could be demonstrated with coronary artery reperfusion at 3 hours after occlusion [104]. Bush et al. [54], measuring systolic wall thickening during occlusion and reperfusion for 4 weeks in conscious dogs, found that reperfusion after 2 hours of occlusion improved the contractile function in zones of moderate and severe dysfunction. However, reperfusion after 4 hours of occlusion did not restore function in either zones of moderate or severe dysfunction. Thus, the weight of evidence indicates that in conscious dogs, the crucial time for reperfusion occurs between 1 and 3 hours after coronary artery occlusion, with insignificant functional salvage with reperfusion at later times. Just as occurred with brief occlusions, reperfusion after 1 to 3 hours of occlusion resulted in delayed recovery of regional contractile function. Regional function improved insignificantly with reperfusion thereafter [45, 54, 102, 103]. Coronary artery reperfusion in conscious, chronically instrumented baboons was even less successful in salvaging regional myocardial function [105]. In those experiments coronary artery reperfusion after 3 hours of coronary artery occlusion was associated with impaired reflow, which could be the mechanism responsible for the ultimate failure of regional function to recover [105].

It is tempting to extrapolate these findings to the clinical setting of thrombolytic or surgical reperfusion, but the differences between animal models and humans in terms of degree of collateral flow and chronicity of coronary obstruction make comparisons hazardous. This may account for the belief that a beneficial effect can be seen with reperfusion greater than 6 hours after the onset of ischemia. Most studies in patients have shown only modest improvement in global ejection fraction between acute and chronic studies in patients successfully recanalized, but Stack et al. [106] found a more consistent improvement in regional contractile function in this group of patients.

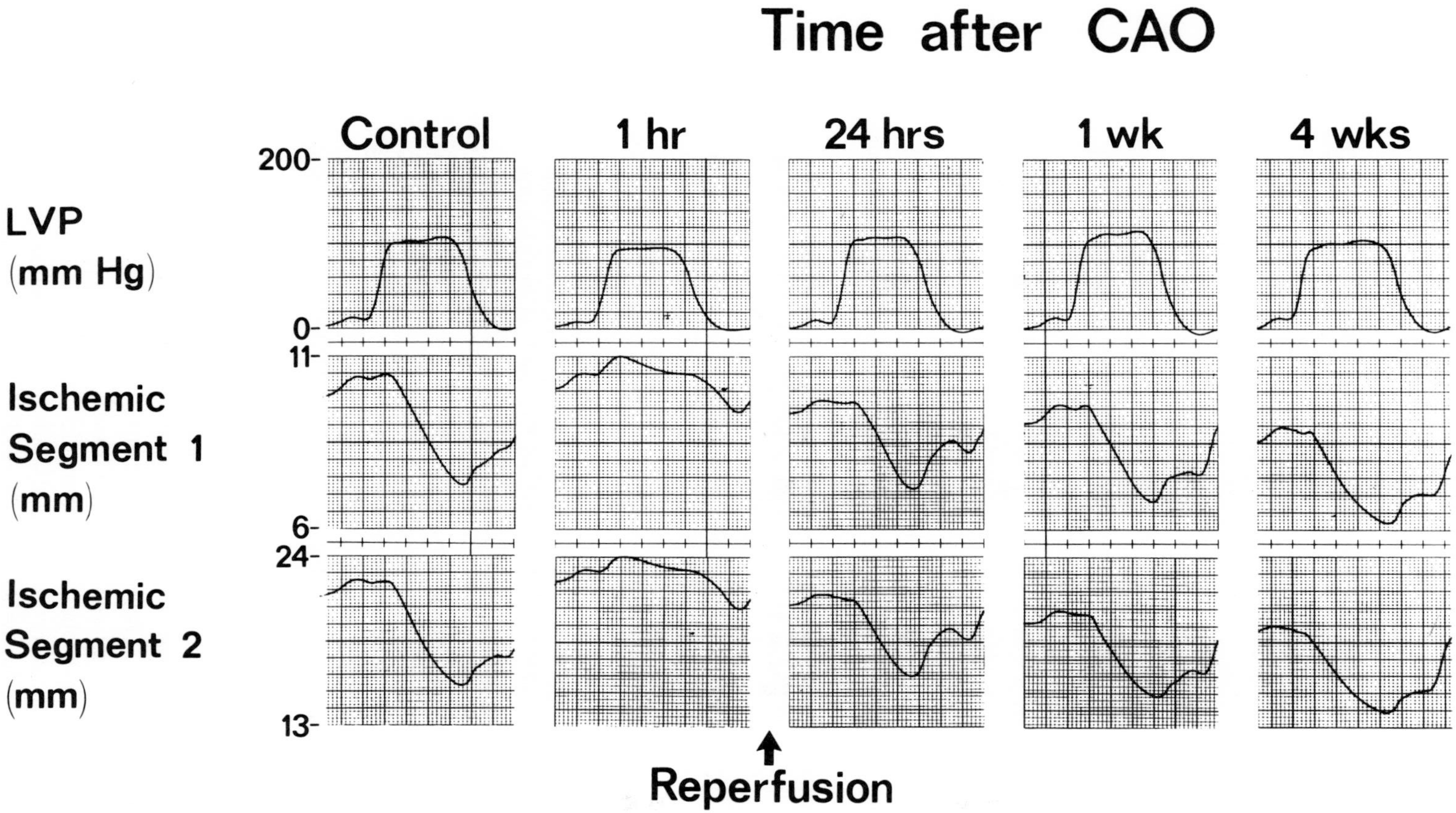

FIGURE 1–9. Phasic recordings of LV pressure and segmental shortening in two severely ischemic segments prior to coronary artery occlusion (CAO), at 1 hour of CAO just before reperfusion, and 24 hours, 1 week, and 4 weeks later. (From Lavallee et al., *European Journal of Cardiology* (in press). Reprinted with permission.)

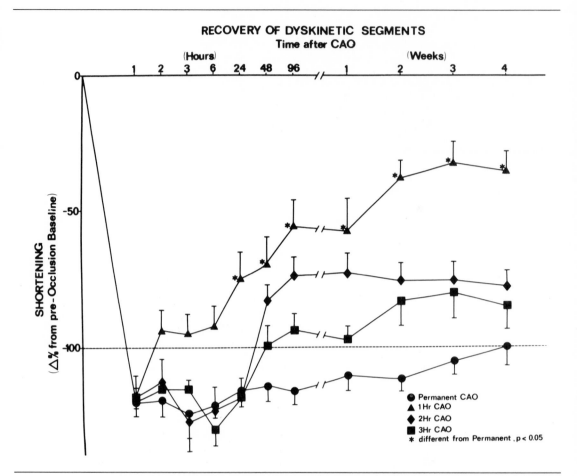

FIGURE 1–10. Time course of systolic shortening in the dyskinetic segments in the P group (circles) or 1-hour group (triangles), 2-hour group (diamonds), and 3-hour group (squares). Systolic shortening is expressed as percentage of change from precoronary artery occlusion (CAO) baseline. Values depressed by over 100 percent represent paradoxical systolic motion. The asterisks represent responses different from those in the P group. (From Lavallee, M. et al. Salvage of myocardial function by coronary artery reperfusion 1, 2, and 3 hours after occlusion in conscious dogs. *Circulation Research* 53:235, 1983.)

Currently, potential methods are being intensively investigated for extending the critical time period of coronary artery occlusion after which reperfusion is no longer beneficial. Since several hours generally elapse between the onset of coronary artery occlusion and the opportunity for induction of therapy, this is one of the most important problems facing clinical cardiology. Investigations are directed at methods for inducing thrombolysis more rapidly, on the one hand, and delaying the development of necrosis, on the other. It is conceivable that administration of therapeutic agents to alleviate the necrotic process at the time of coronary artery reperfusion may be potentially useful. Clearly, the most important goal of coronary artery reperfusion is to recover the contractile properties of ischemic myocardium. If that cannot be accomplished effectively, the long-term beneficial effects of

coronary artery reperfusion will be less significant.

## References

1. See, G. Bochefontaine et Roussy. Arret rapide des contractions rhythmiques des ventricules cardiaques sous l'influence de l'occlusion des arteres coronaires. *Comtes. rendus.* 92:86, 1881.

2. Porter, T. On the results of ligation of the coronary arteries. *J. Physiol.* (Lond) 15:121, 1894.
3. Tennant, R. and Wiggers, C.J. The effect of coronary occlusion on myocardial contraction. *Am. J. Physiol.* 112:351, 1935.
4. Prinzmetal, M., Schwartz, L.L. Corday, E., Spritzler, R., Bergman, H.C., and Kruger, H.E. Studies on the coronary circulation. VI. Loss of myocardial contractility after coronary artery occlusion. *Ann. Intern. Med.* 31:429, 1949.
5. Sayen, J.J, Sheldon, W.F. Pierce, G. and Kuo, P.T. Polarographic oxygen, the epicardial electrocardiogram and muscle contraction in experimental acute regional ischemia of the left ventricle. *Circ. Res.* 6:779, 1958.
6. Heikkila, J., Tabakin B.S., and Hugenholtz P.G. Quantification of function in normal and infarcted regions of the left ventricle. *Cardiovasc. Res.* 6:516, 1972.
7. Tatooles, C.J. and Randall, W.C. Local ventricular bulging after acute coronary occlusion. *Am. J. Physiol.* 201:451, 1961.
8. Schelbert, H.R., Covell, J.W., Burns, J.W., Maroko, P.R. and Ross, J. Jr. Observations on factors affecting local forces in the left ventricular wall during acute myocardial ischemia. *Circ. Res.* 29:306, 1971.
9. Banka, V.S., Chadda, K.D. and Helfant, R.H. Limitations of myocardial revascularization in restoration of regional contraction abnormalities produced by coronary occlusion. *Am. J. Cardiol.* 34:156, 1974.
10. Puri, P.S. and Bing, R.J. Effect of drugs on myocardial contractility in the intact dog and in experimental myocardial infarction: Basis for their use in cardiogenic shock. *Am. J. Cardiol.* 21: 886, 1968.
11. Hood, W.B., Covelli, V.H., Abelmann, W.H. and Norman, J.C. Persistence of contractile behavior in acutely ischaemic myocardium. *Cardiovasc. Res.* 3:249, 1969.
12. Hawthorne, E.W. Asynergy of cardiac contraction—experimental. In *Therapeutic Advances in the Practice of Cardiology,* C.P. Bailey, A.G. Shapiro, and S. Gollub. New York: Grune & Stratton, 1970, p. 227.
13. Goldstein, S. and DeJong, J.W. Changes in left ventricular wall dimensions during regional myocardial ischemia. *Am. J. Cardiol.* 34:56, 1974.
14. Bugge-Asperheim, Leraand, S. and Kul, F. Local dimensional changes of the myocardium by ultrasonic technique. *Scand. J. Clin. Lab. Invest.* 24:361, 1969.
15. Theroux, P. Franklin, D., Ross, J., Jr., and Kemper, W.S. Regional myocardial function during acute coronary artery occlusion and its modification by pharmacologic agents in the dog. *Circ. Res.* 35:896, 1974.

16. Gallagher, K.P., Kumada, T., Koziol, J.A., McKown, M.D., Kemper, W.S., and Ross, J., Jr. Significance of regional wall thickening abnormalities relative to transmural myocardial perfusion in anesthetized dogs. *Circulation* 62:1266, 1980.
17. Gallagher, K.P., Osakada, G. Hess, O.M., Koziol, J.A., Kemper, W.S., and Ross, J., Jr. Subepicardial segmental function during coronary stenosis and the role of myocardial fiber orientation. *Circ. Res.* 50:352, 1982.
18. Heyndrickx, G.R., Millard, R.W., McRitchie, R.J., Maroko, P.R., and Vatner, S.F. Regional myocardial function and electrophysiological alterations after brief coronary artery occlusion in conscious dogs. *J. Clin. Invest.* 56:978, 1975.
19. Sasayama, S., Franklin, D., Ross, J., Jr., Kemper, W.S., and McKown, D. Dynamic changes in left ventricular wall thickness and their use in analyzing cardiac function in the conscious dog. A study based on a modified ultrasonic technique. *Am. J. Cardiol.* 38:870, 1976.
20. Roan, P., Scales, F., Saffer, S., Buja, M., and Willerson, J.T. Functional characterization of left ventricular segmental responses during the initial 24 h and 1 wk after experimental canine myocardial infarction. *J. Clin. Invest.* 64:1074, 1979.
21. Vatner, S.F. Correlation between acute reductions in myocardial blood flow and function in conscious dogs. *Circ. Res.* 47:201, 1980.
22. Ross, J., Jr. and Franklin, D. Analysis of regional myocardial function, dimensions, and wall thickness in the characterization of myocardial ischemia and infarction. *Circulation* 53 (Suppl I):I-88, 1976.
23. Kerber, R.E., and Abboud, E.M. Echocardiographic detection of regional myocardial infarction. An experimental study. *Circulation* 47: 997, 1973.
24. Kerber, R.E., Marcus, M.L., Ehrhardt, J., Wilson, R., and Abboud, E.M. Correlation between echocardiographically demonstrated segmental dyskinesis and regional myocardial perfusion. *Circulation* 52:1097, 1975.
25. Lieberman, A.N., Weiss, J.L., Jugdutt, B.I., Becker, L.C., Bulkley, B.H., Garrison, J.G., Hutchins, G.M., Kallman, C.A., and Weisfeldt, M.L. Two-dimensional echocardiography and infarct size: Relationship of regional wall motion and thickening to the extent of myocardial infarction in the dog. *Circulation* 65:739, 1981.
26. Wyatt, H.L., Meerbaum, S., Heng, M.K., Rit, J., Gueret, P. and Corday, E. Experimental evaluation of the extent of myocardial dyssynergy and infarct size by two-dimensional echocardiography. *Circulation* 63:607, 1981.
27. Weyman, A.E., Franklin, T.D., Jr., Hogan,

R.D., Gillam, L.D., Wiske, P.S., Newell, J., Gibbons, E.F., and Foale, R.A. Importance of temporal heterogeneity in assessing the contraction abnormalities associated with acute myocardial ischemia. *Circulation* 70:102, 1984.

28. Meister, S.G., Casey, P.R., Jacobs, L., and Banett, M.J. 2D echo definition of endocardium (abstr). *Circulation* 62 (Suppl III):III–132, 1980.

29. Hirzel, H.O., Sonnenblick, E.H., and Kirk, E.S. Absence of a lateral border zone of intermediate creatine phosphokinase depletion surrounding a central infarct 24 hours after acute coronary occlusion in the dog. *Circ. Res.* 41:673, 1977.

30. Factor, S.M., Okun, E.M., and Kirk, E.S. The histological lateral border of acute canine myocardial infarction. A function of microcirculation. *Circ. Res.* 48:640, 1981.

31. Murdock, R.H., Harlan, D.M., Morris, J.J., Pryor, W.W., Jr., and Cobb, F.R. Transitional blood flow zones between ischemic and nonischemic myocardium in the awake dog. Analysis based on distribution of the intramural vasculature. *Circ. Res.* 52:451, 1983.

32. Cox, D.A., and Vatner, S.F. Myocardial function in areas of heterogeneous perfusion after coronary artery occlusion in conscious dogs. *Circulation* 66:1154, 1982.

33. Streeter, D.D., Spotnitz, H.M., Patel, D.P., Ross, J., Jr., and Sonnenblick, E.H. Fiber orientation in the canine left ventricle during diastole and systole. *Circ. Res.* 24:339, 1969.

34. Genain, C., Theroux, P., Thuillez, C., Bourassa, M.G., and Waters, D.D. The interrelationships between function and flow in the subendocardial and subepicardial regions of the left ventricle (abstr). *Circulation* 60 (Suppl II): II–28, 1979.

35. Theroux, P., Ross, J., Jr., Franklin, D., Kemper, W.S., and Sasayama, S. Regional myocardial function in the conscious dog during acute coronary occlusion and responses to morphine, propranolol, nitroglycerin, and lidocaine. *Circulation* 53:302, 1976.

36. Tyberg, J.V., Forrester, J.S., Wyatt, H.L., Goldner, S.J., Parmley, W.W., and Swan, H.J.C. An analysis of segmental ischemic dysfunction utilizing the pressure-length loop. *Circulation* 49:-748, 1974.

37. Forrester, J.S., Wyatt, H.L., DaLuz, P.L., Tyberg, J.V., Diamond, G.A., and Swan, H.J.C. Functional significance of regional ischemic contraction abnormalities. *Circulation* 54:64, 1976.

38. Pagani, M., Vatner, S.F., Baig, H., and Braunwald, E. Initial myocardial adjustments to brief periods of ischemia and reperfusion in the conscious dog. *Circ. Res.* 43:83, 1978.

39. Kumada, T., Karliner, J.S., Pouleur, H., Gallagher, K.P., Shirato, K., and Ross, J., Jr. Effects of coronary occlusion on early ventricular diastolic events in conscious dogs. *Am. J. Physiol.* 237:H542, 1979.

40. Weigner, A.W., Allen, G.J., and Bing, O.H.L. Weak and strong myocardium in series: Implications for segmental dysfunction. *Am. J. Physiol.* 235:H776, 1978.

41. Tyberg, J.V., Yeatman, L.A., Parmley, W.W., Urschel, C.W., and Sonnenblick, E.H. Effects of hypoxia on mechanisms of cardiac contraction. *Am. J. Physiol.* 218:1780, 1970.

42. Hefner, L.L., Sheffield, L.T., Cobbs, G.C., and Klip, W. Relation between mural force and pressure in the left ventricle of the dog. *Circ. Res.* 11:654, 1962.

43. Wyatt, H.L., DaLuz, P.L., Forrester, J., Diamond, G., Chagrasulis, R., and Swan, H.J.C. Depression of function in nonischemic myocardium after coronary occlusion (abstr). *Circulation* 49 (Suppl III):III–119, 1974.

44. Amano, J., Lavallee, M., Randall, W.C., Vatner, S.F., and Thomas, J.X. Relative importance of cardiac nerves and the Frank-Starling mechanism on regional ventricular function following acute coronary occlusion in conscious dogs (abstr). *Circulation* 70 (Suppl II):II–180, 1984.

45. Lavallee, M., Cox, D., Patrick, T.A., and Vatner, S.F. Salvage of myocardial function by coronary artery reperfusion 1, 2, and 3 hours after occlusion in conscious dogs. *Circ. Res.* 53:235, 1983.

46. Salisbury, P.F., Cross, C.E., and Rieben, P.A. Acute ischemia of the inner layers of the ventricular wall. *Am. Heart J.* 66:650, 1963.

47. Buckberg, G.D., Fixler, D.E., and Archie, J.P. Experimental subendocardial ischemia in dogs with normal coronary arteries. *Circ. Res.* 30:67, 1972.

48. Banka, V.S., Bodenheimer, M.M., and Helfant, R.H. Relation between progressive decreases in regional coronary perfusion and contractile abnormalities. *Am. J. Cardiol.* 40:200, 1977.

49. Waters, D.D., Daluz, P., Wyatt, H.L., Swan, H.J.C., and Forrester, J.S. Early changes in regional and global left ventricular function induced by graded reductions in regional coronary perfusion. *Am. J. Cardiol.* 39:537, 1977.

50. Wyatt, H.L., Forrester, J.S., Tyberg, J.V., Goldner, S., Logan, S.E., Parmley, W.W., and Swan, H.J.C. Effect of graded reductions in regional coronary perfusion on regional and total cardiac function. *Am. J. Cardiol.* 36:185, 1975.

51. Stowe, D.F., Mathey, D.G., Moores, W.Y., Glantz, S.A., Townsend, R.M., Kabra, P., Chatterjee, K., Parmley, W.W., and Tyberg, J.V. Segment stroke work and metabolism depend on coronary blood flow in the pig. *Am. J. Physiol.* 234:H597, 1978.

52. Weintraub, W.S., Hattori, S., Agarwal, J.B., Bodenheimer, M.M., Banka, V.S., and Helfant, R.H. The relationship between myocardial blood flow and contraction by myocardial layer in the canine left ventricle during ischemia. *Circ. Res.* 48:430, 1981.

53. Savage, R.M., Guth, B., White, F.C., Hagan, A.D., and Bloor, C.M. Correlation of regional myocardial blood flow and function with myocardial infarct size during acute myocardial ischemia in the conscious pig. *Circulation* 64:699, 1981.

54. Bush, L.R., Buja, M., Samowitz, W., Rude, R.E., Wathen, M., Tilton, G.D., and Willerson, J.T. Recovery of left ventricular segmental function after long-term reperfusion following temporary coronary occlusion in conscious dogs. Comparison of 2 and 4 hour occlusions. *Circ. Res.* 53:248, 1983.

55. Becker, L.C., Ferreira, R., and Thomas, M. Mapping of left ventricular blood flow with radioactive microspheres in experimental coronary artery occlusion. *Cardiovasc. Res.* 7:391, 1973.

56. Vokonas, P.S., Malsky, P.M., Paul, S.J., Robbins, S.L., and Hood, W.B., Jr. Radioautographic studies in experimental myocardial infarction: Profiles of ischemic blood flow and quantification of infarct size in relation to magnitude of ischemic zone. *Am. J. Cardiol.* 42:67, 1978.

57. Jugdutt, B.I., Hutchins, G.M., Bulkley, B.H., and Becker, L.C. Myocardial infarction in the conscious dog: Three-dimensional mapping of infarct, collateral flow and region at risk. *Circulation* 60:1141, 1979.

58. Wyatt, H.L., Forrester, J.S., DaLuz, P.L., Diamond, G.A., Chagrasulis, R., and Swan, H.J.C. Functional abnormalities in nonoccluded regions of myocardium after experimental coronary occlusion. *Am. J. Cardiol.* 37:366, 1976.

59. Guth, B.D., White, F.C., Gallagher, K.P., and Bloor CM. Decreased systolic wall thickening in myocardium adjacent to ischemic zones in conscious swine during brief coronary artery occlusion. *Am. Heart. J.* 107:458, 1984.

60. Corday, E., Kaplan, L., Meerbaum, S., Brasch, J., Constantini, C., Lang, T-W., Gold, H., Rubins, S., and Osher, J. Consequences of coronary arterial occlusion on remote myocardium: Effects of occlusion and reperfusion. *Am. J. Cardiol.* 36:385, 1975.

61. Braunwald, E., and Kloner, R.A. The stunned myocardium: Prolonged, postischemic ventricular dysfunction. *Circulation* 66:1146, 1982.

62. Bogen, D.K., Rabinowitz, S.A., Needleman, A., McMahon, T.A., and Abelmann, W.H. An analysis of the mechanical disadvantage of myocardial infarction in the canine left ventricle. *Circulation Res.* 47:728, 1980.

63. Mann, T., Brodie, B.R., Grossman, W., and McLaurin, L.P. Effect of angina on the left ventricular diastolic pressure-volume relationship. *Circulation* 55:761, 1977.

64. Papaietro, S.E., Coghlan, H.C., Zisserman, D., Russell, R.O., Rackley, C.E., and Rogers, W.J. Impaired maximal rate of left ventricular relaxation in patients with coronary artery disease and left ventricular dysfunction. *Circulation* 59:984, 1979.

65. Rousseau, M.F., Veriter, Co., Detry, J–M.R., Brasseur, L., and Pouleur, H. Impaired early left ventricular relaxation in coronary artery disease: Effects of intracoronary nifedipine. *Circulation* 62:764, 1980.

66. Reduto, L.A., Wickemeyer, W.J., Young, J.B., Del Ventura, L.A., Reid, J.W., Glaeser, D.H., Quinnes, M.A., and Miller, R.R. Left ventricular diastolic performance at rest and during exercise in patients with coronary artery disease. Assessment with first-pass radionuclide angiography. *Circulation* 63:1228, 1981.

67. Bonow, R.D., Bacharach, S.L., Green, M.V., Kent, K.M., Rosing, D.R., Lipson, L.C., Leon, M.B., and Epstein, S.E. Impaired left ventricular diastolic filling in patients with coronary artery disease: Assessment with radionuclide angiography. *Circulation* 64:315, 1981.

68. Dwyer, E.M. Left ventricular pressure-volume alterations and regional disorders of contraction during myocardial ischemia induced by atrial pacing. *Circulation* 42:1111, 1970.

69. Barry, W.H., Brooker, J.Z., Alderman, E.L., and Harrison, D.C. Changes in diastolic stiffness and tone of the left ventricle during angina pectoris. *Circulation* 49:255, 1974.

70. Gaasch, W.H., Levine, H.J., Quinones, M.A., and Alexander, J.K. Left ventricular compliance: Mechanisms and clinical implications. *Am. J. Cardiol.* 38: 645, 1976.

71. Hess, O.M., Osakada, G., Lavelle, J.F., Gallagher, K.P., Kemper, W.S., and Ross, J., Jr. Diastolic myocardial wall stiffness and ventricular relaxation during partial and complete coronary occlusions in the conscious dog. *Circ. Res.* 52:387, 1983.

72. Bourdillon, P.D., Lorell, B.H., Mirsky, I., Paulus, W.J., Wynne, J., and Grossman, W. Increased regional myocardial stiffness of the left ventricle during pacing-induced angina in man. *Circulation* 67:316, 1983.

73. Pouleur, H., Rousseau, M.F., van Eyll, C., and Charlier, A.A. Assessment of regional left ventricular relaxation in patients with coronary artery disease: Importance of geometric factors and changes in wall thickness. *Circulation* 69:696, 1984.

74. Glantz, S.A., and Parmley, W.W. Factors which affect the diastolic pressure-volume curve. *Circ. Res.* 42:171, 1978.

75. Mitchell, J.H., Linden, R.J., and Sarnoff, S.L. Influence of cardiac sympathetic and vagal nerve stimulation on the relation between left ventricular diastolic pressure and myocardial segment length. *Circ. Res.* 8:1100, 1960.

76. Weisfeldt, M.L., Armstrong, P., Scully, H.E., Sanders, C.A., and Daggett, W.M. Incomplete relaxation between beats after myocardial hypoxia and ischemia. *J. Clin. Invest.* 53:1626, 1974.

77. Mason S.J., Weiss, J.L., Weisfeldt, M.L., Garrison, J.B., and Fortuin, N.J. Exercise electrocardiography: Detection of wall motion abnormalities during ischemia. *Circulation* 59:50, 1979.

78. Grossman, W., and Barry, W.H. Diastolic pressure-volume relations in the diseased heart. *Fed. Proc.* 39:148, 1980.

79. Theroux, P., Ross, J. Jr., Franklin, D., Covell, J.W., Bloor, C.M., and Sasayama, S. Regional myocardial function and dimensions early and late after myocardial infarction in the unanesthetized dog. *Circ. Res.* 40:158, 1977.

80. Forrester, J.S., Diamond, G., Parmley, W.W., and Swan, H.J.C. Early increase in left ventricular compliance after myocardial infarction. *J. Clin. Invest.* 51:598, 1972.

81. Pirzada, F.A., Ekong, E.A., Vokonas, P.S., Apstein, C.A., and Hood, W.B., Jr. Experimental myocardial infarction. XIII. Sequential changes in left ventricular pressure—length relationships in the acute phase. *Circulation* 53:970, 1976.

82. Hood, W.B., Bianco, J.A., Kumar, R., and Whiting, R.B. Experimental myocardial infarction. IV. Reduction of left ventricular compliance in the healing phase. *J. Clin. Invest.* 49:1316, 1970.

83. Phillips, S.J., Kongtahworn, C., Zeff, R.H., Benson, P.C., Iannone, L., Brown, T., and Gordon, D.F. Emergency coronary artery revascularization: A possible therapy for acute myocardial infarction. *Circulation* 60:241, 1979.

84. Hartzler, G.O., Rutherford, B.D., McConahay, D.R., Johnson, W.L., McCallister, B.D., Gura, G.M., Jr., Conn, R.C., and Crockett, J.E. Percutaneous transluminal coronary angioplasty with and without thrombolytic therapy for treatment of acute myocardial infarction. *Am. Heart. J.* 106:965, 1983.

85. Jennings, R.B., Sommers, H.M., Smyth, G.A., Flack, H.A., and Linn, H. Myocardial necrosis induced by temporary occlusion of a coronary artery in the dog. *Arch. Pathol.* 70:68, 1960.

86. Jennings, R.B. Early phase of myocardial ischemic injury and infarction. *Am. J. Cardiol.* 24:753, 1969.

87. Puri, P.S. Modification of experimental myocardial infarct size by cardiac drugs. *Am. J. Cardiol.* 33:521, 1974.

88. Weiner, J.M., Apstein, C.S., Arthur, J.H., Pirzada, F.A., and Hood, W.B., Jr. Persistence of myocardial injury following brief periods of coronary occlusion. *Cardiovasc. Res.* 10:678, 1976.

89. Heyndrickx, G.R., Baig, H., Nellens, P., Leusen, I., Fishbein, M.C., and Vatner, S.F. Depression of regional blood flow and wall thickening after brief coronary occlusions. *Am. J. Physiol.* 234:H653, 1978.

90. Puri, P. Contractile and biochemical effects of coronary reperfusion after extended periods of coronary occlusion. *Am. J. Cardiol.* 36:244, 1975.

91. Kloner, R.A., Ellis, S.G., Lange, R., and Braunwald, E. Studies of experimental coronary artery reperfusion. Effects on infarct size, myocardial function, biochemistry, ultrastructure and microvascular damage. *Circulation* 68 (suppl I): I-8, 1983.

92. Fox, A.C., Reed, G.E., Meilman, H., and Silk, B.B. Release of nucleotides from canine and human hearts as an index of prior ischemia. *Am. J. Cardiol.* 43:52, 1979.

93. DeBoer, L.W.V., Ingwall, J.S., Kloner, R.A., and Braunwald, E. Prolonged derangements of canine myocardial purine metabolism after a brief coronary artery occlusion not associated with anatomic evidence of necrosis. *Proc. Natl. Acad. Sci. USA* 77:5471, 1980.

94. Swain, J.L., Sabina, R.L., McHale, P.A., Greenfield, J.C., Jr., and Holmes, E.W. Prolonged myocardial nucleotide depletion after brief ischemia in the open-chest dog. *Am. J. Physiol.* 242:H818, 1982.

95. Tomada, H., Parmley, W.W., Fijimura, S., and Mateoff, J.M. Effects of ischemia and reoxygenation on regional myocardial performance of the dog. *Am. J. Physiol.* 221:1718, 1971.

96. Lange, R., Ware, J., and Kloner, R.A. Absence of a cumulative deterioration of regional function during three repeated 5 or 15 minute coronary occlusions. *Circulation* 69:400, 1984.

97. Maroko, P.R., Kjekshus, J.K., Sobel, B.E., Watanabe, T., Covell, J.W., Ross, J., Jr., and Braunwald, E. Factors influencing infarct size following experimental coronary artery occlusions. *Circulation* 43:67, 1971.

98. Reimer, K.A., Lowe, J.E., Rasmussen, M.M., and Jennings, R.B. The wavefront phenomenon of ischemic cell death. I. Myocardial infarct size vs. duration of coronary occlusion in dogs. *Circulation* 56:786, 1977.

99. Maroko, P.R., Libby, P., Ginks, W.R., Bloor, C.M., Shell, W.E., Sobel, B.E., and Ross, J., Jr. Coronary artery reperfusion. I. Early effects of

local myocardial function and the extent on myocardial necrosis. *J. Clin. Invest.* 51:2710, 1972.

100. Mathur, V.S., Guinn, G.A., and Burris, W.H. Maximal revascularization (reperfusion) in intact conscious dogs after 2 to 5 hours of coronary occlusion. *Am. J. Cardiol.* 36:252, 1975.

101. Constantini, C., Corday, E., Lang, T–W., Meerbaum, S., Brasch, J., Kaplan, L., Rubins, S., Gold, H., and Osher, J. Revascularization after 3 hours of coronary arterial occlusion: Effects on regional cardiac metabolic function and infarct size. *Am. J. Cardiol.* 36:368, 1975.

102. Theroux, P., Ross, J., Jr., Franklin, D., Kemper, W.S., and Sasayama, S. Coronary arterial reperfusion. III. Early and late effects on regional myocardial function and dimensions in conscious dogs. *Am. J. Cardiol.* 38:599, 1976.

103. Ellis, S.G., Henschke, C.I., Sandor, T., Wynne, J., Braunwald, E., and Kloner, R.A. Time course of functional and biochemical recovery of myocardium salvaged by reperfusion. *J. Am. Coll. Cardiol.* 1:1047, 1983.

104. Lavallee, M., Cox, D.A., and Vatner, S.F. Effects of coronary after reperfusion on recovery of regional myocardial function in conscious dogs. *Europ. J. Cardiol.*, in press.

105. Heyndrickx, G.R., Patrick, T., Manders, T., Rogers, G., Rosendorff, C. and Vatner, S.F. Relation between hyperemia following coronary reperfusion and subsequent recovery of regional function in conscious baboons (abstr.) *Circulation* 70 (Suppl II):II–259, 1984.

106. Stack, R.S., Phillips, H.R., Grierson, D.S., Behar, V.S., Kong, Y., Peter, R.H., Swain, V., and Greenfield, J.R. Functional improvement of jeopardized myocardium following intracoronary streptokinase infusion in acute myocardial infarction. *J. Clin. Invest.* 72:84, 1983.

# 2. PATHOPHSIOLOGY OF CORONARY ARTERY DISEASE IN HUMANS

Peter F. Cohn

Pantel S. Vokonas

The clinical presentation of coronary artery disease is familiar to most physicians, but the pathophysiologic basis of myocardial ischemia in humans—with its relevant therapeutic implications—has become evident only within the last two decades. There had once been almost no hemodynamic or metabolic information regarding mechanisms of the anginal state in humans, for example, but now there are a great number of such studies in the medical literature. To these have been added new investigations of the coronary circulation. The purpose of the present chapter is to review the important pathoanatomic and pathophysiologic features of coronary artery disease in humans and to relate them to the clinical setting whenever possible.

In the course of this review certain *areas of controversy* will be discussed: theories regarding the pathogenesis of coronary atherosclerosis; the functional significance of collaterals; whether coronary artery thrombosis precedes acute myocardial infarction or vice versa; the significance of myocardial perfusion studies in patients with coronary artery disease; the basis for elevated filling pressures during angina; circulatory dynamics in various angina-provoking situations, such as exertion, cold weather etc., with particular emphasis on the role of coronary vasospasm; the differential diagnosis of congestive heart failure in patients with coronary artery disease; and the genesis of ischemia-related ventricular arrhythmias.

## Pathoanatomy of the Coronary Circulation

### NORMAL CORONARY ANATOMY
Figure 9–1 illustrates normal coronary anatomy in humans: a short left coronary artery bifurcates into left anterior descending and circumflex branches to supply the major part of the left ventricle, and the right coronary artery perfuses the right ventricle and terminates on the inferoposterior surface of the left ventricle near the distal end of the circumflex artery. In about 90 percent of individuals, the posterior descending artery arises from the right system, resulting in a "right dominant system." "Dominance" is strictly an anatomic term and does not imply that the vessel perfuses most of the left ventricle. This perfusion is a function of the left coronary system, even though it alone supplies the crux (posterior base) of the heart in about 10 percent of individuals. (This is also the pattern in many animals, such as the dog.) The major coronary arteries give off small arteries that divide rapidly, become progressively smaller, and terminate in a rich network of arterioles and capillaries. Collateral vessels are part of the arterial network, but because they appear to function only during or as a result of ischemia, they will be discussed later when autopsy findings and coronary arteriographic findings in patients with coronary artery disease are described.

The venous drainage of the left coronary system is via the anterior great cardiac vein and the lateral marginal veins, which empty into the coronary sinus, while the right coronary artery empties mainly into the right atrium via smaller anterior and posterior cardiac veins.

## PATHOGENESIS OF CORONARY ATHEROSCLEROSIS

As discussed in chapter 18, the coronary arteries may be involved with inflammatory processes, degenerative metabolic diseases, or congenital anomalies. The major cause of abnormal coronary anatomy in contemporary Western society, however, is atherosclerosis. The association of coronary artery disease with certain risk factors (e.g., hyperlipidemia, smoking, hypertension, and carbohydrate intolerance) will be discussed at length in chapter 3 and again in chapter 11 in relation to the prevention of coronary artery disease. As both chapters point out, considerable points of controversy remain.

The precise manner in which the atherosclerotic lesions form in the coronary (as well as in other arterial) beds is also unresolved. Ross and Glomset [1] have reviewed this subject extensively, and many of their observations are worth emphasizing. It is generally accepted, for example, that the intima is the cell layer principally involved in atherosclerosis and that three different kinds of lesions may be demonstrated: the fatty streak, the fibrous plaque, and the complicated lesion. The *fatty streak* is found in young people and causes no or only minimal vascular obstruction and no clinical symptoms. The *fibrous plaque* is the most characteristic lesion of advancing atherosclerosis. Unlike the yellowish fatty streak, it is white and elevated and protrudes into the arterial lumen. Cholesterol and cholesterol esters constitute the lipid material that accumulates in smooth muscle cells in the intima of the artery. The cells and the extracellular matrix (also comprised of lipids) form the fibrous cap that covers a deeper deposit of cell debris and free extracellular lipid. Whether the fatty streak is actually a forerunner of the fibrous plaque is uncertain, but there is little question that the *complicated lesion* is a fibrous plaque that has become altered due to hemorrhage, calcification, cell necrosis, and mural thrombosis. This type of lesion is most commonly associated with arterial occlusive disease.

How does the atherosclerotic process begin? Normally, the endothelium forms a barrier to the passage of blood constituents into the arterial wall. When this endothelial barrier is disrupted by mechanical or chemical injury in experimental models (chronic hypercholesterolemia may also be such an injury-inciting agent), the injured tissue is involved in an immediate response that includes local platelet adhesion and aggregation [2]. Smooth muscle cells also migrate across the internal elastic lamina into the intima as part of the tissue response, and there is also increased formation of connective tissue protein. Study of the biologic characteristics of endothelial cells has been greatly aided by the development of techniques that permit their growth in vitro. As Ross and Glomset [1] have noted, these techniques may provide answers to the fundamental questions concerning the pathogenesis of atherosclerosis.

At present, based on the experimental studies cited above as well as on long-standing pathologic observations, the *response-to-injury hypothesis* is one of the more attractive concepts. According to this hypothesis, any number of factors (e.g., hypertension, hyperlipidemia, viruses, and the like) can injure the arterial endothelium and trigger the tissue response described above. Focal desquamation of the endothelium results, exposing the underlying subendothelial connective tissue to platelets as well as to circulating lipids and other elements. Focal deposition of intracellular and extracellular lipids, proliferation of arterial smooth muscle cells, and formation of large amounts of connective tissue matrix result (figure 2–1). If both the injury and the tissue response are limited, the endothelial barrier is restored and the lesion regresses. In contrast, if the injury is continuous or repeated, the lesion can enlarge, undergo internal necrosis and hemorrhage, and result in the kind of luminal obliteration seen in figure 2–2. One of the factors that may contribute to the continuous injury is hyperlipidemia. As noted by Ross and Glomset [1], several questions arise about this hypothesis. Is the relation of risk factors to coronary artery disease based on the endothelial injury, the subsequent response to the injury, or both? What are the characteristics of the platelet (and possibly other) factors that promote cell proliferation? By what "removal" mechanisms do the lesions actually regress? Why

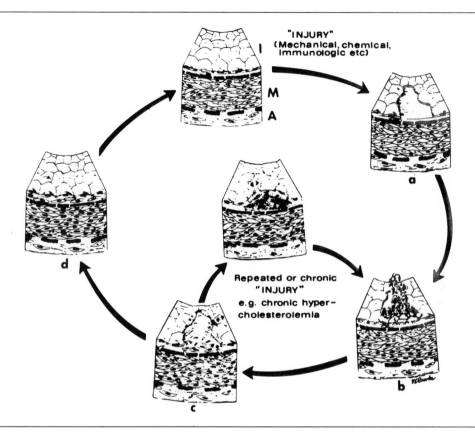

FIGURE 2–1. Two possible different cycles of events according to the response-to-injury hypothesis. The cycles begin in a normal coronary artery (uppermost section). The intima (1), or innermost layer, consists of a narrow region bounded on the luminal side (top of section) by a single continuous layer of endothelial cells and peripherally by the fenestrated elastic fibers of the intimal elastic lamina (broken dark line). The cellular content of the media (M), or middle layer, consists entirely of smooth muscle cells. The adventitia (A), or outermost layer, begins with the external elastic lamina (broken dark line), and the cellular content consists of fibroblasts intermixed with smooth muscle cells. The large cycle of events may represent what occurs in all persons at varying times. Endothelial injury may lead to desquamation (a) and platelet adherence, aggregation, and release (b), which are followed by smooth muscle proliferation and connective tissue formation (c). If the injury is a single event, the lesions may go on to heal and regress, leaving a slightly thickened intima (d). The smaller, inner cycle demonstrates the possible consequences of repeated or chronic injury to the endothelium. Lipid deposition may occur and smooth muscle proliferation may continue after a sequence of proliferation, regression, proliferation, and regression, leading to a complicated lesion that contains newly formed connective tissue and lipids that may eventually calcify. This sequence of events could lead to a complicated lesion that goes on to produce clinical sequelae (e.g., thrombosis and infarction) as depicted in figure 2–2. (From Ross, R. and Glomset, J.A. The pathogenesis of atherosclerosis. Reprinted, by permission of the *New England Journal of Medicine,* 295:369, 1976.

are the lesions often focal in humans, whereas many forms of experimental injury provoke a more generalized response?

An alternative hypothesis has been proposed by Benditt and Benditt [3]. Their *monoclonal (monotypic) hypothesis* suggests that the atherosclerotic lesion is derived from a single smooth mus-

cle cell that acts as a progenitor (clone) of other proliferative cells. Based on biochemical profiling of the cells, it would appear that each atherosclerotic lesion may be a form of benign neoplasm. The original cell could have been transformed into neoplastic growth by one of several mechanical, chemical, or even infectious

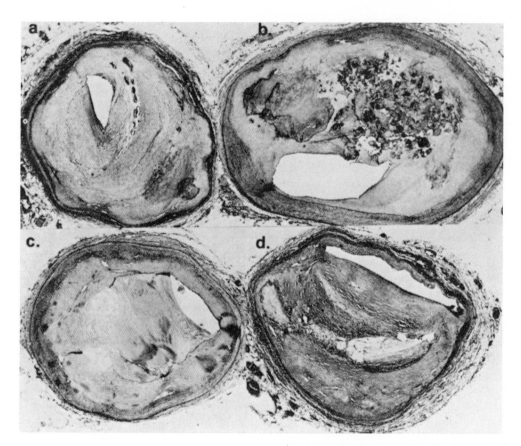

FIGURE 2–2. Sections representing the sites of maximal narrowing by atherosclerosis plaques in the right (a), left main (b), left anterior descending (c), and left circumflex (d) coronary arteries of a 41-year-old man who died suddenly after having had angina pectoris for 7 years. (Sections a, b, and c: elastic Van Gieson's stain; section d; a hematoxylin-eosin stain; magnification of each: × 25.) (From Roberts, W.C. *Cardiovasc. Med.* 2:29, 1977.)

agents. This cell-selection theory represents a new and exciting concept in the pathogenesis of atherosclerotic lesions.

Still another concept in this field is the *clonal-senescence hypothesis* of Martin and Sprague [4]. Instead of initiation of lesion formation by a wildly growing smooth muscle cell, they propose the opposite theory: there may be a decline in activity (i.e., senescence) of the crucial stem cells in the intima and media that control smooth muscle proliferation. A feedback control system with inhibitory substances to prevent undue pre-plication is also proposed. With the breakdown of this control system with age, smooth muscle accumulation may occur in atherosclerotic plaques.

Finally, in addition to factors influencing endothelial cell injury and smooth muscle and fibroblast cell migration and proliferation, there is also the question of lipid accumulation within the atherosclerotic lesion. How do the cholesterol and cholesterol esters that form the major components of the advanced plaque accumulate there? In a review of the cellular mechanisms for lipid deposition, Small [5] noted that a delicate balance of cholesterol uptake, metabolism, and removal is needed to maintain cellular cholesterol homeostasis and that the cells of the arterial intima that are involved in the atherosclerotic process are not in equilibrium, but rather in "positive" cholesterol balance. Defects that may lead to an accumulation of cholesterol in cells include high external levels of low-density (beta) lipoproteins, defective lysosomal function or enzyme deficiencies impairing the breakdown of low-density remnants, defective transport out of the lysosome after the lipoprotein moiety has been broken down, unsuppressed cholesterol synthesis within the cell, deficient high-density (alpha) lipoprotein levels, as well as other defects. A combination of events is most likely involved in the development of advanced plaques.

In summary, storage of lipid in the vessel wall is believed to be due to the presentation of increased levels of serum lipids to the subendothelial arterial spaces as a result of a break in the endothelial barrier, increased levels of cholesterol in the blood itself (i.e., hypercholesterolemia), or both. The entrance of lipids (insudation) into the cells of the arterial wall—whether the cells are present initially or have migrated there—appears to be largely dependent on the low-density lipoprotein (LDL) moiety. Elevated serum levels of total cholesterol, particularly of the LDL fraction, appear to enhance this process [6]. The increased amount of cholesterol in the blood may be due to secondary (mainly dietary) influences, or when primary, it may be due to familial defects in intracellular LDL receptors [7] (figure 2-3). Hypertension facilitates entrance of lipids [8], although few investigators regard it as the major initiating factor in atherosclerosis. Why certain arteries—such as those in the coronary and cerebral circulation—seem particularly prone to the development of obstructive atherosclerotic lesions remains a puzzle. Why women are protected until the menopause is likewise unknown, but recent studies [9] (described further in chapter 3) suggest that in addition to hormonal effects, higher serum levels of "protective" high-density lipoproteins (HDL) may be partly responsible.

A variety of mechanisms have been suggested to explain how the other major risk factors—namely, cigarette smoking and diabetes mellitus—hasten the atherosclerotic process. The ingredients of cigarette smoke thought to be associated with the development of atherosclerotic lesions are carbon monoxide and nicotine, but again the pathophysiologic mechanisms are unclear. These ingredients may contribute to the initial vascular injury, may be responsible for a hemostatic vasospastic effect, or may stimulate higher levels of circulating catecholamines to

the same end. Increased platelet adhesiveness and enhanced platelet aggregability may also be factors. Diabetics have been reported to have circulating substances that stimulate excess proliferation of smooth muscle cells as well as to have arterial walls that show an increased propensity to bind lipoprotein. Increased serum levels of very low density (prebeta or VLDL) lipoprotein are also present in diabetics, although VLDL is not as prevalent in atherosclerotic plaques as is LDL.

## AUTOPSY AND CORONARY ARTERIOGRAPHIC FINDINGS IN PATIENTS WITH CORONARY ARTERY DISEASE

*The Coronary Arteries.* In patients with histories of chronic angina pectoris or previous myocardial infarction, the coronary arteries are usually diffusely involved by the atherosclerotic process at autopsy. During life, when the vessels are distended, some areas are obviously more narrowed by plaques than are others, and this is observed by coronary arteriography (see figures 9–8 to 9–10). In fatal coronary artery disease, two and commonly three of the major coronary arteries are narrowed by more than 50 percent in diameter (corresponding to about 75 percent reduction in cross-sectional area). The lumens can be quite variable in shape when these vessels are examined (see figure 2–2). Roberts[10] has summarized his extensive experience with the pathologic aspects of this disease and has observed that the residual lumen may be located centrally or peripherally and its shape may be circular, oval, slitlike, or "half-moon." The slitlike lumen may appear almost normal on some coronary arteriographic projections when it extends from one side of the vessel to the other, and hence multiple angiographic projections are valuable when coronary artery disease is suspected (see chapter 9). Roberts also emphasized that the atherosclerotic process is limited to the epicardial coronary arteries, and except for the vessels in the papillary muscles, atherosclerosis spares the intramyocardial coronary arteries [10]. The most severe narrowings, particularly when calcified, appear to be located in the proximal portion of the coronary arteries.

The sites of predilection for coronary atherosclerosis in humans appear to be determined by

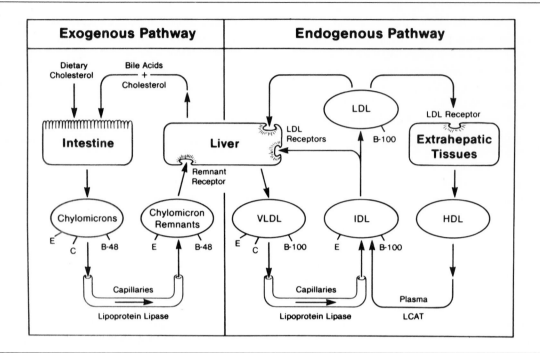

FIGURE 2–3. Separate pathways for receptor-mediated metabolism of lipoproteins carrying endogenous and exogenous cholesterol. HDL denotes high-density lipoprotein, LCAT lecithin:cholesterol acyltransferase, LDL low-density lipoprotein, IDL intermediate-density lipoprotein, and VLDL very low density lipoprotein. The distinction between exogenous and endogenous cholesterol applies to the immediate source of the cholesterol in plasma lipoproteins. After the exogenous cholesterol has been delivered to the liver and has been secreted in VLDL, it is considered endogenous cholesterol. HDL is shown as the lipoprotein that removes cholesterol from extrahepatic cells. The cholesterol is delivered to IDL through the action of plasma LCAT and a cholesteryl ester-transport protein. (From Goldstein, J.L. et al. Defective lipoprotein receptors and alhecosclerosis. Reprinted, by permission from the *New England Journal of Medicine,* 309:288, 1983.)

hydraulic factors. Sites that are especially prone to the development of atheromatous lesions are usually epicardial in location and include the bifurcation of the main left coronary artery itself, the bifurcation of the left anterior descending artery into its first septal and diagonal branches, and the major curves of the right coronary and left circumflex arteries [11]. It should be noted that unlike that of autopsy series, the patient population studied by coronary arteriography represents a more diverse group. Thus, there are usually equal distributions of one-, two-, and three-vessel disease (as defined in chapter 9) in coronary arteriographic studies that correlate clinical and anatomic findings [12, 13]. Greater than 50 percent stenosis of the left main coronary artery is present in 3 to 10 percent of the patients, and they usually have dis-

ease of other vessels as well (see figure 9–10). Total occlusion of the left main coronary artery is rare, but it is not incompatible with survival [14]. Coronary artery ectasia (aneurysmal dilatation) is present in less than 5 percent of patients with coronary artery disease [15]. The clinical significance of ectasia in coronary artery disease is not clear; it most likely represents a form of coronary atherosclerosis that may be associated with a higher frequency of hypertension.

*Coronary Collaterals.* Coronary arteriographic findings in patients with unstable angina, particularly of the new-onset type, may show a lesser frequency of single vessel lesions compared to patients with stable angina, but they are even more remarkable in that there is a relative paucity of collateral vessels [16]. As noted earlier, collateral vessels are considered part of the arterial network; in humans, however, they are essentially unused pathways under normal circumstances, and as a result they are small and not easily demonstrable. If preformed, they rapidly increase in size when chronic (but not acute) myocardial ischemia is present, and in certain circumstances they can actually be formed de novo in response to the ischemic stimulus [17]. *Intracoronary collaterals* connect the right and left system; *intercoronary collaterals* run between the branches of one system. Collateral vessels may be epicardial, intramyocardial (e.g., in the interventricular septum), or subendocardial. Examples of collaterals visualized by coronary angiography are depicted in figures 9–8 and 9–9. Coronary collaterals large enough to be visible on human coronary angiograms are observed only where there is a high-grade (more than 50 percent and usually more than 75 percent) luminal stenosis, but even in 15 to 20 percent of such instances no collaterals are visible [18], for reasons that are not clear.

The functional significance of such collateral vessels in humans is controversial. They do not protect against exercise-induced ischemia, but they may offer some protection against future myocardial infarction [18], and in addition, they may enhance left ventricular wall motion in some circumstances [19, 20]. Although not readily visualized in humans after an acute coronary occlusion, animal experimentation has yielded more definitive evidence that these vessels are functional after such an event [17]. These vessels in animals appear to limit the extent of the ischemic process, thereby reducing mortality. The means of stimulation of collateral flow would appear to be an important goal for future animal and human investigations.

## CONTROVERSIES CONCERNING THE PATHOGENESIS OF ACUTE MYOCARDIAL INFARCTION

Traditionally, coronary thrombosis had been considered to be the major cause of acute myocardial infarction. However, when clinicopathologic studies demonstrated that thrombosis could occur without infarction (in case of well-developed collateral vessels, for example) and that small subendocardial infarcts could occur in

the absence of thrombus-associated coronary occlusions, the role of thrombosis became less well defined. Because of this ambiguity and also because the entire concept of thrombus causing infarcts had been challenged, a workshop on the subject was held at the National Institutes of Health [21] to discuss the subject. *It was accepted that the subendocardial type of infarction could evolve without thrombosis,* and only the etiology of transmural infarctions was discussed. The bulk of the speakers supported the traditional role of coronary thrombosis as a preceding event. For example, Chapman cited his autopsy experience with several hundred transmural infarctions. Over 90 percent had recent coronary artery occlusion. Erhardt and Roberts presented the opposing viewpoint, that coronary thrombosis is a *consequence* of an acute myocardial infarction. In their experience, thrombi were most common in patients with pump failure. Thus, the infarct—whether due to an episode of coronary spasm, hemorrhage into a plaque, or to excess myocardial oxygen requirements in relation to impaired perfusion through chronically stenosed vessels —leads to a period of diminished coronary blood flow. Diminished flow, combined perhaps with endothelial injury and platelet aggregation, could then result in *secondary* formation of an intravascular thrombus. However, as a result of this workshop and other subsequent studies summarized in more recent reviews [22, 23], it is now generally accepted that a transmural myocardial infarction is caused by coronary thrombosis in more than 90 percent of cases, with coronary spasm playing a very minor role.

## PATHOLOGY OF ACUTE MYOCARDIAL INFARCTION

As early as 20 minutes, and especially by 60 minutes, following experimental coronary artery occlusion, irreversible cellular injury occurs. The pathology of the acutely infarcted area involves complex ultrastructural changes that are initially visible only via electron microscopy: peripheral aggregation of nuclear chromatin, disruption of the myofibrillar pattern, development of relaxation bands, loss of mitochondrial matrix density, mitochondrial swelling, and appearance of amorphous dense bodies within the mitochondria. The usual subsequent sequence of events in the uncomplicated infarction is briefly summarized as follows. The first gross changes are minimal, and the infarcted area may be only somewhat paler than surrounding normal myocardium. At about 24 hours, the infarct has become yellow and striking changes in cellular morphology are evident with the light microscope. These changes include clumping of the cytoplasm of the myocardial fibers, alterations of the cross striations, blurring of the nuclei, and interstitial proliferation of leukocytes. Over the course of the next several days, phagocytosis and the removal of fragmented muscle fibers is readily apparent and is initially most marked at the periphery of the infarction, which is now reddish-purple. Two weeks postinfarction, muscle removal is well advanced at the periphery and scar formation is under way. Fibroblasts proliferate and lay down bundles of collagen, and as the scar grows more prominent by the fourth week, the infarcted area becomes noticeably gray. Complete healing usually takes about 6 weeks.

It has been generally accepted that after coronary artery occlusion the ischemic zone presumably contains various amounts of both irreversibly and reversibly injured cells, especially since pathologic studies demonstrated that myocardial necrosis is not completely uniform in the affected area. The subepicardium is often spared, for example, and even when the infarction is transmural, "islands" of viable myocardium are frequently still present, usually at the periphery of the infarct.

The latter observation suggests the presence of a "border zone" of transmural infarction at the lateral periphery; such an intermediate region has been identified by a variety of investigators using different study techniques to evaluate the effects of acute coronary artery occlusion. However, other experimental studies of acute ischemic injury have noted *no* differences in cardiac enzyme depletion between the center and lateral peripheries of the ischemic zone and have raised questions as to whether a border zone exists *at all.* This controversy has important clinical implications, since therapies designed to salvage ischemic myocardium are based on the presence of reversibly damaged, "jeopardized" myocardium. Although the bulk of current evidence favors the theory that there is a continuum

of metabolic flow and electrophysiologic changes between the core of an ischemic area and surrounding normal tissue, the exact nature of this border zone still remains uncertain. There appears to be a growing trend toward acceptance of a *subepicardial* zone of ischemic but viable myocardium. However, the presence, and especially the size, of a *lateral* border zone is open to more disagreement.

## Pathophysiology of Myocardial Ischemia in Humans

As noted at the beginning of the chapter, an appreciation of the pathophysiology of myocardial ischemia is important not only for better understanding but also for treating ischemic heart disease. For example, since myocardial ischemia is related to an *imbalance between myocardial oxygen supply and demand,* the treatment of ischemic heart disease (which in our society is predominantly coronary artery disease) is accordingly directed toward correction of this imbalance, either by increasing the capacity of the coronary arteries to supply blood to the ischemic myocardium or by reducing the myocardial oxygen demand. Specific therapeutic regimens for treating myocardial ischemia in humans are discussed in chapters 12, 13, and 14. In general, *medical treatment* of coronary artery disease is directed primarily toward reducing myocardial oxygen demand; however, recent techniques such as coronary angioplasty and intracoronary thrombolysis directly improve myocardial oxygen supply by increasing blood flow. *Surgical procedures,* and especially direct myocardial revascularization utilizing saphenous vein and internal mammary artery grafts, are designed primarily to improve myocardial oxygen supply by increasing blood flow to areas supplied by obstructed vessels.

### DETERMINANTS OF MYOCARDIAL OXYGEN DEMAND

Mammalian cardiac muscle is unlike skeletal muscle in that it cannot develop an appreciable oxygen debt during vigorous activity and repay it later. The heart cannot be rested in the same manner as an arm or leg. As a consequence of its sustained contractile activity, the heart's oxygen needs are relatively high, even during periods of no stress, and it extracts nearly 75 percent of the available oxygen in the coronary circulation. This oxygen is used to generate high-energy phosphate compounds; since aerobic (oxidative) metabolism is the primary source of cardiac energy generation, the rate of myocardial oxygen consumption ($M\dot{V}o_2$) correlates closely with total cardiac energy requirement.

The $M\dot{V}o_2$ is determined by six factors, three of which may be considered major and three minor (figure 2–4). The three *minor* factors are related to basal metabolism, the activation of contraction, and myocardial fiber shortening (or external cardiac work). Although many of the studies reporting the relative unimportance of these factors in determining the $M\dot{V}o_2$ have been performed in isolated muscle, they appear relevant to the whole heart [24]. The *major* determinants of myocardial oxygen consumption are the systolic wall stress or tension (a function of intraventricular volume, pressure, and wall thickening during systole), the duration of that tension (primarily a function of heart rate and, to a lesser extent, of systolic ejection time), and the contractile state of the myocardium [24]. Therefore, $M\dot{V}o_2$ increases when left ventricular systolic pressure, volume, or wall thickening increases; when the heart rate is elevated; and when the contractile state of the myocardium is enhanced, such as with administration of digitalis.

In the clinical setting, it is not often possible to measure all these factors directly; therefore, indirect measurements or indices of myocardial oxygen consumption must be employed. These indices are limited because they fail to include ventricular volume and the contractile state of the myocardium; they utilize only the product of the systolic blood pressure (which, in the absence of aortic stenosis, is the same pressure as in the left ventricle), the heart rate, and the ejection time [25]. This "triple product" is closely related to the tension-time index, a laboratory measurement of the area under the systolic phase of the left ventricular pressure curve multiplied by the heart rate. The "double product" (systolic blood pressure times heart rate) as an index of $M\dot{V}o_2$ seems equally reliable based on exercise studies [25, 26] and has been used extensively in clinical investigations. For example, two decades ago Robinson [27] studied effort-induced angina and correlated the onset of chest pain with the double product. He found that in the same patient, effort-induced angina could be provoked over a relatively narrow range of heart rate–blood pressure products, and the range could never be significantly exceeded without the development of pain (figure 2–5). These studies, as well as others to be discussed in subsequent sections, have helped to establish the hemodynamic profiles of various specific clinical subsets of coronary artery disease.

## CORONARY BLOOD FLOW: THE MAJOR FACTOR INFLUENCING MYOCARDIAL OXYGEN SUPPLY

Oxygen supply can be considered in terms of oxygen extraction and delivery. Since the amount of oxygen extracted from the blood by the heart is nearly maximal at rest, there is little reserve capacity to meet increased demand; in addition, the oxygen content of the blood cannot be significantly increased under normal atmospheric conditions. Only by increasing the delivery of oxygen (e.g., by augmenting coronary blood flow) are increased myocardial demands met. There are certain instances (e.g., during tachycardia in patients with myocardial hypertrophy, especially when due to aortic stenosis) in which the subendocardium may be underperfused in the absence of coronary arterial obstruction [28], but the major cause of re-

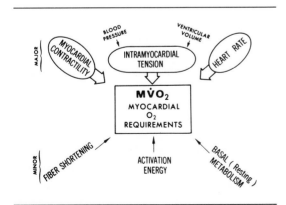

FIGURE 2–4. Major and minor determinants of myocardial oxygen consumption ($M\dot{V}o_2$). (From Amsterdam, E.A. et al. *Am. J. Cardiol.* 33:737, 1974.)

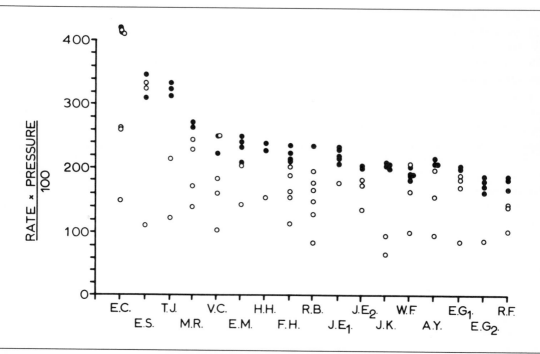

FIGURE 2–5. Products of heart rate and systolic blood pressure achieved during periods of exercise in 15 patients (J.E. and E.G. were studied twice). Solid dots denote episodes in which pain occurred, and open circles, those in which there was no pain. The lowest open circle for each patient shows a representative resting level. Each patient had a relatively narrow range of rate-pressure products in which angina could be provoked. This range is never significantly exceeded without development of pain. (From Robinson, B.F. Relation of the heart rate and systolic blood pressure to the onset of pain in angina pectoris. *Circulation* 35:1073, 1967. Reproduced by permission of the American Heart Association, Inc.)

stricted delivery of oxygenated blood to the myocardium is atherosclerotic obstruction of the coronary arteries. To understand how the heart "adapts," or tries to adapt, to this restriction of flow, the factors that regulate coronary blood flow must be considered.

*Regulation of Coronary Blood Flow.* Coronary blood flow is directly related to both the perfusion pressure (essentially the aortic diastolic pressure) and the duration of diastole (during which most of the myocardial flow is delivered) and inversely related to the resistance of the coronary vascular bed.

Resistance can be affected by active changes in the tone of the smooth muscle of the vessel wall (intrinsic factors) or by extravascular mechanical compression of the coronary arteries (extrinsic factors). Intrinsic factors include autoregulation, metabolic factors (increased $M\dot{V}_{O_2}$), neural factors, and the influence of various pharmacologic agents [29]. The basis for autoregulation (i.e., the ability of the coronary circulation to maintain relatively constant blood flow despite large changes in coronary arterial perfusion pressure) is not completely understood, but it is probably related to the action of tissue metabolites as well as to that of neurogenic and humoral agents. In fact, autoregulation may be related mostly to one specific product of cardiac metabolism: the vasodilator substance, adenosine [30].

Whatever the mechanism of the autoregulatory phenomenon, the site of action appears to be the arteriole, the resistance vessel. When the larger arteries are obstructed by atheroma or by spasm, their narrowing also contributes significantly to resistance to blood flow. In this situation, the arteriolar bed distal to the site of obstruction is maximally vasodilated (as a result of autoregulation), and there is too little vasodilatory reserve to meet increasing myocardial oxygen requirements. The result is myocardial ischemia, with the subendocardial region particularly vulnerable, as has been well demonstrated by animal studies [31, 32].

Much of what we know about the coronary circulation is derived from such animal studies because there are technical and ethical limits to what can be done in human investigations. Creating coronary artery disease in animals, especially in dogs, by means of mechanical constriction of the vessels is not directly analogous to the human situation. In addition, dogs have a much better developed collateral system, which must be considered in interpreting the effects of therapeutic interventions. Nevertheless, data applicable to the clinical setting can often be obtained from such studies.

For example, Gould and associates have addressed the problem of the hemodynamic significance of various degrees of stenosis of the coronary arteries [33, 34]. In their studies they employed the increased coronary blood flow response (coronary hyperemia) caused by intracoronary injections of sodium diatrizoate (a commonly used radiographic contrast agent). Under experimental conditions this agent causes a transient, maximal vasodilatation comparable to a 10-second occlusion of a coronary artery. Results in dogs (figure 2–6) show that (1) pressure gradient-flow characteristics, or hydraulic resistance, of stenoses do not become abnormal enough to alter resting coronary blood flow when the stenoses are less than 60 percent of the vessel diameter (equivalent to about 85 percent reduction in cross-sectional area); (2) with lesions of between 60 and 85 percent of the vessel diameter, compensatory vasodilatation of the distal coronary vascular beds maintains near normal resting flow, but adaptive vasodilatation fails to compensate for lesions of greater than 85 percent; and (3) some vasodilatory reserve is still present (probably in the subepicardium) when coronary artery flow is reduced below normal by a stenosis of the vessel.

The *length* of the narrowed segment may also contribute to the hemodynamic significance of the lesion. An experimental model has been devised to calculate the contribution of several variables (diameter, length, exit angle, etc.) to

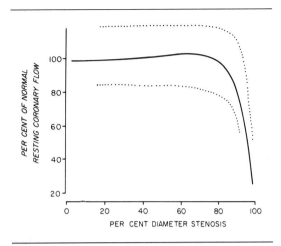

FIGURE 2–6. Relation between varying, experimentally induced degrees of stenosis of the diameter of the left circumflex coronary artery in dogs (abscissa) and the percentage of normal (control) resting coronary flow in that vessel (ordinate). (From Gould, K.L., et al. Compensatory changes of the distal coronary vascular bed during progressive coronary constriction. *Circulation* 51:1085, 1975. Reproduced by permission of the American Heart Association, Inc.)

the hemodynamic significance of a coronary arterial stenosis [35].

*Studies of Coronary Blood Flow in Patients with Coronary Artery Disease.* One of the problems in evaluating alterations in coronary blood flow in humans has been the necessity for using *indirect* methods, since, as noted, flowmeters cannot be attached to the coronary arteries nor can other techniques applicable to experimental animals be used in clinical settings.

Over the past 30 years a variety of studies have employed a wide range of techniques for quantitating coronary blood flow in humans. These include three basic types: (1) methods using diffusible inert gases (some of them radioactive) [36, 37], (2) continuous coronary sinus thermodilution [38], and (3) radioclearance techniques [39]. Methods are described in detail in the references cited. Despite the number of studies, there was no consensus on whether absolute reduction in flow exists, either at rest or during interventions that can provoke angina. Rowe and co-workers [40], for example, studied 31 patients with angina pectoris, and they measured coronary blood flow using the nitrous oxide method. All subjects had undergone coronary arteriography and the extent of disease had been "scored," yet there was no correlation between these scores and the mean coronary blood flow values in the left ventricle. Klocke and Wittenberg [41] noted similar results with nitrous oxide and hydrogen gas techniques, as did Cohen and associates [12], who used radioactive xenon and krypton washout techniques, respectively, and Ganz and colleagues [38], who measured coronary sinus blood flow with a thermodilution technique.

Data that indicate a reduction in myocardial blood flow at rest in patients with coronary artery disease have recently been provided by Klocke [36]. This investigation evaluated mean left ventricular blood flow in 20 normal subjects and in 26 patients with angina pectoris and arteriographically documented coronary artery disease. Significantly lower flows in the patients with coronary artery disease were noted. In this study, helium was used as a tracer (rather than nitrous oxide or hydrogen gas, as had been used previously [41]); in addition, more sensitive arterial and coronary sinus desaturation techniques were used to detect these differences, which were not obvious with simultaneous measurements using traditional nitrous oxide and krypton desaturation curves. Other investigators have also noted lower flows in patients with coronary artery disease [39] by measuring myocardial blood flow with intravenous bolus injections of rubidium-84 and a coincidence counting technique. Although such differences were present in the control (rest) state [42], they could be accentuated with right atrial pacing or atropine infusion. Knoebel and co-workers [43, 44], for example, demonstrated decreases in myocardial blood flow in subjects with coronary artery disease during these later interventions. The coronary sinus flow technique has also been used [45] to demonstrate that adrenergically mediated coronary vascular tone (precipitated by a cold pressor stimulus) can reduce coronary blood flow in patients with chronic angina and, therefore, may contribute to ischemic episodes.

*Evaluation of Regional Myocardial Perfusion.* One of the reasons that no consensus existed as

to alterations in myocardial blood flow in coronary artery disease was that the methods described above measure the *average* myocardial blood flow (i.e., the inert gas techniques) or the *total* myocardial blood flow (i.e., the rubidium-84 clearance and coronary sinus thermodilution techniques). At rest, values for normal subjects and coronary patients overlap considerably, although, as we have noted, several studies have reported mean differences between groups. However, techniques to evaluate *regional* myocardial perfusion have further added to the data that indicate patients with chronic ischemic heart disease *do* have abnormalities of coronary blood flow. For example, Wilson and associates [46], using coronary sinus thermodilution measurements of great cardiac vein flow combined with atrial pacing, have recently demonstrated that some patients with angina and left anterior descending coronary artery disease had a marked restriction in their ability to increase coronary blood flow during stress. Because the great cardiac vein selectively drains the distribution of the left anterior descending artery, this can be considered an example of regional flow. Other studies performed both at rest and after various interventions have employed a scintillation camera and either intracoronary injections of xenon-133 or of radioactive microspheres or the intravenous injections of an isotope of potassium or one of its analogs. Such techniques will be described further in chapter 8. In particular, the measurement of regional myocardial flow using intracoronary injection of xenon-133 and the scintillation camera has provided interesting data on *quantitative* flow measurements [37].

In these studies [37] flow differences between areas subserved by stenosed coronary arteries and areas that are normally perfused have been demonstrated (figure 2–7). In other studies using krypton-81m, subnormal flow responses in coronary patients could be accentuated by atrial pacing [47]. Cannon and co-workers [48] have also shown differences in *mean* left ventricular flow in patients with multivessel disease; these differences were related in part to lower levels of hemodynamic variables that determine myocardial oxygen consumption and were similar to

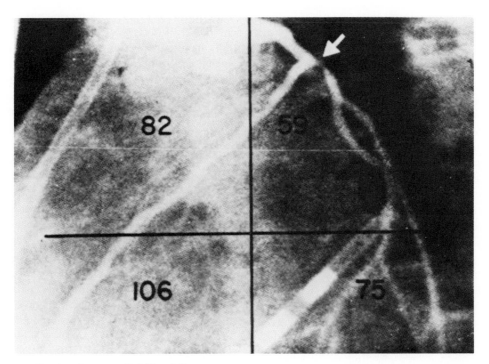

FIGURE 2–7. Regional myocardial blood flow measurements (ml/min/100g) obtained from our regions of the heart are superimposed on the left coronary arteriogram (left anterior oblique projection) of a patient with a high-grade lesion in the proximal left circumflex artery (arrow). Flow is lowest in regions distal to the lesion (59, 75) compared to the normally perfused regions supplied by the left anterior descending artery (82, 106). The regional flow values were obtained by recording the washout of xenon-133 following injection of the radioisotope (in saline) into the left main coronary artery. (From Cohn, P.F. *Adv. Cardiol.* 23:57, 1978.)

those observed in Klocke's study [36] using the helium technique. Coronary blood flow measured by the regional xenon-133 technique has also been shown to be diminished in areas of subnormal ventricular wall motion, both at the site of previous infarction [49] and in noninfarcted regions [50]. This reduction in flow in areas of subnormal wall motion can be due to the effects of the coronary arterial stenosis, to reduced myocardial oxygen requirements in a noncontracting region of scar, or to both. A combination of intervention ventriculography (discussed later in this chapter and again in chapter 9) and measurement of regional wall motion is necessary to evaluate the regional blood flow

values in such instances. Evaluation of collateral flow using the xenon-133 technique has provided mixed results. In some but not all patients with coronary artery disease, the expected fall in regional perfusion occurring with atrial pacing does not occur in the presence of adequate collaterals. The relation of collateral vessels to augmentation of flow, however, is still not settled [52]. The xenon-133 technique has also been used to confirm—on a regional basis [53]—the effect of the cold pressor test [45] on altering coronary blood flow.

In another "invasive" technique for evaluating regional myocardial perfusion, several groups have injected macroaggregated serum albumin microspheres labeled with iodine-131, technetium-99m, or indium-113m directly into the coronary arteries of patients with and without coronary artery disease [54]. Scintillation camera myocardial perfusion images were obtained, and they have been reported to demonstrate perfusion abnormalities, mainly in areas of prior infarction. Although such images cannot be used to quantitate myocardial blood flow, they complement the results of studies using inert gas techniques. Patients with significant coronary artery disease but without previous infarction, for example, usually demonstrate abnormalities in flow distribution on the scintigram during contrast-agent hyperemia [55]. Such flow abnormalities are similar to those observed with contrast-agent hyperemia and the xenon-133 technique [56].

The use of the scintillation camera (or rectilinear scanner) for quantitative and qualitative studies of regional myocardial perfusion in coronary artery disease is not limited to the catheterization laboratory. Zaret and co-workers [57] initially reported the use of intravenously administered potassium-43, for example, to delineate areas of myocardial infarction as well as regions that became transiently ischemic during angina pectoris. These regions corresponded to areas supplied by stenosed coronary arteries on the arteriogram. Using the same technique, potassium-43 distribution has been shown to be homogeneous both at rest and during exercise in 12 normal subjects. Three hundred subsequent patient studies with potassium and its analogs have confirmed these initial impressions, and the value of noninvasive perfusion studies is generally accepted. Thallium-201 has now replaced potassium-43 as the tracer of choice for this type of study (see chapter 8). In patients without prior infarction, identification of underperfused areas resulting from significant coronary artery stenosis is aided by the use of exercise scintigrams (see figure 8–4). Pharmacologic coronary vasodilation with dipyridamole has also been used with thallium-201 imaging, in a manner similar to that of contrast-agent hyperemia, to assess the significance of coronary artery stenoses [58]. Thus, areas supplied by vessels with hemodynamically significant lesions will show new or increased image defects compared to areas supplied by normal vessels, since the latter can still demonstrate vasodilatory reserve. Another monovalent cation that is currently used for regional myocardial perfusion studies (with position tomography) is rubidium-82 [59].

To summarize, invasive and noninvasive techniques for the study of regional myocardial perfusion are useful in demonstrating impaired myocardial flow either at rest or during stress in many patients with coronary artery disease.

## CIRCULATORY DYNAMICS IN SPECIFIC ANGINA-PROVOKING SITUATIONS

Angina pectoris is the most common subjective expression of myocardial ischemia. It is not the only subjective expression of the ischemic process, and indeed some persons have no symptoms associated with myocardial ischemia (see The Phenomenon of Silent Myocardial Ischemia in chapter 4). The clinical presentation of angina —and its subgrouping into chronic (stable), unstable, and variant (Prinzmetal's) types—is discussed in chapter 4. The present discussion is concerned with the pathophysiologic basis of the anginal episodes themselves.

Angina pectoris may be provoked by physical exertion (with sexual activity being considered in this category), emotional stress, exposure to cold weather, and the consumption of large meals. Angina can also develop at rest or during arrhythmias, and it can be provoked by other less specific situations (i.e., anemia or fever). Common to all these states is the development or worsening of abnormal left ventricular function *during* angina, manifested as elevated filling pressures, reduced cardiac output, abnormal wall motion, or a combination of these factors. In the last decade it has become apparent, however, that what is not common to all these states is the *genesis* of the particular anginal episodes.

When the circulatory dynamics of angina were first investigated in depth during the 1960s, the consensus of these studies was that transient episodes of myocardial ischemia were due to an increase in myocardial oxygen needs in the presence of an oxygen supply that was limited because of a fixed atheromatous lesion. Thus, angina was considered *secondary* to the increased oxygen demand rather than due to *primary* dynamic alterations in the coronary circulation. In the 1970s, however, alterations in coronary vascular tone were demonstrated directly via angiography and indirectly via myocardial perfusion studies. Therefore, different anginal mechanisms could be invoked in different clinical states, with coronary vasospasm being increasingly implicated in many of them in addition to Prinzmetal's angina [60]. Figure 2–8 illustrates the concept of dynamic coronary obstruction. In this schema, increased (or decreased) vascular tone superimposed on an

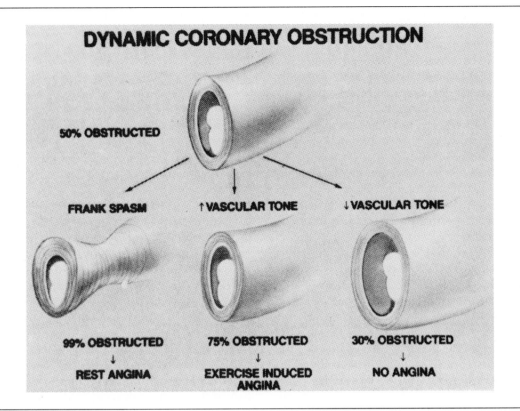

FIGURE 2–8. How a 50 percent atherosclerotic lesion can cause angina at rest, exercise-induced angina, or no angina, depending on the underlying tone of the coronary vessel. (From Epstein, S.E. and Talbot, T.L. *Am. J. Cardiol.* 48:797, 1981.)

atherosclerotic lesion could cause varying degrees of stenosis. At most, this could range from complete obstruction (with ST segment elevation indicating transmural ischemia) to incomplete obstruction (with ST segment depression indicating subendocardial depression). Evidence for this concept is supplied by the studies cited earlier of myocardial blood flow during cold stimuli [45, 53], as well as the recent studies of Crea et al. [61] using ergonovine to precipitate ST segment depression in patients with chronic, effort-induced angina.

*Exertion, or Effort-induced, Angina.* The blood pressure–heart rate product has been mentioned earlier in this chapter as providing a rough approximation of myocardial oxygen requirements, and most patients with angina have a pre- dictable, constant, and reproducible anginal threshold for this product during exertion (see figure 2–5). As noted previously, studies detailing abnormalities of regional myocardial perfusion *during* exercise have been reported using noninvasively administered radioisotopes [57, 58]. Such studies cannot differentiate between primary and secondary changes in perfusion, that is, changes due to vascular spasm versus changes due to imbalance between myocardial oxygen demand and fixed, restricted supply. However, the latter mechanism is believed to predominate in most, but not all, instances of effort angina, since as noted above, vasospastic stimuli can also produce the typical ST segment depression of effort-induced angina [61].

*Angina Due to Emotional Stress.* Emotional stress is a very common antecedent to the development of angina. It need not be accompanied by shouting or other manifestations of anxiety, as theatrical productions suggest. A patient reported by Robinson [27], for example, developed chest pain while doing mental arithmetic and was noted to have increases in both heart rate and blood pressure. Elevations of one or both of these indices may have the same effect and may be brought about by central nervous system stimulation, increased catecholamine release, or both. Lown reported one patient who was "conditioned" to develop angina when he reached a certain number of steps on a two-step exercise protocol; when the patient was told he had reached that number but in fact was not yet near it, he still developed angina and ECG changes. Whether development of angina of this type also involves coronary spasm is uncertain since results are conflicting [62, 63].

*Angina Due to Cold Weather.* Effort-induced angina might not occur in some patients during the performance of certain tasks at moderate temperatures, yet it may occur during the *same* level of exertion at cold temperatures. Several groups, most recently Lassvik and Areskog [64], have reported that peripheral resistance is increased acutely by exposure to a cold environment. The consequent rise in arterial pressure augments the $MVo_2$ and provokes angina, especially when the patient then exercises. As noted earlier, however, the response to a cold pressor stimulus (e.g., ice water) has been used to document changes in myocardial blood flow in patients with a history of chronic angina [45, 53]. Normal control subjects did not show this alteration. Because the effect occurred too soon to be accounted for purely by the rise in blood pressure and because it was blocked by the $\alpha$-adrenergic antagonist phentolamine, a primary alteration in coronary vascular tone was suspected, which perhaps is partly mediated via cardiac reflexes. The alteration in tone appears to be at the arteriolar level, since large coronary arteries show no significant change in luminal size [65].

*Angina Due to Ingestion of Meals.* The deleterious effect of meals on exercise capacity is a well-recognized phenomenon in patients with coronary artery disease, but it is not well understood. The decrease in exercise capacity during or after meals has been explained by the occurrence of a more rapid *rise* in heart rate and blood pressure than what is observed preprandially, but without

any change in the absolute levels of the triple product [66]. By contrast, postprandial angina at rest has been attributed to coronary spasm [67].

*Angina at Rest (Spontaneous Angina).* It is now generally accepted that coronary vasospasm is the cause of Prinzmetal's form of spontaneous, or rest, angina (figure 2–9). This form of rest angina (also termed "variant angina") is characterized by ST segment elevations on the electrocardiogram and no preceding elevation in blood pressure or heart rate. The more common type of rest angina (a part of the unstable angina complex described in chapter 4) that is associated with ST segment depression, and may or may not have associated heart rate and blood pressure elevations, is now also believed to have a large vasospastic component. As Maseri and Chierchia [60] have commented, the idea that angina pectoris can be due totally to "transient spasm of the coronary arteries was put forward about one hundred years ago, became accepted at the beginning of this century, was questioned in the late twenties, fell into complete disrepute in the forties, was reproposed in the sixties, was conclusively demonstrated in the early seventies, and became accepted as pathophysiologic concept in the late seventies." Much of the credit for this dramatic reversal of scientific opinion is due to the studies from Maseri's laboratory. As shown by the example in figure 2–10, this group clearly showed that a primary reduction in coronary blood flow could be responsible for spontaneous myocardial ischemia and preceded hemodynamic alterations. That these episodes were not merely minor alterations in coronary blood flow was documented by thallium-201 studies showing large regional reductions in myocardial perfusion.

What is responsible for this inappropriate focal constriction of large coronary arteries that occurs both in normal areas and areas of critical atherosclerotic narrowing? The answer to this question is still uncertain. Possible mechanisms include increased $\alpha$-adrenergic tone and an imbalance in the blood between those prostaglandins with vasoconstricting and those with vasodilating properties. Because platelets release thromboxane $A_2$, their aggregation in the lumens of coronary arteries has been carefully

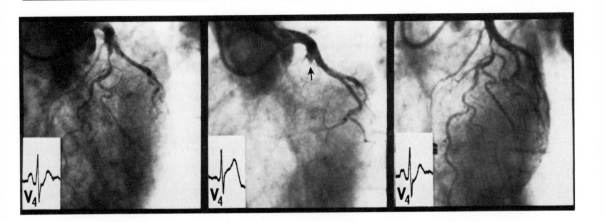

FIGURE 2–9. Cineangiographic frames of the left coronary artery in the right anterior oblique projection and ECG (insert). Patient was a 60-year-old male with unstable angina. During a pain-free interval (left panel), a high-grade proximal lesion in the anterior descending artery is present. Later, during an episode of spontaneous pain (middle panel), ST elevation was observed in leads $V_{-4}$, with total occlusion (arrow) of the anterior descending artery in the area of the high-grade proximal lesion. Following sublingual nitroglycerin administration, pain and ST changes resolved, and the anterior descending artery was again visualized (right panel).

studied. Since the release of thromboxane $A_2$ (as measured in coronary venous blood) is much greater during spontaneous angina than during pacing in induced angina, it has been linked to the genesis of this type of angina [68]. However, Maseri's group has shown that reduction of platelet thromboxane $A_2$ by aspirin to neglible levels failed to reduce the number of ischemic episodes. Whatever the "triggering" mechanism for the spasm—be it increased α-adrenergic tone (which has also been recently questioned by Maseri's group [69]) or thromboxane $A_2$ or other vasoactive substances—it still is unclear why there is variable susceptibility to spasm in different individuals and in different regions of the coronary bed in the same individual. A spastic element may also contribute to angina occurring during sleep, although this is usually attributed to either an increase in heart rate or blood pressure due to dreaming, or to an increase in venous return due to the recumbent position.

*Less Specific Situations.* Anemia lowers the oxygen-carrying capacity of the blood and can precipitate or aggravate angina, as can tachycardias of whatever cause (including fevers) because the increase in heart rate increases myocardial oxygen requirements. Cardiac arrhythmias (even frequent ectopic beats) have also been reported to reduce coronary blood flow both in experimental animals and in humans. The increased myocardial oxygen demands due to the hyperthyroid state or to certain drugs, especially digitalis and catecholamines, can also precipitate or aggravate angina.

In any of the situations noted above, the onset of angina can be hastened by cigarette smoking, because nicotine increases heart rate and blood pressure and exposure to carbon monoxide produces carboxyhemoglobin, thereby reducing oxygen supply [70]. Inhalation of fumes from *other* people's cigarettes in smoke-filled rooms or of polluted air (especially from car exhausts) may also increase carbon monoxide exposure.

## *Effect of Myocardial Ischemia on Cardiac Metabolism, Performance, and Electrical Activity in Humans: Basic Concepts*

### CARDIAC METABOLISM

*Normal Cardiac Metabolism.* Normally, glucose and fatty acids are the major fuel sources of the heart, but other substances that can be used

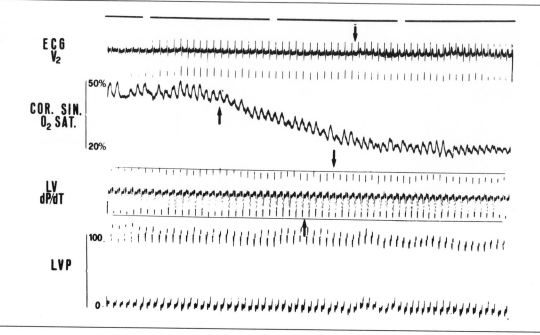

FIGURE 2–10. High-speed playback (paper speed 10 mm/sec) of an ischemic episode characterized by peaking of T-waves, denoting reduction in coronary blood flow in this patient. Arrows indicate the onset of change for each recorded parameter. A drop in coronary sinus oxygen saturation (CSO$_2$S)—denoting reduction in coronary blood flow—precedes the onset of ECG and hemodynamic changes, i.e., a fall in left ventricular (LV) dp/dt and rise in LV end-diastolic pressure. (From Chierchia, S. et al. *Circulation* 61:759, 1980. Reproduced by permission of the American Heart Association, Inc.)

include pyruvate, acetate, ketone bodies, and amino acids. Lactate formed in skeletal muscle during muscular exercise can also provide a useful substrate for cardiac metabolism, but the myocardium does not produce lactate under normal circumstances. The rate of utilization of glucose and fatty acids is related to the production and use of high-energy phosphate compounds by oxidative metabolism, and the latter process is linked to the mechanical activity of the myocardium. Almost all the high-energy phosphate (adenosine triphosphate, or ATP) production is linked to oxidative metabolism within the mitochondria, and normally ATP production by cytoplasmic glycolysis is relatively unimportant (figure 2–11). In the presence of hypoxia or ischemia, however, glycolysis may become a more important source of ATP. It is important to stress that ischemia and hypoxia are *not* synonymous, although reduced oxygen supply to the tissues is common to both. Hypoxia exists *despite* adequate perfusion, whereas in ischemia, oxygen deprivation is *due* to inadequate perfusion.

*Effect of Ischemia.* The effect of ischemia on myocardial metabolism has been extensively studied in animal preparations after coronary ar-

tery ligation [71]. After ischemia has persisted for 20 to 60 minutes, the ultrastructural changes in myocardial cells become irreversible [72]; these changes are associated with metabolic alterations that lead to a loss of ATP production. When myocardial oxygen tension falls (e.g., as a result of depletion of myocardial oxygen reserves), high-energy phosphate levels become reduced, and lactate is now produced. The utilization of tissue glycogen and exogenous glucose is increased at the same time, while there is an inhibition of the oxidative metabolism of fatty acids. Thus, there is a marked increase in glycolytic flux during the transition from aerobic to anaerobic energy production. The effect of this increasing flux is to slow the rate of decline of the level of myocardial high-energy phosphate

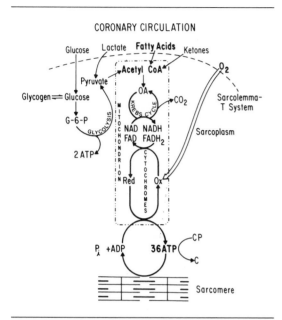

FIGURE 2–11. Metabolic pathways of energy (adenosine triphosphate) production within the cardiac cell. Complete oxidation of a substrate such as glucose that is present in the coronary circulation yields a total of 38 moles of adenosine triphosphate per mole of glucose, whereas glycolysis alone provides only 2 moles of adenosine triphosphate per mole of glucose, and whereas glycolysis alone provides only 2 moles of adenosine triphosphate. ADP = adenosine diphosphate: ATP = adenosine triphosphate; C = creatine; CP = creatine phosphate; CoA = coenzyme A; FAD and $FADH_2$ = flavin adenine dinucleotide and its reduced form, respectively; G-6-P = glucose-6-phosphate; NAD and NADH = nicotinamide adenine dinucleotide and its reduced form, respectively; OA = oxaloacetic acid; Ox = oxidation; $P_i$ = inorganic phosphate; Red = reduction. (From Amsterdam, E.A. *Am. J. Cardiol.* 32:461, 1973.)

compounds and *temporarily* arrest the mechanical deterioration of the anoxic heart. This can be considered only a stop-gap mechanism because persistence of ischemia will cause the heart to undergo irreversible injury.

Myocardial ischemia has metabolic "markers" that aid in its detection both clinically and experimentally. As we have noted, lactate is normally consumed through oxidation by the heart, so the systemic and coronary arterial lactate concentration exceeds the coronary venous concentration. The acceleration of glycolysis in ischemia, however, is characterized by the

*production* of lactate. Lactic acid production can be recognized in the intact heart by the presence of higher concentrations in the coronary sinus (venous) blood than in arterial blood. This determination is useful in establishing or confirming the diagnosis of myocardial ischemia in patients with ambiguous clinical, electrocardiographic, or coronary arteriographic findings [73]. When a catheter is placed in the coronary sinus, coronary lactate measurements may be obtained at rest and after suitable stress, such as isoproterenol administration or pacing. The regional lactate pattern, when combined with coronary cinearteriography, is helpful in localizing areas of myocardial ischemia and significant coronary artery lesions [73]. Other metabolic markers of ischemia that have been utilized in this type of study are amino acids [74] and adenosine metabolites [75].

## CARDIAC PERFORMANCE

*The Myocardial Contractile Unit.* The ventricular myocardium is composed of interconnecting cells (fibers) that contain numerous cross-banded bundles (fibrils or myofibrils) that traverse the length of the cell [76]. It is the fibrils that contain the contractile proteins actin and myosin, arranged as myofilaments within the serially repeating units called *sarcomeres.* The sarcomere also contains other proteins—troponin and tropomyosin—that help to regulate the contractile process. Surrounding the entire myocardial cell (with its fibrils, nucleus, and cytoplasmic structures) is a membrane (sarcolemma). Because the sarcolemma plays an important role in ion exchange, it is involved in several functions related to the electrophysiologic properties of the cell, including generation of the action potential. These are summarized in a subsequent section, Cardiac Electrical Activity.

One of the ions involved in transmembrane fluxes (calcium) also serves as the link between the electrical activity of the cell and its mechanical activity (i.e., contraction). Calcium apparently can be stored within the cell until it is needed for contraction. An important site of storage is the sarcoplasmic reticulum, a complex network of anastomosing channels within the cytoplasm of the myocardial cell. The fundamental mechanism of myocardial cell contraction appears to involve an increase in intracellular calcium concentration (from both extracellular fluid influx and release from intracellular storage sites). The increased calcium ion concentration, in the presence of ATP and magnesium ion, interacts with the regulatory proteins so that the filaments of actin and myosin "slide" over one another, producing shortening of the fiber [76]. The biochemical basis of relaxation appears to involve the reaccumulation of calcium ions within the sarcoplasmic reticulum, but many questions regarding this process remain unanswered.

*Effect of Ischemia.* At the cellular level, myocardial function may be adversely affected in ischemia by both oxygen deprivation and lack of substrates necessary for energy production, but the changes due to acute versus prolonged ischemia may differ. The initial deterioration of myocardial contractile activity observed during ischemia may be due to factors other than simply the depletion of ATP, the major energy source. It may be partly due to alterations in ion transport across the cell membrane with disruption of the excitation-contraction coupling mechanism described previously. Studies in isolated cardiac muscle have demonstrated that *acute* ischemia results in a depression of myocardial contractility that is associated with shortening of the plateau of the action potential, suggesting an abnormality in the inward movement of calcium ions [76]. With *prolonged* ischemia, there is marked binding of calcium by the sarcoplasmic reticulum, perhaps because of the development of intracellular acidosis, which causes calcium to be displaced from sites on the contractile protein [77]. This binding of calcium further reduces contractility. In this setting, one of the possible ways to improve cardiac performance is through correction of acidosis.

In addition to the deficiency of oxygen and substrates necessary for energy production, there is an accumulation of metabolic endproducts from damaged cells. These endproducts include not only hydrogen ions, but also potassium ions and lysozymal enzymes. Excessive extracellular potassium may prevent electrical activation of the cell, whereas lysozy-mal enzymes may directly change cell structure.

*Abnormalities of Left Ventricular Function in Patients with Coronary Artery Disease.* As opposed to experimental studies described in chapter 1 in which isolated cardiac muscle or the intact ventricle can be evaluated extensively without regard to the survival of the animal, studies of left ventricular performance in humans must utilize technology that carries minimal risk for the patient and, if possible, is part of the diagnostic protocol. Among the noninvasive methods included are echocardiography (chapter 7), radionuclide ventriculography (chapter 8), and exercise testing (chapter 6) and among the invasive techniques, cardiac catheterization and angiography (chapter 9).

MEASUREMENTS OF LEFT VENTRICULAR FUNCTION. In the cardiac catheterization laboratory or coronary care unit, standard hemodynamic measurements are useful in evaluating left ventricular function in patients with coronary artery disease, but the pathophysiologic basis of the abnormal measurements is not always clear. Although the frequency of abnormally elevated ventricular filling pressures or reduced cardiac output increases with the severity and extent of vessel disease and the presence of a new or old infarction [78, 79], there is a great deal of overlap in such values among patients with one-, two-, or three-vessel disease. In angina pectoris, the elevation in ventricular filling pressure may be related to reduced compliance (distensibility), to transient left heart failure, or to both [80–84]. The phenomenon of incomplete or altered left ventricular relaxation can also be observed in patients with ischemic heart disease under conditions of rapid atrial pacing [85] when the ventricle becomes stiffer [86]. Shortening of the diastolic filling period by decreasing ventricular filling may further depress left ventricular performance.

In the cardiac catheterization laboratory the hemodynamic abnormalities observed in the resting state usually reflect prior myocardial infarctions; in those patients with normal resting hemodynamics, abnormalities of left ventricular function can often be elicited by various interventions. Dynamic leg exercise is commonly used to induce ischemia and precipitate left ventricular dysfunction, such as alterations in the left ventricular end-systolic pressure-volume relationship [87], but isometrics have also been used for this purpose. Atrial pacing is particularly well suited for combined hemodynamic-metabolic-ventriculographic studies [88].

Contrast and radionuclide left ventriculograms may reveal localized regions of abnormal wall motion during systole, termed *asynergy* by Herman and Gorlin [89]. Asynergy includes reduced movement (hypokinesis). Fibrosis is most likely to occur in association with dyskinesis [90]. (The term "asynchrony" is sometimes used to refer to a disordered sequence of contraction.) Asynergy may occur in 60 to 70 percent of patients, usually in conjunction with abnormal hemodynamic findings, and it is often also demonstrable by echocardiography. As determined by serial cineangiographic studies [91], the evolution and frequency of asynergy reflects, to a large extent, the frequency of myocardial infarctions, and in such instances, dysfunction is mostly due to scar tissue. It is not surprising, therefore, to find a good correlation between ECG evidence of local infarction (i.e., Q-waves) and corresponding regional asynergy [92]. Many other patients, however, will have areas of abnormal wall motion that become apparent only after ischemia is induced, again by techniques such as atrial pacing [93] or exercise [94], in the cardiac catheterization laboratory. Exercise during radionuclide ventriculography or echocardiography [95] can also accentuate these abnormalities (see chapters 7 and 8). In such patients, the asynergy is "reversible"; that is, wall motion reverts to normal when the ischemic episode ceases. The more proximal the lesion the greater the area of transient dysfunction with exercise [96].

The reversibility of asynergy in regions that already show evidence of damage on the resting contrast ventriculogram has recently been the center of intensive investigation using intervention ventriculography (see chapter 9). The purpose of such studies has been to devise techniques to differentiate those areas that are permanently damaged (being composed mainly of scar tissue as a result of infarction) from those that are temporarily ischemic or "stunned" [97]. These techniques employ the use of inotropic

stimulation with epinephrine (see figure 9–4) [98] and postextrasystolic potentiation (figure 2–12) [99], or they use pharmocologic agents such as nitroglycerin (figure 2–13) [100]. The mechanism of action of the inotropic agents is different from that of nitroglycerin, which primarily reduces preload. The effect of inotropic agents has also been correlated with prognosis, particularly after cardiac surgery (see figure 2–12). Histopathologic studies (done at the time of open-heart surgery) in patients in whom either of these techniques has been employed at cardiac catheterization have demonstrated that the responsive asynergic segments are generally made up of histologically intact myocardium, whereas the nonresponsive segments have marked muscle loss and replacement by fibrous tissue [96, 101]. The more responsive areas are generally associated with less severe degrees of coronary artery stenosis, are better collateralized, and have a lower frequency of Q-waves on the ECG [102, 103]. A relation between the sum of the R-waves on the scalar ECG and the left ventricular angiographic ejection fraction was determined both at rest and after augmentation [104]. The applica-

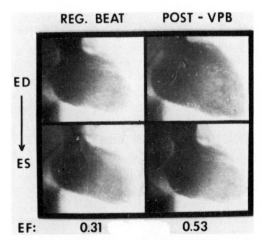

FIGURE 2–12. Marked augmentation of left ventricular function in a patient who subsequently underwent successful myocardial revascularization. Left ventriculograms in the right anterior oblique view at both end-diastole (ED) and end-systole (ES) are shown. The sequence on the left occurred during a regular beat, and the sequence on the right followed a ventricular premature beat (post-VPB). The systolic ejection fraction (EF) was 0.31 and increased to 0.53 following a VPB. (From Cohn, L.H. et al. *J. Thorac. Cardiovasc. Surg.* 72:835, 1976.)

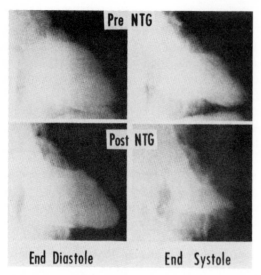

FIGURE 2–13. Effect of nitroglycerin (NTG) on ventricular wall motion. Prior to administration of NTG (top panel), the left ventriculogram in the right anterior oblique projection demonstrated impaired wall motion with an ejection fraction of 0.42. Following NTG (lower panel), there was a marked increase in contractility of the ventricle and the ejection fraction rose 0.56. (From Conti, C.R. *Circulation* 5:227, 1977. Reproduced by permission of the American Heart Association, Inc.)

tion of this technique is described in figure 2–14.

In addition to better defining the histopathologic basis of the asynergic regions, such studies have prognostic and even therapeutic implications, as will be discussed further in chapter 12. Whether they can be adapted to noninvasive techniques for evaluating left ventricular wall motion remains to be determined. One approach that appears potentially valuable uses an external mechanical stimulator (developed by Zoll) to induce ventricular extrasystoles during M-mode echocardiography (figure 2–15). This technique can be used to evaluate both overall [105] and local [106] contractile reserve in patients with coronary artery disease.

Contrast left ventriculography may also show evidence of *mitral valve prolapse*. In one series, 15 of 92 patients with coronary artery disease had this finding [107], and in another series it was observed in 30 of 95 patients [108]. The basis for the prolapse in coronary artery disease is complex and is probably related to impaired contractility of the ventricular myocardium and papillary muscles. Some would argue that the two entities occur coincidentally, because mitral valve prolapse is also found in many patients without coronary artery disease.

CONGESTIVE HEART FAILURE. The clinical syndrome of congestive heart failure may be based on several mechanisms. In the absence of ischemia-induced mitral regurgitation, clinical evidence of congestive heart failure usually occurs only when regional asynergy is so severe and extensive that the uninvolved myocardium cannot compensate adequately. When contraction ceases in 20 to 25 percent of the left ventricle, hemodynamic evidence of left ventricular failure is usually present, whereas with the loss of 40 percent or more of the left ventricular myocardium, clinically severe pump failure or cardiogenic shock may develop [109]. The subject is discussed further in chapter 13.

A *left ventricular aneurysm* is usually defined as a paradoxical (dyskinetic) systolic expansion of a portion of the ventricular wall, but many cardiologists also interpret the term to include akinetic as well as dyskinetic abnormalities [110]. The aneurysm may be composed totally of fibrous tissue or various mixtures of fibrous and muscle tissue. In vitro length-tension studies of tissue taken from human ventricular aneurysms by Parmley and associates [111] have demonstrated that chronic fibrous aneurysms appear to produce their primary mechanical disadvantage through a loss of contractile tissue, and they show only minimal systolic paradox. By contrast, aneurysms made up largely of muscle tissue produce mechanical disadvantages by significant paradoxical expansion as well as by loss of effective contraction.

In autopsy studies the frequency of ventricular aneurysm following myocardial infarction is varied, as is the frequency observed during left ventriculography. As many as 35 percent of patients with coronary artery disease have this finding [112]. The aneurysms also vary in size and can involve from 5 to 35 percent of the left ventricular surface [113]. The usual clinical manifestation is congestive heart failure, although many patients with aneurysms will *not* have this finding. Others may present with angina, arrhythmias, or systemic embolization with or without congestive heart failure.

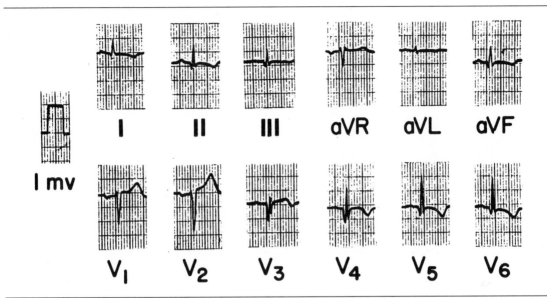

FIGURE 2–14. The electrocardiogram of a 54-year-old patient showing old anterolateral and diaphragmatic myocardial infarction. The sum of R-waves in aVL, aVF, and $V_1$ to $V_6$ (R) is 3.9 mV. The resting ejection fraction (EF) after a sinus beat was 0.29, and the augmented EF after a premature ventricular contraction was 0.49. Using the following equations (1) resting EF = 6.6 R(mV) + 9.4, and (2) augmented EF = 8.6 R(mV) + 11.0, a good correlation was observed between R and EF in 73 patients with coronary artery disease. (From Askenazi, J. et al. *Am. J. Cardiol.* 41:494, 1978.)

Specific diagnostic clues to the presence of an aneurysm include persistent ST segment elevation and an abnormal contour of the silhouette of the left ventricle on the chest roentgenogram. Only nonspecific abnormalities may be found when phonocardiography, apexcardiography, and M-scan echocardiography are used to evaluate left ventricular function, and thus such methods cannot confirm the diagnosis. The radionuclide ventriculogram, however, can graphically demonstrate aneurysms, as can two-dimensional echocardiographic techniques [114] (see also chapters 7 and 8). Cases of left ventricular aneurysm in the absence of coronary artery disease but with prior infarction have been reported; in these cases, recanalization of the coronary artery lumen is suggested.

In addition to aneurysm formation, mitral regurgitation secondary to *papillary muscle rupture or dysfunction* may be the basis for the congestive heart failure [115] in patients with coronary artery disease. There is a high prevalence of prior myocardial infarctions in such patients, but the frequency of the syndrome (as with aneurysm) varies. One group reported a 31 percent frequency of mitral regurgitation on angiography [116]. Clinical features that help identify this syndrome as the cause of acute pulmonary edema or of the milder symptoms of left-sided failure include the murmur, a small left atrium on echocardiography, and demonstration of the abnormal mitral valve leaflet on echocardiography. The echocardiographic findings are especially important, since the timing and duration of the murmur are more variable than originally thought [117]. The ECG is nonspecific; most patients have angiographic evidence of multivessel coronary artery disease [117].

Burch and co-workers [118] used the term *ischemic cardiomyopathy* to describe the condition when coronary artery disease results clinically in severe myocardial dysfunction that is indistinguishable from the manifestations of primary disease of the myocardium. The most systemic study of such patients was by Yatteau et al. [119] and by Dash et al. [120]. In both studies, patients with isolated ventricular aneurysm were excluded, but all patients had generalized abnormalities of left ventricular wall motion and some

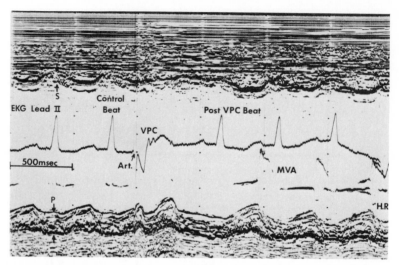

FIGURE 2–15. Echocardiogram demonstrating augmentation of septal (S) and posterior (P) wall motion following a noninvasive, externally induced ventricular premature contraction (VPC). In this patient, the systolic
dimensional shortening and the ejection fraction of the control beat preceding the VPC were 14 percent and
0.27, respectively, and these values increased to 19 percent and 0.38 in the potentiated beat following the VPC.
MVA = mitral valve apparatus; Art. = artifact indicating external mechanical stimulus and onset of VPC.
Arrows (from top to bottom) = right septum, left septum, posterior endocardium, and posterior epicardium.
(From Cohn, P.F., et al. A new, noninvasive technique for inducing postextrasystolic potentiation during
echocardiography. *Circulation* 56:598, 1977. Reproduced by permission of the American Heart Association,
Inc.)

had mitral regurgitation. Prior infarctions were
very common, but a minority of patients did not
have any chest pain, past or present. Whether
the clinical picture of cardiomegaly and congestive heart failure can develop in a *totally* silent
way (with neither a history of angina nor of
symptomatic infarction) is not clear from these
studies, but in patients without an anginal history, the clinical presentation and physical
findings suggest only congestive heart failure
due to left ventricular dysfunction. In individuals presenting in this manner, cardiomyopathy
(due to causes *other* than ischemic heart disease)
should be considered first. Cardiac catheterization may be necessary to diagnose this disorder.

Any condition in which there is stasis of blood
in the left ventricle, whether it be due to aneurysm or ischemic cardiomyopathy, or acute myocardial infarction, will increase the chance of left
ventricular mural thrombi forming. Because
these thrombi may embolize to the arterial circulation with potentially catastrophic results, a variety of noninvasive methods for detecting them
have been tested. Two-dimensional echocardi-

ography and the indium-111 labeled platelet
technique appear the best methods for identifying such thrombi [121].

## CARDIAC ELECTRICAL ACTIVITY

*Electrophysiology of the Heart.* Our understanding of the electrophysiology of the heart has
been greatly enhanced by the use of intracellular
microelectrodes to record the electrical activity
of individual cardiac fibers in experimental
preparations [122]. With this technique, one
can measure the transmembrane potential during diastole as well as the changes in transmembrane potential that occur during depolarization
and repolarization, that is, the action potential
(figure 2–16). Thus, as measured with a micro-
electrode, during diastole the interiors of these
cells are negatively charged with respect to the
extracellular fluid. This transmembrane potential is largely due to the concentration gradient
of potassium maintained by the cell across a
membrane, which in its resting state is permea-
ble to potassium ions but relatively impermeable
to other cations. In some cells, such as those of

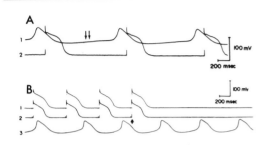

FIGURE 2–16. Action potentials of cardiac cells. The upstroke denotes activation (depolarization), the downstroke indicates repolarization, and the baseline represents the resting (polarized) state. These action potentials illustrate abnormal automaticity, entrance block, and exit block in Purkinje fibers that survive acute myocardial infarction (AMI). The anterior descending coronary artery was ligated in dogs. About 24 hours later, the heart was removed, dissected to yield a preparation composed of both infarcted and noninfarcted ventricular tissues, placed in a tissue bath, and superfused with Tyrode's solution. Intracellular recordings were made with glass microelectrodes. **(A)** Abnormal automaticity in AMI. The upper tracing (1) is from an automatic subendocardial Purkinje fiber (PF) in the infarct; the lower tracing (2) is from a subendocardial PF in a noninfarcted area. The PF in the infarct (1) has a low maximum diastolic (resting) voltage; and a slowly rising, low-amplitude action potential. Spontaneous diastolic depolarization (double arrow) is present; this activates the cell and propagates slowly to activate the entire preparation. The PF action potential recorded from the cell outside the infarct (2) is normal. **(B)** Entrance block and exit block in AMI. The upper two tracings (1 and 2) are from PF in noninfarcted regions; the lower tracing (3) is from a PF in an infarcted zone. To the left of the single arrow, the preparation is stimulated vis surface of the preparation; to the right of the arrow, stimuli are not applied. During stimulation, there is entrance block into the infarcted zone, indicated by the lack of relationship between activation in the normal PF and those in the infarct. When stimulation stops, exit block from the infarct is revealed, that is, spontaneous action potentials in the infarct (3) do not propagate to sites 1 and 2 outside the infarct. (From Bigger, J.T., Jr. et al. Ventricular arrythmias in ischemic heart disease: mechanics, prevalence, significance and management. Reprinted, by permission from *Prog. Cardiovasc. Dis.,* 19:255, 1977.)

the sinus node, membrane potential during diastole is not constant but declines spontaneously to a level at which a full-fledged action potential is generated. This phenomenon of spontaneous diastolic depolarization, or *automaticity,* is a characteristic of the pacemaker cells of the sinus node as well as other latent cardiac pacemakers, including certain specialized atrial fibers, some cells in the atrioventricular (AV) junction, and, during the ischemia, Purkinje fibers (see figure 2–16). In other fibers, such as normal ventricular muscle cells, membrane potential during diastole remains constant; action potentials arise in these cells only in response to threshold stimuli.

Regardless of cell type, the depolarization that occurs in response to a threshold stimulus and the process of repolarization that follows are due to ion fluxes across the cell membrane. These fluxes are controlled by variations in membrane permeability, ion concentration gradients, and a sodium pump mechanism. The contributions of each of the various membrane channels for ion conductance are not identical for all cardiac cells and partly account for the differences in the morphology of the action potential [122]. Thus, Purkinje fibers, ventricular muscle cells, and atrial muscle cells are characterized by a relatively high potential across the cell membrane during diastole as well as extremely rapid rates of depolarization. In addition, the action potentials are large and exhibit prominent plateau phases prior to repolarization. Such cells have been termed *fast-response fibers.* Evidence from voltage clamp studies suggests that depolarization in these fibers results from a sudden, large *inward* current of ions (predominantly sodium ions) through the so-called fast membrane channel. Current flow through this channel is initially of a large magnitude, but declines quickly after the onset of depolarization as the fast membrane channel becomes inactivated or closed.

During the latter part of the sodium-dependent rapid depolarization phase, a second membrane conductance channel begins to open. Although this second so-called slow channel accounts for very little of the initial rapid phase of depolarization, it remains open longer than the fast channel. The *additional inward* current flow through this slow channel is carried predominantly by calcium ions and, to a lesser extent, by sodium ions. Current that flows during this slow channel is responsible for the plateau phase of the action potential. (The calcium, which enters the cell during this time, also plays an important role in coupling excitation to myocardial contraction.) Toward the end of the plateau phase, *outward* currents through the cell membrane are activated. These currents are carried largely by potassium ions and repolarize the membrane to its resting (diastolic) potential.

Sinus node cells, certain AV node cells, and diseased depolarized Purkinje fibers or ventricular muscle cells generate action potentials with low amplitudes and low rates of depolarization. Because this is unlike the normal fast-response fibers noted above, these action potentials have been termed *slow responses* and may depend predominantly on calcium currents flowing through the slow membrane channel.

*The Surface Electrocardiogram.* The genesis of the surface electrocardiogram is related to the depolarization and repolarization of individual cardiac cells that are electrically connected to one another. As the wave of depolarization spreads across the heart following stimulus, it causes differences in extracellular electrical potential recorded between the areas that are depolarized (negative) and the polarized areas (positive) ahead of the advancing wavefront. As described by Kupersmith [123], these differences in electrical potential can be expressed as vectors that are oriented from depolarized to polarized areas; thus, the QRS *complex* of the surface electrocardiogram reflects the sum of the vectorial forces of the ventricles. Forces from the left ventricle predominate because of its greater mass. When depolarization is complete, there are no longer any potential differences within the heart, and the surface electrocardiogram becomes isoelectric *(ST segment).* Potential differences again occur within the ventricles when some ventricular cells become completely repolarized ahead of others; these differences are represented by the *T-wave.* With the subsequent complete repolarization of the ventricles, the surface electrocardiogram again becomes isoelectric *(T-P interval)* prior to the beginning of atrial depolarization. The QRS complex and T-wave vectors are usually oriented in the same direction on the electrocardiogram. This is due to the fact that depolarization and repolarization occur in different directions. The wave of depo-

larization spreads down the bundle branches to the distal Purkinje fibers and thence to ventricular muscle, spreading from endocardium to epicardium. However, since action potential duration in ventricular muscle cells is shorter than in the Purkinje fibers, the wave of repolarization spreads from epicardium to endocardium.

Soon after experimental coronary artery occlusion, certain biochemical changes in ischemic myocardium dramatically affect cellular membrane permeability. These include (1) loss of sodium pump activity, resulting in intracellular sodium and water accumulation; (2) subsequent extracellular hyperkalemia; and (3) intracellular acidosis due to the accumulation of lactate from anaerobic metabolism. Thus, as a consequence of myocardial ischemia and infarction, the action potential of ventricular cells is altered and characteristic changes occur in ventricular depolarization and repolarization. These changes affect the morphology of the QRS complex, the ST segment, and the T-wave of the surface electrocardiogram, depending on whether the injury is predominantly transmural (and involves the subepicardial region of the ventricle) or nontransmural (involving predominantly the subendocardial region). The changes also affect impulse formation and conduction. These various effects are summarized in the following sections.

*Transmural Injury Patterns.* When necrosis occurs, the involved cells can no longer be depolarized. As a result, there is an imbalance in vectorial forces, and unopposed forces from the noninjured wall of the heart become apparent in the initial portion of the QRS complex. In general, this effect can be masked by left bundle branch block and left hemiblocks, but not by right bundle branch block. These vectors are oriented away from the infarcted zone, and either Q-waves appear or R-waves lessen or disappear on the surface electrocardiogram over the area of necrosis. In the case of a posterior infarct, new R-waves appear in the anterior leads opposite the area of necrosis.

There is generally a good correlation between the electrocardiographic localization of healed myocardial infarction and autopsy studies, but for a variety of reasons (remoteness of surface leads from certain areas of the heart, multiple infarctions, etc.), the electrocardiogram tends to underestimate the extent of infarction, particularly in the lateral and inferobasal regions of the left ventricle [124].

In acute transmural infarcts, ST segment abnormalities associated with subepicardial ischemia are usually present. Characteristic ST segment elevation in leads overlying the infarct area are attributed to the net result of systolic and diastolic injury currents. Whether the systolic or diastolic injury current is the main cause of ST segment alteration is not clear, because shifts in the baseline (which are affected by diastolic injury current) are not detected as isolated events on conventional ECG recordings. Ischemia also alters the normal sequence of ventricular repolarization, causing flattening or inversion of the T-waves.

The earliest changes in acute myocardial infarction may be "hyperacute" T-waves similar to those occurring in hyperkalemia. (Local elevation of potassium, due to cellular necrosis, may be the basis for many of the ST-T abnormalities noted early in the infarction, and similar transient alterations in membrane fluxes of potassium may explain the ECG findings of ischemia.) More commonly, the earliest recorded stage of the infarction is ST segment elevation in surface leads overlying the infarcted area accompanied by ST segment depressions in reciprocal leads. Usually Q-waves develop and T-waves become inverted *before* the ST segment returns to the baseline. The sequence of surface ECG changes during an acute anterior wall infarction is depicted in figure 13–3. Figure 10–2 is an example of a healed posterior wall infarct, and figure 2–11 an example of combined anteroinferior infarctions.

Transmural ischemia without infarction is characterized by the ST and T-wave abnormalities (although these are reported rarely) and by reversibility of the ECG abnormality and no significant cardiac enzyme elevation. Although transmural ischemia is sometimes associated with typical exertion-related angina, its occurrence usually indicates Prinzmetal's angina.

*Nontransmural Injury Patterns.* In general, nontransmural infarctions are not associated with QRS abnormalities, but there are enough

exceptions [124] that the clinician should be aware of the possibility that extensive or even strategically placed small nontransmural infarcts can cause abnormal Q-waves. Because the subepicardial region is normal, the typical ST segment abnormality is *depression* in the ECG lead over the injured area rather than elevation. Again, this ST segment abnormality is the net result of injury currents in systole and diastole. T-wave flattening or inversion is also seen with this type of healed infarct.

The characteristic site of myocardial ischemia *without* infarction is the subendocardium. The ST segment vector on the surface ECG is similar except the changes are transient and there is no significant elevation of cardiac enzymes. Figure 4–1 is an example of this type of myocardial ischemia; it is also the most common type of ischemic response during exercise tests, as discussed in chapter 6.

*Similar ECG Findings in Other Disease States.* ST segment elevation is not unique to acute myocardial infarction and may occur with pericarditis or development of a left ventricular aneurysm. Similarly, a variety of disorders may result in ST depression and T-wave inversion: electrolyte imbalance, myocarditis, drug effect, etc. Abnormal Q-waves may also be seen with other disorders, especially primary or secondary cardiomyopathy, and trauma. For these reasons, the physician should relate the ECG to the clinical situation whenever possible before definitely assigning a diagnosis.

*Abnormalities of Impulse Formulation and Conduction.*

VENTRICULAR ARRHYTHMIAS. Ventricular arrhythmias are the most common disturbances of heart rhythm associated with myocardial ischemia. Their genesis has been ascribed to abnormal reentry (i.e., disturbances of impulse conduction in ischemic areas), enhanced automaticity of Purkinje fibers (i.e., disturbances of impulse formation), or both. The following discussion summarizes some of the current concepts concerning these rhythm disturbances [125] (treatment is discussed in chapter 15).

Based on experiments in dogs in which the left anterior descending coronary artery is suddenly occluded, ventricular arrhythmias related to myocardial ischemia and infarction in this setting occur in two distinct phases. The *early phase* begins immediately following coronary occlusion and may last from 15 minutes to a few hours followed by a relatively nonarrhythmic period, after which ventricular arrhythmias again supervene at about 6 to 9 hours. The second, or *late phase,* may last from 24 to 48 hours. A similar bimodal distribution of ventricular arrhythmias is not apparent from studies in the clinical setting of acute myocardial infarction in humans. However, complete information regarding ventricular arrhythmias, particularly those occurring during the very early phases of acute ischemic injury, is often difficult if not impossible to obtain.

Action potentials from ventricular fibers in the ischemic zone immediately following coronary occlusion characteristically show a slow initial phase of depolarization. Such slow-response action potentials in acutely ischemic myocardium are believed to promote reentrant activation and possibly ventricular fibrillation soon after acute coronary occlusion. Thus, bipolar electrograms recorded from ischemic myocardium immediately following coronary occlusion show a decrease in QRS amplitude and an increase in QRS duration. Conduction velocities through the ischemic region slow markedly, and long delays occur between the activation of endocardium and epicardium in the ischemic zone. Later, intramural bipolar electrograms in the central ischemic zone demonstrate progressive lingering of electrical activity after each QRS. This fragmented electrical activity is believed to result in premature ventricular depolarization, ventricular tachycardia, and ventricular fibrillation. In addition, ventricular arrhythmias may occur when activation of the ischemic epicardium is sufficiently delayed so that secondary waves of excitation reach the nonischemic margins of the infarct after these tissues have already repolarized. As a result, "circus movements" of electromotive waves are created, and these may in turn lead to reentrant arrhythmias.

Ventricular arrhythmias that arise during the late phase following coronary occlusion in experimental ischemia are believed to be related to certain changes in the electrophysiologic behav-ior of Purkinje fibers in the ischemic region. Since subendocardial Purkinje fibers derive metabolic substrates and oxygen from blood within the ventricular cavity, they contain an abundance of intracellular glycogen and perform less mechanical work than other ventricular fibers. Therefore, they can resist ischemic damage during the early period following coronary occlusion. When ischemic damage does occur, it is characterized by progressive accumulation of intracellular lipid droplets 6 to 10 hours following coronary occlusion. Significant alterations in the electrophysiologic properties of these fibers closely parallel the time-course of accumulation of this intracellular lipid material. Diastolic transmembrane potential, amplitude of the action potential, and the rate of initial depolarization are all reduced at 24 hours following coronary occlusion, with the development of spontaneous diastolic depolarization and spontaneous activation (i.e., *enhanced automaticity*) (see figure 2–16). This spontaneous depolarization of Purkinje fibers underlying the infarct and the propagation of impulses to the ventricular myocardium surrounding the infarct zone may initiate either premature ventricular beats or other ventricular arrhythmias. These spontaneously depolarizing fibers may sometimes be protected by entrance block and may exhibit various degrees of *exit block* (see figure 2–16). Ventricular arrhythmias resulting from abnormal Purkinje automaticity include noncoupled premature ventricular depolarizations, nonparoxysmal ventricular tachycardia, and accelerated idioventricular rhythm, all of which are known to occur commonly during the first few days following clinical acute myocardial infarction. Reentry occurring in abnormal Purkinje fibers within an infarct has also been demonstrated as a cause of ventricular arrhythmias during the late phase of arrhythmias after coronary occlusion. This mechanism may be one cause of coupled ventricular premature contractions or ventricular tachycardia due to the "R-on-T" phenomenon.

*Release arrhythmias* occur when blood is suddenly restored to a temporarily ligated coronary artery; they are most likely due to chemical and electrical gradients caused by the washout of metabolites and electrolytes that have accumulated in the ischemic area. Fatal arrhythmias in the absence of pathologic evidence of infarction, or those occurring after coronary spasm or thrombolysis may be clinical manifestations of these arrhythmias also termed reperfusion arrhythmias.

Clinical and experimental studies [126, 127] suggest that the magnitude and extent of acute ischemic injury, the infarct size, and the degree of subsequent fibrosis are important in determining the type and severity of ventricular arrhythmias. Although the precise mechanisms are not known, it is hypothesized that significant changes in regional mechanical function and geometry produced by ischemia influence the magnitude and duration of reentrant pathways generated at the margins of the ischemic zone.

OTHER ARRHYTHMIAS AND CONDUCTION DISTURBANCES. Aside from ventricular ectopy, bradyarrhythmias and atrioventricular (AV) and interventricular (IV) conduction disturbances may occur in acute myocardial ischemia [128]. The arrhythmogenic mechanisms can be directly due to ischemia of the sinus node (supplied by the right coronary artery in about 50 percent of humans and by the left main or left circumflex arteries in the other 50 percent), ischemia of the AV node (supplied by the right coronary artery in almost 90 percent of instances), or ischemia of the left and right bundle branches of the conducting system (supplied by septal branches of the left anterior descending artery). Arrhythmias can also be indirectly induced by ischemia. Thus, in *acute inferior wall myocardial injury,* there may be enhanced local release of acetylcholine from autonomic postganglionic fibers in the atria and adjacent to the AV node. This intense but spurious vagotonic state may result in a dramatic inhibition of sinus node automaticity and decreased conduction velocities through the atrial musculature and AV junction, leading to sinus bradycardia and/or progressive degrees of disturbances in AV conduction (first-degree, Wenchebach-type second-degree, and even third-degree AV block). At times, the cardiac rhythm may be usurped by a subsidiary His-Purkinje or idioventricular pacemaker.

In contrast, *acute anterior wall myocardial injury* is characterized by increased sympathetic tone, resulting in enhanced automaticity of all cardiac pacemakers and accelerated conduction velocities through all nonischemic cardiac tissues. Therefore, *supraventricular tachycardias* are common in this setting and may be related to incipient power failure, perhaps due to systolic aneurysmal bulging of the ischemic region and increased secretion of catecholamines. Liberthson et al. [129] have questioned this association of supraventricular arrhythmias with anterior myocardial infarction and power failure. Their study found a similar distribution of supraventricular arrhythmias with anterior and inferior infarction, but noted a higher-than-expected frequency of pericardial inflammation in these patients. Irritation of atrial tissue (rather than pump failure) was postulated as the cause of the arrhythmias.

Atrioventricular and interventricular conduction disturbances in extensive anterior myocardial infarction are usually due to direct ischemic damage to His bundle and proximal bundle branches. Conduction disturbances such as Mobitz-type-2AV block may be sudden or may be heralded by a right bundle branch block, left anterior hemiblock, or both.

## Conclusions

One of the more attractive concepts to explain the pathogenesis of coronary artery disease in humans is the response-to-injury hypothesis, in which injury to the arterial endothelium caused by a variety of factors initiates desquamation, platelet adherence, smooth muscle proliferation, and connective-tissue formation. The delicate equilibrium needed to maintain normal cellular cholesterol homeostasis is somehow altered, and cholesterol and cholesterol esters accumulate in the arterial intima. When the coronary arteries are examined in patients with clinical coronary artery disease, the end results of such processes are observed: fibrous, lipid-filled plaques are transformed into mural thrombi via hemorrhage, calcification, and cell necrosis, often obliterating the vessel lumen. With extensive large-vessel involvement, smaller collateral vessels develop and may or may not offer protection against myocardial ischemia. There is now generalized agreement that a transmural myocardial infarction is preceded by an intravascular thrombosis.

The physiologic and anatomic basis of myocardial ischemia is best understood in the context of a dynamic imbalance between myocardial oxygen demand and supply. Circulatory dynamics in angina-provoking situations vary. A predominant, "primary" cardiac effect (coronary vasospasm) is attributed to certain types of rest angina and suspected in some episodes of emotionally induced angina; it is also felt at present to probably be a contributory factor in typical, exertion-related angina, but incrased myocardial oxygen demands due to systemic hemodynamic factors are still believed to be most important in this type of angina.

Studies of coronary blood flow in humans, while complicated by a number of technical and theoretical limitations, suggest that regional abnormalities of perfusion exist during ischemia. These abnormalities are most apparent under the conditions of external stress produced in the cardiac laboratory by pacing tachycardia, exercise, the use of pharmacologic agents, or by induction of vasospasm.

In humans, the elevated ventricular filling pressures associated with the anginal state have been ascribed to transient heart failure, reduced compliance, or both. Intervention ventriculography has proved useful in differentiating wall motion abnormalities due to fibrosis from those due to ischemia. In syndromes of coronary heart disease that are not predominantly associated with acute ischemia, congestive heart failure is usually due to left ventricular aneurysm, papillary muscle dysfunction with mitral regurgitation, or both.

The genesis of ventricular arrhythmias observed in myocardial ischemia is most likely related to the size of the ischemic area and the alterations in the extracellular environment and intracellular composition caused by ischemia. Both abnormal automaticity and reentrant activation have been postulated as mechanisms for the electrical instability of the ischemic region.

## References

1. Ross, R. and Glomset, J.A. The pathogenesis of atherosclerosis. *N. Engl. J. Med.* 295:369, 420, 1976.
2. Niewiarowski, S. and Rao, A.K. Contribution of thrombogenic factors to the pathogenesis of atherosclerosis. *Prog. Cardiovasc. Dis.* 26:197, 1983.
3. Benditt, E.P. and Benditt, J.M. Evidence for a monoclonal origin of human atherosclerotic plaques. *Proc. Natl. Acad. Sci. U.S.A.* 70:1753, 1973.
4. Martin, G.M. and Sprague, C.A. Symposium on in vitro studies related to atherogenesis: Life histories of hyperplastoid cell lines from the aorta and skin. *Exp. Mol. Pathol.* 18:125, 1973.
5. Small, D.M. Cellular mechanisms for lipid deposition in atherosclerosis. *N. Engl. J. Med.* 297:873, 294, 1977.
6. Walton, K.W. Pathogenetic mechanisms in atherosclerosis. *Am. J. Cardiol.* 35:542, 1975.
7. Goldstein, J.L., Kita, T., and Brown, M.S. Defective lipoprotein receptors and atherosclerosis: Lessons from an animal counterpart of familial hypercholesterolemia. *N. Engl. J. Med.* 309:288, 1983.
8. Chobanian, A.V. The influence of hypertension and other hemodynamic factors in atherogenesis. *Prog. Cardiovasc. Dis.* 26:177, 1983.
9. Kannel, W.B. High-density lipoproteins: Epidemiologic profile and risks of coronary artery disease. *Am. J. Cardiol.* 92:9B, 1983.
10. Roberts, W.C. Coronary heart disease: A review of the abnormalities observed in the coronary arteries. *Cardiovasc. Med.* 2:29, 1977.
11. Gorlin, R. Coronary Anatomy. In *Coronary Artery Disease.* Philadelphia: Saunders, 1976, p. 56.
12. Cohen, L.S., Elliott, W.C., Klein, M.D., and Gorlin, R. Coronary heart disease: Clinical, cinearteriographic and metabolic correlations. *Am. J. Cardiol.* 17:152, 1966.
13. Proudfit, W.L., Shirey, E.K., Sheldon, W.C., and Sones, F.M., Jr. Certain clinical characteristics correlated with extent of obstructive lesions demonstrated by selective cine coronary arteriography. *Circulation* 38:947, 1968.
14. Goldberg, S., Grossman, W., Markis, J.E., Cohen, M.V., Baltaxe, H.A., and Levin, D.C. Total occlusion of the left main coronary artery: A clinical hemodynamic and angiographic profile. *Am. J. Med.* 64:3, 1978.
15. Markis, J.E., Joffe, C.D., Cohn, P.F., Feen, D.J., Herman, M.V., and Gorlin, R. Clinical significance of coronary arterial ectasia. *Am. J. Cardiol.* 37:217, 1976.
16. Oliva, P.B. Unstable rest angina with ST-segment depression: Pathophysiologic considerations and therapeutic implications. *Ann. Int. Med.* 100:424, 1984.
17. Cohen, M.V. The functional value of coronary collaterals in myocardial ischemia and therapeutic approach to enhance collateral flow. *Am. Heart J.* 95:396, 1978.
18. Gorlin, R. Coronary Collaterals. In *Coronary Ar-

*tery Disease.* Philadelphia: Saunders, 1976, p. 65.

19. Levin, D.C. Pathways and functional significance of the coronary collateral circulation. *Circulation* 50:831, 1974.
20. Goldberg, H.L., Goldstein, J., Borer, J.S., Moses, J.W., and Collins, M.B. Functional importance of coronary collateral vessels. *Am. J. Cardiol.* 53:694, 1984.
21. Chandler, A.B., Chapman, I., Erhardt, L.R., Roberts, W.C., Schwartz, C.J., Sinapius, D., Spain, D.M., Sherry, S., Ness, P.M., and Simon, T.L. Coronary thrombosis in myocardial infarction: Report of a workshop on the role of coronary thrombosis in the pathogenesis of acute myocardial infarction. *Am. J. Cardiol.* 34:823, 1974.
22. Oliva, P.B. Pathophysiology of acute myocardial infarction, 1981. *Ann. Int. Med.* 94:236, 1981.
23. Dalen, J.E., Ockene, I.S., and Alpert, J.S. Coronary spasm, coronary thrombosis, and myocardial infarction: A hypothesis concerning the pathophysiology of acute myocardial infarction. *Am. Heart J.* 104:1119, 1982.
24. Braunwald, E., Ross, J., Jr., and Sonnenblick, E.H. Myocardial Energetics. In *Mechanisms of Contraction of the Normal and Failing Heart* (2nd ed.). Boston: Little, Brown, 1976, p. 171.
25. Amsterdam, E.A., Hughes, J.L., DeMaria, A.N., Zelis, R., and Mason, D.T. Indirect assessment of myocardial oxygen consumption in the evaluation of mechanisms and therapy of angina pectoris. *Am. J. Cardiol.* 33:737, 1974.
26. Gobel, F.L., Nordstrom, L.A., Nelson, R.R., Jorgensen, C.R., and Wang, Y. The rate-pressure product as an index of myocardial oxygen consumption during exercise in patients with angina pectoris. *Circulation* 57:549, 1978.
27. Robinson, B.F. Relation of heart rate and systolic blood pressure to the onset of pain in angina pectoris. *Circulation* 35:1073, 1967.
28. Hoffman, J.I.E. and Buckberg, G.D. The myocardial supply: demand ratio. A critical review. *Am. J. Cardiol.* 41:327, 1978.
29. Braunwald, E., Ross, J.J., Jr., and Sonnenblick, E.H. Regulation of Coronary Blood Flow. In *Mechanisms of Contraction of the Normal and Failing Heart* (2nd ed.). Boston: Little, Brown, 1976, p. 208.
30. Rubio, R. and Berne, R.M. Regulation of coronary blood flow. *Prog. Cardiovasc. Dis.* 18:105, 1975.
31. Ball, R.M. and Bache, R.J. Distribution of myocardial blood flow in the exercising dog with restricted coronary artery inflow. *Circ. Res.* 38:60, 1976.
32. Archie, J.P., Jr. Intramyocardial pressure: Effect of preload on transmural distribution of systolic coronary blood flow. *Am. J. Cardiol.* 35:904, 1974.
33. Gould, K.L., Lipscomb, K., and Hamilton, G.W. Physiologic basis for assessing critical coronary stenosis. Instantaneous flow response and regional distribution during coronary hyperemia as measures of coronary flow reserve. *Am. J. Cardiol.* 33:87, 1974.
34. Gould K.L., Lipscomb, K., and Calvert, C. Compensatory changes of the distal coronary vascular bed during progressive coronary constriction. *Circulation* 51:1085, 1975.
35. Lipscomb, K. and Hooten, S. Effect of stenotic dimensions and blood flow on the hemodynamic significance of model coronary artery stenoses. *Am. J. Cardiol.* 42:781, 1978.
36. Klocke, F.J. Coronary blood flow in man. *Prog. Cardiovasc. Dis.* 19:117, 1976.
37. Cannon, P.J., Sciacca, R.R., Fowler, D.L., Weiss, M.B., Schmidt, D.H., and Casarella, W.J. Measurement of regional myocardial blood flow in man: Description and critique of the method using xenon-133 and a scintillation camera. *Am. J. Cardiol.* 36:783, 1975.
38. Ganz, W., Tamura, K., Marcus, H.S., Donoso, R., Yoshida, S., and Swan, H.J.C. Measurement of coronary sinus blood flow by continuous thermodilution in man. *Circulation* 44:181, 1971.
39. Cohen, A., Gallagher, J.R., Luebs, E.D., Vargo, A., Yamanaka, J., Zaleski, E.J., Bluemchen, G., and Bing, R.J. Quantitative determination of coronary flow with positron emitter (rubidium-84). *Circulation* 32:636, 1965.
40. Rowe, G.G., Thomsen, J.H., Stenlund, R.R., McKenna, D.H., Sialer, S. and Corliss, R.J. A study of hemodynamics and coronary blood flow in man and its relation to the coronary arteriogram. *Circulation* 39:139, 1969.
41. Klocke, F.J. and Wittenberg, S.M. Heterogeneity of coronary blood flow in human coronary artery disease and experimental myocardial infarction. *Am. J. Cardiol.* 24:872, 1969.
42. Cowan, C., Duran, P.V.M., Corsin, G., Goldschlager, N., and Bing, R.J. The effects of nitroglycerin on myocardial blood flow in man: Measured by coincidence counting and bolus injection of 84-rubidium. *Am. J. Cardiol.* 24:154, 1969.
43. Knoebel, S.B., McHenry, P.L., Bonner, A.J., and Phillips, J.F. Myocardial blood flow in coronary artery disease. Effect of right atrial pacing and nitroglycerin. *Circulation* 47:690, 1973.
44. Knoebel, S.B., McHenry, P.L., Phillips, J.F., and Widlansky, S. Atropine-induced cardioacceleration and myocardial blood flow in subjects with and without coronary artery disease. *Am. J. Cardiol.* 33:327, 1974.
45. Mudge, G.H., Jr., Grossman, W., Mills, R.M.,

Jr., Lesch, M., and Braunwald, E. Reflex increase in coronary vascular resistance in patients with ischemic heart disease. *N. Engl. J. Med.* 295:1333, 1976.

46. Wilson, J.R., Martin, J.L., Untereker, W.J., Laskey, W., and Hirshfeld, J.W. Sequential changes in regional coronary flow during pacing-induced angina pectoris: Coronary flow limitation precedes angina. *Am. Heart J.* 107:269, 1984.

47. Selwyn, A.P., Forse, G., Fox, K., Jonathan, A., and Steiner, R. Patterns of disturbed myocardial perfusion in patients with coronary artery disease: Regional myocardial perfusion in angina pectoris. *Circulation* 64:83, 1981.

48. Chen, P.H., Nichols, A.B., Weiss, M.B., Sciacca, R.R., Walter, P.D. and Cannon, P.J. Left ventricular myocardial blood flow in multivessel coronary artery disease. *Circulation* 66:537, 1982.

49. Dwyer, E.M., Jr., Dell, R.B., and Cannon, P.J. Regional myocardial flow in transmural myocardial infarction. *Circulation* 48:924, 1973.

50. See, J.R., Cohn, P.F., Holman, B.L., Roberts, B.H., and Adams, D.F. Angiographical abnormalities associated with alterations in regional myocardial blood flow in coronary artery disease. *Br. Heart J.* 38:1278, 1976.

51. See, J.R., Cohn, P.F., Holman, B.L., Adams, D.F., and Maddox, D.E. Significance of reduced regional myocardial blood flow in asynergic areas evaluated with intervention ventriculography. *Am. J. Cardiol.* 43:179, 1979.

52. Cohn, P.F., Maddox, D.E., Holman, B.L., and See, J.R. Effect of coronary collateral vessels on regional myocardial blood flow in patients with coronary artery disease: Relation of collateral circulation to vasodilatory reserve and left ventricular function. *Am. J. Cardiol.* 46:359, 1980.

53. Malacoff, R.F., Mudge, G.H., Jr., Holman, B.L., Idoine, J., Bifolck, L., and Cohn, P.F. Effect of the cold pressor test on regional myocardial blood flow in patients with coronary artery disease. *Am. Heart J.* 106:78, 1983.

54. Hamilton, G.W., Ritchie, J.L., Allend, D., Lapin, E., and Murray, J.A. Myocardial perfusion imaging with $^{99m}$Tc or $^{113m}$ In macroaggregated albumin: Correlation of the perfusion image with clinical, angiographic, surgical and histologic findings. *Am. Heart J.* 89:708, 1975.

55. Ritchie, J.L., Hamilton, G.W., Gould, K.L., Allen, D., Kennedy, J.W., and Hammermeister, K.E. Myocardial imaging with indium-113m- and technetium-99m-macroaggregated albumin. New procedure for identification of stress induced regional ischemia. *Am. J. Cardiol.* 35:380, 1975.

56. Holman, B.L., Cohn, P.F., Adams, D.F., See,

J.R., Roberts, B.H., Idoine, J., and Gorlin, R. Regional myocardial blood flow during hyperemia induced by contrast agent in patients with coronary artery disease. *Am. J. Cardiol.* 38:416, 1976.

57. Zaret, B.L., Strauss, H.W., Wells, H.P., Jr., and Flamin, M.D. Noninvasive regional myocardial perfusion with radioactive potassium: Study of patients at rest, with exercise and during angina pectoris. *N. Engl. J. Med.* 288:809, 1973.

58. Albro, P.C., Gould, K.L., Westcott, R.J., Hamilton, G.W., Ritchie, J.L., and Williams, D.L. Noninvasive assessment of coronary stenoses by myocardial imaging during pharmacologic coronary vasodilation. III. Clinical trial. *Am. J. Cardiol.* 42:751, 1978.

59. Selwyn, A.P., Allan, R.M. and L'Abbate A. Relations between regional myocardial uptake of rubidium-82 and perfusion. *Am. J. Cardiol.* 50:112, 1982.

60. Maseri, A. and Chierchia, S. Coronary artery spasm: Demonstration, definition, diagnosis and consequences. *Prog. Cardiovasc. Dis.* 25:169, 1982.

61. Crea, F., Davies, G., Romeo, F., Chierchia, S., Bugiardini, R., Kaski, J.C., Freedman, B., and Maseri, A. Myocardial ischemia during ergonovine testing: Different susceptibility to coronary vasoconstriction in patients with exertional and variant angina. *Circulation* 69:690, 1984.

62. Schiffer, F., Hartley, L.H., Schulman, C.L., and Abelmann, W.H. Evidence for emotionally-induced coronary arterial spasm in patients with angina pectoris. *Br. Heart J.* 44:62, 1980.

63. Bassan, M.M., Marcus, H.S., and Ganz, W. The effect of mild-to-moderate mental stress on coronary hemodynamics in patients with coronary artery disease. *Circulation* 62:933, 1980.

64. Lassvik, C.T. and Areskog, N.H. Angina in cold environment: Reactions to exercise. *Br. Heart J.* 42:396, 1979.

65. Feldman, R.L., Whittle, J.L., Marx, J.D., Pepine, C.J., and Conti, C.R. Regional coronary hemodynamic responses to cold stimulation in patients without variant angina. *Am. J. Cardiol.* 49:665, 1982.

66. Goldstein, R.E., Redwood, D.R., Rosing, D.R., Beiser, G.D., and Epstein, S.E. Alterations in the circulatory response to exercise following a meal and their relationship in postprandial angina pectoris. *Circulation* 44:90, 1971.

67. Figueras, J., Singh, B.N., Ganz, W., and Swan, H.J.C. Haemodynamic and electrocardiographic accompaniments of resting postprandial angina. *Br. Heart J.* 42:402, 1979.

68. Mehta, J., Mehta, P., Feldman, R.L., and Horalek, C. Thromboxane release in coronary artery disease: Spontaneous versus pacing-induced angina. *Am. Heart J.* 107:286, 1984.

69. Chierchia, S., Davies, G., Berkenboom, G., Crea, F., Crean, P., and Maseri, A. α-Adrenergic receptors and coronary spasm: An elusive link. *Circulation* 69:8, 1984.

70. Aranow, W.S. Smoking, carbon monoxide, and coronary heart disease. *Circulation* 48:1169, 1973.

71. Brachfield, N. Metabolism of Myocardial Ischemia. In E Donoso and R. Gorlin (eds.), *Current Cardiovascular Topics,* Vol. III: Angina Pectoris. New York: Grune & Stratton, 1977, p. 1.

72. Jennings, R.B. Early phase of myocardial ischemic injury and infarction. *Am. J. Cardiol.* 24:753, 1969.

73. Herman, M.V., Elliott, W.C., and Gorlin, R. An electrocardiographic, anatomic, and metabolic study of zonal myocardial ischemia in coronary heart disease. *Circulation* 35:834, 1967.

74. Mudge, G.H., Jr., Mills, R.M., Jr., Taegtmeyer, H., Gorlin, R. and Lesch, M. Alterations of myocardial amino acid metabolism in chronic heart disease. *J. Clin. Invest.* 58:1185, 1976.

75. Vrobel, T.R., Jorgensen, C.R., and Bache, R.J. Myocardial lactate and adenosine metabolite production as indicators of exercise-induced myocardial ischemia. *Circulation* 66:555, 1982.

76. Braunwald, E., Ross, J., Jr., and Sonnenblick, E.H. Structure and Function of the Myocardial Cell. In *Mechanisms of Contraction of the Normal and Failing Heart* (2nd ed.). Boston: Little, Brown, 1976, p. 28.

77. Katz, A.M. Effects of ischemia on the contractile processes of heart muscle. *Am. J. Cardiol.* 32:456, 1973.

78. Cohn, P.F., Herman, M.V., and Gorlin, R. Ventricular dysfunction in coronary artery disease. *Am. J. Cardiol.* 33:307, 1974.

79. Moraski, R.E., Russell, R.O., Jr., Smith, M., and Rackley, C.E. Left ventricular function in patients with and without myocardial infarction and one, two or three vessel coronary artery disease. *Am. J. Cardiol.* 35:1, 1975.

80. Cohn, P.F. and Gorlin, R. Abnormalities of left ventricular function associated with the anginal state. *Circulation* 46:1065, 1972.

81. McCans, J.L. and Parker, J.O. Left ventricular pressure-volume relationships during myocardial ischemia in man. *Circulation* 48:775, 173.

82. Barry, W.H., Brooker, J.Z., Alderman, E.L., and Harrison, D.C. Changes in diastolic stiffness and tone of the left ventricle during angina pectoris. *Circulation* 49:255, 1974.

83. Mann, T., Goldberg, S., Mudge, G.H., and Grossman, W. Factors contributing to altered left ventricular diastolic properties during angina pectoris. *Circulation* 59:114, 1979.

84. Sharma, B., Behrens, T.W., Erlein, D., Hodges, M., Asinger, R.W., and Francis, G.S. Left ventricular diastolic properties and filling characteristics during spontaneous angina pectoris at rest. *Am. J. Cadiol.* 52:704, 1983.

85. Carroll, J.D., Hess, O.M., Hirzel, H.O., and Krayenbuehl, H.P. Exercise-induced ischemia: The influence of altered relaxation on early diastolic pressures. *Circulation* 67:521, 1983.

86. Bourdillon, P.D., Lorell, B.H., Mirsky, I., Paulus, W.J., Wynne, J., and Grossman, W. Increased regional myocardial stiffness of the left ventricle during pacing-induced angina in man. *Circulation* 67:316, 1983.

87. Dehmer, G.J., Lewis, S.E., Hillis, L.D., Corbett, J., Parkey, R.W., and Willerson, J.T. Exercise-induced alterations in left ventricular volumes and the pressure-volume relationship: A sensitive indicator of left ventricular dysfunction in patients with coronary artery disease. *Circulation* 63:1008, 1981.

88. Helfant, R.H., Forrester, J.S., Hampton, J.R., Haft, J.I., Kemp, H.G., and Gorlin, R. Coronary heart disease. Differential hemodynamic, metabolic, and electrocardiographic effects in subjects with and without angina pectoris during atrial pacing. *Circulation* 42:601, 1970.

89. Herman, M.V. and Gorlin, R. Implications of left ventricular asynergy. *Am. J. Cardiol.* 23:538, 1969.

90. Ideker, R.E., Behar, V.S., Wagner, G.S., Starr, J.W., Starmer, C.F., Leff, K.L., and Hackel, D.B. Evaluation of asynergy as an indicator of myocardial fibrosis. *Circulation* 57:715, 1978.

91. Markis, J.E., Joffee, C.D., Roberts, B.H., Ransil, B.J., Cohn, P.F., Herman, M.V., and Gorlin, R. Evolution of left ventricular dysfunction in coronary artery disease: Serial cineangiographic studies without surgery. *Circulation* 62:141, 1980.

92. Bodenheimer, M.M., Banka, V.S., and Helfant, R.H. Q waves and ventricular asynergy: Predictive value and hemodynamic significance of anatomical localization. *Am. J. Cardiol.* 35:615, 1975.

93. Pasternac, A., Gorlin, R., Sonnenblick, E.H., Haft, J.I., and Kemp, H.G. Abnormalities of ventricular motion induced by atrial pacing in coronary artery disease. *Circulation* 45:1195, 1972.

94. Sharma, B. and Taylor, S.H. Localization of left ventricular ischemia in angina pectoris by cineangiography during exercise. *Br. Heart J.* 37:963, 1975.

95. Crawford, M.H., Petru, M.A., Amon, K.W., Sorensen, S.G., and Vance, W.S. Comparative value of 2-dimensional echocardiography and radionuclide angiography for quantitating changes in left ventricular performance during exercise limited by angina pectoris. *Am. J. Cardiol.* 53:42, 1984.

96. Leong, K-H and Jones, R.H. Influence of the location of left anterior descending coronary artery stenosis on left ventricular function during exercise. *Circulation* 65:109, 1982.

97. Braunwald, E. and Kloner, R.A. The stunned myocardium: Prolonged, post-ischemia ventricular dysfunction. *Circulation* 66:1146, 1982.

98. Horn, H.R., and Teichholz, L.E., Cohn, P.F., Herman, M.V., and Gorlin, R. Augmentation of left ventricular contraction pattern in coronary artery disease by inotropic catecholamines: The epinephrine ventriculogram. *Circulation* 49:1063, 1974.

99. Dyke, S.H., Cohn, P.F., Gorlin, R., and Sonnenblick, E.H. Detection of residual myocardial function in coronary artery disease using postextrasystolic potentiation. *Circulation* 50:694, 1974.

100. McAnulty, J.H., Hattenhauer, M.T., Rosche, J., Kloster, F.E., and Rahimtoola, S.H. Improvement in left ventricular wall motion following nitroglycerin. *Circulation* 51:140, 1975.

101. Bodenheim, M.M., Banka, V.S., Hermann, G.A., Trout, R.G., Pasdar, H., and Helfant, R.H. Reversible asynergy: Histopathologic and electrographic correlations in patients with coronary artery disease. *Circulation* 53:792, 1976.

102. Banka, V.S., Bodenheimer, M.M., and Helfant, R.H. Determinants of reversible asynergy: Effect of pathologic Q waves, coronary collateral and anatomic location. *Circulation* 50:714, 1974.

103. Banka, V.S., Bodenheimer, M.M., and Helfant, R.H. Determinants of reversible asynergy: The native coronary circulation. *Circulation* 52:810, 1975.

104. Askenazi, J., Parisi, A.F., Cohn, P.F., Freedman, W.B., and Braunwald, E. Value of the QRS complex in assessing left ventricular ejection fraction. *Am. J. Cardiol.* 41:494, 1978.

105. Cohn, P.F., Angoff, G.H., Zoll, P.M., Sloss, L.J., Markis, J.E., Graboys, T.B., Green, L.H., and Braunwald, E. A new, noninvasive technique for inducing postextrasystolic potentiation during echocardiography. *Circulation* 56:598, 1977.

106. Cohn, P.F., Angoff, G.H., and Sloss, L.J. Noninvasively-induced postextrasystolic potentiation of ischemic and infarcted myocardium in patients with coronary artery disease. *Am. Heart J.* 97:187, 1979.

107. Verani, M.S., Carroll, R.J., and Falsetti, H.L. Mitral valve prolapse in coronary artery disease. *Am. J. Cardiol.* 37:1, 1976.

108. Aranda, L.M., Befeler, B., Lazzaro, R., Embi, A., and Machado, H. Mitral valve prolapse and coronary artery disease. Clinical, hemodynamic and angiographic correlations. *Circulation* 52:245, 1975.

109. Swan, H.J.C., Forrester, J.S., Diamond, G., Chatterjee, K., and Parmley, W.W. Hemodynamic spectrum of myocardial infarction and cardiogenic shock: A conceptual model. *Circulation* 45:1097, 1972.

110. Gorlin, R., Klein, M.D., and Sullivan, J.M. Prospective correlative study of ventricular aneurysm. Mechanistic concept and clinical recognition. *Am. J. Med.* 42:512, 1967.

111. Parmley, W.W., Chuck, L., Kivowitz, C., Matloff, J.M., and Swan, H.J.C. In vitro length-tension relations of human ventricular aneurysms. Relation of stiffness to mechanical disadvantage. *Am. J. Cardiol.* 32:889, 1973.

112. Cheng, T.O. Incidence of ventricular aneurysm in coronary artery disease. An angiographic appraisal. *Am. J. Med.* 50:340, 1971.

113. Klein, M.D., Herman, M.V., and Gorlin, R. A hemodynamic study of left ventricular aneurysm. *Circulation* 35:614, 1967.

114. Visser, C.A., Kan, G., David, G.K., Lie, K.I., and Durrer, D. Echocardiographic-cineangiographic correlation in detecting left aneurysm: A prospective study of 422 patients. *Am. J. Cardiol.* 50:337, 1982.

115. Burch, G.E., DePasquale, N.P., and Phillips, J.H. The syndrome of papillary muscle dysfunction. *Am. Heart J.* 75:399, 1968.

116. Gahl, K., Sutton, R., Pearson, M., Caspari, P., Lairet, A., and McDonald, L. Mitral regurgitation in coronary heart disease. *Br. Heart J.* 39:13, 1977.

117. Shelburne, J.C., Rubeinstein, D., and Gorlin, R. A reappraisal of papillary muscle dysfunction. Correlative, clinical and angiographic study. *Am. J. Med.* 46:862, 1969.

118. Burch, G.E., Giles, T.D., and Colcolough, H.L. Ischemic cardiomyopathy. *Am. Heart J.* 79:291, 1970.

119. Yatteau, R.F., Peter R.H., Behar, V.S., Bartel, A.G., Rosati, R.A., and Kong, Y. Ischemic cardiomyopathy: The myopathy of coronary artery disease. Natural history and results of medical versus surgical treatment. *Am. J. Cardiol.* 34:520, 1974.

120. Dash, H., Johnson, R.A., Dinsmore, R.E., and Harthorne, J.W. Cardiomyopathic syndrome due to coronary artery disease. I. Relation to angiographic extent of coronary disease and to remote myocardial infarction. *Br. Heart J.* 39:733, 1977.

121. Starling, M.R., Crawford, M.H., Sorensen, S.G., and Grover, F.L. Comparative value of invasive and noninvasive techniques for identifying left ventricular mural thrombi. *Am. Heart J.* 106:1143, 1983.

122. Fozzard, H.A. and DasGupta, D.S. Electrophysiology and the electrocardiogram. *Mod. Conc. Cardiovasc. Dis.* 44:29, 1975.

123. Kupersmith, J. Electrophysiologic and Electrocardiographic Aspects of Myocardial Ischemia, Including Stress Testing. In *Current Cardiovascular Topics* (Vol. III), E. Donoso and R. Gorlin (eds.), *Angina Pectoris.* New York: Stratton, 1977, p. 28.

124. Sullivan, W., Vlodaver, Z., Tuna, N., Long, L., and Edwards, J.E. Correlation of electrocardiographic and pathologic findings in healed myocardial infarction. *Am. J. Cardiol.* 42:724, 1978.

125. Bigger, J.T., Jr., Dresdale, R.J., Heissenbuttel, R.H., Weld, F.M., and Wit, A.C. Ventricular arrhythmias in ischemic heart disease: Mechanics, prevalence, significance and management. *Prog. Cardiovasc. Dis.* 19:255, 1977.

126. Gang, E.S., Bigger, J.T., Jr., and Livelli, F.D., Jr. A model of chronic ischemic arrhythmias: The relation between electrically inducible ventricular tachycardia, ventricular fibrillation threshold and myocardial infarct size. *Am. J. Cardiol.* 50:469, 1982.

127. Califf, R.M., Burks, J.M., Behar, V.S., Margolis, J.R., and Wagner, G.S. Relationship among ventricular arrhythmias, coronary artery disease, and angiographic and electrocardiographic indicators of myocardial fibrosis. *Circulation* 57:725, 1978.

128. Rotman, M., Wagner, A.S., and Wallace, A.G. Bradyarrhythmias in acute myocardial infarction. *Circulation* 45:703, 1972.

129. Liberthson, R.R., Salisbury, K.W., Hutter, A.M., Jr., and DeSanctis, R.W. Atrial tachyarrhythmias in acute myocardial infarction. *Am. J. Med.* 60:956, 1976.

# 3. THE EPIDEMIOLOGY OF CORONARY ARTERY DISEASE

William B. Kannel
Joseph Stokes III

Atherosclerosis is the dominant epidemic disease of all developed societies. Its most common and serious clinical manifestation is coronary artery disease, or, as we prefer, coronary heart disease (CHD), which currently accounts for more than a third of all deaths in the United States and causes more patients to seek the help of physicians than any other disease. It also ranks third behind accidents and cancer as the most important cause of years-of-potential-life-lost before age 65 in the United States [1].

The terms used to identify the various ways in which CHD manifests itself clinically are listed in table 3–1. Our understanding of the pathogenesis of both atherosclerosis and CHD has made extraordinary advances over the last 35 years, and we are no longer laboring under the misconceptions of the nineteenth century pathologists when Virchow concluded that the disease was inflammatory and Rokitansky considered it thrombogenic. It is now feasible both for physicians in their practice and those engaged in public health to identify individuals at high risk of developing CHD in whom modification of one or more risk factors can prevent the disease [2].

This chapter is organized according to McKeown's model of disease pathogenesis [3], which assumes that all health and disease are determined by (1) our genetic inheritance; (2) factors in our physical, biological, and social environment; (3) the health behaviors that we use to cope with these genetic and environmental con-

straints; and finally (4) the accessibility and quality of our medical care, which, in the case of CHD, includes preventive and rehabilitative services as well as those related to the diagnosis and treatment of its various clinical manifestations.

Physicians and other health professionals are playing an increasingly important role in interrupting this chain of pathogenesis, not only by advising patients as to what they should do but also by setting a good example (i.e., optimizing their own personal health behavior). They also have available to them an array of potent antihypertensive and serum lipid-modifying drugs, as well as surgery (such as gastric plication and small-bowel bypass) to control stubborn cases of obesity and dyslipidemia. However, the pathogenesis of CHD is complex, and even the biostatistical techniques of multivariate analysis that have been widely applied by both analytic and experimental epidemiologists still leave a substantial residual variance, indicating that we have as yet been unable to unravel fully the web of causation and end all controversy.

At least 35 factors, most of which will be reviewed in this chapter, have been suggested by one or more studies to be associated with increased risk of CHD. Dyslipidemia, hypertension, and cigarette smoking are now known to be *causative,* since their modification either individually or in concert (see chapter 11) reduces the morbidity and mortality from CHD. However, risk factors vary in relation to particular manifestations of the disease, which are listed in table 3–1. For example, the risk factors for sudden death (SD) differ substantially from those

Cohn, P.F. (ed.), Diagnosis and Therapy of Coronary Artery Disease. Copyright © 1985 by Martinus Nijhoff Publishing. All rights reserved.

TABLE 3–1. Major clinical manifestations of coronary heart disease

---

*Angina pectoris* (AP)
  Stable
  Unstable

*Dysrhythmias*
  Atrial
  Ventricular

*Myocardial infarction (MI)*
  Recognized
  Unrecognized
    Symptomatic
    Silent

*Congestive heart failure (CHF)*

*Death*
  Sudden (SD)
  Nonsudden

---

for angina pectoris (AP) and for myocardial infarction (MI). Susceptibility to atherosclerosis undoubtedly varies from person to person and from one population to another, for many reasons that remain obscure. Also, we can usually detect only overt disease, which can be far advanced before becoming symptomatic. Furthermore, risk factors measured only a short time prior to an attack may poorly reflect their true causative relationship.

Some have suggested that because of the difficulty of preventing CHD, a better strategy would be to improve the methods of its diagnosis and treatment. The problem with this approach is that the pooled data from the several prospective studies of CHD undertaken over the past 35 years indicate that a significant number of patients will die suddenly before the disease has been identified and treatment begun. Even though it may be possible for modern coronary care to salvage some patients who may die from dysrhythmias, even the best of emergency medical services cannot save many of those who may die suddenly out of hospital. Treating a disease whose first symptom is too often the last is not easy; for this reason both primary and secondary prevention of coronary heart disease is being promoted as the strategy of controlling the disease [4, 5].

A risk factor is defined as a factor associated with the development of a condition and suspected to be causative [6]. If one factor (Factor A) is reported to be associated with another (Factor B), only four explanations of the association are possible. It can be due to either (1) chance, (2) the fact that Factor A *causes* Factor B, (3) vice versa, or (4) that both Factors A and B are caused by some third factor. The strength and consistency of the association may help to decide whether it is likely to be etiologic. Since a cause must always precede an effect, the temporal relationship between A and B may also help to suggest the pathogenic pathway. Consistent with conventional biological wisdom, it is also necessary to trace a plausible causal pathway from a cause to an effect. The best "proof" of causality is through experimental intervention, which accounts, in large part, for the huge investment made by the National Institutes of Health and other research agencies in the United States and abroad in randomized, clinical trials over the past 15 years [7, 8]. Although experiments can be done with much greater ease and less expense in the laboratory using either animal, cellular, or biochemical models, generalizability to man from such experiments is always hazardous. Therefore, despite their cost, complexities, and other difficulties, a clinical trial may still be warranted if proof of causation is required.

## The Causes of Coronary Heart Disease
Table 3–2 lists the standardized multivariate coefficients for the major risk factors of CHD and total cardiovascular disease based upon 14 years of follow-up of the original Framingham Heart Study cohort aged 35 to 64.

GENETIC
It has been recognized for many years that CHD "runs in families." The important genetic factors include not only age, sex, and race, but also the genetic determinants of serum lipids, both juvenile (Type I) and adult-onset (Type II) diabetes mellitus, and primary hypertension. Although CHD clearly is a familial disease, disagreement still persists as to how much of this aggregation is due to genetic factors and how much derives

TABLE 3–2. Net effect of major risk factors on incidence of coronary heart disease and total cardiovascular disease

| Risk factors | Standardized Multivariate Coefficients | | | |
| | Coronary heart disease | | Total cardiovascular disease | |
| | Men | Women | Men | Women |
|---|---|---|---|---|
| Physical activity index | −.127 | .135 | −.184* | .043 |
| Systolic blood pressure | .169* | .358* | .271* | .414* |
| Cigarettes | .206* | .006 | .247* | .137 |
| Cholesterol | .374* | .283* | .305* | .212* |
| Glucose | .130* | .158* | .200* | .145* |
| ECG-LVH | .085 | .049 | .143* | .169* |
| Age | .340* | .471* | .442* | .505* |

*P = <.05.
Men and women 35–64. Framingham Study. 14-Year follow-up.

from the fact that family members usually eat at the same table and otherwise share the same home environment [9].

Age still remains the best single predictor of both death and the development of CHD, since it usually takes many years for occlusive atherosclerosis to evolve. However, the disease usually begins in childhood, especially for those unfortunate victims of homozygous familial hypercholesterolemia [10] and others at unusually high risk. Otherwise, symptomatic disease usually does not become manifest until either the fourth or fifth decades of life.

Premenopausal women have only a quarter the CHD risk of men, although it is still unclear as to how much of this "protection" is due to genetically determined humoral effects on physiologic risk factors (such as the level of HDL-cholesterol) and how much can be explained by the substantially different health behaviors of the two sexes. For example, until recently cigarette smoking was far less socially acceptable for women than for men.

Many studies have suggested that certain races are unusually susceptible to the development of CHD. Blacks and Orientals have a higher prevalence of hypertension than do Caucasians, but no excess of CHD. Here again it is difficult to dissect the genetic components free from dietary behavior and environmental factors known to influence the level of blood pressure and CHD.

In addition to age, sex, and race, the genetic factors that have been most intensively studied are those that affect the levels of serum lipids, arterial blood pressure, and the development of diabetes mellitus. As Goldstein and Brown [10] point out, familial hypercholesterolemia is one of the most common genetic diseases of man, with about one in every 500 individuals throughout the world inheriting at least one gene of this autosomal dominant condition. The defect is in the cell receptor of low-density lipoprotein cholesterol (LDL-C). The most common mutations lead to a reduction of receptor protein required for internalization of LDL-C. Fortunately, it appears that heterozygotes can increase the number of LDL receptors by the use of bile-acid-binding resins and other drugs.

Genetic studies of hypertension have demonstrated that the more closely two individuals are related, the closer is the concordance between their blood pressures [11]. It has also been suggested that the mechanism for this concordance is genetically determined membrane transport of sodium [12]. This latter finding has given rise to the hope that it may be possible to identify salt-sensitive individuals prior to a rise in blood pressure, whereby hypertension could be prevented by restricting the dietary intake of salt and by employing other preventive hygienic measures in such individuals.

The genetics of both the juvenile (Type I) and

adult-onset (Type II) diabetes mellitus is complex. Also, it is still unclear whether it is the level of blood sugar or some other manifestation of diabetes that explains the high prevalence of the macrovascular lesions associated with the disease. Epidemiologic studies have established that even though diabetes is associated with dyslipidemia, these unfavorable lipid patterns cannot entirely explain the increase in risk of CHD associated with diabetes [13].

## ENVIRONMENTAL FACTORS

In the strictest sense, every factor involved in the pathogenesis of any disease that is not genetic must be environmental. Therefore, it is usually useful to distinguish between factors in the macroenvironment (of particular concern to public health and environmental hygiene) and those of the microenvironment, over which the patient and physician have more control. The most pervasive environmental factor that has contributed to the current epidemic of CHD is the "good life," which is associated with too much food and too many labor-saving devices. Some also claim that our lives may be more continuously stressful than were those of our forebears, who lived in less complex societies.

The fact that CHD and other manifestations of atherosclerosis are most prevalent in developed societies has given rise to the concept that the disease is caused by the availability of foods dense in calories and with a high content of saturated fatty acids [14]. This, combined with the development of labor-saving devices such as the elevator and the motor vehicle, has encouraged a slothful pattern of living more closely associated with coronary risk than that of less developed contemporary societies. Indeed, geopathologic studies today indicate a close correlation between death rates from CHD and per capita income [15]. Inferences have also been drawn that it is the stress of modern societies that produces a social environment conducive to the development of CHD [16]. This idea is at best an unproved hypothesis. This issue will probably remain unresolved, as it is difficult to define and study certain kinds of coronary-prone behavior. To date, it has been virtually impossible to define uniformly and consistently what is meant by a

"stressful event"; not even the death of a spouse can always be assumed to be stressful to the surviving marriage partner. One possible exception to this rule is a study by Trichopoulos and his associates, who analyzed both the total and cause-specific mortality immediately following the 1981 Athens earthquake. They observed a significant excess of deaths due to heart disease, in addition to those due to the trauma of the earthquake itself [17].

Two elements of the physical environment have attracted particular attention. Clinicians have suggested for many years that snow shoveling and other types of severe physical exertion during cold weather increase the risk of sudden death from CHD, for which they have also developed a physiologic rationale. Epidemiologists have also confirmed the existence in temperate climates of a significant seasonal swing in CHD mortality that peaks during the coldest months of the year. It has also been suggested that extremely hot weather can also represent an environmental risk.

Schroeder [18] first suggested that trace metal toxicity might play a role in the pathogenesis of hypertension and other forms of cardiovascular disease. However, his initial studies in Japan, and other subsequent investigations, have not only failed to confirm his original hypothesis but have shown, instead, a generally *inverse* relationship between the hardness of drinking water and cardiovascular mortality when comparisons are made between various geographic regions within the United States [19]. In general, these correlations have *not* held true when more detailed analyses have been undertaken within any given area, thus suggesting that the observed macrocorrelations may be due to more fundamental geopathologic confounders. Intense interest in the subject is stimulated by the hope that it might provide a clue to an efficient means of controlling cardiovascular disease. The removal of pathogenic microorganisms from community water supplies still stands as the most cost-effective public health measure yet devised. Unfortunately, hope is fading that history will be repeated, since there is no clear evidence that either trace-metal deficiency or toxicity plays a role in the pathogenesis of CHD.

## HEALTH BEHAVIORS*

Despite genetic and environmental constraints, the individual can still affect his or her health by means of the personal choices involved in dietary, exercise, smoking, drinking, and other behaviors that influence health. Indeed, it has been estimated that at least half of preventable disease, disability, and untimely death in the United States today could be controlled by modifying one or more of these important health behaviors [20].

At least seven behaviors have been incriminated as major influences on the risk of CHD. Most attention has been paid to dietary habits because of their effect on body weight, serum lipids, blood pressure, and diabetes. However, increasing attention has also been paid to physical exercise, cigarette smoking, the consumption of alcohol and caffeine-containing beverages, and to a behavior pattern that has been defined by Rosenman and his associates. Finally, coronary risk is also presumably related to the willingness of the individual to seek the advice of health professionals and to adhere to preventive and therapeutic drug regimens such as those prescribed in the stepped-care of hypertension.

*Diet.* Almost all nutritionists would now agree that the percentage of calories derived from fat, the ratio of saturated to polyunsaturated fatty acids, and the cholesterol content of the diet all have independent effects on the concentration of serum lipids—particularly on the triglycerides and the cholesterol carried by the low-density lipoproteins [21–24]. Indeed, the relationship is so predictable that formulas have been derived to predict the effect of these three factors on the level of serum total cholesterol. Few would also deny that dyslipidemia is the most important modifiable physiologic risk factor in the pathogenesis of CHD. It is virtually impossible to experimentally produce atherosclerosis in animals without either raising or otherwise altering the pattern of serum lipids. There have also been a host of international studies correlating the level of serum cholesterol and the fat content of the

diet with death rates from CHD. Despite this evidence, controversy continues to plague what is often referred to as the "diet-heart hypothesis" [25]. These doubts stem primarily from the difficulties that epidemiological studies have encountered in demonstrating a close relationship between diet and CHD morbidity and mortality within a population sample. The data from intervention studies regarding the value of alteration of the diet in reducing the incidence of CHD and other cardiovascular events have also been mixed [9].

Salt as a precursor of hypertension is likewise still embroiled in controversy [26]. Here again, international and intercultural comparisons have shown that blood pressure tends to be higher and to rise more rapidly with increasing age among those peoples whose diet contains a lot of salt than among those who use less. It is also true that the blood pressure of almost any subject or patient can be raised or lowered either by restricting or increasing the salt content of the diet. However, in many cases the restriction required may be as severe as a daily intake of less than a gram of sodium chloride. On the other hand, some individuals seem to be able to consume as much as 15 grams of salt a day without experiencing a significant rise of blood pressure.

The most recent source of dietary controversy concerns fiber, which has been proposed as a means of controlling diverticulosis and colorectal cancer as an adjuvant to the regulation of blood sugar and as a means of reducing levels of serum LDL-cholesterol. Fiber, particularly pectin, has the capacity to bind bile acids in the bowel, thus diverting cholesterol to the synthesis of these acids and reducing enterohepatic recycling of cholesterol. However, the effect is not striking. But because of the inverse correlation between the fiber and fat content of most diets, it has been difficult to design epidemiologic studies to determine the independent effect of each of these two constituents. Storage of calories also seems to play a role in promoting dyslipidemia. The evidence incriminating refined carbohydrate as a promoter of either dyslipidemia or cardiovascular sequelae is unconvincing [22].

The results of the Lipid Research Clinic intervention trial of cholestyramine are encouraging,

---

*Defined as those behaviors that have a significant impact on health [6].

and the Oslo Heart Study Trial of dietary modification of serum cholesterol and control of cigarette smoking has demonstrated that decreasing serum lipids reduces risk [28]. Fears about the hazards of such dietary changes would seem to be unfounded, since what is being advocated is only a Mediterranean or Oriental type of diet. Such diets have been consumed by generations of peoples without apparent harm and do not appear to be a gastronomic nightmare, since these styles of eating are not without their advocates among gourmets.

*Exercise.* Exercise appears to be beneficial both in the primary and secondary prevention of CHD [29] and in reducing the case-fatality rate of patients hospitalized with acute myocardial infarction. Its role in the rehabilitation of patients following a coronary event is less well defined and will be explored in chapter 16. Various mechanisms have been suggested as to how exercise exerts its effect. It plays a role in maintaining optimum body weight and in the treatment of obesity. Systematic exercise also lowers the heart rate, and probably resting blood pressure, and plays a role in raising the level of HDL-C. Although several prospective studies have demonstrated an association between an increased level of physical activity and low risk of CHD [30], it has not been possible as yet to conduct a controlled primary intervention trial and thus demonstrate a truly causal relationship between exercise and the reduction of CHD risk. Early British social-class data showed that the professional and business class exhibited almost twice as much coronary mortality as did unskilled workers [31]. Morris and co-workers interpreted this as reflecting their sedentary lifestyles and supported the contention by showing that a higher mortality rate from coronary heart disease existed among the London bus drivers than among the more active conductors. Such occupational activity findings have now been extended to postal and telephone workers. Exercise has been invoked to explain why coronary mortality is greater in more highly developed countries as well as in urban populations. Autopsy data have been inconsistent, some showing, and others failing to show, a relation of job activity to coronary atherosclerosis [32]. The

fact that men commonly work at jobs suited to their vigor, strength, health, wants, and aspirations makes it difficult, because of either self-selection or assignment, to draw conclusions from occupational activity data. This is especially true if such data are retrospective. The subject is discussed further in chapter 12.

An examination of the health consequences of physical inactivity in the relatively sedentary Framingham cohort revealed that both overall and cardiovascular mortality were inversely related to the level of physical activity as assessed (figure 3–1) [33]. This effect, however, was rather modest compared to the other risk factors examined, but it did persist when these factors were taken into account. For women, the effect was negligible after correcting for age. Because the impact of physical inactivity is considerably weaker than that of other major risk factors, it does not seem likely that exercise programs alone would make as great an impact on cardiovascular disease incidence as would either the control of blood pressure, the cigarette habit, obesity, or hyperlipidemia. Data from eastern Finland, where physical activity levels are high, show the highest coronary incidence that has yet been observed anywhere in the world. These data suggest that other factors can overwhelm any protective effect of exercise. Physical exer-

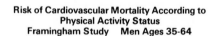

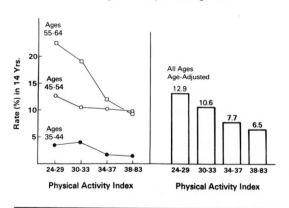

FIGURE 3–1. Risk of cardiovascular mortality according to physical activity status: Men ages 35–64. (From the Framingham Study.)

cise and conditioning are best employed in a comprehensive multiple risk factor intervention program, especially since experimental information is inadequate regarding the benefit of changes in the state of physical conditioning, either on risk factors or on cardiovascular health. Problems in recruiting, operating, gaining long-term adherence, controlling for other risk factors, and analyzing a primary prevention study of the efficacy of physical conditioning are so formidable that definitive information from such a study is unlikely to be provided in the foreseeable future.

In summary, mounting epidemiologic evidence supports an association between physical inactivity and increased risk of coronary heart disease in men. This is based on a sizable body of information about the generally favorable relation of physical activity, particularly leisure activity, on the risk of coronary heart disease. The evidence for exercise benefits for other cardiovascular diseases—such as stroke, occlusive peripheral arterial disease, and congestive failure —is far weaker.

*Cigarette Smoking.* The case against cigarette smoking in CHD is far stronger [34–36]. As illustrated in figure 3–2 there is a consistent, dose-related relationship between cigarette smoking and the risk of developing CHD. Its effects vary, with little impact on the incidence of angina pectoris, but cigarette smoking shows an impressive relationship to sudden death and myocardial infarction, particularly in men. It is one of the most powerful, modifiable risk factors that exerts an independent effect in a multivariate analysis. The effect in women is smaller, which has usually been ascribed to the fact that women may not inhale cigarette smoke as regularly or as deeply as men and to the fact that angina pectoris is their dominant CHD manifestation.

Uncertainty still exists as to whether carbon monoxide, nicotine, or perhaps even tar in cigarette smoke, alone or in concert, is responsible. Despite the overwhelming evidence that cigarette smoking is bad for one's health, the cigarette manufacturers have consistently denied the dangers, using the elliptical logic that "there is nothing harmful in cigarette smoke, but you should filter it out." Unfortunately, the evidence to date indicates that the filters may actually *increase* the risk of cardiovascular sequelae because they raise the concentration of carbon monoxide in cigarette smoke [37]. In any case, smoking filter cigarettes did not appear to reduce the risk of CHD among men less than 55 years in the Framingham cohort, as illustrated in figure 3–2.

Evidence incriminating the cigarette habit in coronary artery disease and occlusive peripheral arterial disease is now substantial. Why its relationship to brain infarction is so weak is hard to explain. Also obscure is why the influence of smoking on peripheral arterial disease is so strong compared with its influence in coronary heart disease. We also do not know why cigarette smoking is so weakly related to development of angina pectoris.

Although risk (figure 3–3) has been related to the number of cigarettes smoked each day, whether risk is related to the duration of the habit is not entirely clear. Giving up cigarette smoking may be associated with a prompt reversal to lower risk as well as with a further gradual decline in risk over the ensuing years. The evidence is substantial that those who quit promptly reduce their risk to half that of those who continue to smoke (see figure 3–3). Why the benefits of quitting smoking regarding coronary *morbidity* do not extend beyond age 65 is unclear. Are these persons the survivors who have put themselves to a severe test and demonstrated

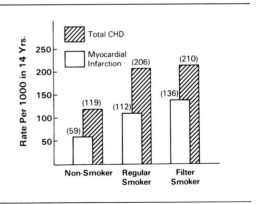

FIGURE 3–2. Risk of coronary heart disease according to cigarette smoking: Filter vs. nonfilter: Men under age 55. (From the Framingham Study.)

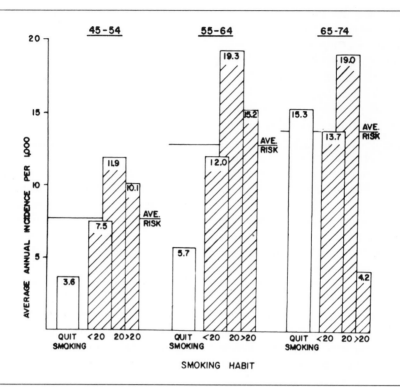

FIGURE 3–3. Incidence of coronary events among cigarette smokers according to subsequent cigarette habit in men age 45 to 74 years at initial examination. Average (ave.) risk increases with increasing number of cigarettes smoked, but there is no appreciable difference between smoking 20 cigarettes daily and smoking more than 20. The apparent marked decline in risk at over 20 cigarettes per day in the 65- to 74-year-old age group is probably not statistically valid, because there were a small number of heavy smokers and wide confidence limits in the over-65 age group. Quitting smoking reduces risk dramatically, except in the 65- to 74-year-old group. (From the Framingham Study.)

that they have a patent coronary circulation? Why women seem relatively immune is also not clear. Except for peripheral arterial disease, the contribution of the cigarette habit to cardiovascular risk in women has been thought to be relatively feeble. However, recent evidence does appear to link cigarette smoking to myocardial infarction in women, especially in those under the age of 40 [38]. The independent contribution of the cigarette habit to risk is most ominous in those persons with other established risk factors, but the *risk ratio* does not appear to increase with quantitative increases in other risk factors. While most affluent societies show a strong association, there are some low-incidence areas that show a lack of effect of cigarettes.

It thus appears that there is an independent transient, noncumulative effect of cigarette smoking that triggers lethal attacks but that is reversible. Very likely, there is also a long-term, chronic, only partially reversible, atherogenic effect. The more potent, acute effect appears to operate mainly in persons with an already compromised arterial circulation that favors sudden occlusions in the circulation to the head, heart,

or limbs and in those that may also promote lethal arrhythmias.

*Alcohol.* Alcohol appears to have a mixed effect with a "U-shaped" relationship to the incidence of CHD. The direct relationship that several studies have reported between alcohol and blood pressure and the fact that heavy drinkers clearly run the risk of developing cardiomyopathy and serious dysrhythmias tempers the advice that drinking is beneficial [39, 40].

The widespread and often excessive use of

alcohol justifies a careful consideration of its possibly harmful cardiovascular influences. Studies using modern methods do not substantiate the old concept of a beneficial effect of alcohol on coronary blood flow. Hazards of alcohol on the cardiac apparatus have long been recognized and have often been attributed to coexisting malnutrition. More recent evidence supports a direct, cardiotoxic role for alcohol when taken in large amounts. There is ample evidence that alcohol abuse can cause cardiomyopathy, and it has been associated with dysrhythmias and deterioration of left ventricular performance. Mechanisms for such cardiotoxic action are still speculative and involve cumulative effects of chronic ethanol ingestion per se, intensified drinking episodes, simultaneous exposure to trace metals, nutritional deficiency, and superimposed infection.

The data linking alcohol to coronary morbidity and mortality have been inexplicably inconsistent. Findings of a possible beneficial effect, based on prospective data, have been noted. Although heavy alcohol use is clearly toxic to the heart muscle, this does not preclude a beneficial effect of more moderate intakes on the coronary vessels. The latter possibility certainly warrants further prospective investigation, taking into account the type of alcoholic beverage, the amount and pattern of drinking, and the associated risk factors, which should include the levels of triglycerides, HDL, and blood pressure particularly. Also, the relation of alcohol use to cardiovascular disease appears to differ between cultures, and these effects must be sorted out. All such studies must distinguish alcohol abuse from alcohol use in moderation. The induction of hypertriglyceridemia by alcohol is well documented, but such abnormalities are transient and appear to have no lasting ill effects on the cardiovascular system. While VLDL-C levels are increased, those of HDL-C (which has a protective effect) are also raised. The implications of these lipid changes induced by alcohol are currently unclear. Alcohol intake also is weakly related to hypertension and gout. Despite this and its strong association with cigarette and coffee use, the use of alcohol does not appear to contribute to peripheral arterial disease and, in some studies, even shows a beneficial effect. Resolution of

the remaining issues about alcohol usage probably will require further prospective studies. Until then, those interested in protecting patients against atherosclerotic cardiovascular disease have no good reason to restrict social drinking. What data there are show, if anything, a lower incidence in those who drink in moderation.

The alcohol data from the Framingham Heart Study are summarized in figure 3–4. The beneficial effect shown may possibly be mediated through its effect on increasing HDL-C concentration. The evidence to date suggests that unless one has a personal or family history of alcohol abuse, one or two drinks a day (up to 30 ounces of absolute alcohol per day) would seem to be prudent. However, it is well to remember that the 30 grams of ethanol in two ounces of a 100-proof distilled liquor provides 210 calories in addition to those that may be contained in the vehicle with which they may be mixed. Beer and wine also provide additional "empty" carbohydrate calories, which may more than match those derived from the ethanol itself.

*Coffee and Caffeine Beverages.* Although case-control studies of coffee and other caffeine-containing beverages have suggested coffee as a cause of CHD [41], the data from prospective studies—including the Framingham Heart Study, which is summarized in figure 3–5, and the Pooling Project—have failed to show any consistent relationship between coffee consumption and the risk of CHD.

Prospective data have been developed that

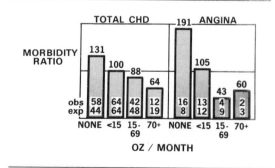

FIGURE 3–4. Risk of coronary heart disease and angina according to alcohol intake: Mean 50–62; 18-year follow-up. (From the Framingham Study.)

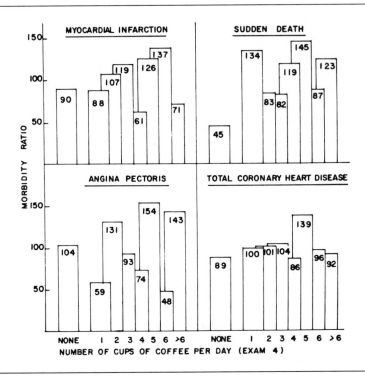

FIGURE 3-5. Risk of developing manifestations of coronary heart disease is apparently unrelated to coffee intake in men age 38 to 74 (12-year follow-up). (From the Framingham Study.)

provide some encouragement in that they show no evidence that coffee in moderation is harmful. Although many unresolved issues remain, most prospective data on the possible relation of coffee intake to coronary attacks support the hypothesis of a lack of relationship when cigarette smoking is adequately taken into account. An apparent relation to overall mortality was attributable to coincident cigarette usage. An examination of the relation between coffee intake and risk factors has revealed no important connection except for the associated tendency to cigarette smoking.

*Stress and Type A/B Behavior.* Although it seems likely that an emotional upheaval may precipitate a coronary attack in vulnerable persons, the role of social and emotional factors in the evolution of coronary heart disease remains speculative. Research efforts on psychosocial factors, though numerous, have been inconsistent. In particular, it is usually not clear whether the psychosocial state precedes or follows the onset of coronary heart disease. Serious methodologic problems must be solved before the

role of emotional stress in the development of coronary heart disease can be evaluated. Such problems include better definition of the phenomenon of stress and more precise measures to quantitate it.

Status incongruity, social mobility, and certain behavioral characteristics have been implicated as factors in the development of cardiovascular disease [16]. In patients with clearly established coronary heart disease, a pattern of goal-directed, strongly aggressive, overachieving personalities has been noted. Also, inadequate vacation periods have been implicated. The Western Collaborative Study has shown prospectively that behavior characterized by excessive competitive drive, preoccupation with deadlines, chronic impatience, a strong sense of time urgency, and excessive aggressive ambition (Type A behavior) is associated with an increased risk of coronary attacks independently of other risk factors [42]. This conclusion awaits further confirmation. It is alleged that our contemporary life-style promotes Type A patterns of behavior by regarding highly those who perform aggressively and rapidly. It is not clear whether the risk of coronary heart disease can be favorably influenced by modifying such behavior, nor is it certain that the behavior pattern can be modified. Until these questions can be resolved, it would appear prudent to focus upon the modification of correctable risk factors in Type A individuals.

A cross-sectional study of 1,822 persons age 45 to 74 at Framingham indicated that women with coronary heart disease scored significantly higher on Type A behavior, emotional lability, aging worries, tension, and anxiety symptoms than did women free of coronary heart disease. The prevalence of coronary heart disease was significantly higher among working women and housewives, who, based on a questionnaire, were classified as Type A, than among those classified as Type B, the antithesis of Type A. Although the prevalence of coronary heart disease was substantially greater in Type A women, this increase was not found in men, in whom only a trivial and statistically nonsignificant relationship was noted. It will be interesting to observe whether further prospective data will support these prevalence observations on men and women in the Framingham cohort. The biologic pathway remains to be determined for the psychosocial attributes related to cardiovascular disease. Testing in the Western Collaborative Study appears to indicate that the Type A behavior pattern exerts some influence independently of and not mediated through the conventional risk factors. For example, a recent analysis by Shekelle and his associates failed to demonstrate that the Jenkins Activity Survey (a measure of Type A behavior) could predict risk in the Western Collaborative Study. Rosenman and his colleagues still insist that Type A/B behavior can be identified reliably only by trained interviewers, while others have selected a few key questions as an element of a structured interview as the more efficient means of determining coronary-prone behavior patterns. These uncertainties have at least delayed, and perhaps have eliminated, any large-scale intervention trial to determine causality and to test the feasibility and efficiency of such modification as a means of preventing CHD.

*Health-Care-Seeking Behavior.* Finally, various studies continue to suggest that patient delay in seeking help after the onset of the chest pain, which usually heralds a myocardial infarction, remains one of the clear causes of prehospitalization mortality from acute myocardial infarction. On the other hand, as reviewed below, despite the current sophisticated electrocardiographic and enzymatic diagnosis of acute MI, a remarkable number of symptomatic myocardial infarctions still elude detection, which combined with the truly asymptomatic attacks allow conservative estimates of unrecognized MI as between 25 to 35 percent of all episodes.

The failure of many patients to heed their physician's advice, and most particularly their inability to adhere to the drug regimens that are essential to the stepped-care of hypertension and for the prevention of recurrence of myocardial infarction, remains a troublesome problem to which the adverse side effects of these potent and expensive drugs also make a contribution.

HEALTH CARE SERVICES

Physicians and other health professionals, including cardiologists, are playing an increasingly important role, not only in performing coronary risk assessment, but also in planning and implementing risk reduction programs. Increasingly, they are encouraging their patients to undertake the difficult tasks of modifying their dietary, exercise, smoking, and other important health behaviors that contribute to coronary risk. They currently can prescribe one or more of five categories of antihypertensive drugs and a smaller but growing number of drugs that favorably modify the pattern of serum lipids [27]. Indeed, systematic health maintenance of adults by internists and other primary care physicians is fast becoming as much an accepted aspect of their role as well child care has been for the pediatrician.

Unfortunately, not all physicians accept their preventive role and thereby they become part of the problem. Also, whether or not they recognize their preventive responsibilities, many health professionals still fail to set a good example by practicing good personal health behavior themselves, and thereby provide a poor role model for their patients. An ashtray filled with cigarette butts on the doctor's desk may speak far louder than the most passionate antismoking appeal.

Some coronary risk is iatrogenic. For example, particular care must also be taken in prescribing birth control pills, for it is now well established that oral contraceptives are capable of contributing to the risk of cardiovascular disease, including hypertension, acute myocardial infarction, stroke, and thromboembolism, particularly in women over 35 years of age who smoke cigarettes [43]. Although these risks may be acceptable for younger, nonsmoking women, a recent UK Royal College Study [44] determined that age, cigarette smoking, and oral contraceptives all escalated risk of cardiovascular mortality. Smokers were at higher risk than nonsmokers in every age group, 15 through age 45, and the relative risk of acute myocardial infarction among oral contraceptive users who smoked 25 cigarettes or more per day was 39 times that of nonsmokers who were not on "the pill."

The use of oral contraceptives may provoke hypertension and lipid abnormalities, impair glucose tolerance, and affect blood clotting. Such effects could account for the excessive number of atherothrombotic and thromboembolic catastrophes reported in retrospective studies. Because of the low incidence of cardiovascular disease in women in their reproductive years, the prospective data are also sparse, and there is little likelihood of developing adequate data in the near future. The UK Royal College Study also illustrated that there are five times as many deep vein thromboses and four times as many strokes in women using oral contraceptives as in controls.

With a substantial and growing percentage of the female population taking oral contraceptives regularly for most of their reproductive life, it is conceivable that we could be headed for an escalation of female cardiovascular morbidity and mortality during the child-bearing years. The combined effects on risk factors and enhancement of clotting could eventually erode the female cardiovascular risk advantage over men.

Although comparison of recent trends in coronary mortality between the two sexes shows nothing alarming to date, secular trends in the incidence of coronary heart disease in women, who are increasingly taking up smoking and using the contraceptive pill, need to be monitored. We need better guidelines for monitoring women on contraceptive pills to detect alarming worsening of atherogenic traits and changes in blood coagulation. The indications, the contraindications, and the time to prescribe alternative methods of contraception need to be more explicitly defined. More research is needed to determine the smallest amount of estrogen effective in protecting against pregnancy, the safest estrogen compound, and the optimal estrogen-progestin combination. In the meantime, women who are prescribed oral contraceptives should be made aware of the risk and should be monitored periodically for any deterioration in their cardiovascular risk profile. Those who are most susceptible to such effects can be prescribed alternative contraceptives before trouble ensues. Since smoking seems to aggravate the problem, those using oral contraceptives should be strongly advised not to smoke.

PHYSIOLOGIC RISK FACTORS

Except for age and sex, all of the physiologic risk factors of coronary disease are modifiable. However, intervention trials have shown how difficult it may be for many (even for those at highest risk) to actually make the changes required.

*Obesity.* Confusion surrounds the role of obesity as a risk factor for CHD [45]. The fact that some studies demonstrate that obesity makes little, if any, *independent* contribution to CHD incidence obscures the fact that it reflects imprudent dietary and exercise habits and that it has unfavorable effects on at least four other powerful physiologic predictors of coronary risk, i.e., blood pressure, LDL-C, HDL-C, and blood sugar [46]. Indeed, some contend that the control of obesity constitutes the most important public health priority in the United States today.

Although most obesity in humans is environmentally produced, the determinants of obesity are poorly understood. Secular trends in the prevalence of obesity in the general population over the past two decades clearly indicate that life-style plays a role. Obesity is very much a family affair, in which spouses as well as siblings and offspring share, also indicating an environmental influence. Finally, the correlation of lower weights with higher education that was noted in the original Framingham cohort and elsewhere also supports the contention that there are important socioeconomic influences.

Despite extensive insurance data and epidemiological evidence, some investigators question its hazard. Insurance company statistics suggest that obesity adversely affects cardiovascular mortality and that life expectancy improves with weight reduction. Because of possible selective bias, however, generalization from such data is considered imprudent.

Few quarrel with the evidence that obesity promotes glucose intolerance, hypertriglyceridemia, hypertension, and raised LDL-C and reduced HDL-cholesterol levels [22]. Although many of these factors are established precursors of coronary heart disease, some doubt that obesity is an important contributor to atherosclerotic disease. Apparently, the basis for this skepticism is the lack of some *independent* contribution of obesity to cardiovascular disease that is not mediated through established risk factors.

It is quite true that moderate obesity, when unaccompanied by any of the major risk factors, carries little risk of cardiovascular disease. However, few people can gain weight without a worsening of the atherogenic traits that frequently accompany obesity. These atherogenic physiologic accompaniments of obesity predispose to coronary heart disease as documented at Framingham and elsewhere. Data from the Framingham Heart Study clearly indicate that weight gain influences blood lipids, raising both the cholesterol-rich LDL and the triglyceride-rich VLDL levels as well as lowering the protective HDL-cholesterol level. Obese persons in the Framingham cohort also tended to develop higher blood pressures, more diabetes, and a greater prevalence of gout. Combinations of such atherogenic traits are known to be associated with a pronounced risk of coronary heart disease.

Unless such traits have a different connotation when promoted by obesity, it is difficult to see how obesity can be considered a noncontributor to cardiovascular disease. An examination of the regression of cardiovascular disease incidence on the various risk factors in lean and obese persons at Framingham showed no indication that the risk factors are better tolerated in the obese. Longitudinal data convincingly attest to the atherogenic potential of obesity. These data indicate that observed changes in weight are mirrored by equivalent changes in certain atherogenic traits (figure 3–6). On the average, each 10-pound weight gain is accompanied by a 6.5 mmHg increase in systolic blood pressure, an 11 mg/dl increase in serum cholesterol, a 2 mg/dl increase in blood sugar, and a small change in serum uric acid. For men these effects hold at all ages and at any level of obesity; in women they are roughly half this order of magnitude. Of preventive importance is the fact that weight loss is accompanied by a corresponding reduction in the levels of these risk factors.

Some have questioned the importance of elevated blood pressure in the obese, claiming that it is a "fat arm" artifact. This is clearly *not* the case. Blood pressures taken in the forearm and by direct, intra-arterial measurement have been shown to be as well correlated with relative weight as are those taken in the obese upper arm. There is also no evidence that high blood pressure is a less ominous finding in the obese than it is in the lean; an examination of the incidence of cardiovascular disease in different weight classes shows no evidence that the risk related to high blood pressure is any less in the obese than in the lean.

The distinct excess incidence of cardiovascular morbidity and mortality in the obese is largely explained by the accompanying worsening of atherogenic traits. Why obesity is particularly related to angina pectoris and sudden death and is inversely related to occlusive peripheral arterial disease is not clear. The cardiovascular hazards of obesity in women seem greatest for congestive heart failure and atherothrombotic brain infarction, whereas in men they are roughly equivalent for all types of cardiovascular disease. In women, the triad of obesity, diabetes, and low HDL-cholesterol levels appears to be especially ominous. Significant net contri-

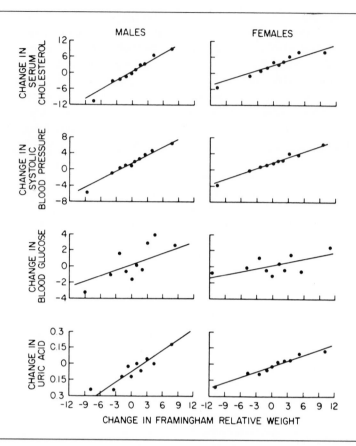

FIGURE 3–6. Changes in values for serum cholesterol (mg/dl), systolic blood pressure (mmHg), blood glucose (mg/dl), and uric acid (mg/dl) associated with changes in relative weight. The latter is defined as the ratio of body weight to median weight for the particular sex-height group. Increasing weight adversely affects the factors cited. (From the Framingham Study.)

butions suggesting some unique effect of obesity per se are found only for coronary heart disease in men and for congestive heart failure in women.

In summary, although obesity ranks low compared to other risk factors for cardiovascular disease (as judged by the size of standardized regression coefficients), it is nevertheless important because it reversibly promotes traits such as alterations in LDL-C and HDL-C levels, blood sugar, and blood pressure. This reversibility makes the correction of obesity one of the most important hygienic measures (aside from the avoidance of cigarettes) that is available for the control of cardiovascular disease.

*Physical Fitness.* Physical fitness, as measured on the treadmill and bicycle ergometer, is gaining acceptance as a new index of physiologic risk. Both the Lipid Research Clinics Prevalence Study and the Framingham Heart Study are cur-

rently assessing its independent contribution to risk. Whether or not objective measures of fitness contribute more information than that obtained from a questionnaire about the exercise habits reported by individuals is unknown.

*Hyperglycemia.* The problem of diabetes has changed from one that has been primarily concerned with the acute metabolic consequences of ketoacidosis, coma, and early death to one concerning the cardiovascular sequelae in later life. Despite the availability of more sensitive diagnostic procedures and more effective treatment for hyperglycemia, physicians continue to encounter an excessive incidence of coronary disease, strokes, cardiac failure, renal failure, neuropathy, and retinopathy in their diabetic patients. Debate continues as to whether close control of hyperglycemia is helpful in avoiding either the macro- or microangiopathy associated with diabetes. It is not clear whether the risk of vascular sequelae is proportional to the level of blood sugar or whether some critical value of blood sugar characterizes the diabetic candidate for cardiovascular disease. Also not certain is to what extent the vascular complications of diabetes are attributable to the coexistent atherogenic traits, such as hypertension, hyperlipidemia, or the obesity that often accompanies diabetes. Whether or not diabetics are particularly sensitive to the adverse effects of the major cardiovascular risk factors remains to be answered.

The adult-onset, ketoresistant, hyperinsulinemic diabetes so common in the general population appears to genuinely contribute to cardiovascular disease. Based on 20 years of surveillance of the Framingham cohort in which subsequent cardiovascular disease was related to prior evidence of diabetes, a two- to threefold increased risk of clinical atherosclerotic disease has been documented, particularly in women [47]. Studies at Framingham and elsewhere have shown that the impact of diabetes is greatest for occlusive peripheral arterial disease. The reason for this is obscure, considering that the lesions in the head, heart, and limbs of the diabetic appear to be the same. It may be that the combination of large- and small-vessel disease in the diabetic makes the limbs more susceptible.

It is also unclear why the impact of diabetes is greatest in women, in whom the disease virtually eliminates the female advantage over men regarding cardiovascular mortality. Cardiovascular morbidity and mortality are higher in diabetic women than among nondiabetic men. On the average, diabetic men and women both have higher blood pressures, blood lipid levels, and relative weights than nondiabetics, but multivariate analysis of data of the Framingham Study reveals that the impact of diabetes on cardiovascular risk cannot be attributed solely to their higher level of atherogenic traits. Also, there is no evidence that risk factors have a greater impact in diabetics than in nondiabetics.

The regression coefficients for the incidence of cardiovascular sequelae on the various risk factors are no different in the diabetic than in the nondiabetic individual.

Whether or not oral hypoglycemic agents are harmful in the diabetic, they certainly fail to prevent its cardiovascular sequelae. The risk of cardiovascular sequelae in the diabetic varies over a wide range, depending on the level of other cardiovascular risk factors (see table 3–2). Thus, those in most jeopardy can be identified, since not all diabetics are at great risk. Possibly because of a lower burden of risk factors, diabetics in less affluent societies have fewer cardiovascular complications. The diabetic with multiple risk factors is a high-risk candidate who deserves even more attention than the comparable nondiabetic. Some unique feature of diabetes is operative that is apparently neither an altered ability to contend with risk factors nor entirely mediated through them. Alleviation of associated risk factors by the correction of hypertension and lipid abnormalities, weight reduction, and the avoidance of cigarettes should substantially reduce risk. Reliance solely on the correction of hyperglycemia would appear to be imprudent. We can expect specific interventions against diabetes to work only after we have delineated more precisely the mechanisms involved so that more specific corrective measures can be conceived.

*Arterial Blood Pressure.* Figure 3–7 illustrates the interrelationship between blood pressure and other important risk factors in promoting CHD. This pathogenic relationship is graduated and independent of cigarette smoking, glucose intolerance, serum lipids, and left ventricular hypertrophy by electrocardiogram. Therefore, obesity, serum lipids, blood pressure, blood sugar, and cigarette smoking are all linked together in a complex pathogenic web [48]. Although women in general are at lower risk prior to the age of menopause than men, the same multivariate risk factor relationships hold for them except that cigarette smoking is of less importance.

Hypertension is now acknowledged to be the most prevalent and powerful contributor to cardiovascular and cerebrovascular disease. The

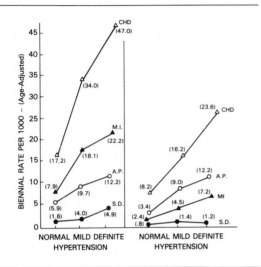

FIGURE 3–7. Risk of clinical manifestations of coronary heart disease by hypertensive status at each biennial exam: 26-year follow-up; Subjects 35–84. (From the Framingham Study.) (Men are in the left panel, women in the right.)

high prevalence of hypertension continues despite the introduction of increasingly effective antihypertensive agents. Gross undertreatment of the hypertensive population, which is now less pervasive, appears to stem from difficulties with adherence to treatment and a number of misconceptions about hypertension. Casual high blood pressure is strikingly related to subsequent cardiovascular morbidity and mortality. The lowest pressure recorded on a subject is not a valid reason for deferring treatment if the average pressure is high. At any age and for either sex, the risk of major cardiovascular events is proportional to the height of the blood pressure, systolic (figure 3–8) or diastolic, casual or basal.

There is no evidence to support the contention that the cardiovascular sequelae of hypertension derive solely from the diastolic component or that isolated systolic hypertension is innocuous [49]. The risk associated with any implied critical hypertensive blood pressure varies over a wide range, depending not only on evidence of target organ involvement, but also on the number of associated cardiovascular risk factors. The height of the blood pressure is also of critical importance. High blood pressure is definitely a major factor in the evolution of

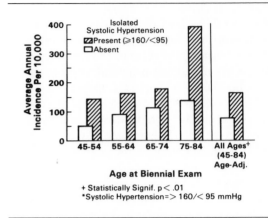

FIGURE 3–8. Risk of myocardial infarction with isolated systolic hypertension: 24-year follow-up; men 45–84. (From the Framingham Study.)

atherosclerosis, and women and the elderly do not tolerate hypertension well. To wait for the appearance of target organ involvement is not safe, since half the cardiovascular events occur before such evidence becomes evident. Treatment of hypertension, even in an atherosclerotic individual, is not necessarily hazardous and usually prolongs life. Hypertension is best viewed as an important component of a cardiovascular risk profile, and, as such, all hypertension should be treated, even borderline elevations accompanied by other risk factors.

*Serum Lipids.* Prospective epidemiologic studies of the evolution of cardiovascular disease have firmly established that high serum total cholesterol levels are precursors of coronary heart disease [50–53]. This evidence has stimulated considerable research into the transport and intermediary metabolism of the blood lipids. Our understanding of the role of cholesterol and the lipids that transport it in the development of coronary heart disease has been further enhanced by epidemiologic studies from Framingham and elsewhere. Prospective data have now firmly linked fraction of the serum total cholesterol transported on the low-density lipoprotein fraction to the development of coronary heart disease. Attention has been focused on the partitioning of the serum total cholesterol in the various lipoprotein fractions and examining the individual atherogenic potential of each component. Independent contributions of very low density lipoprotein cholesterol and its triglyceride content have not been found. Prospective data now available from various sources [54] indicate a strong inverse relationship between the HDL-cholesterol content in the serum and the subsequent risk of coronary heart disease.

Thus, further detailed study of the lipid-related risk of coronary heart disease has revealed that the contribution of the serum total cholesterol is not homogeneous. Serum total cholesterol is comprised of four components: LDL-cholesterol, which promotes atherogenesis; HDL-cholesterol, which is protective; and IDL-C and VLDL cholesterol, which are probably neutral (see also chapter 2). Within the range of values that most laboratories characterize as "within normal limits," the risk associated with the serum total cholesterol level has been found to increase over a fivefold range (figure 3–9). The impact of the serum cholesterol level on risk has been shown to be augmented in youth and by other coronary risk factors. Its impact also varies in relation to the partitioning of cholesterol among the various lipoprotein fractions; a large amount of cholesterol in the HDL fraction is protective, whereas a large amount in the LDL fraction is atherogenic. Thus, at any level of serum total cholesterol, the risk varies over a fourfold range, depending on the associated HDL-value. The previous position that all the predictive information pertaining to coronary heart disease may be obtained from the serum total cholesterol value must be accordingly modified. The demonstrated protective effect of HDL-cholesterol is at least as strong as the disease-promoting effect of LDL-cholesterol (figure 3–10). Also, the HDL-C effect is independent of other lipids as well as of other major risk factors.

Triglycerides have been incriminated in coronary atherogenesis by a number of investigators. Most prospective and case-control studies do indeed show that higher triglyceride levels, taken alone, are associated with higher coronary heart disease rates. However, mounting evidence from prospective epidemiologic studies at Framingham and elsewhere has served to deemphasize triglyceride as an *independent* contributor to atherosclerotic cardiovascular disease. Using appropriate multivariate analysis, little net effect of the triglyceride level can be demonstrated when the associated serum LDL-C and HDL-C levels, glucose tolerance, and weight are taken into account [54]. Thus, where rigorous statistical analysis designed to assess the net contribution of cholesterol and triglyceride levels to risk has been carried out, the triglyceride level has been found to provide little useful predictive information when the cholesterol-lipoprotein values are available. Triglyceride appears to derive its predictive power largely, if not entirely, from other associated risk factors. Also, to date, lesions have not been produced in animals by selectively increasing their triglyceride levels alone. Further, persons in many parts of the world with low mortality due to coronary heart disease have substantially higher triglyceride values than do those in high-incidence areas.

Triglyceride values can be helpful in approximating the LDL-C values without having to resort to ultracentrifugation; that is, the total cholesterol minus HDL-cholesterol minus triglyceride divided by 5 represents a close estimate of low-density lipoprotein cholesterol. Knowledge of triglyceride elevation should trigger concern about glucose tolerance, overweight, and alcohol intake. There is evidence that the VLDL fraction, which carries the bulk of triglyceride, consists of a complex lipoprotein with intricate metabolic functions and a close relationship to HDL and LDL. Conceivably, further investigation may uncover some reason for treating high triglyceride levels to reduce risk. For the present, the value of such an intervention appears meager, unless there is an associated chylomicronemia, a depressed HDL-C, or an elevated LDL-C.

No intervention studies are presently available that demonstrate the efficacy of raising the HDL-C levels to reduce risk. However, in the search for an optimal therapy for ameliorating atherosclerosis, the prudent treatment would appear to be that which raises the HDL-C and lowers LDL-C. Fortunately, many of the recommendations for the control of coronary heart disease, such as avoidance of smoking, weight reduction, and physical exercise, should accomplish both.

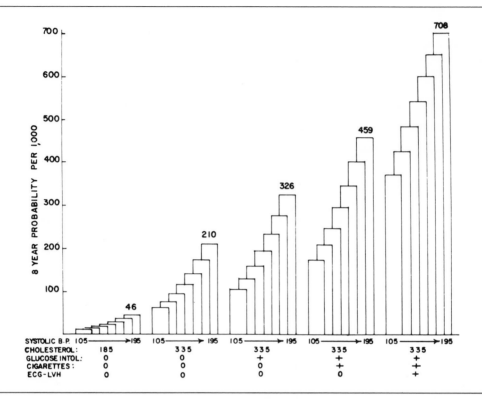

FIGURE 3–9. Risk of cardiovascular disease in 40-year-old men according to systolic blood pressure (BP, in mmHg) at specified levels of other risk factors (18-year follow-up). Increasing BP directly affects risk. Values for serum cholesterol in milligrams per deciliter. ECG-LVH = left ventricular hypertrophy on the electrocardiogram; intol.-intolerance. (From the Framingham Study.)

*Menopause.* Evidence implicating menopause in the loss of protection against coronary heart disease that women enjoy during their reproductive years has been inconsistent [13]. Case-control, autopsy, and even prospective population studies have not all uniformly shown the anticipated loss of relative immunity in women with premature menopause. Also, female hormones, particularly estrogen, have, if anything, been implicated as atherogenic rather than protective agents. Therefore, the question arises as to whether the 10-year female advantage over men in the incidence of coronary heart disease stems from a biologic or from life-style advantage.

In the United States, there is little to suggest that living habits such as diet and physical activity are sufficiently different between the sexes to explain the sex difference in incidence of coronary heart disease. There is also little to indicate that differences in the level of risk factors during adult life explain most of the difference. At any level of risk factors, singly or combined, women have a distinct advantage over men. Conceiva-

bly, however, lower levels of blood pressure and serum lipids in early life could play a larger role in protecting women than these data imply. Women do smoke less than men, and smoking has less impact on cardiovascular disease in women than in men, which could account for some of the difference. However, even among nonsmokers, women have a distinct advantage over men. Only diabetes and low HDL-C levels seem to cancel the female advantage over men, but this is true only for cardiovascular mortality and not for morbidity. The population prevalence of diabetes is only 4 percent, and generally equal in men and women. Thus, there is little likelihood that the distribution of risk factors between the sexes favors a lower incidence of coronary heart disease in females.

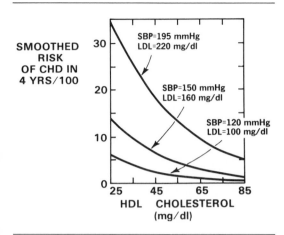

SMOOTHED
RISK
OF CHD IN
4 YRS/100

SBP=195 mmHg
LDL=220 mg/dl

SBP=150 mmHg
LDL=160 mg/dl

SBP=120 mmHg
LDL=100 mg/dl

HDL   CHOLESTEROL
(mg/dl)

FIGURE 3–10. Risk of coronary heart disease according to levels of HDL-cholesterol. Men aged 55; 24-year follow-up. (From the Framingham Study.)

In the original Framingham cohort, a dramatic rise in the incidence of coronary heart disease was observed in postmenopausal women, and more severe manifestations of the disease were observed. In the cohort of 2,873 women who were followed for 24 years, no premenopausal women developed a myocardial infarction or died of coronary heart disease, whereas in women under 55 after either natural or surgical menopause, 40 percent of those presenting with coronary disease presented with myocardial infarction or death rather than with angina pectoris.

The incidence of premenopausal coronary heart disease was very low in the 40- to 45-year-old age group. It was significantly higher at that age after the menopause. In the age groups 45 to 49 and 50 to 54, cardiovascular disease incidence rates, in general, in those undergoing the menopause were more than double those in the premenopausal state. This was true whether the menopause was natural or surgical, and the coronary heart disease was no more severe in the surgical group. In the group with surgical menopause, the excess incidence of coronary heart disease was noted whether the ovaries were removed or not.

Thus, as regards atherosclerotic cardiovascular disease, women are clearly the biologically superior sex. The essence of this superiority and its biochemical nature have yet to be elucidated. However, among women as well as men risk varies greatly in relation to their individual burden of risk factors.

*Hematologic Factors.* Pathologists have long been aware of the fact that although atherosclerosis can be found in almost every major artery of the systemic circulation, it spares the pulmonary arteries except when there is a pathologic increase in pulmonary arterial pressure. It usually begins in areas of turbulence where the smooth, laminar flow of blood is disturbed, occurring either at the bifurcation of the vessel or where the arterial anatomic configuration encourages turbulence. This includes that which is caused by large atherosclerotic plaques themselves, possibly explaining why the disease may accelerate rapidly after a long period of latency. A vicious, self-perpetuating cycle is thus possible where a plaque produces turbulent flow, which, in turn, encourages the further growth of the plaque. Some believe that it is the chaotic nature of the coronary arterial blood flow, with end-systolic reversal, that makes the coronary arteries particularly vulnerable. Other investigators are still pursuing the Rokitansky hypothesis that atherogenesis is basically a thrombotic process. Recent studies of platelets, prostaglandins, and the early phases of clotting have encouraged this line of research. Blood hematocrit is the most important determinant of blood viscosity, but it is uncertain whether increased viscosity explains the independent contribution that high hematocrit makes to coronary risk in women and to the risk of stroke in both sexes[55].

The Paris Prospective Study of CHD has also recently drawn attention to the fact that there is a direct relationship between the white blood cell count and the risk of developing a myocardial infarction. Those with counts greater than 10,000 per cubic millimeter in that study experienced about 6 times the risk of MI as those with counts less than 5,000 per cubic millimeter [56]. Other studies [57] suggest that this finding is confounded by the fact that cigarette smoking causes leukocytosis. The Kaiser-Permanente Study, however, indicates an independent effect and possible interaction with cigarette smoking.

Although antithrombins were first described by Brinkhous et al. in 1939 [58], antithrombin III (AT III) has only recently attracted special attention. This is because it is depressed by estrogen-containing oral contraceptives. Further, more than 100 families throughout the world are afflicted with an autosomal dominant AT III deficiency, about half of whom experience venous thromboembolism at one time or another throughout their lives. However, whether they are at increased risk of either atherosclerosis or arterial thrombosis is unclear.

*Humoral Factors.* Other humoral factors in coronary risk have also been scrutinized. Deficiency of thyroid hormones has been suggested as a cause of coronary disease by virtue of their effect on serum lipids. Also, a recent case-control study on the survivors of the original Framingham Heart Study cohort found serum estradiol levels to be significantly higher in subjects with CHD than among controls, except in those subjects who were 75 years of age or older.

## Other Pertinent Considerations

### CARDIOVASCULAR RISK PROFILES

Predictive equations based upon decades of follow-up of the 5,209 men and women who participated in the Framingham Study since 1948 have synthesized the major risk factors into a composite score, or cardiovascular risk profile. The multivariate profiles detect a higher percentage of susceptible individuals than is possible using single-risk-factor assessments [59]. The composite score also provides a less misleading approach since it tends to overlook fewer persons with multiple marginal abnormalities who are also at high risk. These formulations have been shown to have wide application in the United States and to foretell accurately the extent of disease to be expected in a community from its burden of risk attributes.

In the Framingham Study, the chance of developing cardiovascular disease by age 65 was found to be 37 percent for a man and 18 percent for a woman. The gravity of the situation has stimulated interest in identifying, in advance, those persons who are at substantial risk of developing cardiovascular disease and in specifying the characteristics that place them in such jeopardy. The major risk factors have been identified through the Framingham and similar studies. Any of these factors can be used individually to separate high- from low-risk persons, but the efficacy of such an approach varies with the characteristic chosen and the cardiovascular disease for which risk is being assessed.

Efficient risk characterization requires that we take into account the exact value of the risk attributes, because for major risk factors such as blood pressure and the serum cholesterol level, risk is proportional to the level of the risk attribute, and no critical values (i.e., arbitrary cutoff levels) are discernible. Also, a single-risk-factor approach is neither logical nor effective for screening high-risk persons for cardiovascular disease. At any level of blood pressure or serum cholesterol, the risk of cardiovascular disease varies widely, depending on the level of other risk factors that contribute to the occurrence of disease. To be efficient, risk evaluations must synthesize the major contributors to cardiovascular disease quantitatively into a composite score. This has been accomplished using a multiple-logistic formulation that estimates the conditional probability of any major cardiovascular event for any set of risk factors. This formulation employs the actual level of each of the factors, their regression coefficients, and constants for the intercepts. An efficient set of risk factors for this purpose includes those cited earlier, that is, the serum cholesterol level, systolic blood pressure, glucose tolerance, presence of LVH on the ECG, and the cigarette habit. Using these data, handbooks have been developed and distributed by the American Heart Association (AHA) and the National Heart, Lung and Blood Institute (NHLBI) [60]. Therefore, physicians, in their office practice, can identify high-risk persons according to the combination of such risk factors.

Determinations of such variables can be obtained in an unprepared patient, atraumatically, at modest cost, and using only ordinary office procedures and simple laboratory tests. Thus, knowing the person's age and sex, cardiovascular events can be predicted over a very wide range [61]. An example of this calculation is given in figure 3–11. In this way, physicians can identify that one-tenth of the general population from which 22 percent of coronary heart disease, 31 percent of the occlusive peripheral arterial disease, 43 percent of the brain infarction, and 40 percent of the congestive heart failure will evolve.

These risk formulations can be further improved by taking into account high-density lipoprotein cholesterol (HDL-C) values, and a multiplier has been tabulated in the AHA-NHLBI handbook to adjust such risk formulations. Although the pathogenesis may differ from one cardiovascular disease to another, there is apparently a sufficiently common process to warrant considering the incidence of atherosclerotic cardiovascular risk function has been devised on that assumption that is fairly efficient for predicting all cardiovascular disease with a common hypertensive and atherosclerotic basis.

Finally, the utility of many of the proposed prophylactic measures for reducing the risk of cardiovascular disease requires a rational method of identifying high-risk persons so as to focus attention properly on them while avoiding needlessly alarming persons at lower risk because of single stigmata. Also, it is important not to provide false reassurance to persons with multiple marginal risk factors who may be at greater than average risk. Cardiovascular risk profiles provide an effective instrument for avoiding both pitfalls. Such profiles do assist in the search for, and care of, persons at high risk of cardiovascular disease.

## RISK-FACTOR EVALUATION IN THE ELDERLY

The cohorts of epidemiologic studies such as that at Framingham have now entered the geriatric age group, which has provided an opportunity to determine whether the same cardiovascular risk factors that operate for young adults are also relevant for the aged. This determination is important, not as a quest for immortality, but for the goal of improving the quality of the later years of life.

Even more so than in the young, cardiovascular disease is the major cause of disability and death in the aged. It is not, however, an inevitable result of senescence, but related to identified risk factors. Using a set of risk attributes, each of

which exerts an independent effect in advanced age, it is possible to estimate the risk of a cardiovascular event in the elderly over a wide range. Thus, one-tenth of the elderly population can be identified in which about a third of the future coronary events and half the brain infarctions will occur [61]. Using multiple-logistic-risk formulations, it is possible to identify as high a percentage of potential cases of cardiovascular disease in the elderly as in the young.

High-density lipoprotein cholesterol, low-density lipoprotein cholesterol, systolic blood pressure, diabetes, and ECG evidence of LVH are all associated with a risk of coronary disease in the aged. HDL-C is inversely related; the rest are positively related. Hypertension is the key remediable contributor to cardiovascular morbidity and mortality in the elderly, for which prophylactic treatment is grossly deficient. This is probably because of the patients' difficulties in adhering to recommended treatment and because of misconceptions about the role of hypertension in promoting cardiovascular disease in the elderly. Hypertension is not an inevitable, physiologic, compensatory, or innocuous phenomenon in the aged. The relative, absolute, and attributable risks of hypertension are just as great in the elderly as in the young.

Although the impact of many of the major risk factors does wane with advancing age, it is clearly possible to identify high-risk elderly persons and the predisposing factors that may be correctable. The ability to predict cardiovascular disease in the elderly from identified risk factors, however, is no guarantee that intervention to eliminate such factors will be fruitful.

## RISK FACTORS IN SUDDEN DEATH

Because sudden death (within an hour of the onset of symptoms) is a prominent feature of coronary mortality, there is considerable interest in factors that predispose specifically to its occurrence. Persons highly vulnerable to death from coronary attacks can be identified from their coronary risk profile well in advance of sudden demise. The risk profile of candidates for sudden death, however, is indistinguishable from that of persons who will manifest coronary heart disease in general, although for the former, obesity, the cigarette habit, and intraventricular con-

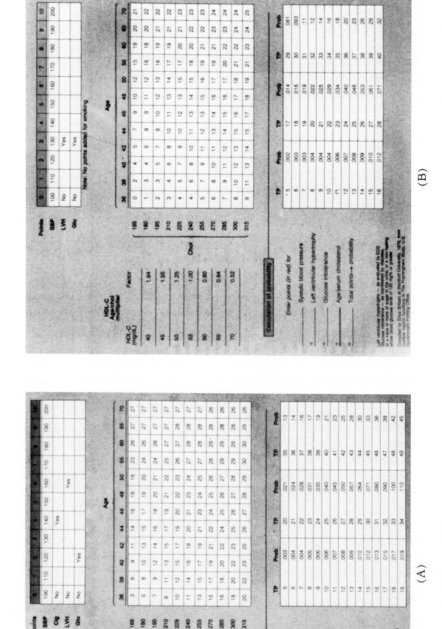

FIGURE 3–11. (A) Probability of developing coronary heart disease in 6 years: Men (Aged 35–70) (B) Probability of developing coronary heart disease in 6 years: Women (Aged 35–70). (© 1984. Reproduced from *Hospital Medicine*, February 1984, with permission of Hospital Publications, Inc.)

duction disturbances have greater effects [62, 63]. Risk profiles constructed from some of these ingredients allow an estimate of risk over a 14-fold range and identify that tenth of the population from which a third of the sudden deaths will evolve.

Although the same precursors are generally found to be present in persons whose coronary attacks are fatal as in those whose are not, a number of coronary risk factors are positively related to the proportion of coronary deaths that were suddenly fatal. These include level of general physical activity, obesity, intraventricular block, and the cigarette habit. The other major coronary risk factors are not specifically related to the suddenness of coronary fatalities.

Persons with premature ventricular contractions have about a threefold increase of risk of sudden death. Virtually all the sudden deaths associated with premature contractions are also associated with evidence of an ischemic myocardium, which is usually manifested by other ECG abnormalities (see chapter 5). The proportion of coronary deaths that are sudden is no greater among those persons with premature ventricular contractions than among those without them; this fact was well illustrated in the Coronary Drug Project [64]. Ventricular premature contractions seem, in general, to reflect the severity of the ischemic damage to the myocardium, and they do not seem likely to be a direct cause of sudden death due to ventricular fibrillation in the late postinfarction period, as they are in the acute phase of the myocardial infarction.

Thus, factors associated with an increased incidence of sudden death are not necessarily related to the suddenness of coronary fatalities. While control of risk factors will not specifically reduce the risk of sudden death, such control can reduce the occurrence of coronary attacks and hence indirectly reduce the likelihood of sudden death. Thus far, the potential sudden death victim cannot be confidently discriminated from the person destined for a less precipitous coronary death. Sudden coronary deaths would appear to be more a consequence of the nature of the ischemic disease in the heart than of the factors that predispose to coronary atherosclerosis. The inescapable conclusion seems to be that the prevention of sudden coronary death requires the prevention of coronary attacks by avoidance or correction of coronary risk factors.

## Conclusions

Despite some continued skepticism, the concept of the cardiovascular risk profile has been thoroughly validated in a variety of population samples. Although major undiscovered cardiovascular risk factors undoubtedly still remain to be uncovered, those already established provide a sound basis for effective prophylaxis.

The utility of conventional risk factors in assessing the prognosis in those with already established coronary heart disease remains to be demonstrated convincingly. Existing data are too inconsistent to render a sound judgment. The problem is complicated by the fact that the cardiovascular event may alter the risk factors. Only a controlled intervention trial can provide the needed answers. At present, only relief of hypertension, dyslipidemia, and quitting cigarettes seem of proved benefit.

Despite considerable pessimism, risk factors have been found to operate powerfully in the elderly and allow the identification of as high a percentage of potential cardiovascular disease cases in them as in the young. It would thus seem worthwhile to ascertain whether controlling risk factors that operate in advanced age can improve the quality of life in the aged.

Specific risk factors for sudden death have not been clearly identified, although physical activity, obesity, intraventricular block, and the cigarette habit may be such factors. Ventricular premature contractions per se may not be a direct cause of sudden death in the coronary candidate, as they are in the acute phase of a myocardial infarction. Control of conventional risk factors will not *specifically* reduce the risk of sudden death; however, such prophylaxis may still, by virtue of a reduction in the risk of coronary attacks, result in fewer suddenly fatal events.

There is a growing conviction that atherosclerotic cardiovascular disease is chiefly a product of a faulty life-style or adverse environmental influences, but only the cigarette habit, dyslipidemia, and hypertension are clearly causative. The level of physical activity required is still speculative, as is the minimal effective frequency and duration. Evidence for the role of the typical American diet is less direct but quite substantial. This evidence is broadly based on animal experiments, metabolic studies in humans, autopsy data, tracer studies of lipid metabolism, and prospective epidemiologic studies relating blood lipid levels to the development of atherosclerotic diseases. The final link in the chain of evidence, in which it is shown that alteration in the diet does in fact reduce the potential for disease, is now emerging [8]. It has been determined, however, that it will not be feasible to obtain definitive evidence, because of cost, the sample size needed, problems of adherence, and secular changes in the control group. We are thus forced to make decisions based on the incomplete information available. We may arrive at conclusions about the efficacy of diet modification by inference, however, after sizable proportions of the population have changed their diet for a decade or more. Whatever the cause of the recent 33 percent decrease in cardiovascular mortality since 1968 [65], it is clear that it is environmentally related and that the change in life-style required is neither drastic nor unacceptable to most Americans.

There is no evidence to support a recommendation to restrict coffee and moderate alcohol intake to help prevent coronary heart disease. Prescription of oral contraceptives without monitoring the cardiovascular risk profile for any alarming changes would appear imprudent on the basis of the evidence available. This is especially true for women who smoke and are over age 35.

Since the protective effect demonstrated for HDL-cholesterol is at least as strong as the disease-promoting influence of LDL-cholesterol, attention to the partition of the serum cholesterol between these lipoprotein fractions appears imperative. This is true both for the selection of preventive measures and for the estimation of risk. Less concern about VLDL-cholesterol and triglyceride levels would seem in order, although many would still dispute this statement.

Correction of misconceptions about the importance of labile and systolic hypertension, casual high blood pressure, and hypertension in the elderly and in women will be required be-

fore further inroads against the sequelae of this most powerful risk factor can be made.

Specific interventions against diabetes as a cardiovascular risk factor will evolve only after we better delineate the mechanisms involved. Meanwhile, attention to other risk factors would appear to be paramount, and preoccupation with correction of hyperglycemia alone seems to be a shortsighted approach.

Determination of the reason for the relative immunity of the premenopausal woman to atherosclerotic cardiovascular disease may be important, not only so that this protection can be extended beyond the reproductive years, but also because some hope may be offered for men as well.

## References

1. *Morbidity and Mortality Weekly Report* 32:583, November 11, 1983.
2. Kannel, W.B. and Schatzkin, A. Risk factor analysis. *Prog. Cardiovasc. Dis.* 26:309, 1983.
3. McKeown, T. *Medicine in a Modern Society.* New York: Hafner, 1966.
4. Borhani, N.O. Primary prevention of coronary heart disease: A critique. *Am. J. Cardiol.* 40:259, 1977.
5. Whereat, A.F. Prevention of heart disease. *Am. J. Cardiol.* 37:449, 1976.
6. Stokes, J., III, Noren, J., and Shindell, S. Definition of terms and concepts applicable to clinical preventive medicine. *Journal of Community Health* 8:33, 1982.
7. Hypertension Detection and Follow-Up Program Cooperative Group. Five-year findings of the Hypertension Detection and Follow-Up Program. *JAMA* 242:2562, 1979.
8. Multiple Risk Factor Intervention Trial Research Group. Multiple Risk Factor Intervention Trial: Risk factor changes and mortality results. JAMA 248:1465, 1982.
9. Kannel, W.B., Feinleib, M., McNamara, P.M., et al. An investigation of coronary disease in families: The Framingham Offspring Study. *Am. J. Epid.* 110:281, 1979.
10. Goldstein, J.L., and Brown, M.S. Familial Hypercholesterolemia. In J.B. Stanbury, J.B. Wyngaarden, D.S. Frederickson, et. al (eds), *The Metabolic Basis of Inherited Disease,* (5th ed.). New York: McGraw-Hill, 1983, pp. 672–712.
11. Rose, R.J., Miller, J.Z., Grim, C.E., and Christian, J.C. Aggregation of blood pressure in the families of identical twins. *Am. J. Epidemiol.* 109:503, 1979.
12. Canessa, M., Adragna, N., Solomon, H.S., Con-

nolly, T.M., and Tosteson, D.C. Increased sodium-lithium countertransport in red cells of patients with essential hypertension. *N. Engl. J. Med.* 302:772, 1980.

13. Wingard, D.L., Barrett-Connor, E., Criqui, M. Suarez, L. Clustering of heart disease risk factors in diabetic compared to nondiabetic adults. *Am. J. Epidemiol.* 117:19, 1983.

14. Miettinen, M., Turpeinen, O., Karvonen, M.J., Eluosa, R., and Paavilainen E. Effect of cholesterol-lowering diet on mortality from coronary heart disease and other causes: A twelve-year clinical trial in men and women. *Lancet* 2:835, 1972.

15. Keys, A. Coronary heart disease in seven counties. *Circulation* 41 (Suppl 1):1, 1970.

16. Jenkins, C.D. Psychological and social precursors of coronary disease (II). *N. Engl. J. Med.* 284:-307, 1971.

17. Trichopoulos, D., Katsouyanni, K., Zavitsanos, X., Twonou, A., and Dalla-Vorgia, P. Psychological stress and fatal heart attack: The Athens (1981) earthquake natural experiment. *Lancet* 1:-441, 1983.

18. Schroeder, H.A. Relation between mortality from cardiovascular disease and treated water supply. *JAMA* 172:98, 1960.

19. Sharrett, A.R., and Feinleib, M. Water constituents and trace elements in relation to cardiovascular disease. Preventive Medicine 4:20, 1975.

20. *Healthy People.* The Surgeon General's Report on Health Promotion and Disease Prevention. DHEW/PHS, 79-55071A, 1979.

21. Yudkin, J. and Roddy, L. Levels of dietary sucrose in patients with occlusive atherosclerotic heart disease. *Lancet* 2:6, 1964.

22. Little, J.A., Birchwood, B.L., Simmons, D.A., Antar, M.A., Kallos, A., Buckley, G.C., and Csima, A.: Interrelationship between the kinds of dietary carbohydrate and fat in hyperlipoproteinemic patients. *Atherosclerosis* 11:173, 1970.

23. Dayton, S., Pearce, M.L., Hashimoto, S., Dixon, W.J., and Tomiyasu, U. A controlled clinical trial of a diet high in unsaturated fat in preventing complications of atherosclerosis. *Circulation* 40 (Suppl 2):1, 1969.

24. Sacks, F.M., Castelli, W.P., Donner, A., and Kass, E.H. Plasma lipids and lipoproteins in vegetarians and controls. *N. Engl. J. Med.* 292:-1148, 1975.

25. Diet and Ischaemic heart disease—agreement or not? *Lancet* 2:317, 1983.

26. Michell, A.R. Salt appetite, salt intake, and hypertension: A deviation of perspective. *Pers. Biol.* Med. 21:335, 1978.

27. The Lipid Research Clinics Coronary Prevention Trial Results: I. Reduction in incidence of coronary heart disease. *JAMA* 251:351, 1984.

28. Hjermann, I., Velve Byre, K., Holme, I., and Leren, P. Effect of diet and smoking intervention on the incidence of coronary heart disease: Report from the Oslo Study Group of a randomized trial in healthy men. *Lancet* 2:1303, 1981.

29. Froelicher, V.F., and Oberman, A. Analysis of epidemiologic studies of physical inactivity as risk factor for coronary artery disease. *Prog. Cardiovasc. Dis.* 15:41, 1972.

30. Kannel, W.B. High-density lipoproteins: Epidemiologic profile and risks of coronary artery disease. *Am. J. Cardiol.* 52:9B, 1983.

31. Morris, J.N., Heady, J.A., Raffle, P.A.B., Roberts, C.G., and Parks, J.W. Coronary heart disease and physical activity of work. *Lancet* 2:1053, 1953.

32. Spain, D.M., and Bradess, V.A. Occupational physical activity and the degree of coronary atherosclerosis in "normal" men: A post-morten study. *Circulation* 22:239, 1960.

33. Kannel, W.B., and Sorlie, P.D. Some health benefits of physical activity: The Framingham Study. *Arch. Intern. Med.* 139:857, 1979.

34. Kannel, W.B., McGee D.L. and Castelli W.P. Latest perspectives on cigarette smoking and cardiovascular disease: The Framingham Study. J. Cardiac Rehab. 4:267, 1984.

35. Kannel, W.B., and Castelli, W.P. Significance of nicotine, carbon monoxide and other components in the development of cardiovascular disease. In Proceedings of the Third World Conference on Smoking and Health, Vol 1: *Modifying the Risk for the Smoker.* Washington D.C.: U.S. Department of Health, Education and Welfare, DHEW Publ. No. (NIH) 76, 1975.

36. Astrup, P., Kjeldsen, K., and Wanstrup, J. Enhancing influence of carbon monoxide on the development of atheromatosis in cholesterol-fed rabbits. *J. Atheroscler. Res.* 7:343, 1967.

37. Benowitx, N.L., Hall, S.M., Herning, R.I., Jacob, P., Jones, R.T., and Osman, A.L. Smokers of low-yield cigarettes do not consume less nicotine. *N. Engl. J. Med.* 309:139, 1983.

38. Surgeon General of the United States. The Health Consequences of Smoking for Women: A report of the Surgeon General. Rockville, MD: Office on Smoking and Health, Public Health Service. U.S. Department of Health and Human Services, 235–249, 1980.

39. Kannel, W.B. Coffee, cocktails and coronary candidates. *N. Engl. J. Med.* 297:443, 1977.

40. Yano, K., Rhoads, G.G., and Kagan, A. Coffee, alcohol and risk of coronary heart disease among Japanese men living in Hawaii. *N. Engl. J. Med.* 297:405, 1977.

41. Jick, H., Meittinen, O.S., Neff, R.K., Shapiro, S., Heinonen, O.P., and Slone, D. Coffee and myocardial infarction. *N. Engl. J. Med.* 289:63, 1973.

42. Rosenman, R.H., Brand R.J., Sholtz, R.I., and

Friedman, M. Multivariate prediction of coronary heart disease during 8½ years of follow-up in the Western Collaborative Group Study. *Am. J. Cardiol.* 37:903, 1976.

43. Kannel, W.B. Oral contraceptive hypertension and thromboembolism. *Int. J. Gynaecol. Obstet.* 16:466, 1979.

44. Royal College of General Practitioners' Oral Contraception Study. Further analyses of mortality in oral contraceptive users. *Lancet* 1:541, 1981.

45. Gordon, T., and Kannel, W.B. Obesity and cardiovascular disease: The Framingham Study. *Clin. Endocrinol. Metabol.* 5:367, 1976.

46. Ashley, F.W., Jr. and Kannel, W.B. Relation of weight change to changes in atherogenic traits: The Framingham Study. *J. Chronic. Dis.* 27:103, 1974.

47. Kannel, W.B. and McGee, D.L. Diabetes and cardiovascular risk factors: The Framingham Study. *Circulation* 59:8, 1979.

48. Kannel, W.B. and Sorlie, P. Hypertension in Framingham. In O. Paul (ed.), *Epidemiology and Control of Hypertension.* Miami, FL: Symposia Specialists, pp. 553–592, 1975.

49. Kannel, W.B., Dawber, T.R., and McGee, D.L. Perspectives on systolic hypertension: The Framingham Study. *Circulation* 61:1179, 1978.

50. Gordon, T., Castelli, W.P., Hjortland, M.C., Kannel, W.B., and Dawber, T.R. Predicting coronary heart disease in middle-aged and older persons: The Framingham Study. *JAMA* 238:497, 1977.

51. Castelli, W.P., Doyle, J.T., Gordon, T., James, C.G., Hjortland, M.C., Hulley, S.B., Kagan, A., and Zukel, W.J. HDL cholesterol and other lipids in coronary heart disease: The cooperative lipoprotein phenotyping study. *Circulation* 55:767, 1977.

52. Hjermann, I., Enger, S.C., Helgeland, A., Holme, I., Leren, P., and Trygg, K. The effect of dietary changes on high density lipoprotein cholesterol. The Olso Study. *Am. J. Med.* 66:105, 1979.

53. Gordon, T., Kannel, W.B., Castelli, W.P., and Dawber, T.R. Lipoproteins, cardiovascular disease and death: The Framingham Study. *Arch. Intern. Med.* 141:1128, 1981.

54. Castelli, W.P., Abbott, R.D., and McNamara, P.M. Summary estimates of cholesterol used to predict coronary heart disease. *Circulation* 67:730, 1983.

55. Kannel, W.B., Gordon, T., Wolf, P.A., and McNamara, P.M. Hemoglobin and the risk of cerebral infarction: The Framingham Study. *Stroke* 3:409, 1972.

56. Zalokar, J.B., Richard, J.L., and Claude, J.R. Leukocyte count, smoking and myocardial infarction. *N. Engl. J. Med.* 304:465, 1981.

57. Prentice, R.J., Szatrowski, T.P., Fukikura, T., Kato, H., Mason, M.W., and Hamilton, H.H. Leukocyte counts and coronary heart disease in a Japanese cohort. *Am. J. Epidemiol.* 116:496, 1982.

58. Brinkhous, K.M., Smith, H.P., Warner, E.D., and Seegers, W.H. Inhibition of blood clotting and unidentified substances which act in conjunction with heparin to prevent the conversion of prothrombin to thrombin. *Am. J. Physiol.* 125:683, 1939.

59. McGee, D.L. The probability of developing certain cardiovascular diseases in eight years at specified values of some characteristics. In *The Framingham Study.* Section 28. Washington D.C.: U.S. Department of Health, Education and Welfare, DHEW Publ No (NIH) 74–618, 1973.

60. Sorlie, P. Cardiovascular diseases and death following myocardial infarction and angina pectoris: Framingham Study, 20-year follow-up. In *The Framingham Study.* Section 32. Washington, D.C.: U.S. Department of Health, Education and Welfare, DHEW Publ No. (NIH) 77–1247, 1977.

61. Brittain, E. Probability of coronary heart disease developing. *West. J. Med.* 136:86, 1982.

62. Kannel, W.B., Doyle, J.T., McNamara, P.M., Quickenton, P., and Gordon, T. Precursors of sudden coronary death: Factors related to the incidence of sudden death. *Circulation* 51:606, 1975.

63. Doyle, J.T., Kannel, W.B., McNamara, P.M., Quickenton, P., and Gordon, T. Factors related to suddenness of death from coronary disease: Combined Albany-Framingham studies. *Am. J. Cardiol.* 37:1073, 1976.

64. Coronary Drug Project Research Group. The prognostic importance of premature ventricular complexes in the late post-infarction period: Experience in the Coronary Drug Project. *Acta. Cardiol* (Brux) Suppl, 18:33, 1974.

65. Havlik, R.J., and Feinleib, M., eds. Proceedings of the Conference on the Decline in Coronary Heart Disease Mortality. U.S. Department of HEW, PHS, NIH Publ No, 79–1610, 1979.

# II. DIAGNOSIS AND EVALUATION OF CORONARY ARTERY DISEASE

# 4. EVALUATION OF ANGINAL SYNDROMES USING STANDARD CLINICAL PROCEDURES

Peter F. Cohn

A common theme that runs through the entire spectrum of clinical coronary artery disease is the presence of chest pain or chest discomfort. The pain or discomfort may be typical or atypical of classic (Heberden's) angina, and for that reason many cardiologists prefer to use "anginal syndrome" (or "chest pain syndrome") as a general descriptive term for the varieties of chest pain and related complaints. It is fair to say that chest pain and its equivalents—arm, neck, or jaw pressure, burning, or numbness—represent the *predominant* symptoms in four of the most important clinical subsets of this disease: acute myocardial infarction, chronic (stable) angina pectoris, unstable angina, and Prinzmetal's variant angina. An anginal syndrome may also be present to some degree in patients with coronary artery disease who present with cardiac arrhythmias or in those with congestive heart failure due to left ventricular aneurysm, ischemic cardiomyopathy, or papillary muscle dysfunction. Only in the small subset of patients with totally "silent" or asymptomatic myocardial ischemia is it absent.

Chest pain may be due to cardiac disorders other than coronary artery disease (aortic valvular disease, for example), and although such disorders may often be readily diagnosed by standard clinical procedures (i.e., history, physical examination, chest roentgenogram, and electrocardiogram), one cannot always be certain that coronary artery disease is not *also* present. By contrast, in patients without other cardiac disease, chest pain due to coronary artery disease can often be distinguished from that due to non-cardiac disorders (musculoskeletal or gastrointestinal disease, for example) by means of the standard clinical tools available to physicians. In many instances, not only can the presence of coronary artery disease be strongly suspected, but its severity can also be estimated.

The purpose of this chapter is to discuss the clinical procedures listed in the preceding paragraph that are routinely employed for the evaluation of patients with anginal syndromes. Impressions obtained from such procedures will be compared to the results of invasive procedures (i.e., hemodynamic studies, coronary arteriography, and left ventriculography) in order to demonstrate how the patient's signs and symptoms (as demonstrated by the clinical evaluation) relate to the underlying pathophysiology. Attention will be focused primarily on patients in whom an acute myocardial infarction is *not* suspected, since diagnosis of an acute myocardial infarction will be the subject of a separate chapter (see chapter 10).

In the course of this chapter, several areas of controversy will be discussed. Traditional teachings, for example, have primarily emphasized the value of the clinical history in making a diagnosis. Is this approach still valid in light of newer clinical-coronary arteriographic correlations? Other areas of controversy include the diagnostic significance of "typical" versus "atypical" angina pectoris; how unstable angina differs from stable angina; the relationship between specific features of the anginal syndrome and specific lesions in the coronary vasculature; the value of the physical examination; the significance (or lack of it) of the fourth heart sound; what can be learned from routine blood tests, especially in relation to hyperlipidemias; the significance of a normal electrocardiogram (ECG) at rest; the role of the exercise test as an office (or clinic) screening procedure; and what are reasonable guidelines for the differential diagnosis of chest pain. A summary of these controversial points will be offered at the conclusion of the chapter.

## The Clinical History

The importance of taking an adequate history cannot be overemphasized, even in light of the valuable noninvasive and invasive diagnostic tools at the disposal of the contemporary physician. What is the nature of the pain? Does it radiate? What relieves it? Has the patient experienced a prior myocardial infarction, or is there a family history of heart disease—particularly coronary artery disease—in family members under 55 years of age? Has the patient been told he or she has hypertension, diabetes, or a hyperlipidemia? As Sampson and Cheitlin [1] have noted in their excellent review, trying to obtain answers to these and other questions can be complicated by problems inherent in the physician-patient relationship: namely, the failure of the physician to ask the questions and pursue the answers and the failure of the patient to reply adequately, whether due to a disordered mental state or merely the inability to remember accurately or to verbalize.

When the history is properly taken, however, a clear picture of the patient's complaints can be obtained. Based on this profile, the physician can usually decide if the patient's chest pain syndrome is typical or atypical of classic (Heberden's) angina pectoris. Although angina pectoris is not specific for coronary artery disease, the term is most often associated with pathologic evidence of atherosclerosis of of the large coronary arteries.

### ORIGIN AND IMPLICATIONS OF THE TERM "ANGINA PECTORIS"

The syndrome of angina pectoris that Heberden described in 1768 is still a useful clinical model. Furthermore, his description also dates the onset of the clinical recognition of this syndrome, and the subsequent reports of its occurrence serve as an indirect commentary on the incidence of coronary artery disease.

Unlike the word *dolor,* which means pain, *angina* was meant to indicate a sense of strangling. Heberden noted that fear of death *(angor animi)* often accompanied this chest (or rather, "breast") pain. In his original report, he described many of the other features that are still associated with this symptom complex: episodes of pain that are paroxysmal in nature, pain occurring with walking or after heavy meals, relief with rest, and increased incidence of sudden death. These are the features that are now considered typical of angina pectoris. Today, many physicians would probably add the accompanying sensation of breathlessness, which Heberden did not mention. Although Heberden's description applies to the majority of anginal episodes, it should be stressed that many patients with coronary artery disease present with some or none of these features in an atypical or variant form. This will be discussed more fully later in the chapter.

Following Heberden's original account of angina pectoris [2], relatively few publications dealt with this syndrome before the onset of the twentieth century. Paul Dudley White described some of these reports [3]. Austin Flint, for example, in analyzing over 150 cases of organic heart disease, found only seven patients with angina pectoris. No cases *at all* occurred in his practice in the years 1860 to 1865. As White commented, it seems very probable that Austin Flint recognized angina pectoris when he encountered it, and because he represented the majority of better-educated internists in the country at that time, there would appear to have been far less coronary artery disease 100 years ago than now. It seems hard to believe that if acute myocardial infarction and sudden death occurred often in young and middle-aged men, as it does in the present era, it could have escaped attention, even in the absence of the kind of clinical-pathologic correlations that are common today.

The reasons for the lower incidence are, of course, speculative. Many patients with lesser degrees of angina pectoris would not seek medical attention as they would today. White has theorized that in the nineteenth century, the people admitted to hospitals were more impoverished than "better-off" citizens who were treated at home, and, since coronary artery disease is a condition that we now recognize as accompanying affluence rather than poverty, such selection also may have played a part in the lower incidence reported from hospital surveys.

In the mid-nineteenth century, renewed interest in angina pectoris was stimulated by Brunton's report [4] on the use of amyl nitrate for treating angina pectoris, yet as White [3] has noted, by the time William Osler published his textbook in 1892, he still referred to it as a rare disease associated "particularly with sclerosis of the root of the aorta and changes in the coronary arteries." To confirm the rare nature of this syndrome, White reviewed the hospital records of 800 patients who were under his care when he was an intern in the wards of the Massachusetts General Hospital from 1912 to 1913. Of these patients, 700 were males, mostly between the ages of 20 and 60. Only eight of these were diagnosed as having angina pectoris; three clearly had syphilitic aortitis as the cause of the pain, and another had rheumatic aortic regurgitation. Thus, as Osler reported, coronary artery disease at the beginning of the twentieth century was certainly uncommon in the United States.

In the 1920s, more interest was centered on coronary artery disease, and there were increasing reports of the frequency of angina pectoris. Wearn [5], for example, reported 19 cases of myocardial infarction at the Peter Bent Brigham Hospital and commented that there might be a premonitory chest pain syndrome before the actual infarction occurred (a forerunner of the currently named syndrome of unstable or preinfarction angina). White [6] and his associates wrote a series of reports on the variable prognosis in angina pectoris and coronary thrombosis, confirming the work done by MacKenzie [7]. With the development of cardiology as a specialty in the 1920s, interest in this syndrome grew rapidly. The value of the electrocardiogram was appreciated, as was the importance of chest pain and the ECG abnormalities brought out by exercise. Perhaps the most important next step in understanding the pathophysiology of angina pectoris was the clinical-pathologic correlations of Blumgart and his associates [8]. Their studies were particularly important because they demonstrated the different histopathologic findings in angina pectoris and myocardial infarction and stressed the role of collateral circulation. Not long after the work of Blumgart and associates the modern era of studying coronary artery disease began with the introduction of coronary arteriography, which allowed the evaluation of coronary anatomy in vivo in patients with chest pain syndromes. Today, we also employ a variety of increasingly sophisticated noninvasive procedures, such as radioisotopic-exercise studies, to assist in the functional assessment of lesions seen on the coronary arteriogram and in the selection of patients for arteriography.

## SPECIFIC HISTORICAL FEATURES OF THE ANGINAL SYNDROME

*Quality and Duration of the Pain.* Heberden's initial report concerning the syndrome of angina pectoris described the chest discomfort as conveying a sense of "strangling and anxiety." This description is still remarkably pertinent today [9, 10], although adjectives used to describe this distress now include viselike, constricting, suffocating, crushing, heavy, and squeezing. Some patients make a clenched fist over their precordium to indicate what their discomfort is like. In other patients the quality of pain is even more vague in nature, and it may be described as only a mild, pressurelike discomfort or an uncomfortable, numbing sensation. Anginal equivalents of breathlessness, faintness, or fatigue have also been reported by some patients. Whatever the quality of the pain, the anginal syndrome usually begins gradually and reaches a maximum intensity before dissipating over a period of minutes. Dissipation of the feeling usually is a result either of cessation of the activity that precipitated it or of complete rest. Longer periods of pressurelike pain suggest unstable angina (or myocardial infarction), but on the other hand, if the pain persists steadily for days *without* development of an infarction, it is unlikely that it is due to myocardial ischemia. Sharp, stabbing chest pain that comes and goes in a matter of seconds or dull, continuous discomfort should make one consider other causes of chest pain besides myocardial ischemia, particularly musculo-skeletal and gastrointestinal disorders (to be discussed shortly). Similarly, changes in posture do not usually affect the pain of myocardial ischemia, and these thus serve to distinguish it from pericardial disease or hiatus hernia.

*Radiation of the Pain.* The site of the pain is usually retrosternal, but radiation is common. The pain usually radiates down the inner surface of the left arm, and, not infrequently, the right arm and the outer surfaces of both arms are also involved. Sampson and Cheitlin [1] have documented the wide number of regions that can be other sites of radiation, with neck, jaw, tooth, and throat pain observed most commonly (table 4–1).

*Precipitation and Relief of the Pain.* In typical (Heberden's) angina, the pain is usually related to effort or to emotion, but it must be stressed again that not all patients with coronary artery disease have typical angina, nor is their pain always diagnostic. Sexual intercourse and eating can also precipitate the discomfort, as can a variety of other factors, including the excessive metabolic demands of fever, thyrotoxicosis, tachycardia from whatever cause, severe ane-

mia, hypoglycemia, cigarette smoking, and exposure to cold air. In all these conditions, underlying coronary artery obstruction is usually present, and most of the other factors serve merely to increase the mechanical work of the heart and thus precipitate ischemia and subsequent chest pain. It is becoming increasingly apparent, however, that increases in coronary vascular tone (and in some cases frank spasm) also play a role in the genesis of angina. This is especially true in cold- or emotion-induced angina, and in many instances of angina at rest. Some of the specific hemodynamic and other pathophysiologic derangements have been considered in detail in chapter 2.

Although many activities will reproducibly evoke symptoms in many patients, there may be a lack of such reproducibility and predictability in other patients. In these latter individuals, performing a specific activity may cause angina one day but not the next because there is a complex interplay of factors relating to the physcologic and emotional "set" of the patient and to the level of vascular tone in the coronary arteries. Some patients are able to "walk through" their pain until it is dissipated. In general, however, relief of pain is usually afforded by rest or by cessation of the particular activity that incited it, rather than by "walking through." When nitroglycerin is successfully used, relief can occur within several minutes, and the response to the drug is often a useful diagnostic tool. In the study by Horwitz and co-workers [11], for example, 90 percent of the patients with angina who exhibited a prompt response to nitroglycerin had angiographically documented coronary artery disease. Although some patients with severe disease were *not* relieved by nitroglycerin, a longer duration of time before relief is obtained (if at all) usually suggests that the pain is not ischemic in origin, especially if the drug's side effects (headache and flushing) are experienced soon after the medication is taken, indicating that it has not lost its potency. Carotid sinus pressure can also bring about alleviation of pain when there is slowing of the heart rate, but in some patients the pain may not be *consistently* relieved by any one or combination of these agents. This does not rule out coronary artery disease; indeed, unstable angina is often

TABLE 4–1. Sites of anginal pain in 150 successive ambulatory patients

| Location of pain | % sole involvement | % involvement at any time |
| --- | --- | --- |
| Anterior chest | 34.0 | 96.0 |
| Left arm (upper) | 0.7 | 30.7 |
| Left arm (lower) | 1.3 | 29.3 |
| Right arm (upper) | 0 | 10.0 |
| Right arm (lower) | 0 | 13.3 |
| Back | 0.7 | 16.7 |
| Epigastrium | 0.7 | 3.3 |
| Forehead | 0 | 6.0 |
| Neck | 2.0 | 22.0 |
| Chin and perioral area | 0 | 8.7 |

From Sampson, J. J. and Cheitlin, M. D. Pathophsiology and differential diagnosis of cardiac pain. *Prog. Cardiovasc. Dis.* 13:507, 1971. Reprinted by permission.

characterized by the inability of the usual therapeutic agents to relieve the chest pain.

*Differentiation of Stable Angina from Unstable Angina and Variant Angina.* The definition of unstable angina pectoris is not without controversy, but as noted in chapter 12, it currently depends on the presence of one or another of the following historical features: (1) chest pain syndrome (usually typical of angina pectoris) of new onset, that is, usually within one month and brought on by moderate or minimal exertion; (2) development of crescendo (more severe) pain superimposed on a pre-existing pattern of exertion-related angina; or (3) pain at rest. There is also a new fourth category: pain in the immediate postmyocardial infarction period. Use of this latter category is more limited; thus, most of the earlier studies to be discussed subsequently (including the National Cooperative Group study) used only the first three categories. This definition is a broad one, and some cardiologists might emphasize certain features over others. Episodes of pain may be discrete as well as multiple, and the three most commonly used categories enumerated above may overlap. Strictly speaking, the pain should *not* be related to obvious precipitating factors, such as anemia or arrhythmias. A more rigorous definition has been proposed that includes only protracted pain of at least 20 to 30 minutes' duration with incomplete or no relief on administration of nitrates [12].

As noted in the definition, the characteristics of the chest pain in this syndrome are similar to those of classic, effort-induced angina, although the pain is usually more intense and prolonged. In addition, it may appear at rest, occasionally waking the patient from sleep. In addition to the pain being more protracted in nature, only incomplete relief can be obtained by the usual therapeutic regimen of nitroglycerin administration or rest. Scheidt and co-workers [13] have pointed out several clues that may alert the clinician to a changing angina pattern: abrupt decrease in tolerance for physical activity in patients with previously stable angina; increase in the frequency, severity, and duration of the angina; radiation of pain to a new site such as the jaw; onset of new features associated with the

pain, such as diaphoresis, nausea, or palpitation; and decreased relief of pain afforded by nitroglycerin in doses that were previously effective.

What proportion of patients with unstable angina have new-onset angina, rest angina, or a crescendo pattern superimposed on stable angina depends on the series of patients studied as well as on how the investigators defined the syndrome at the time of the study. In the few studies where breakdowns are possible (i.e., where there is more than one type of pain pattern and large numbers of patients), Fulton and associates [14] reported 88 patients with new-onset angina versus 79 with crescendo or rest angina or both, and the National Cooperative Group study [15] reported 69 patients with new-onset angina versus 81 with a crescendo pattern, rest angina, or both. Gazes and co-workers [16] reported 27 patients with new-onset angina versus 109 with the crescendo type (four others had "prolonged" pain at rest). The most extensive breakdown of these patterns can be found in the review article by Cairns et al. [17].

Whether *variant angina pectoris* should be considered a type of unstable angina is moot, but it is so considered in this text (see chapter 12). In 1959, Prinzmetal and co-workers [18] first described this unusual syndrome of coronary artery disease. The pain occurred almost exclusively at rest, was not precipitated by physical exertion or emotional stress, and was associated with a current of injury pattern on the ECG that featured pronounced ST evaluation rather than depression. The incidence of the syndrome was then, and is still, unknown. This syndrome can be associated with severe cardiac conduction disturbances and arrhythmias, including bradyarrhythmias, ventricular tachycardia, and ventricular fibrillation, as well as sudden death.

As noted, the historical features of variant angina are different from those of typical angina in that there is usually no exertion-related component. Unlike most patients with rest pain due to unstable angina, the pain has not followed a crescendo pattern that requires lesser and lesser levels of effort to induce the pain until finally it occurs at rest. Although exercise capacity is usually well preserved, some patients will experience their typical pain (and ECG) patterns during treadmill tests [19].

*Summary.* The finding of typical angina is helpful in indicating the presence of coronary artery
disease when other cardiac disease is not present. Even in such instances, typical angina does
not *always* indicate coronary artery disease, and,
as the section Differential Diagnosis of Chest
Pain will discuss, a small but definite number of
patients with typical angina will have normal
coronary arteriograms. Atypical chest pain suggests the absence of coronary artery disease, but
there are enough exceptions that many cardiologists are careful not to rule out the diagnosis on
the basis of the history.

The difference among stable, unstable, and
variant angina is important for prognostic and
therapeutic reasons (see chapter 12), and these
terms should continue to be used. However, it
is becoming apparent that in some patients with
stable angina, attacks come at variable (rather
than fixed) levels of exertion. In these patients,
the episodes at minimal effort are presumably
due to increased coronary vasomotor tone, as in
patients with unstable or variant angina. This
subgroup of patients with typical stable angina
but variable anginal thresholds is best thought of
as having *mixed angina,* a term that will become
increasingly popular as more reports document
its prevalence.

RELATION OF HISTORICAL FEATURES TO
CORONARY ARTERIOGRAPHIC FINDINGS
Before the era of coronary arteriography, it was
difficult to relate the anginal history clearly to
the underlying anatomy, since patients with angina pectoris often come to necropsy *because*
they had suffered fatal acute myocardial infarctions. Thus, the well-known studies of Blumgart
and associates [8] could establish only the extent
of atherosclerosis and the degree of luminal narrowing in patients in whom a terminal event was
*superimposed* on chronic or recent-onset angina.
A study from the National Institutes of Health
has managed to circumvent this problem partially. In this group of 27 patients reported by
Roberts [20], 24 died during or shortly after
cardiac operations designed to relieve severe angina pectoris and 3 died during catheterization.
During life, none of the patients had clinical
evidence of acute myocardial infarction or
congestive failure. At necropsy, each of these

patients had diffuse and extensive coronary
atherosclerosis with severe luminal narrowing of
at least two and often three or four major epicardial coronary arteries. Despite the severe coronary narrowing, there was little myocardial damage in these patients, who had no previous
history of infarction. The left ventricular cavity
was of normal size, and the hearts were of normal weight. Roberts concluded that clinically
isolated and severe angina pectoris is associated
with severe, diffuse, luminal narrowing but relatively little myocardial damage. In this study no
attempt was made to relate pathologic to specific
clinical features.

The advent of coronary arteriography has resulted in extensive correlations between many of
the clinical features of ischemic heart disease and
the in vivo pathoanatomy of patients with chest
pain syndromes, both with and without a prior
myocardial infarction. Limitations in interpreting coronary arteriograms are recognized, especially in the vast middle zone of "borderline"
lesions of 50 to 70 percent stenosis (see chapter
9). Nevertheless, the clinical-arteriographic correlations made by several groups are worth describing. Two of the early studies were from the
Peter Bent Brigham Hospital [21, 22], and they
indicated that multivessel coronary artery disease was more common in patients with severe
angina pectoris compared to single-vessel disease. They noted, however, that even those patients with only single-vessel disease could have
severe angina. These investigators also found
that the number of sites of anginal pain correlated both with the duration of symptoms and,
in general, with the extent of coronary artery
disease; in other words, the greater the extent of
anatomic disease, the longer was the duration of
clinical symptoms. Post-prandial angina, nocturnal angina, and angina without inciting cause
were usually associated with triple-vessel disease. This triad, however, was not seen in all
patients with multivessel disease, again emphasizing the variability, alluded to earlier, in predicting patterns from one patient to another.

In a subsequent study by Proudfit and associates [23], a group of 337 patients with angina
pectoris were studied at the Cleveland Clinic.
The distribution of the pain, the factors precipitating the pain, and the duration and history of

the angina were *not* found to be of any predictive value in relation to the extent of obstructive lesions demonstrated by selective coronary arteriography. These authors concluded that the division of patients who have anginal syndromes into groups on the basis of duration of history did *not* clarify the natural history of symptomatic obstructive coronary arterial disease. In both the Peter Bent Brigham Hospital and Cleveland Clinic series, the pattern of anatomic disease (i.e., the number and specific vessels involved) appeared similar in patients with and without prior myocardial infarction.

Other, more recent clinical-arteriographic studies have also dealt with the relation of historical features to the extent of disease. Fuster and colleagues [24] studied 300 patients within 1 year of the onset of their symptoms; of these, 164 had angina without infarction. Within the purely anginal group, there were similar anatomic patterns in patients with effort, rest, and nocturnal angina. Banks and co-workers [25] could not find a correlation between the extent of vessel disease and the duration of angina in 107 patients. Similarly, Walsh and associates [26] studied 50 patients under the age of 50 and found the duration of symptoms was not significantly reduced in patients with single-vessel disease. Welch and co-workers [27] noted that the percentage of women with coronary artery disease and *atypical* anginal symptoms was close to 50 percent, a figure higher than that noted in young men in previous studies from their institution [28].

Thus, there does not appear to be any consensus regarding a relationship among the historical features of angina (i.e., location, duration, and means of precipitation of pain) compared to the extent or specificity of vessel involvement.

## THE PHENOMENON OF SILENT MYOCARDIAL ISCHEMIA

Epidemiologic studies of unexpected sudden death as well as clinical and postmortem studies of silent myocardial infarction suggest that there may be many individuals with extensive coronary artery obstruction who do not have angina pectoris in any of its recognized forms. In a sense, such individuals are without the benefits of an anginal warning system [29], and ischemic

attacks may go unnoticed until a fatal event ensues or evidence of a prior infarction is detected on routine ECG. In many other patients a myocardial infarction is the first clinical manifestation of ischemic heart disease, although necropsy or angiographic studies indicate the coronary atherosclerosis was of chronic duration. Little is known about the clinical state of such patients *prior* to the morbid event, and discussion of the findings at physical examination, laboratory results, and the like are limited. Yet, at the same time, these individuals are too important *not* to be included in a discussion of chest pain syndromes.

Detection of totally asymptomatic persons with coronary artery disease is fortuitous. Some of these individuals can be identified prior to such an event because of cardiac arrhythmias or abnormal ECGs, or they may also be identified when cardiac catheterization is performed because of a markedly positive exercise test in the setting of coronary risk factors [30, 31]. The cost-to-benefit ratio of exercising large numbers of asymptomatic individuals is not clear, and the specificity of the test in asymptomatic patients is questioned [32, 33]. The most extensive study in this field to this date was performed by Erikssen and associates [34] in Norway. These investigators used a combination of screening techniques (questionnaires, resting ECGs, and exercise-tolerance tests) to study over 2,000 presumably healthy and asymptomatic 40- to 59-year-old men. Over 100 men were subsequently referred for coronary arteriography, and 67 had evidence of coronary artery disease. Thus, approximately 3 to 4 percent of the total group had more than 75 percent stenosis of one or more coronary arteries, and most of these had multivessel disease.

Silent myocardial ischemia can also be demonstrated in individuals who are asymptomatic following a myocardial infarction, as well as in those who *do* have an anginal history. In these latter persons, the pain pattern is variable and cannot always be correlated with objective evidence of myocardial ischemia, especially ST segment depression. Thus, in a series of patients reported by Bartel and co-workers [35], 17 percent of the patients with an anginal history, coronary artery disease documented on angiography, and positive ECG responses to treadmill testing had neither angina nor its equivalents during or within several minutes after the tests. In our initial study of patients with this syndrome [36], we noted similar results using the two-step test. We compared the patients with and without chest pain during positive exercise tests, but could find no clinical, hemodynamic, or angiographic features that separated the two groups. In our most recent study we evaluated the fall in radionuclide ejection fractions during exercise and again could not distinguish between patients with asymptomatic versus symptomatic myocardial ischemia [37]. Others, however, have reported that, in general, asymptomatic episodes are shorter and cause less left ventricular dysfunction than do symptomatic episodes [38]. Silent ischemia can also be demonstrated during ambulatory ECG monitoring [39] in patients with documented coronary artery disease (Figure 4–1), but because of the problem of artifacts, there is still some controversy as to the reliability of this technique in demonstrating minor degrees of ST segment depression.

The ischemia-angina interrelation is a complex one, and not unexpectedly, there are individuals whose subjective symptoms are either not present or are too vague to be clearly defined by the patient or the physician. Several explanations can be offered to explain this difference in the reporting of symptoms; they include not only different thresholds of central or peripheral pain sensitivity or perception [40], but also psychological "denial" and the influence of cultural and subcultural norms concerning the "acceptability" of symptoms in otherwise healthy people. Since metabolic, humoral, neurologic, and psychological factors are all involved in the sensation of pain, the great variability from individual to individual is not surprising. At this point, it might be useful to review what is known about the subjective sensation of myocardial ischemia.

Generation of the myocardial pain impulse is very complex, and not all the mechanisms are clearly understood. For example, the substance that actually stimulates the nerve endings and begins the series of interactions that culminates in a sensation of pain is not known. Lewis [41]

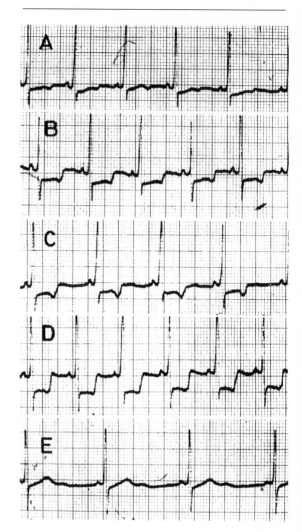

FIGURE 4–1. An example of the ST-T changes observed during 24-hour ambulatory ECG monitoring in a 56-year-old man. (A) Slight ST-T abnormalities were noted during most of the day; (B) increasing degrees of ST segment depression were observed after meals; (C) at rest; and (D) during walking. (E) Only during sleep at night was the ECG normal. Although the patient had apparent evidence of myocardial ischemia as shown in panels B, C, and D, he experienced pain only while walking (panel D). (From Stern, S. and Tzivoni, D. The dynamic nature of the ST-T segment in ischemic heart disease. *Am. Heart J.* 91:820, 1976.)

called this a "P factor" in describing the pain of both skeletal muscle and myocardial ischemia. A host of substances have been suggested as being the P factor, but most recent evidence favors peptide substances that are related as a result of *transient* ischemia; these include kallikrein and kinins [42]. Acidosis or hyperkalemia in the surrounding tissue bed may trigger the release of these peptides, and the sensory end-plates of the intracardiac sympathetic nerves appear to be particularly sensitive to them. The end-plates are receptors in a network of unmyelinated nerves that lie between the cardiac muscle fibers and are also found around coronary blood vessels. These nerve fibers travel to the cardiac plexus and then ascend to the sympathetic ganglia (C7-T4). The impulses are transmitted to corresponding spinal ganglia and then are conveyed via the spinal cord to the thalamus and finally the cerebral cortex.

Whether coronary vasoconstriction itself can cause pain on a purely vascular (as opposed to ischemic) basis is unclear, nor is there any convincing evidence that stretching of the myocardium—as in an aneurysmal segment—can cause episodes of chest pain. Malliani and Lombardi [43] have emphasized that "afferent cardiac symptomatic fibers can signal both mechanical and chemical events and we are still unable to predict when nocioception (a receptive process) will give rise to pain (a conscious experience)." They conclude that the "intensity" of the stimuli from the heart, rather than their "specifity" (for pain), may be the key to understanding cardiac pain.

The pain of myocardial ischemia is perceived in various regions of the chest because it is "referred" to the corresponding peripheral dermatomes, which supply afferent nerves to the same segment of the spinal cord that the heart does. The mechanism of such pain referral is not completely understood. Some impulses mediated by the sympathetic pathway appear to converge with impulses from somatic thoracic structures on the same nerves ascending the spinal cord. Pain impulses can be referred to the medial aspects of the arm via common connections to the brachial plexus, and they can be referred to the neck via common connections with the cervical roots. Jaw pain is not as easily explained, since the fifth cranial nerve would have to be involved.

This explanation of the generation of the pain impulse is incomplete in several areas. For exam-

ple, in addition to the fact that the pain-producing substance itself is not clearly identified, there is no ready explanation as to why angina-like pain is not felt more commonly in other situations where there is inflammation and presumably ischemia of the myocardium, such as in myocarditis. Also, as noted earlier, some patients with clear-cut evidence of coronary disease and ischemia have no chest pain whatsoever, and others have chest pain that disappears after myocardial infarction, even though the ischemia may be persisting. It is postulated that in the latter patients, the nerve endings have been damaged or destroyed as a result of the infarction. Destruction of nerve endings may also explain painless ischemia in diabetics.

## The Physical Examination

### GENERAL EXAMINATION

General physical examination of the patient with a chest pain syndrome may reveal abnormalities that suggest (but are not specific for) coronary artery disease. The blood pressure may be elevated chronically or acutely during an anginal attack. Evidence of vascular disease in the carotid, iliac, or peripheral leg vessels suggests widespread atherosclerosis, as do abdominal aortic aneurysms. These aneurysms do not prove that the cause of the chest pain is due to coronary artery disease, but they can raise the level of suspicion. Similarly, xanthomas suggestive of hyperlipidemia, particularly hypercholesterolemia, may be present on the hands, elbows, ankles, and especially the eyelids, where they are termed xanthelasma [44]. Arcus senilis in whites under the age of 50 also suggests the presence of this metabolic abnormality, whereas it is a less specific indication in the older age group and in blacks. Abnormal pulsation of the sternoclavicular joint may indicate an aneurysm, including the dissecting type.

One of the more interesting general physical findings that has been recently reported as indicative of coronary artery disease is the diagonal ear-lobe crease (figure 4–2), which was initially reported by Frank [45] and subsequently shown by Elliott [46] to be more prevalent in patients with coronary artery disease than in a control

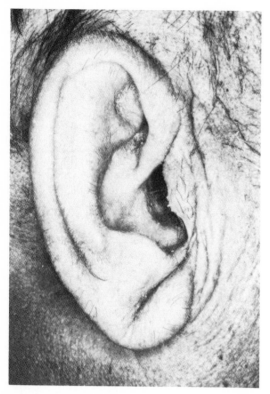

FIGURE 4–2. Ear with a typical diagonal ear-lobe crease. (From Elliott WJ. *Am. J. Med.* 75:1024, 1983.)

group. What the basis for this relationship is (if present) is obscure, and at present the controversy remains unresolved.

The general physical examination can also reveal abnormalities that suggest another cause for the chest pain, including nonatherosclerotic forms of coronary artery disease. Marfan's syndrome, for example, is associated with a number of cardiac abnormalities (including dissection of the aorta), and it can be recognized by its characteristic skeletal and occular abnormalities. (These other forms of coronary artery disease are discussed in chapter 18.) Factors that can exacerbate angina of whatever cause may also be detected by physical examination (for example, anemia or thyroid abnormalities).

During an anginal attack, the findings on general physical examination often are strikingly different from those at rest. Thus, the patient's complexion may become pale; he complains of a cold sweat, appears anxious with labored breathing, and is frequently immobile in a sitting or standing position. Except in cases of cardiac spasm, the heart rate, blood pressure, or both are elevated. Equally striking are changes in the cardiac examination.

## CARDIAC EXAMINATION

Cheng [47] has pointed out that the cardiac examination—long considered to be noncontributory in coronary artery disease, especially in patients whose only evidence of cardiac disease is a history of chest pain—may actually supply useful clues (table 4–2) to the diagnosis of coronary artery disease in patients with anginal syndromes as well as to the functional state of the myocardium in other individuals with a more clear-cut ischemic basis for their pain (evidence of prior infarction on ECG, for example).

Examination of the anterior precordium by inspection and palpation can be extremely valuable, yet many physicians do not fully utilize this procedure to search for abnormal impulses. The sustained apical pulsation of aortic regurgitation may be particularly vigorous. With the patient supine or lying on the left side, dyskinetic bulges at the apex of the heart may also be found on palpation of the chest or recorded with a variety of techniques; these correspond to aneurysms of the left ventricle and often complement the ausculatory findings of diastolic filling sounds [48]. (In some patients, dyskinetic bulges may be present only during the anginal attacks.) Atrial and ventricular gallops may often be palpable, as may the thrills associated with significant aortic stenosis or mitral regurgitation.

Murmurs of idiopathic hypertrophic subaortic stenosis or aortic valvular stenosis suggest that the cause of the chest pain may be conditions other than, or in addition to, coronary artery disease. Differentiation between aortic and subaortic stenosis is aided by Valsalva's maneuver, since a louder murmur during this maneuver is indicative of muscular rather than valvular obstruction. Examination of the carotid pulse is also helpful. It is characteristically brisk and often bifid in idiopathic hypertrophic subaortic stenosis, whereas in patients with valvular aortic stenosis the pulse is small and the upstroke is delayed and often exhibits prominent anacrotic notch or shudder.

TABLE 4–2. Cardiac findings in patients with coronary artery disease

| Sign | Clinical significance | Frequency |
|------|----------------------|-----------|
| Abnormal precordial systolic bulge | Left ventricular wall motion abnormality | Not usually present unless patient has sustained a prior myocardial infarction (especially anterior wall) or is experiencing angina at time of examination |
| Decreased intensity of first heart sound | Decrease in left ventricular contractility | Difficult to evaluate in resting state, but can be commonly demonstrated during angina |
| Paradoxical splitting of second sound | Left ventricular wall motion abnormality | Very uncommon, but occasionally noted during angina |
| Third heart sound (ventricular gallop) | Increased left ventricular diastolic pressure, with or without clinical congestive heart failure | Not usually present unless patient sustained an extensive myocardial infarction; may occasionally be present during angina |
| Fourth heart sound (atrial gallop) | Reduced ventricular compliance ("stiff heart") | Common; very common if patient sustained a prior myocardial infarction as well as during angina |
| Apical systolic murmur (in absence of rheumatic mitral regurgitation or Barlow's syndrome) | Papillary muscle dysfunction | Not usually present unless patient has sustained a prior myocardial infarction; may occasionally be present during angina |
| Diastolic murmur (in absence of aortic regurgitation) | Coronary artery stenosis | Rare |

In the absence of aortic and subaortic lesions, the indirect carotid pulse recordings can be used to obtain systolic time intervals. Abnormalities in these parameters have been reported to be more common in patients with coronary artery disease than in control patients [49], but such results are not always found and the value of this measurement has been questioned [50].

The murmur of mitral regurgitation may be indicative of coronary artery disease, because such murmurs can be due to papillary muscle dysfunction [48]. The murmur may assume a variety of configurations from early systolic to late systolic, and it may be accentuated with exertion or during an acute anginal attack. Midsystolic clicks suggestive of mitral valve prolapse may also be present in coronary artery disease [51], although they obviously can also suggest another cause for the chest pain (i.e., Barlow's syndrome).

The diastolic murmur and characteristic pulses of aortic regurgitation raise important diagnostic considerations. A *well-localized* diastolic murmur (in the absence of aortic regurgitation) is a rare finding, however, and it has been attributed to stenosis in the coronary artery. In one patient undergoing successful revascularization surgery, this diastolic murmur disappeared [52].

In a study of 22 patients with coronary artery disease and 32 controls, the amplitude of the first heart sound in patients increased less with exercise than it did in the normal controls, suggesting left ventricular dysfunction [53]. Similar results have recently been reported using atrial pacing to induce ischemia [54]. The second heart sound has also been studied, and one of the more intriguing cardiac findings at rest, particularly during an anginal attack, is the paradoxical splitting of this sound. Its frequency is uncertain, but when present it is apparently related to asynergy of left ventricular contraction [48, 55].

Both third and fourth heart sounds (or, as some prefer, ventricular and apical gallops) are common in coronary artery disease, as demonstrated by several groups [48, 56, 57]. These investigations employed both auscultatory and phonocardiographic procedures, often with complementary apexcardiographic recordings of abnormal filling waves. The relation of the auscultatory findings to *both* hemodynamic and coronary arteriographic data was initially provided in a study of 93 patients with coronary disease at the Peter Bent Brigham Hospital [56]. Third or fourth heart sounds or apexcardiographic equivalents were present on the phonocardiogram in 42 patients. A subsequent study from the same institution demonstrated that the frequency of such findings could be increased during handgrip exercise [58], even when angina pectoris was not precipitated by that intervention. Other groups have noted an increase in prevalence during episodes of unstable angina [59] or with dynamic exercise [48].

At the Peter Bent Brigham Hospital, 75 percent of the patients with coronary artery disease were demonstrated to have third or fourth heart sounds at rest or after handgrip exercise, compared to only 22 percent of controls. The pathologic basis for these findings is apparently related to the functional state of the left ventricle and particularly to the pressure during diastole (figure 4–3) [56, 60]. Therefore, the absence of any of these diastolic filling sounds or impulses does not rule out the possibility of significant coronary atherosclerosis; it merely indicates the absence of significant left ventricular dysfunction. Since they are also present in hypertension, aortic valvular disease, and cardiomyopathy, these signs are not specific for coronary artery disease.

The significance of the fourth heart sound in patients being evaluated for coronary artery disease (or other cardiac diseases, for that matter) has been questioned by Spodick and Quarry [61] and others [62] in a series of reports indicating a very high frequency of such findings in normal subjects, particularly in the older age groups. It is often difficult to reconcile some of the conflicting communications in this controversy, since several groups cited earlier [48, 56–58, 60] have noted that only a minority of patients with coronary artery disease have fourth heart sounds at rest, and their presence in such patients appears related to abnormal ventricular dynamics. In these studies, patients with coronary artery disease and normal left ventricular performance appear to have a lesser prevalence of such sounds, as do control subjects. In contrast, other groups [61, 62] report that they hear (or record) these sounds in nearly *all* subjects, diseased or otherwise. Part of the problem may be due to differing definitions of a fourth heart sound, because some vibrations can usually be recorded on the phonocardiogram at low-frequency ranges. Many investigators would not consider such vibrations abnormal unless they had greater amplitude and pitch and could be readily recorded even at medium-frequency ranges. Because of this controversy, there is no consensus as to the significance of the fourth heart sound per se, although Travel [63] has concluded that most observers would regard *clearly audible* fourth heart sounds accompanied by *palpable* (or abnormally large apexcardiographic) A-waves as pathologic.

SUMMARY
The physical examination is not as limited in patients with chest pain as previously held; there is no question that it can be of value, especially with appropriate application of the necessary recording techniques and particularly during the course of the anginal attacks.

## The Electrocardiogram

The resting electrocardiogram (ECG) in patients with chest pain syndromes due to coronary artery disease has been normal in 25 to 50 percent of the reported series, depending on the prevalence of patients with myocardial infarctions in the respective series [55]. Patients with a history of severe angina pectoris may have normal ECG tracings when free of pain; however, significant left ventricular asynergy has been reported to be rare without some abnormalities of the resting ECG [64].

When the ECG is abnormal, the most common findings are nonspecific ST-T changes with or without evidence of prior transmural infarction, but a variety of conduction disturbances

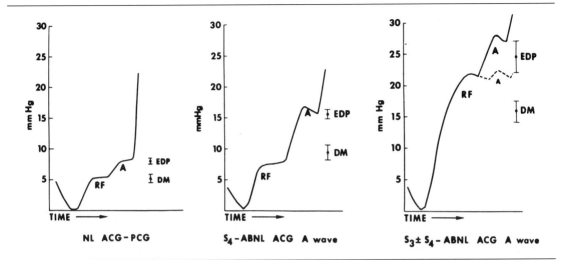

FIGURE 4-3. Relationship between left ventricular (LV) diastolic pressure tracings and average values of LV diastolic mean (DM) and end-diastolic pressures (EDP) in 130 selected patients with anginal syndromes who underwent coronary arteriography and hemodynamic studies. Bars indicate mean values and standard errors of the mean. Left panel: The 85 patients with normal apex- and phonocardiographic (ACG-PCG) results, as defined in this study, usually had normal rapid filling (RF) and atrial filling (A) phases during ventricular diastole. Mean LVEDP and LVDMP were also normal in this group. Center panel: Most of the 34 patients with isolated fourth heart sounds ($S_4$) or abnormal ACG A-waves had elevated LVEDP, primarily due to a prominent atrial filling phase. LVDMP was only minimally elevated (normal is less than 8 mmHg). Right panel: All 11 patients with third heart sounds ($S_3$) had marked elevations of both EDP and DM. Rapid filling phases were prominent with either normal or prominent atrial filling phases. (From Cohn, P.F. et al. Diastolic heart sounds and filling waves in coronary heart disease. *Circulation* 44:196, 1971. Reprinted by permission of the American Heart Association, Inc.)

have also been observed. It must be emphasized that left bundle branch block and left anterior hemiblock are *not* specific for coronary artery disease and are, in fact, more common in cardiomyopathies or as a manifestation of fibrotic or degenerative diseases of the conducting system (Lev's disease and Lenegre's disease). Even in the presence of typical anginal symptoms, such findings do not always indicate coronary artery disease [65]. In addition to conduction defects, a variety of arrhythmias, especially ventricular premature beats, may be present and are also nonspecific. Ventricular ectopic activity that is precipitated by exertion and associated with pain, however, should be regarded with more concern. The finding of left ventricular hypertrophy is uncommon in uncomplicated coronary artery disease and suggests other causes for the chest pain (e.g., valvular heart disease, idiopathic hypertrophic subaortic stenosis, or hypertension).

The P-wave on the ECG tracing also may contain helpful diagnostic information. Chronic intermittent increases in left atrial pressure in association with left atrial hypertrophy during episodes of angina pectoris may result in increased magnitude of the P terminal force in lead V in some patients with coronary artery disease [66]. In fact, Bethell and Nixon [67] consider the development of P-waves more negative than −0.02 mm sec as an early ECG indicator of coronary disease. Others [68] disagree. In apparently normal ECGs at rest, newer analytic techniques, such as the high-frequency ECG [69], are said to demonstrate abnormalities in patients with coronary artery disease. The practicality of such techniques for widespread use is unproved. Like the bizarre notching of the QRS complex sometimes seen on otherwise normal ECGs, however, the abnormalities recorded by these techniques may be additional subtle signs of coronary artery disease.

Because of the nonspecific nature of the ECG findings (except for Q-waves indicative of myocardial infarction), the resting ECG is not a reliable predictor of coronary artery disease unless spontaneous angina is occurring and ST abnormalities can be documented. Therefore, obtaining an ECG during or after some form of stressful intervention (especially if angina can be precipitated) is a valuable adjunct in the office (or clinic) evaluation of patients with chest pain syndromes who are suspected of having coronary artery disease. Techniques for exercise testing will be described in chapter 6. Very positive responses in symptomatic individuals (2 mm or more of ST segment depression, exertional hypotension, reduced exercise tolerance, etc.) have been found to be invariably associated with coronary artery disease, usually of the multivessel type [70]. Although these kinds of responses occur in less than 40 percent of patients with coronary artery disease, they are extremely valuable because they are so specific. Less positive tests or negative tests are of less diagnostic value. In interpreting exercise tests, it must be remembered that false-positive responses can occur; these may be due to valvular or other forms of heart disease (especially if left ventricular hypertrophy is present), digitalis use, or electrolyte disturbances (especially hypokalemia in a patient taking diuretics).

The most striking finding in the syndrome of *unstable angina* involves the resting ECG. Marked ST depression or elevation, with or without associated T-wave inversion, is the rule. In the National Cooperative Group study [15], for example, only 19 of 150 patients with documented coronary artery disease did not have ST segment changes during angina, and these 19 had T-wave inversions. These ST-T changes may completely or partially clear with relief of the pain. Normalization of abnormal T-waves during rest pain has been reported to be an indication of myocardial ischemia [71]; however, this response during an exercise test is usually *not* considered diagnostic of coronary artery disease by itself. Some series have reported a small number of patients with angiographically determined coronary artery disease who do not have ECG changes during ischemia [72]. In general, however, this is more characteristic of patients

who are subsequently found *not* to have coronary artery disease.

The resting ECG is also the key to the diagnosis of the *variant angina* syndrome. Characteristic ST segment elevations develop with pain. The ST segment elevation is of the concave type; it may be present in any lead, especially in the inferior ones, and disappears with subsidence of the pain. Transient Q-waves have been observed in isolated cases [73], and arrhythmias and conduction disturbances are not uncommon.

Another form of "resting" ECG that has been reported to demonstrate arrhythmias and other forms of myocardial ischemia in patients with coronary artery disease is the 12- to 24-hour ambulatory monitor [38]. The monitor records cardiac activity during the subject's work and leisure time and enables the physician to document when and how often the patient is experiencing ischemia (see figure 4–1) as well as the effectiveness of antiarrhythmic or antianginal preparations. Although, as we have previously noted, the problem of artifacts raises questions as to the reliability of some ST changes, Stern and co-workers [74] reported good correlation between the ST segment depression occurring during normal activity and arteriographic findings. As noted earlier in the chapter, pain need not accompany the ST depression, and as with exercise testing, false-positive responses can occur in patients with chest pain due to other forms of heart disease, in patients who are taking digitalis preparations, and so on.

No discussion of ECG examination is complete without some mention of vectorcardiography. This technique is particularly useful in depicting infarction patterns when the findings on the scalar ECG are equivocal. In addition, Young and associates [75, 76], in combined vectorcardiographic-ventriculographic studies, have recently demonstrated that some of the abnormal vector patterns indicate not only infarction but also severe abnormalities of left ventricular function.

Thus, the ECG remains a key feature in the diagnosis of coronary artery disease, especially when it can be obtained during an episode of chest pain and demonstrates ischemic changes. The resting ECG is limited because a significant minority of patients with coronary artery disease

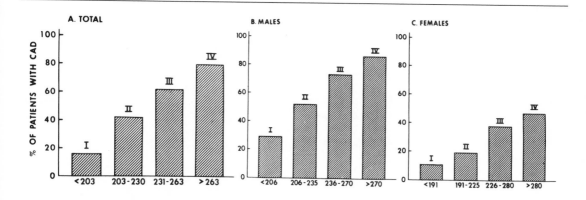

FIGURE 4–4. Relationship between the frequency of angiographically documented coronary artery disease (CAD) and the serum cholesterol levels (according to quartile distribution) in a total group (panel A) of 200 patients (half with and half without CAD) and in the subgroups of 134 men (panel B) and 66 women (panel C). Cholesterol levels are represented on the abscissa (mg/dl). The observed trend of increasing association with CAD as cholesterol levels rise is similar to that reported in the Framingham Study (see chapter 3), in which the development of clinical coronary artery disease in asymptomatic persons was related to cholesterol level. (From Cohn, P.F. et al. *Ann. Intern. Med.* 84:241, 1976.)

will have normal tracings and because of the nonspecific nature of many of the arrhythmic conduction and repolarization abnormalities.

## Standard Laboratory Tests

Most routine laboratory tests are within normal limits in patients with anginal syndromes due to coronary artery disease, but there are exceptions that aid in diagnosis and management. Thus, anemia may be detected and may be contributing to the chest pain; the same may be true of thyroid abnormalities. Cardiac enzymes are normal, and their levels serve to differentiate patients with chest pain (especially the unstable angina form) from those with acute myocardial infarctions.

One of the striking features of all types of coronary artery disease is the frequency with which certain metabolic abnormalities are detected. Since hyperlipidemia and carbohydrate intolerance are recognized as risk factors for the development of coronary artery disease, this is

not unexpected, yet the prevalence of these abnormalities, particularly in young patients (i.e., under the age of 50 years), can be impressive. Heinle and co-workers [77] noted that 95 percent of patients under the age of 50 had either carbohydrate intolerance or Type II (increase in low-density lipoproteins) or Type IV (increase in very low-density lipoproteins) hyperlipoproteinemias. Similar findings have been reported by others, including Banks and colleagues [25]. In considering the serum lipids themselves (rather than the lipoprotein patterns), the relative importance of total serum cholesterol levels versus triglyceride levels has been documented in a study of 200 subjects (figures 4–4, 4–5), half with and half without coronary artery disease [78]. Furthermore, association with *multivessel disease* (not noted in these figures) was particularly striking in patients with serum cholesterol levels above 280 mg/dl (80 percent) compared to those with levels below 203 mg/dl (4 percent). Both the importance of rising cholesterol levels and the relative lack of importance of the triglyceride levels have been confirmed by Gotto and associates [79] in an even larger number of patients. High-density lipoprotein–cholesterol levels have been shown to correlate in an *inverse* manner with presence of angiographically determined coronary artery disease, which further confirms the epidemiologic data discussed in chapter 3.

Specialized tests of platelet function and reactivity have also been reported to be abnormal in many patients with coronary artery disease [81], which suggests that increased platelet aggrega-

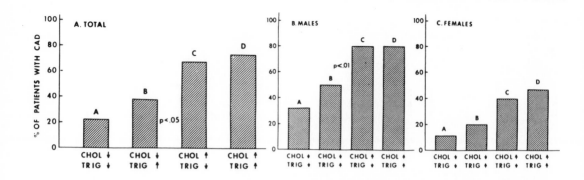

FIGURE 4-5. Relationship between the frequency of CAD and various combinations of cholesterol and triglyceride levels (based on their quartile distribution) for the same patient population as shown in figure 4-4. For lipid levels, ↑ = quartiles III and IV and ↓ = I and II as defined in figure 4-4. Again, the total group of patients (panel A) and the subgroups of males (panel B) and females (panel C) are depicted. Elevated cholesterol levels appeared to be more significantly associated with CAD whether or not triglyceride levels were elevated, whereas the opposite was not true. These results are again similar to the epidemiologic data obtained in the Framingham Study and described in chapter 3. (From Cohn, P.F. et al. *Ann. Intern. Med.* 84:241, 1976.)

tion may play a role in certain types of myocardial ischemia. At the present time, however, such tests cannot be considered routine.

The chest roentgenogram is usually normal in coronary artery disease. In one series, only 16 percent of 207 patients with coronary artery disease had cardiomegaly on standard chest roentgenograms [82]. Cardiomegaly is much more common in patients with coronary artery disease who have congestive heart failure symptoms or who have experienced a myocardial infarction. The chest roentgenogram can be helpful if it shows either aortic valve calcification (adding to the suspicion that significant aortic stenosis is present) or a frank left ventricular aneurysm.

The presence of coronary arterial calcification is another helpful clue to the diagnosis of coronary artery disease, although it is found in only a minority of such patients. Fluoroscopy is the preferred method of reliably detecting this abnormality. In addition to being present in patients with angina, coronary arterial calcification has also been reported to be present in asymptomatic subjects with positive exercise tests [83].

The newest cardiac imaging procedure, nuclear magnetic resonance, after initial animal experiments, is now beginning to be used for cardiac evaluation in humans. Unlike computed tomography, it can be gated to the cardiac cycle and is particularly useful for demonstrating abnormalities of left ventricular function associated with myocardial infarction [84]. At present, however, it cannot be considered a routine part of the laboratory evaluation.

## Differential Diagnosis of Chest Pain

### NONCARDIOVASCULAR DISEASE

Because the pain response to true myocardial ischemia is not uniform and because other entities can mimic angina in one way or another, the differential diagnosis of chest pain is often difficult. Chest pain can accompany a variety of noncardiac disease, ranging from purely psychogenic disorders to carcinoma of the lung. More common ones are listed in table 4-3. The differential diagnosis usually involves either disturbances of the gastrointestinal tract or musculoskeletal abnormalities of the chest wall and adjoining structures. Differentiating the chest pain of noncardiac disorders from that of angina pectoris is usually, but not always, possible when the quality of the pain, its duration, the precipitating factors, and associated symptoms are all taken into consideration [85, 86]. The digestive tract is often a cause of chest pain [87, 88]; typical abnormalities are described in the subsequent paragraph.

TABLE 4–3. Spectrum of disorders to consider in the differential diagnosis of chest pain

*Noncardiovascular disorders*
  Neuromuscular
    Costochondritis and other chest wall syndromes
    Radicular syndromes
    Inflammatory syndromes of the shoulder joint
  Gastrointestinal
    Esophageal disease and hiatal hernia
    Peptic ulcer or gastritis
    Gallbladder disease
  Psychologic
    Psychoneuroses
    Psychosomatic complaints

*Cardiovascular and pulmonary disorders*
  Coronary artery disease (atherosclerotic versus nonatherosclerotic diseases)
  Aortic valve disease
  Idiopathic hypertrophic subaortic stenosis
  Primary myocardial disease
  Pericarditis
  Dissecting aortic aneurysm
  Mitral valve prolapse syndrome
  Pulmonary embolus-infarction
  Pulmonary hypertension, right ventricular strain, or both
  Pneumothorax
  Pleuritis
  Intrathoracic tumor

*Disorders of Unknown Cause*
  Chest pain with normal coronary arteriograms

*Esophagitis* or other abnormalities of esophageal motility with spasm can produce pain that mimics that of myocardial ischemia because the pain is usually substernal in character and may have a burning component to it. When there is an element of esophagospasm, the pain may be alleviated not only by nitroglycerin (like angina), but also by milk or antacids (unlike angina). In addition, acid infusion studies can often confirm the diagnosis of this disorder, particularly if the perfusion test reproduces the patient's usual complaints; otherwise, it is of limited value. Gastric reflux is often associated with *hiatal hernia,* which can be diagnosed radiographically. With hiatal hernia, postprandial distress is most marked when the patient lies down, and this feature helps to differentiate it from true exertion-related angina. *Peptic ulcer* and *gallbladder disease* can also cause diagnostic difficulties,

but again the response to milk (which relieves ulcer distress and aggravates gallbladder disease) serves to differentiate these disorders from true angina, as does the presence of localized abdominal tenderness.

The major *musculoskeletal disorders* that can mimic angina include cervical radiculitis, subacromial bursitis, and, of course, costochondritis. Cervical radiculitis is often present as a constant, continuous ache and often results in neurologic deficit. The pain may be related to motion of the neck, just as motion of the shoulder will trigger attacks of pain that are due to bursitis. Whereas the classic Tietze's syndrome (painful swelling of the costochondral junctions) is uncommon, tender costochondral joints appear to be rather frequent [89]. Physical examination can be useful in revealing their presence. Physical examination may also detect pain brought about by movement of an arthritic shoulder joint, a calcified shoulder tendon, and so on. Occasionally, pain mimicking that of angina can be due to compression of the brachial plexus by the cervical rib.

The possibility of true angina pectoris, therefore, can usually be excluded on the basis of the specific features of the pain. Thus, with gastrointestinal disorders, the brief episodes of sharp, stabbing pain or continual, dull aches of a burning or boring quality are not characteristic of angina, nor is the response to milk or antacid. Relief of pain with eructation is more common with these disorders, although it can occur with true angina. On the other hand, with musculoskeletal disorders the major point in differential diagnosis in most cases is related to some abnormality—e.g., tenderness either on palpation or on movement of the affected part—that may be found on physical examination. It must be stressed, however, that coronary artery disease can coexist with any of these other disorders (including psychoneurosis) and that occasionally exacerbations of noncardiac disease can trigger a true angina attack.

Finally, the importance of the physical examination and the description of the symptoms *during* an episode of pain should be emphasized. If the pain is not exertion-related, immediate suspicion is directed toward noncardiac causes. If an ECG can be obtained during a spontaneous

episode of pain (or as part of an exercise protocol) and there are no ST segment changes or
arrhythmias, then this suspicion is enhanced.
Failure of the blood pressure or heart rate to
increase or of diastolic heart sounds to appear
also provides important negative evidence, although this does not rule out coronary spasm as
a cause of this pain. Observation of the patient
by the physician during an exercise test is often
helpful in evaluating whether the patient's complaints are related to ECG changes. The response of pain to therapeutic maneuvers such as
the administration of nitroglycerin is of obvious
importance, as is the response to milk and antacids.

The response of the pain to regular meals (as
opposed to test doses of milk and antacids) may
be more variable; when the pain is due to peptic
ulcer, the pain may be relieved, but while a regular meal may precipitate gallbladder distress if
that is the underlying problem, it can also exacerbate true angina by as yet unclear mechanisms.

CARDIOVASCULAR AND PULMONARY
DISEASE
The pain of certain cardiovascular diseases may
also mimic that of angina pectoris (see table 4–
3). In addition to dissecting aneurysm of the
aorta (which usually is characterized by a sharp
retrosternal pain with radiation to the back), pulmonary hypertension (either primary or secondary, as with mitral stenosis) may also be a problem in differential diagnosis. In the latter
instance, the history of dyspnea and the associated findings of right ventricular enlargement on roentgenography or of hypertrophy on
the ECG are extremely helpful. Acute pneumothorax and intrathoracic tumors usually require
roentgenography for definite diagnosis, although the former can be suspected from the
pain pattern and clinical examination. The pain
of acute pleuritis or pulmonary embolus-infarction often has a clear-cut relation to respiration,
but it may resemble that of angina at times. The
associated findings (fever and recent upper respiratory infection in the former condition or ta-
chypnea, hemoptysis, and often thrombophlebitis in the latter) serve to differentiate these
diseases from coronary artery disease in many

patients, even before the roentgenographic and
lung scan results are known.

Primary myocardial disease sometimes has a
pain component that can be differentiated only
by cardiac catheterization. In acute pericarditis
the pain is usually increased in severity by lying
backward and is relieved by bending forward.
When it is accompanied by characteristic, diffuse
ST elevations on the ECG, the diagnosis
becomes considerably easier to make.

Other common cardiac diseases that cause
chest pain and must be differentiated from coronary artery disease are aortic stenosis, aortic regurgitation, and idiopathic hypertrophic subaortic stenosis. In these instances, an examination of
the heart and peripheral pulses (with ancillary
graphic techniques) offers the necessary clues to
correct diagnosis, although coronary artery disease may coexist with such disorders, and in
many cases only coronary arteriography can accurately diagnose the presence or absence of significant coronary obstructions. Coronary artery
disease may also coexist with Barlow's syndrome
(mitral valve prolapse). The majority of these
cases are found in otherwise healthy young
women in whom the incidence of coronary artery disease is low. Characteristic auscultatory
and echocardiographic findings in such women
usually rule out coronary artery disease as the
cause of the pain.

One must also consider nonatherosclerotic
causes of coronary artery disease in the differential diagnosis. Perloff [90] has argued that there
is a stereotyped concept of coronary artery disease because of the prevalence and clinical importance of *atherosclerotic* coronary artery disease
in the adult population, and that there are many
other disorders of these vessels to be considered
in constructing a comprehensive differential diagnostic scheme. Is any condition present (e.g.,
atrial fibrillation, endocarditis, mural thrombi,
tumors, or prosthetic heart valves) that could
have resulted in coronary emboli? Are there any
systemic diseases present (e.g., polyarteritis
nodosa, systemic lupus erythematosus, congenital connective-tissue disorders, arteriopathies, or
various malignancies) that could result in inflammatory or infiltrative lesions of the vascular bed?
Has the patient received blunt or penetrating
trauma to the precordium? Has the patient taken

oral contraceptive agents? Is there evidence of syphilitic aortitis? Finally, is there any possibility of congenital abnormalities of the coronary arteries themselves (fistulas or anomalous origin of the vessels) in younger patients suspected of having premature coronary atherosclerosis? While keeping these considerations in mind (see chapter 18), it is still evident that making a diagnosis of coronary artery disease will usually entail a diagnosis of atherosclerotic disease of the large coronary arteries in the overwhelming majority of cases.

UNEXPLAINED CAUSES OF CHEST PAIN

In patients without evidence of obvious cardiac or noncardiac diseases to account for their chest pain, an increasingly common diagnosis involves *chest pain with normal coronary arteriograms* [91–93]. A small number of patients may be shown to have a true coronary spastic component and are considered to have a form of Prinzmetal's variant angina (these patients are discussed further in chapter 12), but for the vast majority the cause of such chest pain is still unknown. Herman and co-workers [93] have discussed at length some of the unproven theories: small-vessel disease of the myocardium, oxyhemoglobin dissociation defects, misinterpretation of coronary arteriograms, occult cardiomyopathy, and psychogenic factors. Whatever the cause of this syndrome in the patients without variant angina, their prognosis is usually good [91–94], though not all patients will return to work [95, 96]. Subsequent coronary artery disease is unlikely to develop [94]; hence, the correct diagnosis is important. Although many cardiologists feel they can easily recognize such persons based on clinical experience, these patients can constitute 10 to 20 percent of individuals undergoing coronary arteriography for stable as well as unstable angina, depending on the reporting institution.

One of the distinguishing characteristics of this syndrome is the higher percentage of female patients; this is in contrast to coronary artery disease, which is uncommon before menopause. Nearly half the patients will have symptoms of typical angina, and the remainder will have a variety of atypical chest pains. As noted earlier, the response to nitroglycerin may be associated with more side effects (headache, flushing, and

so on) in this group of patients than in those with coronary artery disease [11].

Prevalence rates of cigarette smoking and hypertension among these patients are similar to those found in patients with coronary artery disease, but there is a lesser frequency of carbohydrate intolerance and hyperlipidemia. Prevalence rates of possible noncardiac causes of pain (such as gallbladder disease, hiatus hernia, and cervical disc disease) are similar to those of patients with coronary artery disease. The cardiac examination is usually normal. The resting ECG may be abnormal, usually showing nonspecific ST-T abnormalities. Approximately 20 percent of the patients will have positive exercise tests, some will produce lactate with stress, and others will have abnormalities of left ventricular function [97, 98] or of myocardial perfusion [97, 98]. Whether these abnormalities are due to histologic alterations in myocardial mitochronia is unclear [99].

Because of the increasing number of patients being seen with this syndrome in referral centers and because the prognosis is good, intensive effort has been directed at diagnosing the condition without the need for coronary arteriography. Reliance on history alone may be misleading, especially for those patients evaluated at referral centers, since a significant minority of such patients have complaints indistinguishable from those of typical angina pectoris, which is one of the reasons for their referral. Perhaps because these are difficult diagnostic problems referred for consultation, there are enough "false-positive" findings in each of the areas of standard clinical evaluation (some of which were noted above) to make differentiation from true coronary artery disease annoyingly difficult at times. (Whether this is also the case in nonhospital practice is not clear, since—ironically—it is performing the arteriographic procedure that finally determines the absence of coronary artery disease.) A certain number of these patients, for example, will have hypercholesterolemia or positive exercise tests. They may even have family histories suggestive of premature coronary artery disease, and when combined with an anginal syndrome, there is immediate concern on the part of the patients' physicians that coronary artery disease is indeed present.

In dealing with such patients, one approach is to proceed as though they do not have coronary artery disease, another is to manage the patients as if they did (even though atypical features may be present), and yet a third (and the preferred) approach is to refer them for a radioisotopic study such as the thallium-201 exercise test (see chapter 8) or exercise radionuclide ventriculogram (see chapter 8). If these tests are negative, coronary arteriography need not be performed. The advent of these radioisotopic procedures has rendered obsolete the multifactorial noninvasive indices devised in the 1970s [100, 101]; newer approaches based on these tests and pre- and post-test probability analyses are currently in use [102, 103].

## Additional Tests of Cardiac Performance: An Overview

The procedures described in this chapter are those that are commonly employed for the evaluation of patients with anginal syndromes. In addition to these procedures, other tests of cardiac performance can also be utilized. Some have been mentioned briefly; they are described in more detail in chapters 5 to 8. At what point in the future one will be able to say that some of these procedures will become "routine" is moot, although this is already the case at many centers. Chapter 6 discusses the indications, techniques, uses, and complications of exercise testing. If combined with radioisotope imaging (as with thallium-201, discussed in chapter 8), the chances of detecting myocardial ischemia become even greater. When the patient's presentation involves possible arrhythmias (with or without an anginal component), either exercise testing or ambulatory ECG monitoring, or both are useful in providing more data. They are discussed at length in chapter 5.

There are also tests of left ventricular function that can be performed. These include echocardiography—both standard M-mode and two-dimensional scanning—described in chapter 7, as well as radionuclide ventriculography (discussed in chapter 8). These procedures can detect wall motion abnormalities in the resting state, especially when a prior myocardial infarction has occurred. When combined with some form of stressful intervention, they may also reveal "latent" abnormalities of wall motion in patients suspected of having coronary artery disease but without prior myocardial infarctions and wall motion abnormalities at rest. In considering echocardiography and radionuclide left ventriculography, it should be emphasized that it is perfectly reasonable for patients to be referred for these latter procedures in order to obtain *additional* information about their left ventricular function, even when the diagnosis of coronary artery disease seems certain from the standard procedures described earlier in this chapter. This is also true of the exercise test when exercise *tolerance* prior to treatment rather than ECG changes per se is to be determined.

The most definite procedure for diagnosing coronary artery disease—or in discovering the locations of lesions when the diagnosis is established—is still cardiac catheterization and angiography. Unlike the other procedures discussed, this is invasive and has a definite morbidity and mortality—and is in no way routine. Thus, the patient subjected to cardiac catheterization invariably proceeds through a standard clinical work-up, plus one or another of the additional tests noted above, before proceeding to the cardiac catheterization laboratory. The catheterization procedure is discussed in detail in chapter 9.

## Conclusions

The preceding review has highlighted the pertinent historical features, the abnormalities of physical examination, and the various routine laboratory tests (including chest roentgenography and ECG) that help to diagnose anginal syndromes. The ideal diagnostic scheme is one that combines these various procedures because each alone has its deficiencies. Thus, we have seen that the typical anginal symptoms usually, but not always, signify coronary artery disease (in the absence of aortic valvular disease or of idiopathic hypertrophic subaortic stenosis), although many patients with coronary artery disease have atypical features.

There is no agreement as to whether a specific feature of the angina pain (e.g., its location and radiation or its precipitating factor) can be related to the location or extent of the stenotic lesion as demonstrated by coronary arteriography. On physical examination, the significance of the fourth heart sound remains uncertain, and many physicians now seek additional findings (e.g., palpable gallop sound or large apexcardiographic A-wave) before maintaining that what they are hearing is indeed "pathologic." By contrast, there is general agreement that the finding of a normal resting ECG bears little relationship to whether coronary artery disease is present. The definite noninvasive test involves the exercise ECG combined with one (or more) types of radioisotopic procedures.

## References

1. Sampson, J.J. and Cheitlin, M.D. Pathophysiology and differential diagnosis of cardiac pain. *Prog. Cardiovasc. Dis.* 13:507, 1971.
2. Heberden, W. Some account of a disorder of the breast. *Med. Trans. Roy. Coll. Physicians* (Lond.) 2:59, 1772.
3. White, P.D. The Prevalence of Coronary Heart Disease. In H.L. Blumgart (ed.), *Symposium on Coronary Heart Disease* (2nd ed.). New York: American Heart Association, 1968, pp. 1–5.
4. Brunton, T.L. On the use of nitrate of amyl in angina pectoris. *Lancet* 2:97, 1867.
5. Wearn, J.T. Thrombosis of the coronary arteries, with infarction of the heart, *Am. J. Med. Sci.* 165:250, 1923.
6. White, P.D. Coronary Insufficiency, Angina Pectoris. In *Heart Disease.* New York: Macmillan, 1937.
7. MacKenzie, J. *Angina Pectoris.* London: Oxford University Press, 1923, pp. 115–118.
8. Blumgart, H.L., Schlesinger, M.J., and Davis, S. Studies in the relation of the clinical manifestations of angina pectoris, coronary thrombosis, and myocardial infarction to the pathological findings. With particular reference to the significance of the collateral circulation. *Am. Heart J.* 19:1, 1940.
9. Herman, M.V. The clinical picture of ischemic heart disease. *Prog. Cardiovasc. Dis.* 14:321, 1971.
10. Fowler, N.O. Clinical diagnosis. *Circulation* 46:1079, 1972.
11. Horwitz, L.D., Herman, M.V., and Gorlin, R. Clinical response to nitroglycerin as a diagnostic test for coronary artery disease. *Am. J. Cardiol.* 29:149, 1972.
12. Fowler, N.O. "Preinfarctional" angina. A need for an objective definition and for a controlled clinical trial in its management. *Circulation* 44:755, 1971.
13. Scheidt, S., Wolk, M., and Killip, T. Unstable angina pectoris. Natural history, hemodynamics, uncertainties of treatment, and the ethics of clinical study. *Am. J. Med.* 60:409, 1976.
14. Fulton, M., Lutz, W., Donald, K.W., Kirby, B.J., Duncan, B., Morrison, S.L., Kerr, F., Julian, D.G., and Oliber, M.F. Natural history of unstable angina. *Lancet* 1:860, 1972.
15. National Cooperative Group to Compare Medical and Surgical Therapy. Unstable angina pectoris. 1. Report of protocol and patient population. *Am. J. Cardiol.* 37:896, 1976.
16. Gazes, P.C., Mobley, E.M. Jr., Faris, H.M., Jr., Duncan, R.C., and Humphries, G.B. Preinfarctional (stable) angina—a prospective study—ten-year follow-up: Prognostic significance of electrocardiographic changes. *Circulation* 48:331, 1973.
17. Cairns, J.A., Fantus, I.G., and Klassen, G.A. Unstable angina pectoris. *Am. Heart J.* 92:373, 1976.
18. Prinzmetal, M., Kennamer, R., Merliss, R., Wada, T., and Bor, N. A variant form of angina pectoris. *Am. J. Med.* 27:375, 1959.
19. Waters, D.D., Szlachcic, J., Bourassa, M.G., Scholl, J.M., and Theroux, P. Exercise testing in patients with variant angina: Results, correlation with clinical and angiographic features and prognostic significance. *Circulation* 65:265, 1982.
20. Roberts, W.C. The coronary arteries and left ventricle in clinically isolated angina pectoris. A necropsy analysis. *Circulation* 54:388, 1976.
21. Cohen, L.S., Elliott, W.C., Klein, M.D., and Gorlin, R. Coronary heart disease: Clinical, cinearteriographic, and metabolic correlations. *Am. J. Cardiol.* 17:153, 1966.
22. Elliott, W.C. and Gorlin, R. The coronary circulation, myocardial ischemia and angina pectoris. *Mod. Concepts Cardiovasc. Dis.* 35:111, 1966.
23. Proudfit, W.L., Shirey, E.K., Sheldon, W.C., and Sones, F.M., Jr. Certain clinical characteristics correlated with extent of obstructive lesions demonstrated by selective cine-coronary arteriography. *Circulation* 38:947, 1968.
24. Fuster, V., Frye, R.L., Connolly, D.C., Danielson, M.A., Elveback, L.R., and Kurland, L.T. Arteriographic patterns early in the onset of the coronary syndrome. *Br. Heart J.* 37:1250, 1975.
25. Banks, D.C., Raftery, E.B., and Oram, S. Clinical significance of the coronary arteriogram. *Br. Heart J.* 33:863, 1971.
26. Walsh, W., Richards, A.F., and Balcon, R. Coronary arteriographic study of mild angina. *Br. Heart J.* 37:752, 1975.
27. Welch, C.C., Proudfit, W.L., and Sheldon, W.C. Coronary arteriographic findings in 1000 women under age 50. *Am. J. Cardiol.* 35:211, 1975.
28. Welch, C.C., Proudfit, W.L., Sones, F.M., Jr.,

Shirey, E.K., Sheldon, W.C., and Razani, M. Cinecoronary arteriography in young men. *Circulation* 42:647, 1970.

29. Kannel, W.B., Doyle, J.T., McNamara, P.M., Quickenton, P., and Gordon, T. Precursors of sudden coronary death. Factors related to the incidence of sudden death. *Circulation* 51:606, 1975.

30. Hopkirk, J.A.C., Uhl, G.S., Hickman, J.R., Jr., Fischer, J., and Medina, A. Discriminant value of clinical and exercise variables in detecting significant coronary artery disease in asymptomatic men. *J. Am. Coll. Cardiol.* 3:887, 1984.

31. Cohn, P.F. Asymptomatic coronary artery disease: Pathophysiology, diagnosis, management. *Mod. Conc. Cardiovasc. Dis.* 50:55, 1981.

32. Froelicher, V.F., Yanowitz, F.G., Thompson, A.M., and Lancaster, M.C. The correlation of coronary angiography and the electrocardiographic response to maximal treadmill testing in 76 asymptomatic men. *Circulation* 48:597, 1973.

33. Borer, J.S., Brensike, J.D., Redwood, D.R., Itscoitz, S.B., Passamani, E.R., Stone, N.J., Richardson, J.M., Levy, R.I., and Epstein, S.E. Limitations of the electrocardiographic response to exercise in predicting coronary artery disease. *N. Engl. J. Med.* 293:367, 1975.

34. Erikssen, J., Enge, I., Forfang, K., and Storstein, O. False positive diagnostic tests and coronary angiographic findings in 105 presumably healthy males. *Circulation* 54:371, 1976.

35. Bartel, A.G., Behar, V.S., Peter, R.H., Orgain, E.S., and Kong, Y. Graded exercise tests in angiographically documented coronary artery disease. *Circulation* 49:348, 1974.

36. Lindsey, H.E. and Cohn, P.F. "Silent" ischemia during and after exercise testing in patients with coronary artery disease. *Am. Heart J.* 95:441, 1978.

37. Cohn, P.F., Brown, E.J., Wynne, J., Holman, B.L., and Atkins, H.L. Global and regional left ventricular ejection fraction abnormalities during exercise in patients with silent myocardial ischemia. *J. Am. Coll. Cardiol.* 1:931, 1983.

38. Chierchia, S., Lazzari, M., Freedman, B., Brunelli, C., and Maseri, A. Impairment of myocardial perfusion and function during painless myocardial ischemia. *J. Am. Coll. Cardiol.* 1:924, 1983.

39. Stern, S. and Tzivoni, D. The dynamic nature of the ST-T segment in ischemic heart disease. *Am. Heart J.* 91:820, 1976.

40. Droste, C. and Roskamm, H. Experimental pain measurement in patients with asymptomatic myocardial ischemia. *J. Am. Coll. Cardiol.* 1:940, 1983.

41. Lewis, T. Pain in vascular ischemia: Its relation to anginal pain. *Arch Intern. Med.* 49:713, 1932.

42. Del Banco, P.L., Del Bene, E., and Sicuteri, F. Heart Pain. In J.J. Bonica (ed.), *Advances in Neurology* (Vol. 4). New York: Raven Press, 1974, pp. 375–381.

43. Malliani, A. and Lombardi, F. Consideration of the fundamental mechanisms eliciting cardiac pain. *Am. Heart J.* 103:57, 1982.

44. Wagner, R.F., Jr. and Wagner, K.D. Cutaneous signs of coronary artery disease. *Int. J. Dermatol.* 22:215, 1983.

45. Frank, S.T. Aural sign of coronary artery disease. *N. Engl. J. Med.* 289:327, 1973.

46. Elliott, W.J. Ear lobe crease and coronary artery disease. *Am. J. Med.* 75:1024, 1983.

47. Cheng. T.O. Physical diagnosis of coronary artery disease. *Am. Heart J.* 80:716, 1970.

48. Martin, C.E., Shaver, J.A., and Leonard, J.J. Physical signs, apexcardiography, phonocardiography and systolic time intervals in agina pectoris. *Circulation* 46:1098, 1972.

49. Lewis, R.P., Boudoulos, H., Welch, T.G., and Forester, W.F. Usefulness of systolic time intervals in coronary artery disease. *Am. J. Cardiol.* 37:787, 1976.

50. Parker, M.E. and Just, H.G. Systolic time indices in coronary artery disease as indices of left ventricular function: Fact or fancy? *Br. Heart J.* 36:368, 1974.

51. Steelman, R.B., White, R.S., Hill, J.C., Nagle, J.P., and Cheitlin, M.D. Midsystolic clicks in arteriosclerotic heart disease: A new facet in the clinical syndrome of papillary muscle dysfunction. *Circulation* 44:503, 1971.

52. Sangster, J.F. and Oakley, C.M. Diastolic murmur of coronary artery stenosis. *Br. Heart J.* 35:840, 1973.

53. Bergman, S.A., Jr. and Blomquist, C.G. Amplitude of the first heart sound at rest and during exercise in normal subjects and in patients with coronary heart disease. *Am. Heart J.* 90:714, 1975.

54. Clarke, W.B., Austin, S.M., Shah, P.M., Griffen, P.M., Dove, J.T., McCullough, J., and Schreiner, B.F. Spectral energy of the first heart sound in acute myocardial ischemia: A correlation with electrocardiographic, hemodynamic and wall motion abnormalities. *Circulation* 57:593, 1978.

55. Gorlin, R. *Coronary Artery Disease.* Philadelphia: Saunders, 1976, p. 177.

56. Cohn, P.F., Vokonas, P.S., Williams, R.A., Herman, M.V., and Gorlin, R. Diastolic heart sounds and filling waves in coronary artery disease. *Circulation* 44:196, 1971.

57. Bethell, H.J.N. and Nixon, P.G.F. Atrial gallop in coronary heart disease without overt infarction. *Br. Heart J.* 36:682, 1974.

58. Cohn, P.F., Thompson, P., Strauss, W., Todd, J., and Gorlin, R. Diastolic heart sounds during

static (handgrip) exercise in patients with chest pain. *Circulation* 47:1217, 1973.

59. Fischl, S., Gorlin, R., and Herman, M.V. The intermediate coronary syndrome: Clinical, angiographic and therapeutic aspects. *N. Engl. J. Med.* 288:1193, 1973.

60. Voight, G.C. and Friesinger, G.C. The use of apexcardiography in the assessment of left ventricular diastolic pressure. *Circulation* 41:1015, 1970.

61. Spodick, D.H. and Quarry, V.M. Prevalence of the fourth heart sound by phonocardiography in the absence of cardiac disease. *Am. Heart J.* 87:11, 1974.

62. Benchimol, A. and Desser, K.B. The fourth heart sound in patients without demonstrable heart disease. *Am. Heart J.* 93:398, 1977.

63. Travel, M.E. The fourth heart sound—a premature requiem? *Circulation* 49:4, 1974.

64. Swartz, M.H., Pichard, A.D., Meller, J., Teichholz, L.E., and Herman, M.V. The normal electrocardiogram as a predictor of left ventricular function in patients with coronary artery disease. *Br. Heart J.* 39:208, 1977.

65. Haft, J.I., Herman, M.V., and Gorlin, R. Left bundle branch block: Etiologic, hemodynamic, and ventriculographic considerations. *Circulation* 43:279, 1971.

66. Shettigar, U.R., Barry, W.H., and Hultgren, H.N. P wave analysis in ischemic heart disease: An echocardiographic hemodynamic and angiographic assessment. *Br. Heart J.* 39:894, 1977.

67. Bethell, H.J.N. and Nixon, P.G.F. P wave of electrocardiogram in early ischemic heart disease. *Br. Heart J.* 34:1170, 1972.

68. Forfang, K. and Erikssen, J. Significance of P wave terminal force in presumably healthy middle-aged men. *Am. Heart J.* 96:739, 1978.

69. Anderson, G.J. and Bleiden, M.F. The high frequency electrocardiogram in coronary artery disease. *Am. Heart J.* 89:349, 1975.

70. Young, S.G. and Froelicher, V.F. Exercise testing: An update. *Mod. Conc. Cardiov. Dis.* 52:5, 1983.

71. Noble, R.J., Rothbaum, D.A., Knoebel, S.B., McHenry, P.L., and Anderson, G.J. Normalization of abnormal T waves in ischemia. *Arch. Intern. Med.* 136:391, 1976.

72. Haiat, R., Desoutter, P., and Stoltz, J. Angina pectoris without ST-T changes in patients with documented coronary heart disease. *Am. Heart J.* 105:883, 1983.

73. Meller, J., Conde, D.A., Donoso, E., and Dack, S. Transient Q waves in Prinzmetal's angina. *Am. J. Cardiol.* 35:691, 1975.

74. Stern, S., Tzivoni, D., and Stern, Z. Diagnostic accuracy of ambulatory ECG monitoring in ischemic heart disease. *Circulation* 52:1045, 1975.

75. Young, E., Cohn, P.F., Gorlin, R., Levine, H.D., and Herman, M.V. Vectorcardiographic diagnosis and electrocardiographic correlation in left ventricular asynergy due to coronary artery disease. I. Severe asynergy of the anterior and apical segments. *Circulation* 51:467, 1975.

76. Young, E., Angoff, G.H., Steelman, R.B., Levine, H.D., and Cohn, P.F. Vectorcardiographic correlations in left ventricular asynergy due to coronary artery disease. II. Inferior segment. *Am. J. Cardiol.* 41:444, 1978.

77. Heinle, R.A., Levy, R.I., Frederickson, D.S., and Gorlin, R. Lipid and carbohydrate abnormalities in patients with angiographically documented coronary artery disease. *Am. J. Cardiol.* 24:178, 1969.

78. Cohn, P.F., Gabbay, S.I., and Weglicki, W.B. Serum lipid levels in angiographically-defined coronary artery disease. *Ann. Intern. Med.* 84:241, 1976.

79. Gotto, A.M., Gorry, G.A., Thompson, J.R., Cole, J.S., Trost, R., Yeshurun, D., and DeBakey, M.E. Relationship between plasma lipid concentration and coronary artery disease in 496 patients. *Circulation* 56:875, 1977.

80. Swanson, J.O., Pierpont, G., and Adicoff, A. Serum high density lipoprotein cholesterol correlates with presence but not severity of coronary artery disease. *Am. J. Med.* 71:235, 1981.

81. Marcella, J.J., Nichols, A.B., Johnson, L.L., Owen, J., Reison, D.S., Kaplan, K.L., and Cannon, P.J. Exercise-induced myocardial ischemia in patients with coronary artery disease: Lack of evidence for platelet activation or fibrin formation in peripheral venous blood. *J. Am. Coll. Cardiol.* 1:1185, 1983.

82. Aintablian, A., Hamby, R.I., and Garsman, J. Correlation of heart size with clinical and hemodynamic findings in patients with coronary artery disease. *Am. Heart J.* 91:31, 1976.

83. Langou, R.A., Huang, E.K., Kelley, M.J., and Cohen, L.S. Predictive accuracy of coronary artery calcification and abnormal exercise test for coronary artery disease in asymptomatic men. *Circulation* 62:1196, 1980.

84. Higgins, C.B., Lanzer, P., Stark, D., Botvinick, E., Schiller, N.B., Crooks, L., Kaufman, L., and Lipton, M.J. Imaging by nuclear magnetic resonance in patients with chronic ischemic heart disease. *Circulation* 69:523, 1984.

85. Levine, H.J. Difficult problems in the diagnosis of chest pain. *Am. Heart J.* 100:108, 1980.

86. Christie, L.G. and Conti, C.R. Systematic approach to evaluation of angina-like chest pain: Pathophysiology and clinical testing with emphasis on objective documentation of myocardial ischemia. *Am. Heart J.* 102:897, 1981.

87. Henderson, R.D., Wigle, E.D., Sample, K., and

Manyat, G. Atypical chest pain of cardiac and esophageal origin. Chest *73:24,* 1978.

88. Long, W.B. and Cohen, S. The digestive tract as a cause of chest pain. *Am. Heart J.* 100:567, 1980.

89. Wolf, W. and Stein, S. Costosternal syndrome: Its frequency and importance in differential diagnosis of coronary heart disease. *Arch. Intern. Med.* 136:189, 1976.

90. Perloff, J.K. Coronary artery disease—antidote to a stereotype. *Am. J. Cardiol.* 30:437, 1972.

91. Kemp, H.G., Vokonas, P.S., Cohn, P.F., and Gorlin, R. The anginal syndrome associated with normal coronary arteriograms: Report of a six-year experience. *Am. J. Med.* 54: 735, 1973.

92. Bemiller, C.R., Pepine, C.J., and Rogers, A.K. Long-term observations in patients with angina and normal coronary arteriograms. *Circulation* 47:36, 1973.

93. Herman, M.V., Cohn, P.F., and Gorlin, R. Angina-like chest pain without identifiable cause. *Ann. Intern. Med.* 79:445, 1973.

94. Haft, J.I., and Bachik, M. Progression of coronary artery disease in patients with chest pain and normal or intraluminal disease on arteriography. *Am. Heart J.* 107:35, 1984.

95. Ockene, I.S., Shay, M.J., Alpert, J.S., Weiner, B.H., and Dalen, J.E. Unexplained chest pain in patients with normal coronary arteriograms. *New Eng. J. of Med.* 303:1249, 1980.

96. Faxon, D. P., McCabe, C.H., Kreigel, D.E., and Ryan, T.J. Therapeutic and economic value of a normal coronary angiogram. *Am. J. of Med.* 73:500, 1982.

97. Berger, H.J., Sands, M.J., Davies, R.A., Wackers, F.J., Alexander, J., Lachman, A.S., Williams, B.W., and Zaret, B.L. Exercise left ventricular performance in patients with chest pain, ischemic-appearing exercise electrocardiograms, and angiographically normal coronary arteries. *Ann. of Internal Med.* 94:186, 1981.

98. Green, L.H., Cohn, P.F., Holman, B.L., Adams, D.F., and Markis, J.E. Regional myocardial blood flow in patients with chest pain syndromes and normal coronary arteriograms. *Br. Heart J.* 40:242, 1978.

99. Opherk, D., Zebe, H., Weihe, E., Mall, G., Durr, C., Gravert, B., Mehmel, H.C., Schwarz, F., and Kubler, W. Reduced coronary dilatory capacity and ultrastructural changes of the myocardium in patients with angina pectoris but normal coronary arteriograms. *Circulation,* 63:817, 1981.

100. Cohn, P.F., Vokonas, P.S., Williams, R.A., Herman, M.V., and Gorlin, R. A quantitative clinical index for the diagnosis of symptomatic coronary artery disease. *N. Engl. J. Med.* 286:901, 1972.

101. Page, I.H., Benettoni, J.N., Butkus, A., and Sones, F.M., Jr. Prediction of coronary heart disease based on clinical suspicions, age, total cholesterol, and triglyceride. *Circulation* 42:625, 1970.

102. Epstein, S.E. Implications of probability analysis on the strategy used for noninvasive detection of coronary artery disease. *Am. J. of Cardiol.* 46:491, 1980.

103. Diamond, G.A., Staniloff, H.M., Forrester, J.S., Pollock, B.H., and Swan, H.J.C. Computer-assisted diagnosis in the noninvasive evaluation of patients with suspected coronary artery disease. *J. Am. Coll. Cardiol.* 1:444, 1983.

# 5 DETECTION OF CARDIAC ARRHYTHMIAS AND CONDUCTION ABNORMALITIES IN CORONARY ARTERY DISEASE

## Thomas B. Graboys

The detection of sporadically occurring events such as cardiac arrhythmias has led to an ever-burgeoning technology. The clinician, who is now faced with a morass of data, must make management decisions regarding both symptomatic and asymptomatic patient populations. Epidemiologic investigations of persons afflicted with coronary artery disease have resulted in defining certain characteristics of that population that might predispose a given patient to life-threatening arrhythmia or sudden cardiac death. Thus, the potential exists for applying epidemiologic facts to the clinical data obtained using these methods.

This chapter will address primarily the problems of arrhythmia detection and the exposure of arrhythmias in patients with coronary artery disease. It will deal with the utility and limitations of the commonly available methods and describe newer procedures as they apply to the practical management of such patients. Clearly, the prime threat to the coronary patient is electrical instability of the heart; thus, the bulk of this chapter deals with the ventricular arrhythmias. Atrial arrhythmias and conduction abnormalities are included where deemed relevant.

The body of this work is derived from concepts developed in the Cardiovascular Laboratories of the Harvard University School of Public Health under the direction of Dr. Bernard Lown. It is primarily his formulation of an approach to sudden cardiac death that has resulted in the methods detailed in this chapter.

Specific areas of controversy to be discussed in this chapter include the grading system for ventricular arrhythmias, the significance of early-cycle (R-on-T) ectopy, the duration of electrocardiographic (ECG) monitoring with regard to exposure of arrhythmias and as a guide to drug therapy, the utility of exercise to provoke arrhythmia, the significance of exercise-induced arrhythmia, and finally, the use of electrophysiologic modalities to expose electrical vulnerability of the heart.

## Epidemiologic Considerations in a Population with Coronary Artery Disease

### VENTRICULAR ARRHYTHMIAS

*Relation to prognosis.* The advent of the coronary care unit and the use of extensive cardiac monitoring have revealed the ubiquity of the arrhythmias occurring within the acute phase of myocardial infarction of ischemia [1]. It was this experience that drew the attention of the physician to the relations among the ventricular premature beat (VPB), ventricular tachycardia (VT), and ventricular fibrillation (VF) [2]. Current concepts of sudden cardiac death still implicate the VPB as a harbinger of either serious arrhythmia or sudden death, and epidemiologic studies [3–5] have demonstrated that among patients with chronic coronary artery disease, the detection of VPBs portends a greater risk for both subsequent coronary events and sudden death. The experience of the Coronary Drug

Project Research Group [3] indicated that persons exhibiting any VPBs on a baseline, 12-lead ECG were at a twofold greater risk for sudden death than individuals free of such ectopy on a routine tracing. Hinkle et al. [4] reported a detailed follow-up of 811 men between the ages of 35 and 65 who underwent 6-hour ambulatory monitoring, and although they demonstrated that VPBs were a common finding in an aging population, the frequency and complexity (i.e., the multiformity and repetitiveness) of these ectopic beats were found to be closely associated with those of a cohort who exhibited coronary disease. Furthermore, Hinkle and co-workers noted that persons dying suddenly had exhibited a greater frequency of VPBs during previous monitorings.

These data are in accord with the recent Health Insurance Plan of New York (HIP) study by Ruberman and co-workers [6]. These investigators prospectively monitored 1,739 men with recent myocardial infarction for 1 hour and followed them for an average of 24 months. Patients dying suddenly exhibited a characteristic VPB profile. Mortality rates did not differ between patients with unifocal VPBs, regardless of frequency, and those free of ectopy; however, the total mortality for patients exhibiting complex VPBs (multiform, repetitive, and early-cycle ectopy) was nearly two times higher than that of patients with simple VPBs. Early-cycle VPBs (R-on-T) carried a higher probability for sudden death than did either bigeminal or multiform beats. The combination of repetitive arrhythmia and early-cycle VPBs was associated with a 3-year, point-cumulative, sudden death probability of 21 percent, compared to 10.6 percent for those patients with either multiform or frequent ectopic beats.

When carried out to 5 years, mortality was fivefold greater for those individuals with R-on-T or repetitive VPBs. Indeed, these forms of ventricular ectopics carried the highest risk for sudden mortality [7]. Bigger et al. [8] have detailed recently their experience among individuals who demonstrated at least one salvo of ventricular tachycardia (defined as 3 or more successive VPBs), indicating that such individuals experienced greater than a 30 percent annual mortality following acute myocardial infarction.

Among patients with catheterization-documented coronary artery disease, the prognostic import of salvos of ventricular tachycardia occurring either at rest or with exercise has been defined by Califf and co-workers [9]. Patients with salvos of ventricular tachycardia on ambulatory monitoring had a 30 percent annual mortality. The finding of this degree of electrical instability was independent of left ventricular dysfunction. Thus, among comparable groups of patients with ejection fractions less than .40, the presence or absence of VT salvos was the decisive predictor for sudden fatality [9]. The same group assessed the risk for cardiac mortality among CAD patients exhibiting exercise-induced ventricular arrhythmia [10]. Among 620 patients with significant CAD, the finding of repetitive VPBs during exercise was associated with a 25 percent 3-year mortality as compared to a 10 percent mortality in patients free of VPBs during exercise. In both studies, complex or repetitive VPBs carried *no* prognostic significance in those patients *free* of coronary artery disease.

VENTRICULAR DYSFUNCTION AND VPBS. The clinician has been well aware that those patients with severe cardiomyopathy often exhibited a high density of complex VPBs. Among patients with CAD, Calvert et al. [11] examined the relation between complex ventricular ectopy and ventricular dysfunction. Among patients having combined asynergy and elevated left ventricular end-diastolic pressure ( > 19 mmHg), salvos of ventricular tachycardia were noted in 40 percent and ventricular couplets in 67 percent compared to 6 and 12 percent, respectively, in patients without these hemodynamic abnormalities.

IS THE PRESENCE OF REPETITIVE VPBS MERELY AN INDICATOR OF SERIOUS VENTRICULAR DYSFUNCTION, OR DOES IT REPRESENT AN INDEPENDENT RISK FACTOR FOR SUDDEN CARDIAC DEATH? In the previously cited HIP study, Ruberman and co-workers [6] found that the presence of complex VPBs on monitoring carried a higher subsequent cardiac mortality than the subset of patients with congestive failure who did not have these forms of ectopic beats. The highest risk category was those patients with complex VPBs and a history of congestive heart failure.

Schulze and co-workers [12] also found a relation between complex ventricular arrhythmia and sudden death among 81 patients who were followed prospectively for 12 months after they experienced acute myocardial infarction. Implicit in their findings was the role of left ventricular dysfunction. Patients who exhibited a reduced left ventricular ejection fraction, as assessed by gated pool scanning, were at high risk for sudden death, but only if this condition was accompanied by advanced ventricular arrhythmia.

As noted elsewhere, in that subset of CAD patients with left ventricular dysfunction studied by Califf et al. [9], the concomitant finding of ventricular tachycardia salvos carried a nearly sixfold increase in mortality. Follansbee and colleagues [13] retrospectively reviewed a large series of patients with cardiomyopathy undergoing ambulatory ECG monitoring. In that study the finding of any three-beat or more ventricular salvo was associated with an approximate 30 percent annual mortality.

Bigger and co-workers have recently examined the relationships among ventricular arrhythmias, left ventricular dysfunction, and mortality after acute myocardial infarction in 766 patients enrolled in a nine-hospital study [14]. They demonstrated an independent relationship of ventricular arrhythmias and left ventricular dysfunction to subsequent mortality. Runs of ventricular premature beats (VPBs) were associated with a 25 percent 2-year mortality. When ejection fraction (EF) was examined, those patients with VPB runs and an EF less than 30 percent experienced a 42 percent 2-year mortality.

These factors provide one with a formulation for the coronary patient at risk for sudden death: a previous myocardial infarction, ventricular dysfunction with wall motion abnormalities in the presence of advanced forms of ventricular ectopic activity. For the majority of patients, the assessment of ventricular function may be accomplished through history, physical examination, and noninvasive techniques (e.g., chest roentgenography and echocardiography); however, the critical variable in the formulation— the degree of ventricular arrhythmia—requires the application of particular methods designed to expose such ectopy. The presence of the above-mentioned constellation of findings is in our view a mandate for aggressive treatment with antiarrhythmic agents (see chapter 15).

*A Grading System for Ventricular Premature Beats.* In 1971, Lown and Wolf [2] devised a grading system for ventricular arrhythmia that weighted those characteristics of VPBs known or presumed to enhance the risk for sudden death in patients with coronary disease. Although controversy over this grading system has arisen [15, 16], many cardiologists believe that this system does provide a concise, practical amalgam of those features of ventricular ectopy that may portend catastrophic arrhythmia. The grading system divides VPBs into none (grade 0), infrequent (less than one per minute or less than 30 per hour, or grade 1), frequent (more than two per minute or more than 30 per hour, or grade 2), multiform (grade 3), repetitive (grade 4: couplets 4A; VT 4B), and the early-cycle or R-on-T VPBs (grade 5). The grading system may be applied to a 24-hour monitoring period or to grade arrhythmias divulged during exercise testing. This grading system for VPBs is expressed in the following formula:

$$0^3 \ 1^4 \ 2^6_{760} \ 3^6_2 \ 4A^2_3 \ 4B^2_{\underset{(180)}{4-7}} \ 5^1_3.$$

The formula is applied to a 24-hour monitoring period and indicates the number of hours within that period that a patient has VPBs of a particular grade. The translation of this particular formula is as follows: grade 0, none occurred during 3 hours; infrequent VPBs (grade 1) occurred during 4 hours; frequent VPBs (grade 2) occurred during 6 hours to yield a total of 760 VPBs; grade 3 VPBs occurred during 6 hours and exhibited two forms; couplets (grade 4A) occurred during 2 hours, and their greatest frequency in any 1 hour was three per hour; VT (grade 4B) occurred during 2 hours and there were four paroxysms, the longest being seven beats with an average rate of 180 beats per minute; and early VPBs (grade 5) were noted three times in 1 hour.

The above "arrhythmia formula" is intended to allow the clinician to assess rapidly not only the level of ectopy but also its complexity. (This opinion is not shared by Hinkle and co-workers [4], who have emphasized that the risk of future coronary events or sudden cardiac death resides in the quantity of VPBs exhibited by the patient; thus, they contend that an isolated ventricular salvo does not carry the same risk that it would if it occurred in conjunction with frequent extrasystoles.) The proposed formula quantifies VPBs and divides the exposed arrhythmias into relative risk categories. As discussed in chapter 15, the system has been criticized by Bigger and associates [10] for failing to reveal the prevalence of "high and low VPB frequency," yet the issue of the frequency of VPBs is involved, as noted previously, in their "guilt by association" with more advanced grades of ectopy [6, 7]. Indeed, the Health Insurance Plan study by Ruberman and colleagues [6] emphasizes that the mere presence of VPBs, regardless of their frequency, is not a risk factor unless they are accompanied, as is usually the situation, by more complex forms. No one system, whether it defines VPBs quantitatively or describes them as "complex" or "advanced," incorporates all clinical variables into a predictive index. It is again important to emphasize that the significance of VPBs resides in the company they keep. Hence, persons exhibiting complex VPBs without evidence of heart disease are not at enhanced risk.

Despite its obvious advantages, the Lown grading system is weakest in describing that aspect of ventricular arrhythmias that is perhaps the most important: the repetitive forms of VPBs. Frequently, the patient with chronic, stable coronary disease will, when monitored, exhibit a salvo of three or four VPBs. That patient may have minimal ectopy apart from such single bursts of ventricular tachycardia. The grading system classifies the patient as grade 4B, but the salvo is not characterized. Furthermore, the clinical implications of a ventricular salvo of three beats at a rate of 150 beats per minute may differ from those of an accelerating salvo or a six-beat burst of VT at 200 beats per minute.

A second point of controversy concerns the predictive implications of R-on-T or early-cycle ectopy. Engel and co-workers [15] contend that late-cycle VPBs initiate repetitive forms nearly as frequently as early VPBs do, and that often VPBs abut the T-wave without initiating a repet-

itive response. While these statements apply to many patients, the issue lies in the association of the early VPB with more complex forms of ectopy and the lability of the vulnerable period [17, 18]. Indeed, the vulnerable period threshold is not an electrophysiologic constant in the patient with coronary artery disease. Changes in the vulnerable period occur with ischemia, and the patient experiencing frequent episodes of angina may be at risk from an early VPB at one moment and at minimal risk the next. There still appear to be valid reasons for maintaining the early-cycle VPB as a "high-grade" event in the coronary patient.

Recent work from our laboratory documented the increasingly complex forms of VPBs that preceded either ventricular fibrillation or torsade de pointes in a group of patients undergoing ambulatory ECG monitoring [19]. In 11 of 12 patients an increased density of repetitive forms preceded the episode, while in nine patients R-on-T beats initiated the terminal event. These findings were in accord with several other studies that also documented that increasingly complex VPBs are noted just prior to onset of ventricular fibrillation.

## SUPRAVENTRICULAR ARRHYTHMIAS AND BRADYARRHYTHMIAS

Ventricular arrhythmias dominate the rhythm disturbances experienced by patients with chronic coronary artery disease. The appearance of supra-ventricular arrhythmia may reflect changing hemodynamic states, concurrent disease (i.e., pulmonary, pericardial, thyroid, or gastrointestinal disease or valvular involvement), or electrolyte disturbances. Furthermore, patients experiencing paroxysmal atrial tachycardia (PAT) or atrial fibrillation that antedated the clinical manifestations of their coronary artery disease may still continue to experience such arrhythmias.

Symptomatic bradyarrhythmia (atrioventricular or intraventricular conduction disturbances) in the patient with coronary heart disease usually reflects significant myopathy, large areas of infarcted ventricle, or concomitant calcification or sclerotic changes within the heart muscle or conducting system. An estimated 50 percent of patients experiencing the so-called bradycardia-tachycardia syndrome have underlying coronary artery disease [13]. These disturbances complicate many forms of heart disease, however, and reflect the functional state-of-the-heart rather than a specific attribute of ischemic heart disease.

## Methods of Exposing Arrhythmias

### MONITORING

*Overview of In-Hospital and Extended Ambulatory Monitoring.* Arrhythmias are sporadic events; hence, their documentation depends on the duration of monitoring. The Coronary Drug Project Research Group [3] found that 14 percent of those with coronary disease will exhibit some VPBs during the duration of a routine ECG, which is equivalent to approximately 40 seconds of monitoring. If this period is extended to 1 hour of sedentary monitoring, the yield of VPBs is increased to 50 percent [22]. When a coronary patient is continuously monitored for 24 hours, the yield is nearly 90 percent [21].

Monitoring of patients at rest may reduce the yield of ectopy. Thus, to maximize exposure, patients undergoing extended monitoring for reasons other than an acute myocardial infarction should be ambulatory, be encouraged to be physically active, and maintain an accurate diary of daily activities and symptoms.

Extensive technology has been developed for cardiac monitoring. Coronary care unit monitoring now frequently involves computerized systems for automatic rhythm analysis and quantification. Such systems measure prematurity, width, and amplitude of beats, and they may operate with or without operator assistance [23]. An alternative approach to sedentary (coronary care unit) monitoring groups complexes into clusters of QRS signals and compares them to previously stored complexes. This type of system has been reported to provide 95 percent accuracy in VPB detection [24]. The introduction by Holter [25] and associates in 1961 of a practical, portable device that is capable of monitoring for extended periods initiated a technological surge and increased greatly the yield of arrhythmia and conduction disturbance detection. Data reduction for such extended monitorings has evolved at an uneven pace with the monitoring hardware.

In their most basic form, data are qualitatively analyzed by a technician-observer, who assesses the changes in the audiovisual signal that represents the superposition of QRS complexes at 60 to 120 times real time. The problems inherent with this system include variable skills among technicians, boredom or fatigue, inability to quantitate ectopic beats accurately, lack of a qualitative assessment of the trends in either heart rate or ectopic beat frequency, and inattention to correlating the patient's symptoms, as noted in a diary, to observed rhythm or conduction changes. It is, nonetheless, the least expensive method of data reduction.

Computerized systems using QRS algorithms have been applied by a number of investigators with variable reported accuracy [26–28]. Such variability is due in part to false-positive and false-negative findings that result from baseline movement and muscle tremors [28–30]. Hence, quality control and technician interaction are mandatory for all but the most sophisticated computer systems, the cost of which renders them impractical for most community hospitals [31].

An intermediate approach to data reduction integrates the observer with a semiautomated scanning device. This approach provides both quality control and cost accountability as well as accuracy [32, 33]. The system incorporates four basic circuits for the detection of prematurity, amplitude, width, and number of beats. The observer remains an integral element in data interpretation since he or she must preset each circuit, depending on the quality of the printout tape, the degree of artifact, the frequency of arrhythmias, and the configuration of the ectopic beats to be quantified. Once the appropriate degree of sensitivity is programmed by the observer, samples are displayed at fixed time intervals during the tape reading, thus allowing the operator to reject or accept the record of the previous minute's ectopy, which is held on a memory circuit. All VPBs and repetitive (grade 4) forms are quantitated and continuously displayed on an X-Y plotter, where they are superimposed upon the heart rate. The display sheet is divided into a 24-hour time sheet that permits correlation of symptoms, meals, sleep, changes in heart rate, and medications received with the

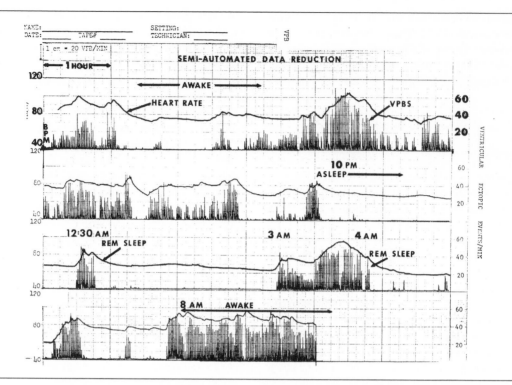

FIGURE 5–1. Data plot from semiautomated scanner that quantitates ectopy from a 24-hour Holter tape. Hourly changes in heart rate and ventricular premature beats (VPBs) are indicated. Specific changes in ectopy are noted during activities, sleep, and rapid eye movement (REM) sleep. (From Armington, R.A., et al. Semiautomated data reduction of ventricular ectopic activity; Methodology and clinical application. *Med. Instrum.* 12:340, 1978 [Copyright Association for the Advancement of Medical Instrumentation]. Used with permission.)

trends in ectopy (figure 5–1). Such observations allow for tailoring of an antiarrhythmic drug program or may reveal important influences on the individual patient's level of arrhythmia.

One additional feature of this system is quality control. It involves taking a printout of an entire hour randomly from the 24-hour tape, which is printed on a single condensed sheet. Thus, all ectopic beats can be quantified and graded, thereby allowing for quality control of both the semiautomated scanning device and the technician reviewing the tape. This type of system has been found to be 96 percent accurate in quantitating ectopic beats over low-, mid-, and high-frequency VPBs (33).

The ability to quantitate and grade arrhythmias allows the clinician to modify or augment therapy in a systematic fashion rather than by intuition. Hence, the efficacy of antiarrhythmic drugs can be judged by comparing pre- and posttreatment monitoring periods [34, 35]. The ideal duration of such monitoring sessions for judging drug efficacy [35, 36] is a subject of controversy and will be discussed later in this chapter.

## Currently Available ECG Analysis Systems.

SUPERIMPOSITION AND PAGING. Superimposing QRS complexes tends to keep the observer's attention focused on one portion of the screen while allowing the observer to see clearly gradual changes in any portion of the QRS complex. For example, changes in RR interval or ST segment are easily seen as "changes in pattern" when viewed as superimposed images. Another example that creates a specific visual cue is atrioventricular dissociation, which appears as a steady QRS pattern with P-waves "sliding" through the cycle. Although instantaneous changes in morphology are readily apparent to the observer, certain temporal relationships may be obscure.

A second method of manual scanning—the paging, or frozen display, method—presents an ECG in segments. Each page displays 1 to 60 minutes of data. During playback the information is displayed on a screen for a period proportional to the amount of information contained in the display, unless the operator stops the system for more detailed analysis. The paging method of displaying several beats at a time allows the operator more time to analyze a specific event than does the superimposition technique; however, if the operator spends a disproportionate amount of time reviewing a particular area of the display, he or she would have less time to notice abnormalities on the rest of the page, assuming a constant paging rate. Nevertheless, depending on the amount of compression, certain temporal relationships may not present strong visual cues. For example, a single APB in a "sea of normals" can easily be overlooked. Thus, it is evident that there are advantages and disadvantages to both superimposition and paging. Some controversy has arisen as to which method gives the operator the best visual cues during high-speed analysis.

CONTINUOUS WRITE-OUT ("FULL DISCLOSURE"). This technique is similar to the concept of paging except that the entire ECG is recorded on hard copy in compressed format. Hard-copy analysis can be as labor intensive as manual scanning techniques if the same information is to be extracted from the recording. In addition, the person reviewing the hard-copy ECG record does not have the advantage of the audio cues provided by manual scanning techniques. Although hard-copy ECG provides a vehicle for beat-to-beat validation of an arrhythmia detector's performance, none of the systems available commercially has included such capability.

REAL TIME. Event recording (real-time ECG processing) has emerged as an alternative to automated high-speed interpretation. These systems make use of the latest microprocessor and memory technology to analyze and store samples of detected arrhythmia and patient-activated events.

On-body processing offers several features not found in passive recording techniques. Nonetheless, one disadvantage is that performance measurements are limited to analysis of the stored samples of detected events. It is important to emphasize that, to date, a rigorous evaluation (real-time analysis versus hard-copy hand count) of real-time recording algorithms has not been undertaken.

Until automated analysis of long-term ECG recordings is more widely accepted, semiautomated analysis will likely be the preferred method. The major objections to semiautomated techniques concern accuracy, reproducibility, and cost effectiveness. Considerable emphasis has been placed on improving detection algorithms and generating computerized trend reports. Methods of verifying performance have not been key elements in the design of currently available ECG analyzers. Nonetheless, the interactive display technique provides an important step in improving the operator's relationships with the machine and is aimed at overcoming some of the problems associated with operator-oriented analysis.

The use of other devices, such as an ambulatory event recorder, has met with variable acceptance, although the results of one system compare favorably to those of extended 24-hour ambulatory monitoring [37]. Similarly, transtelephonic monitoring has been used in the convalescent, postmyocardial infarction patient to identify arrhythmias after hospital discharge. One study by Tuttle and co-workers [38] compared the yield of such arrhythmias provided by a single 24-hour monitoring study recorded prior to hospital discharge with that provided by a daily 1-minute transtelephonic, rhythm strip study carried out for 3 weeks. The systems proved equally effective in disclosing ventricular arrhythmias. The latter form of monitoring may thus have potential in the assessment of drug efficacy.

*Indications for Ambulatory Monitoring in the Patient with Coronary Artery Disease.* The primary purpose of extended 24-hour monitoring is to expose ventricular ectopic activity. In the patient free of arrhythmic symptoms, the factors most likely to render that patient at high risk must be assessed. Left ventricular dysfunction or failure, cardiomegaly, and angina are all variables that are associated with an increased likelihood of VPBs and may augur sudden death [6–12]. This may be particularly true within the initial 6 to 12 months following myocardial infarction.

Patients with chronic, stable coronary artery disease who experience arrhythmic symptoms should undergo ambulatory monitoring. This method will disclose and confirm the presence of VPBs, and it will define those grades of arrhythmia now considered to place the individual coronary patient at risk for sudden death. The finding of other rhythm disturbances (e.g., supraventricular or junctional) or conduction abnormalities may or may not require intervention, depending on the clinical assessment of the patient.

*Trendscription and Other Methods of Monitoring.* Trendscription, devised by Lown and co-workers [39], is an intermediate modality between routine electrocardiography and long-term ambulatory monitoring. The apparatus consists of a radiotelemetry unit and a recording device that presents a hard copy of reduced QRS complexes (figure 5–2). This system is advantageous because it provides the physician with on-line data without delay or third-party (i.e., technician) screening of information. Trendscription has been utilized to detect trends in the arrhythmias of patients within the coronary care unit, during acute drug testing of anti-arrhythmic agents, during exercise stress testing, and in the office setting as a screening method for VPBs. The system can be adapted for telephone transmission by radiotelemetry for the patient with sporadic arrhythmia that is not documented by conventional monitoring.

*Duration of Monitoring.* The optimal duration of monitoring is a subject of controversy. Investigators have noted that hourly or even daily VPB counts fluctuate, and thus longer periods are required to judge drug efficacy or to expose potentially serious arrhythmias [36, 40]. As noted previously, among a coronary disease population, 24-hour ambulatory monitoring will expose VPBs in nearly 90 percent, while a routine ECG will record ectopy in only 14 percent. It is unlikely that extending this costly procedure beyond 24 hours will result in a significant increase in exposed arrhythmias [41]; for epidemiologic purposes, abbreviated monitoring has

proved both effective and cost efficient. The Health Insurance Plan (HIP) study [6] previously cited reflected only 1 hour of sedentary monitoring and demonstrated that this abbreviated period would disclose a high percentage of those at risk for dying suddenly. Graboys and co-workers [43] compared 30 minutes of continuous monitoring (trendscription) to 24-hour ambulatory monitoring records among 145 consecutive patients. They found that the 30-minute period revealed advanced grades of arrhythmia (grades 4 and 5) among 27 (45 percent) of the 60 patients who exhibited these grades in 24-hour monitoring studies. Of importance was that only one patient (0.7 percent of the total) with ventricular tachycardia on 24-hour monitoring failed to display ectopy during the 30-minute recording. Thus, the abbreviated period may serve as a potentially valid screening test for epidemiologic community studies, for screening asymptomatic populations, or in the outpatient assessment of the patient with stable coronary heart disease.

When used to assess antiarrhythmic efficacy, however, the variability of VPB frequency must be considered with regard to the individual patient [40, 42]. The frequency of ectopy may be a function of such diverse factors as the type and extent of underlying heart disease or the physical and psychologic stresses encountered during a particular monitoring session. Nonreproducibility and variability of VPBs are realities of the monitoring method, and they emphasize the limitations of this technique in the assessment of drug efficacy. Hence, our contention has been that monitoring should be but one element of a management program that incorporates other techniques to assess the effectiveness of a given drug [34, 35].

EXERCISE TESTING

Exercise has been utilized for over 50 years in the evaluation of the heart, but the usefulness of this technique extends beyond the assessment of aerobic capacity or ischemic ECG changes. The arrhythmogenicity of exercise has also been appreciated for over 50 years. In 1923 Bourne [44] noted the occurrence of VPBs during exercise in men with coronary artery disease. Only recently, however, has exercise testing been spe-

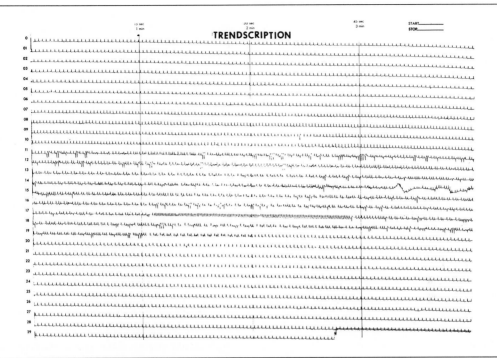

FIGURE 5–2. Trendscription record indicating frequent VPBs and ventricular tachycardia. Each line represents one minute of ECG recording. A striking absence of arrhythmia is noted through 11 minutes of monitoring. The sudden appearance of frequent VPBs, bursts of ventricular tachycardia, and one prolonged bout of ventricular tachycardia during the 18th minute coincided with psychiatric interviewing. (From Graboys, T.B. and Lown, B. *Cardiovasc. Med.* 4:795, 1979.)

cifically employed to expose cardiac arrhythmia [45] as well as to devine antiarrhythmic drug efficacy [34, 35].

The provocation of arrhythmias or conduction abnormalities in patients undergoing exercise is due to acknowledged physiologic changes that occur during exercise. In the patient with coronary heart disease, there is probably a direct relation between the provocation of arrhythmia and myocardial ischemia (figure 5–3). Exercise induces an acute increase in sympathetic tone with a reflex reduction in vagal activity. Accordingly, an increase in myocardial oxygen demand results, which cannot be met because of impaired coronary flow. This results in an altered state of tissue hypoxia and a heterogeneity of refractoriness. Regional areas of ischemia result

in increased cellular automaticity and the emergence of ventricular ectopy [44, 46] (see chapter 2). Atrial arrhythmias may occur by similar mechanisms, particularly if left ventricular filling pressures increase or if transient, ischemia-induced papillary muscle dysfunction produces abrupt, left atrial distention.

Both atrioventricular or intraventricular conduction disturbances may occur during exercise. These may occur on a rate-related basis or because of decremental conduction resulting from ischemia of the atrioventricular junction or bundle of His. Additionally, antiarrhythmic drugs may alter intraventricular or atrioventricular conduction, resulting in either symptomatic bradyarrhythmia or exercise aggravation of ventricular arrhythmia [47]. This is particularly germane in the coronary artery disease population with left ventricular dysfunction. Indeed, this subset of patients may be at highest risk for sudden death and require chronic antiarrhythmic therapy, but they might be at greatest risk for so-called proarrhythmic effects of these agents. In a study carried out at our laboratory we found approximately an 11 percent incidence of antiarrhythmic drug aggrava-

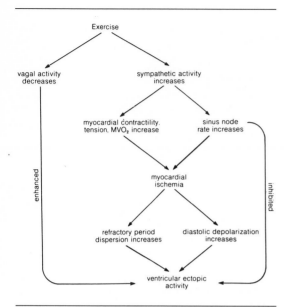

FIGURE 5–3. Mechanism of exercise-induced arrhythmia. (From Lown, B. and Graboys, T.B. *Cardiovasc. Med.* 2:219, 1977.)

tion among patients with malignant ventricular arrhythmia [48].

*Risks of Exercise Testing.* The risks imposed by exercise testing are minimal, providing certain guidelines are adhered to (see chapter 6). The two major complications are the provocation of an acute myocardial infarction or the precipitation of ventricular fibrillation; both these occurrences are rare events. Thus, among 50,000 Master two-step procedures, a single acute infarction occurred [49]. Ventricular fibrillation during exercise is similarly an unusual event. Reported frequencies differ, depending on the patient population undergoing exercise as well as on whether maximal, symptom-limited testing, or submaximal testing is employed. In two extensive series, Doyle and Kinch [51] and Ellestad and associates [52] reported a total of nearly 27,000 exercise tests performed without fatalities or complications. Kattus and McAlpin [53] reported two episodes of VF during testing in a population of 500 patients with coronary heart disease. Irving and Bruce [54] recently detailed six cases of VF drawn from a population of 10,700 persons undergoing maximal exercise

testing. In each case, exertional hypotension preceded the VF, which occurred in the immediate postexercise recovery period.

The most comprehensive review of morbidity and mortality associated with exercise testing is a multicenter study by Rochmis and Blackburn [55]. They culled results of 170,000 exercise studies and found 16 deaths (0.01 percent mortality) that were temporally related to the procedure. This author and co-workers have recently reviewed the occurrence of major dysrhythmic complications (e.g., sustained symptomatic ventricular tachycardia or ventricular fibrillation) in 263 high-risk patients undergoing serial antiarrhythmic drug trials who underwent a total of 1,377 maximal exercise studies [56]. Twenty-four patients (9.1 percent) sustained a complication during 32 tests (2.3 percent), whereas 239 patients (90.9 percent) were free of complication during 1,345 tests (97.7 percent). There were no deaths, myocardial infarctions, or lasting morbid events. An equal number of cardiac arrests occurred on as well as off antiarrhythmic drugs. These findings underscore the need to have all coronary patients being treated with antiarrhythmics undergo exercise testing to assess possible "proarrhythmic" effects [57].

*The Yield of Exercise-Induced Arrhythmia.*

VENTRICULAR ARRHYTHMIA. The extensive review by Jelinek and Lown [45] details the increased yield of VPBs that is obtained during exercise and recovery. They reviewed 1,000 stress tests performed by 625 patients. Ventricular ectopic activity was coded in 610 of the procedures. When the frequency of arrhythmias during and after exercise was compared to that in control ECGs, a nearly threefold increase in frequent ectopics and an eightfold increment in repetitive forms were noted. Of these arrhythmias, 78 percent occurred in the postexercise recovery period. The most common times for the emergence of VPBs were at peak exercise and within the initial 3 minutes of recovery. Indeed, in the absence of an adequate "cooling down" stage, the immediate postexercise recovery period may be most hazardous for the patient with ischemic heart disease. It has been our experience, as well as that of Irving and Bruce

[54], that ventricular fibrillation is most likely to occur at this time. A similar yield of exercise-induced ventricular ectopy was documented by McHenry and colleagues [58], who found that 52 percent of patients with coronary artery disease exhibited VPBs during routine stress testing.

When compared to extended ambulatory monitoring, exercise testing provokes a lower overall yield of ectopy. Ryan et al. [21] compared the prevalence of VPBs among 100 unselected patients with coronary heart disease who underwent 24-hour ambulatory monitoring and exercise testing (table 5–1). Ventricular arrhythmia was demonstrated in 56 percent of those exercise tested and in 88 percent of those monitored. Repetitive beat activity (grade 4) was found in 20 percent during exercise and in 40 percent during monitoring. Furthermore, the occurrence of ventricular tachycardia (grade 4B) was detected more than twice as commonly during monitoring (16 percent) as during exercise testing (7 percent). Of importance, however, was that of the seven patients with exercise-induced ventricular tachycardia, four exhibited this grade during exercise testing but not with ambulatory monitoring. It continues to be our experience that approximately 15 percent of patients undergoing antiarrhythmic drugs will exhibit serious arrhythmia only during the exercise study, thus negating the results of an "acceptable" 24-hour ambulatory monitoring [59] (figure 5–4).

Exercise testing and ambulatory monitoring should be considered complementary methods, and when used conjointly, they will increase the overall yield of arrhythmia. Exercise testing should be an integral element in the management of ventricular arrhythmias, particularly in those patients in whom ectopy is provoked at a critical heart rate. Exercise testing may thus serve as a therapeutic guide to antiarrhythmic control.

ATRIAL ARRHYTHMIA. Patients with coronary artery disease are probably no more likely to develop exercise-induced atrial arrhythmia than are those with a diverse array of disease states, and the occurrence of such arrhythmias may be a

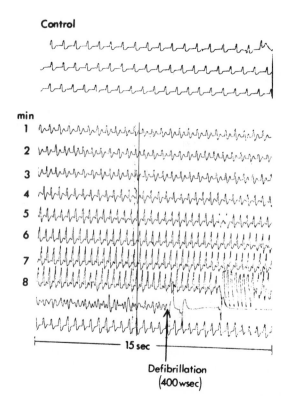

FIGURE 5–4. Excerpt from trendscription record of exercise test. Onset of ventricular fibrillation occurred at peak exercise. Repeated ambulatory monitoring tests failed to show significant ventricular arrhythmia.

TABLE 5–1. Maximum grade of ventricular premature beats (VPB) exposed by ambulatory monitoring and exercise testing among 100 patients with coronary heart disease

| Test | Total with VPBs | VPB grade | | | | | |
|---|---|---|---|---|---|---|---|
| | | 0 | 1 | 2 | 3 | 4A | 4B |
| Exercise | 56 | 44 | 19 | 12 | 5 | 13 | 7 |
| Monitoring | 88 | 12 | 21 | 4 | 23 | 24 | 16 |

function of left ventricular hemodynamics. Among all patients undergoing standard maximal treadmill testing, approximately 25 percent will exhibit some atrial ectopy. Sustained atrial arrhythmias, however, are rare, regardless of the population being exercised. Gooch [60] found only five episodes of sustained atrial tachycardia among 3,000 patients undergoing exercise testing. We have noted 29 episodes of supraventricular tachycardia during 3,000 consecutive treadmill tests (1 percent). Most of these episodes were paroxysmal atrial or junctional tachycardia (75 percent), while the remainder exhibited atrial flutter or fibrillation [61]. When compared to a 3-minute control, exercise increases the occurrence of atrial arrhythmia by a factor of three and the occurrence of supraventricular tachycardia by a factor of two [45]. Patients with a history of atrial arrhythmias will exhibit such arrhythmias more commonly during ambulatory monitoring, yet as with the ventricular arrhythmias, there are patients who are prone to exercise-induced atrial tachyarrhythmias. For example, the author and co-workers found that 18 percent of 22 patients referred with a diagnosis of preexcitation syndrome and a history of symptomatic arrhythmia displayed their supraventricular arrhythmia only during exercise [62].

*Documentation of Arrhythmias During Exercise Testing.* To quantitate precisely all ectopy and to define the nature of the ectopic episodes requires some form of on-line recording system, memory capability, or computer storage and retrieval. The use of a reduced, continuous electrographic recording system—e.g., trendscription, as depicted in figures 5–2 and 5–4—allows identification of arrhythmias or conduction disturbances. Additionally, it permits the physician to detect trends in arrhythmia emergence or suppression. A specific comparison between this type of continuous monitoring system and an intermittent system was carried out by Antman and co-workers from this laboratory [63]. We found that a continuous recording system increased the yield of all VPBs by nearly 20 percent. More importantly, there was an eightfold increase in the yield of complex or repetitive ectopics with continuous recordings compared to intermittent recordings.

It is apparent that casual observations of an oscilloscope with periodic rhythm strips result in a lesser reported or appreciated frequency of ectopy than does continuous recording. This may be particularly relevant for the patient with a brief, exercise-induced ventricular salvo that may reflect significant electrical instability of the ventricle.

*Reproducibility of Exercise-Induced Arrhythmia.* Reproducibility of exercise-induced ventricular arrhythmia is an important consideration if exercise testing is being utilized to assess drug efficacy. Reproducibility is higher among patients exhibiting repetitive forms of VPBs (55 percent) than among those with single VPBs (30 percent) [45]. This may explain the decreased frequency of VPBs during a second treadmill test observed by Lopez and associates [64]. Those authors compared the frequencies of VPBs in two consecutive stress tests; however, the time interval between tests (45 minutes) was inappropriately short. If the intention is to assess antiarrhythmic drug efficacy, a repeat test that is accomplished at the presumed time of peak drug action (1 to 2 hours) would perhaps be more appropriate. Nonetheless, assessing drug efficacy poses a difficult problem. Although nonreproducibility is a reality with both monitoring and exercise testing, these methods used together represent the only procedure commonly available to the practitioner for the management of patients who exhibit significant cardiac arrhythmias [22, 34, 35, 56–59]. Suppression of arrhythmias that occur at peak exercise and during the initial 3 minutes of recovery is an attainable and desired objective.

*Clinical Implications of Exercise-Induced VPBs.* Exercise-induced arrhythmia occurs both in the population that is ostensibly free of heart disease and in those with a variety of underlying cardiac disorders. Extensive experience with exercise testing among asymptomatic Air Force crewmen [65, 66], YMCA populations [45, 67], and other apparently healthy groups [58, 68–70] attest to the spectrum of arrhythmias that may occur during or immediately following exercise (table 5–2). Although many normal individuals may exhibit infrequent VPBs during exercise, a

TABLE 5–2. Exercise-induced ventricular arrhythmias among asymptomatic populations and those with coronary artery disease

| Investigator(s) | Type of population | Number in population | Percentage with any VPBs[a] | Percentage with repetitive VPBs |
|---|---|---|---|---|
| Lamb and Hiss | Asymp. | 851 | 15.7 | — |
| Froelicher et al. | Asymp. | 1,390 | 13.1 | 2.1 |
| McHenry et al. | Asymp. | 295 | 36 | 6.4 |
| Graboys and Lown | Asymp. | 450 | 25 | 2.6 |
| Jelenik and Lown | Asymp. | 163 | 19 | 1.8 |
| Ryan et al. | CAD[b] | 100 | 56 | 35. |
| McHenry et al. | CAD[b] | 73 | 52.1 | 19.2 |

[a]VPB = ventricular premature beat.
[b](CAD) = coronary artery disease.

small subset of healthy persons demonstrate complex ventricular ectopy [58]. Kennedy and Underhill [68] detailed the clinical characteristics of 25 such patients (mean age 49 years) who had had evidence of advanced grades (multiform or repetitive) of VPBs for an average of 6 years. Notably, among 23 subjects exercised, 92 percent demonstrated overdrive suppression of their arrhythmia during the final stage of exercise. Similar findings were noted among a small percentage of asymptomatic YMCA members with repetitive arrhythmia [67].

Certain characteristics of these subjects indicate the benign nature of their arrhythmia: they are asymptomatic, show no evidence of structural heart disease, have normal exercise duration and hemodynamics, and display normal ST segment responses. Our experience has been that such patients usually suppress (overdrive) their VPBs with rapid sinus rates and that frequent or multiform VPBs are the types commonly noted. Certainly, patients with underlying coronary artery disease may also demonstrate overdrive, and this occurrence does not distinguish normal individuals from those with coronary artery disease [71, 72].

Therefore, in terms of predictive implications at the present time, the arrhythmias that occur during exercise must be related to other factors [10]. Udall and Ellestad [73] examined this premise and found that among 569 patients with positive exercise tests and VPBs, there was an 11.4 percent annual incidence of coronary events, compared to only a 1.7 percent incidence

among 1,067 patients who were free of arrhythmias and who had normal ST segment response. Persons exhibiting normal ST segments but exercise-induced VPBs had a 6.4 percent annual incidence of coronary events, and patients with ST segment depression whose ectopy increased during exercise had a 32 percent yearly incidence of new-onset angina, myocardial infarction, or sudden death. Such observations support the findings that advanced grades of ectopy are associated with angiographically severe coronary disease and ventricular wall motion abnormalities [74, 75]. Experience indicates that one can similarly determine a profile of a patient population by employing exercise testing to delineate a high-risk subset: namely, those patients with symptomatic ischemic heart disease and a previous myocardial infarction who develop angina that is associated with VPBs and ST segment depression during exercise, or those patients whose ectopy emerges at peak exercise or the first 3 minutes of recovery, which implies the presence of an unstable reentry focus despite an increased sinus rate. Figure 5–5 illustrates two responses to exercise stress testing: overdrive suppression and rate-related emergence of VPBs.

ELECTROPHYSIOLOGIC STUDIES
Since the first edition of this text, there has been a burgeoning interest in electrophysiologic techniques to expose ventricular arrhythmia and guide antiarrhythmic therapy. It is a technology with many unresolved issues [76]. A full discussion of the technique is beyond the intent of this

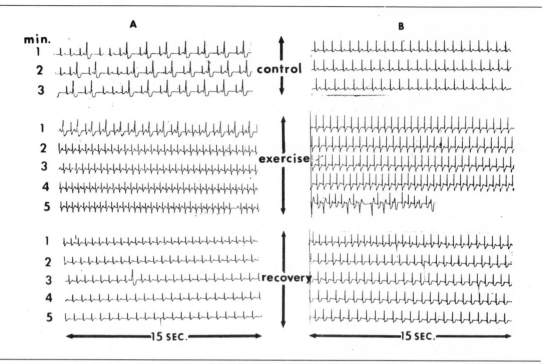

FIGURE 5-5. Excerpts from trendscription records of two patients undergoing maximal treadmill testing. (A) Overdrive suppression. Patient exhibited frequent VPBs during control and in the early stages of exercise; the patient subsequently overdrove all ectopy at peak exercise. (B) Rate-related emergence of VPBs as exercise progressed. Ventricular ectopy persisted into the early phase of recovery and was temporally related to the onset of angina pectoris and ST segment depression.

chapter and is detailed extensively in recent reviews [77–79]. The essentials of programmed stimulation involve placement of a multipolar pacing catheter in the ventricle. Both recording and stimulating functions can then be undertaken at various sites. Premature stimuli are then programmed to fall during electrical diastole. Stimulation protocols vary and may include placement of one to three impulses at energies up to three times the mid-diastolic threshold. Programmed stimulation can be carried out during sinus rhythm or during ventricular pacing at various cycle lengths. The end-points vary from precipitation of sustained ventricular tachycardia (providing it is demonstrated to be the so-called clinical tachycardia) to elicitation of nonsustained ventricular tachycardia [77–81].

An important issue, of course, is the safety of electrophysiologic studies. In the series of Mason and Winkle [79], 52 percent of patients required emergency cardioversion or defibrillation because of hemodynamic compromise. If the end-point of these studies is reproducible nonsustained ventricular tachycardia, the incidence of cardiac arrest is obviously much less [81]. At present it is not clear which protocol or

end-point is ideal. The logic of the technique remains simple: induce a response in the control (off-drug) state and repeat the study during an antiarrhythmic trial. It is the clinical realty that leaves the practitioner bewildered. Specifically, it is not clear which patients should undergo these studies and in which populations a false-positive induction might occur. Recent work from Brugada et al. sheds some light in this area [82]. This group studied 52 patients without a history of symptomatic ventricular tachycardia and 50 patients with symptomatic ventricular tachycardia. In the "non-VT" group, ventricular tachycardia could be induced in 31 of the 52 patients (59 percent). Importantly, five of these patients experienced ventricular fibrillation during this testing. This compared to induction of ventricular tachycardia in 44 of the 50 symptomatic ventricular tachycardia group. The authors emphasize that the nonspecificity of VT induction in select patients may be a result of the aggressiveness of the stimulation protocol.

*Which Patients With Coronary Artery Disease Should Undergo Programmed Ventricular Stimulation?* This author believes that only those patients with malignant ventricular arrhythmia (noninfarction-related ventricular fibrillation; hemodynamically compromising ventricular tachycardia) whose level of ambient ventricular arrhythmia is low or nonreproducible should be subject to invasive study. This may comprise approximately 25 percent of patients of this select subset of the coronary population. In the remainder of patients, anti-arrhythmic drug efficacy can be gauged by the use of ambulatory ECG recordings and exercise stress testing [34, 35].

A recent study by Richards et al. [83] has raised the question of whether all postmyocardial infarction patients should undergo electrophysiologic study. These authors carried out programmed stimulation in 165 patients within 1 month of an acute myocardial infarction. Twenty-three percent of the group exhibited electrical instability defined as either the induction of ventricular fibrillation or ventricular tachycardia lasting at least 10 seconds. The authors calculated that the sensitivity of these findings as a predictor of instantaneous death or spontaneous ventricular tachycardia was 86 percent, and the specificity 83 percent. Unfortunately, no rigorous comparisons were made using noninvasive methods to expose repetitive VPBs (e.g., monitoring and exercise studies), which when incorporated with ventricular function studies may well achieve similar specificity and sensitivity figures. At present there is no justification for routine electrophysiologic studies in postmyocardial infarction patients.

## Detection of Conduction Defects

### EXERCISE TESTING AND CONDUCTION DEFECTS
It is unusual for the patient with hemodynamically stable coronary artery disease to exhibit either atrioventricular or intraventricular conduction disturbance during exercise testing. Their occurrence, then, implies the presence either of structural damage to the atrioventricular junction or to the His-Purkinje system, focal areas of ischemia provoked by exercise, or of a functional disturbance imposed by antiarrhythmic drugs or electrolytes. Exercise increases sympathetic tone and facilitates atrioventricular conduction [84]. Hence, shortening of the PR interval is a common ECG finding. Progression to advanced atrioventricular (AV) block during exercise testing occurs occasionally in patients with normal resting ECGs. Similarly, abolition of first- or second-degree AV block found at rest may be noted during exercise [85]. Rate-related intraventricular conduction disturbances are found both in normal patients and in those with underlying heart disease. In general, the development of exercise-induced left bundle branch block is seen more commonly in patients with heart disease. Occasionally, symptomatic patients who demonstrate bifascicular or trifascicular block on a resting ECG will also display advanced degrees of AV block during exercise or recovery, which thus provides decisive evidence for diagnosis and definitive therapy (figure 5–6).

### ELECTROPHYSIOLOGIC METHODS
The application of basic cardiac electrophysiology to clinical areas has resulted in increased understanding of the various mechanisms that induce both atrioventricular and intraventricular conduction disturbances as well as of the electrophysiology of antiarrhythmic drugs. Those chronic conduction abnormalities that are clinically significant, however, are rarely found in the coronary patient with a heart of normal size and normal ventricular function. Thus, a chronic conduction disturbance reflects the structural state of the myocardium, whereas acute changes in impulse conductivity may be functional or due to ischemia, drug administration, electrolyte imbalance, or changes in sympathetic-parasympathetic tone.

In patients with acute myocardial infarction complicated by bifascicular block, Lichstein and associates [86] utilized His bundle recordings to identify those patients at presumed risk for complete heart block. They based the decision regarding the insertion of a permanent pacemaker

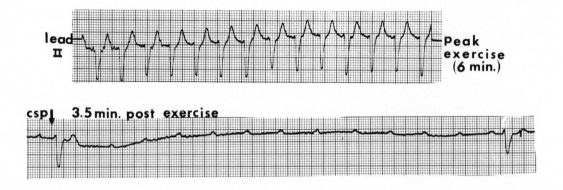

FIGURE 5–6. Record of 78-year-old woman with chronic trifascicular block and history of dizziness who underwent maximal exercise testing. During the third minute following exercise, hyperventilation and carotid sinus pressures (csp) provoked complete heart block with a ventricular escape rhythm of 20 beats per minute. Three previous ambulatory monitoring tests had not demonstrated advanced degrees of atrioventricular (AV) block.

upon the prolongation of the H-V time in this selected group of patients.

Work by Dhingra et al. [87] and Denes et al. [88] has dealt with the issue of chronic bifascicular block, syncope, and, specifically, the utility of His bundle electrocardiography. Dhingra and colleagues studied 186 patients with chronic bifascicular block due to various causes, and they compared those with and without syncope in terms of clinical, ECG, and electrophysiologic indexes. The study did not include patients with acute myocardial infarction. Importantly, the results of electrophysiologic studies were similar in both syncopal and nonsyncopal patients. Those authors emphasized that normal studies "do not preclude subsequent progression of conduction disease" [87]. In a more recent study from this same group, Denes and associates [88] found a low incidence of spontaneous progression to heart block but a significant incidence of sudden death among patients with chronic intraventricular conduction disturbances. Of 277 patients, 68 (24.5 percent) died, of whom 30 were deemed to have suffered sudden cardiac death. Patients who died suddenly had a higher incidence of symptomatic coronary artery disease and ventricular arrhythmias. The use of electrophysiologic data again failed to identify the sudden-death group. The authors emphasized that sudden death in patients with chronic fascicular block results from primary ventricular fibrillation rather than from the abrupt onset of complete heart block or bradyarrhythmia. Thus, although they did not debate the indications for the use of permanent pacemakers in coronary patients who develop

acute, infarct-related intraventricular conduction disturbances, those authors supported the clinican's view that His bundle electrocardiography is of some diagnostic usefulness, but it rarely plays a decisive role in patient management [89]. This subject is discussed further in chapter 15.

## Conclusions

The patient with coronary heart disease may be at risk for sudden death or a future coronary event because of electrical instability of the heart, which is often sporadic and usually asymptomatic. Epidemiologic and pathomorphologic studies have focused on the ventricular premature beat (VPB) as the marker of an electrically unstable ventricle. However, it is not merely the presence of the VPB, but rather the specific characteristics of this form of ectopy that may render the patient with coronary disease vulnerable.

The presence of complex forms of VPBs is associated with both the extent of diseased vessels as well as the state of ventricular function. Monitoring methods are used to disclose asymptomatic, potentially threatening arrhythmias. Extended (24-hour) ambulatory monitoring reveals VPBs among nearly 90 percent of a coronary disease population. Exercise stress testing will yield a lesser frequency of arrhythmias, but it may disclose a subset of patients in whom the arrhythmia is specifically exercise induced. Thus, the two methods prove to be complementary.

Compilation of exercise testing, monitoring, and epidemiologic studies provides a formula for the coronary disease population at high risk for sudden death. Such a patient will have had a recent (within 1 year) myocardial infarction, exhibit reduced left ventricular function, demonstrate repetitive arrhythmias or ventricular tachycardia on monitoring, and have exercise-induced, advanced grades of VPBs with or without ST segment depression. Such patients require an active management program.

## References

1. Lown, B., Klein, M., and Hershberg, P.I. Coronary and precoronary care. *Am. J. Med.* 46:705, 1969.
2. Lown, B. and Wolf, M. Approaches to sudden death from coronary disease. *Circulation* 44:130, 1971.
3. Coronary Drug Project Research Group. Prognostic importance of premature beats following myocardial infarction. *JAMA* 223:1116, 1973.
4. Hinkle, L.E., Carver, S.T., and Argyros, D.C. The prognostic significance of ventricular premature contractions in healthy people and in people with coronary heart disease. *Acta Cardiol.* (Brux.) Suppl. 18:5, 1974.
5. Chiang, B.N., Perman, L.V., Ostrander, L.D., Jr., and Epstein, F.H. Relationship of premature systoles to coronary heart disease and sudden death in the Tecumseh epidemiologic study. *Ann. Intern. Med.* 70:1159, 1969.
6. Ruberman, L.D., Weinblatt, E., Goldberg, J.D., Frank, C.W., and Shapiro, S. Ventricular premature beats and mortality after myocardial infarction. *N. Engl. J. Med.* 279:750, 1977.
7. Ruberman, W., Weinblatt, E., Goldberg, J.D., Frank, C.W., Chaudhary, B.S., and Shapiro S. Ventricular premature complexes and sudden death after myocardial infarction. *Circulation* 64:297, 1981.
8. Bigger, J.T., Weld, F.M., and Rolnitzky, L.M. Prevalence, characteristics and significance of ventricular tachycardia (three or more complexes) detected with ambulatory ECG recording in the late hospital phase of acute myocardial infarction. *Am. J. Cardiol.* 48:815, 1981.
9. Califf, R.M., McKinnis, R.A., Burks, J., Lee, K.L., Harrell, F.E., Jr., Behar, V.S., Pryor, D.B., Wagner, G.S., and Rosati, RA. Prognostic implications of ventricular arrhythmias during 24-hour ambulatory monitoring in patients undergoing catheterization for coronary artery disease. *Am. J. Cardiol.* 50:23, 1982.
10. Califf, R.M., McKinnis, R.A., McNeer, J.F., Harrell, F.E., Jr., Lee, K.L., Pryor, D.B., Waugh, R.A., Harris, P.J., Rosati, R.A., and Wagner, G.S. Prognostic value of ventricular arrhythmias associated with treadmill exercise testing in patients studied with cardiac catheterization for suspected ischemic heart disease. *JACC* 2:1060, 1983.
11. Calvert, A., Lown, B., and Gorlin, R. Ventricular premature beats and anatomically defined coronary heart disease. *Am. J. Cardiol.* 39:327, 1977.
12. Schulze, R., Strauss, H., and Pitt, B. Sudden death in the year following myocardial infarction —relation to ventricular premature contractions in late hospital phase and left ventricular ejection fraction. *Am. J. Med.* 62:192, 1977.
13. Follansbee, W.P., Michelson, E.L., and Morganroth, J. Nonsustained ventricular tachycardia in ambulatory patients: Characteristics and association with sudden cardiac death. *Ann. Intern. Med.* 92:741, 1982.
14. Bigger, J.T., Fleiss, J.L., Kleiger, R. Miller, J.P., Rolnitzky, L.M., and the Multicenter Post-Infarction Research Group. The relationships among ventricular arrhythmias, left ventricular dysfunction, and mortality in the 2 years after myocardial infarction. *Circulation* 69:250, 1984.
15. Engel, T.R., Meister, S.G., and Frankl, W.S. The "R on T" phenomenon: An update and critical review. *Ann. Intern. Med.* 88:221, 1978.
16. Bigger, J.T., Jr., Wenger, T.L., and Heissenbuttel, R.H. Limitations of the Lown grading system for the study of human ventricular arrhythmias. *Am. Heart J.* 93:727, 1977.
17. Axelrod, P.J., Verrier, R.L., and Lown, B. Vulnerability during acute coronary arterial occlusion and release. *Am. J. Cardiol.* 36:776, 1975.
18. Thompson, P.L. and Lown, B. Sequential R on T pacing to expose electrical instability in the ischemic ventricle. *Clin. Res.* 20:401, 1972.
19. Lewis, B.H., Antman, E.M., and Graboys, T.B. Detailed analysis of 24-hour ambulatory electrocardiographic recordings during ventricular fibrillation or torsades de pointes. *JACC* 2:426, 1983.
20. Moss, A.J. and Davis, R.J. Brady-tachy syndrome. *Prog. Cardiovasc. Dis.* 16:439, 1974.
21. Ryan, M., Lown, B., and Horn, H.R. Comparison of ventricular ectopic activity during 24-hour monitoring and exercise testing on patients with coronary heart disease. *N. Engl. J. Med.* 229:224, 1975.
22. Lown, B. and Graboys, T.B. Sudden death: An

ancient problem newly perceived. *Cardiovasc. Med.* 2:219, 1977.

23. Yanowitz, F., Kinias, P., Rawling, D., and Fozzard, H.A. Accuracy of a continuous real-time ECG dysrhythmic monitoring system. *Circulation* 50:65, 1974.

24. Shah, P.M., Arnold, J.M., Haberern, N.A., Bliss, D.T., and McClelland, K.M. Automatic real time arrhythmic monitoring in the intensive care unit. *Am. J. Cardiol.* 39:701, 1977.

25. Holter, N.J. New method for heart studies: Continuous electrocardiography of active subjects over long periods is now practical. *Science* 134:1214, 1961.

26. Oliver, G.C.J., Noble, F.M., Wolff, G.A., Cox, J.R.J., and Amos, H.D. Detection of premature ventricular contractions with a clinical system for monitoring electrographic rhythms. *Comput. Biomed. Res.* 4:523, 1971.

27. Lopes, M.G., Fitzgerald, J., Harrison, D.C., and Schroeder, J.S. Diagnosis and quantification of arrhythmias in ambulatory patients using an improved R-R interval plotting system. *Am. J. Cardiol.* 35:816, 1975.

28. Harrison, D., Fitzgerald, J.W., and Winkle, R.A. Ambulatory electrocardiography for diagnosis and treatment of chronic arrhythmias. *N. Engl. J. Med.* 294:373, 1976.

29. Caceres, C.A. Limitations of the computer in electrocardiographic interpretation. *Am. J. Cardiol.* 38:362, 1976.

30. Knoebel, S.B., Lovelace, D.C., Rasmussen, S., and Wash, S.E. Computer detection of premature ventricular complexes: A modified approach. *Am. J. Cardiol.* 38:440, 1976.

31. Kennedy, H.L. and Caralis, D.G. Ambulatory electrocardiography: A clinical perspective. *Ann. Intern. Med.* 87:729, 1977.

32. Lown, B., Calvert, A.F., Armington, R., and Ryan, M. Monitoring for serious arrhythmias and high risk of sudden death. *Circulation* 52 (Suppl. 3):189, 1975.

33. Armington, R.A., Graboys, T.B., Lown, B., and Lenson, R. Semiautomated data reduction of ventricular ectopic activity: Methodology and clinical application. *Med. Instrum.* 12:340, 1978.

34. Lown, B. and Graboys, T.B. Management of the patient with malignant ventricular arrhythmia. *Am. J. Cardiol.* 39:910, 1977.

35. Graboys, T.B., Lown, B., Podrid, P.J., and DeSilva, R. Long-term survival of patients with malignant ventricular arrhythmia treated with antiarrhythmic drugs. *Am. J. Cardiol.* 50:437, 1982.

36. Morganroth, J., Horowitz, L.N., Josephson, M.E., and Michaelson, Z.L. Limitations of infrequent Holter monitoring in assessing antiarrhythmic efficacy. *Am. J. Cardiol.* 41:401, 1978.

37. Dreifus, L.S. and Pennock, R. Newer technique in cardiac monitoring. *Heart Lung* 4:568, 1975.

38. Tuttle, W.B., Lee, D.W., and Schoenfeld, C.O. Daily transtelephonic electrocardiographic monitoring of convalescent myocardial infarction patients. *Am. J. Cardiol.* 41:399, 1978.

39. Lown, B., Matta, R.J., and Besser, H.W. Programmed trendesciption: A new approach to electrocardiographic monitoring. *JAMA* 232:39, 1975.

40. Winkle, R.A. Spontaneous variability of ventricular ectopy frequently mimics antiarrhythmic drug effect. *Circulation* 57:1116, 1978.

41. Kennedy, H.L., Pescarmona, J.E., Bouchard, R.J., and Caralis, D.G. Asymptomatic healthy persons with frequent complex ventricular ectopy and coronary artery disease. *Am. J. Cardiol.* 41:424, 1978.

42. Morganroth, J., Michelson, E.L., Horowitz, L.N., Josephson, M.E., Pearlman, A.S., and Dunkman, W.B. Limitations of routine long-term electrocardiographic monitoring to assess ventricular ectopic frequency. *Circulation* 58:408, 1978.

43. Graboys, T.B. and Lown, B. Abbreviated electrocardiographic monitoring for exposing ventricular ectopic activity. *Cardiovasc. Med.* 4:795, 1979.

44. Bourne, G. An attempt at the clinical classification of premature ventricular beats. *Q.J. Med.* 20:219, 1923.

45. Jelinek, M.M. and Lown, B. Exercise stress testing for exposure of cardiac arrhythmia. *Prog. Cardiovasc. Dis.* 26:497, 1974.

46. Fortuin, N.J. and Weiss, J.L. Exercise stress testing. *Circulation* 56:699, 1977.

47. Podrid, P.J. and Graboys, T.B. Exercise stress testing in the management of cardiac rhythm disorders. *Medical Clinics of North America* 68:139, 1984.

48. Velebit, V., Podrid, P.J., Lown, B., Cohen, B., and Graboys, T.B. Aggravation and provocation of ventricular arrhythmia. *Circulation* 65:886, 1982.

49. Grossman, L.A. and Grossman, M. Myocardial infarction precipitated by Master step test. *JAMA* 158:179, 1955.

50. Graboys, T.B., DeSilva, R.D., and Lown, B. Exercise stress testing and ambulatory monitoring in patients with malignant ventricular arrhythmia. *Am. J. Cardiol.* 41:400, 1978.

51. Doyle, J.T. and Kinch, S.H. The prognosis of an abnormal electrocardiographic stress test. *Circulation* 41:545, 1970.

52. Ellestad, M.H., Allen, W., Wan, M.C., and Kemp, G.L. Maximal treadmill stress testing for cardiovascular evaluation. Circulation 39:517, 1969.

53. Kattus, A. and McAlpin, R.N. Diagnosis, medical and surgical management of coronary insufficiency. *Ann. Intern. Med.* 69:115, 1968.

54. Irving, J.B. and Bruce, R.A. Exertional hypotension and postexertional ventricular fibrillation in stress testing. *Am. J. Cardiol.* 39:849, 1977.

55. Rochmis, P. and Blackburn, H. Exercise tests: A survey of procedures, safety and litigation experience in approximately 170,000 tests. *JAMA* 217:1061, 1971.

56. Young, D., Lampert, S., Graboys, T.B., and Lown B. Safety of maximal exercise testing in patients at high risk for ventricular arrhythmia. *Circulation* 70:184, 1984.

57. Graboys, T.B. *The Role of Ambulatory Electrocardiographic Monitoring, Exercise Stress Testing* and *Electrophysiologic Studies in the Management of Patients with Malignant Ventricular Arrhythmia.* J. Roelaadt and P. Hugenholtz (eds). The Hague, Netherlands: Martinus Nijhoff, 1982, pp. 79–87.

58. McHenry, P.L., Fisch, C., Jordan, J.W., and Corya, B.R. Cardiac arrhythmias observed during maximal treadmill exercise testing in clinically normal men. *Am. J. Cardiol.* 29:331, 1972.

59. Graboys, T.B. Limitations of Ambulatory Electrocardiographic Recordings to Assess Antiarrhythmic Drug Efficacy. In N. Wenger et al. (eds.), *Ambulatory Electrocardiographic Recording.* Chicago: Year Book Medical Publications, p. 367, 1981.

60. Gooch, A.S. Exercise testing for detecting changes in cardiac rhythm and conduction. *Am. J. Cardiol.* 30:741, 1972.

61. Wright, R.F. and Graboys, T.B. Provocation of supraventricular tachycardia during exercise stress testing. *Cardiovasc. Rev. Reports* 1:57, 1980.

62. Force, T. and Graboys, T.B. Exercise testing and ambulatory monitoring in patients with preexcitation syndrome. *Arch. Int. Medicine* 141:88, 1981.

63. Antman, E., Graboys, T.B., and Lown, B. Comparison of continuous to intermittent electrocardiographic monitoring during exercise testing for exposure of cardiac arrhythmias. JAMA 241:2805, 1979.

64. Lopez, L.V., Conde, C., Castellanos, A., and Myerburg, R.J. Decreased frequency of exercise-induced ventricular ectopic activity in the second of two consecutive treadmill tests. *Circulation* 55:892, 1977.

65. Lamb, C.E. and Hiss, R.G. Influence of exercise on premature contractions. *Am. J. Cardiol.* 10:209, 1962.

66. Froelicher, V.F., Thompson, A.J., Longo, M.R., Triebwasser, J.H., and Lancaster, M. Value of exercise testing for screening asymptomatic men for latent coronary artery disease. *Prog. Cardiovasc. Dis.* 18:265, 1976.

67. Graboys, T.B. and Lown B. Exercise testing among an asymptomatic YMCA population. Unpublished observations.

68. Kennedy, L.H. and Underhill, S.J. Frequent or complex ventricular ectopy in apparently healthy subjects. *Am. J. Cardiol.* 38:141, 1976.

69. McHenry, P.L., Faris, J.V., Jordan, J.W., and Morris, S.N. Comparative study of cardiovascular function and premature ventricular complexes in smokers and nonsmokers during maximal treadmill exercise. *Am. J. Cardiol.* 39:493, 1977.

70. Ekblom, B., Hartley, L.H., and Day, W.C. Occurrence and reproducibility of exercise-induced ventricular ectopy in normal subjects. *Am. J. Cardiol.* 43:35, 1979.

71. Goldschlager, N., Cake, I., and Cohn, K. Exercise-induced ventricular arrhythmias in patients with coronary artery disease. *Am. J. Cardiol.* 31:434, 1973.

72. McHenry, P.L., Morris, S.N., and Kavalier, M. Clinical significance of exercise-induced ventricular arrhythmias. *Am. J. Cardiol.* 33:154, 1974.

73. Udall, J.A. and Ellestad, M.H. Predictive implications of ventricular premature contractions associated with treadmill stress testing. *Circulation* 56:985, 1977.

74. Helfant, R.H., Pine, R., Kabde, V., and Banka, V.S. Exercise-related ventricular premature complexes in coronary heart disease: Correlation with ischemia and angiographic severity. *Ann. Intern. Med.* 80:589, 1974.

75. Zaret, B.L. and Conti, C.R., Jr. Exercise-induced ventricular irritability: Hemodynamic and angiographic correlations. *Am. J. Cardiol.* 29:298, 1972.

76. Graboys, T.B. The stampede to stimulation—numerators and denominators revisited relative to electrophysiologic study of ventricular arrhythmias. *Am. Heart J.* 103:1089, 1982.

77. Horowitz, L.N., Josephson, M.E., and Kastor, J.A. Intracardiac electrophysiologic studies as a method for the optimization of drug therapy in chronic ventricular arrhythmia. *Prog. Cardiovasc. Dis.* 23:81, 1980.

78. Ruskin, J.N., DiMarco, J.P., and Garan, H. Out of hospital cardiac arrest. Electrophysiologic observations and selection of long-term antiarrhythmic therapy. *N. Engl. J. Med.* 303:1073, 1980.

79. Mason, J.W. and Winkle, R.A. Electrode catheter arrhythmia induction in the selection and assessment of antiarrhythmic drug therapy in recurrent ventricular tachycardia. *Circulation* 58:771, 1978.

80. Livelli, F.D., Bigger, J.T, Reiffel, J.A. Gang, E.S., Patton, J.N., Noethling, P.M., Rolnitz Ky, L.M., and Gliklich, J.I. Response to programmed stimulation: Sensitivity, specificity and relation to heart disease. *Am. J. Cardiol.* 50:452, 1982.

81. Podrid, P.J., Schoenberger, A., Lown, B., Lampert, S., Matos, J., Porterfield, J., Raeder, E., and Corrigan, E. Use of nonsustained ventricular tachycardia as a guide to antiarrhythmic drug

therapy in patients with malignant ventricular arrhythmia. *Am. Heart J.* 105:181, 1983.

82. Brugada, P., Green, M., Abdollah, H., and Wellens, H.J.J. Significance of ventricular arrhythmias initiated by programmed ventricular stimulation. *Circulation* 69:87, 1984.

83. Richards, D.A., Cody, D.V., Denniss, A.R. Russell, P.A., Young, A.A., Uther, J.B. Ventricular electrical instability: A predictor of death after myocardial infarction. *Am. J. Cardiol.* 51:75, 1983.

84. Lister, J.W., Stein, E., Kosowsky, B.D., Lau, S.H., and Damato, A.N. Atrioventricular conduction in man: Effect of rate, exercise, isoproterenol, and atropine on the P-R interval. *Am. J. Cardiol.* 16:516, 1965.

85. DeMaria, A.N., Vera, Z., Amsterdam, E.A., Mason, D.T., and Massemi, R.A. Disturbances of cardiac rhythm and conduction induced by exercise. *Am. J. Cardiol.* 33:732, 1974.

86. Lichstein, E., Letavati, A., Gupta, P.K., and Chadda, K.D. Continuous Holter monitoring of patients with bifascicular block complicating anterior wall myocardial infarction. *Am. J. Cardiol.* 40:860, 1977.

87. Dhingra, R.C., Denes, P., Win, D., Chuquimia, R., Amat-y-Leon, F., Syndham, C., and Rosen, K.M. Syncope in patients with chronic bifascicular block. *Ann. Intern. Med.* 81:302, 1974.

88. Denes, P., Dhingra, R.L., Wu, D., Wyndham, C., Amat-y-Leon, F., and Rose, K. Sudden death in patients with chronic bifascicular block. *Arch. Intern. Med.* 137:1005, 1977.

89. Bardol, S.S. and Friedberg, H.D. Second-degree atrioventricular block: A matter of definition. *Am. J. Cardiol.* 33:311, 1974.

# 6. EXERCISE TESTING

Robert A. Bruce

Peter F. Cohn

The current concept of exercise testing is that through the use of a standardized, multistage protocol, an informative, noninvasive extension of the clinical examination of ambulatory persons is provided. Exercise testing generates qualitative and quantitative functional information that aids in the evaluation of the subject's cardiovascular system. Although its diagnostic value is limited to functional mechanisms instead of morphologic causes, it has more prognostic potential than is generally recognized. It supplements the history as well as the physical and electrocardiographic (ECG) examinations of the patient at rest; it can be repeated to evaluate the changes occurring as a result of either the progression of chronic cardiovascular disease or appropriate medical or surgical treatment, physical training, or both. Most important to all physicians, it can easily be incorporated into the routine evaluation of office or clinic patients, even on the initial workup.

Several major controversies, however, warrant review and evaluation. They may be reduced to simple questions regarding whether to test exercise performance, whom to test, and how to test, along with what the results mean. Further controversies include cost effectiveness and whether it has a future in competition with other established and developing noninvasive methods of appraising cardiovascular structure and function. Details abound about criteria for selection or exclusion of persons for testing, methods of testing, adequacy of normal standards of reference, and criteria for interpretation of responses that are also controversial.

Experience with exercise testing has evolved slowly and progressively over the past half-century. Our purpose is not to provide a detailed analysis of an extensive literature that is available elsewhere [1–4], but rather to provide an orientation and perspective that are significantly influenced by our experience with exercise testing, especially as performed by the many physicians who have participated in the prospective community study of the Seattle Heart Watch [5]. This approach is justified by the fact that the study represents a broad spectrum of persons sampled in relation to the cardiovascular problems of coronary heart disease or hypertension, the major causes of mortality and morbidity in the middle-aged sector of the American population. Unlike other population studies, this study uses symptom-limited maximal exercise testing without the potentially hazardous restrictions of arbitrary target heart rates. Equally important, follow-up surveillance for any subsequent cardiovascular morbidity or mortality has been achieved on several thousand men for up to 10 years. New insights about cross-sectional functional differences in relation to disease allow an analysis of the changes in functional limitations with age versus disease, and they clarify the predictive potential of noninvasive clinical and exercise variables. The magnitude of variation in longitudinal observations has also been defined. On the basis of this experience, not as yet duplicated elsewhere to our knowledge, a new frame of reference is provided in which several controversies may be reassessed. No claim is made that the final resolution of any of them has been achieved, but this information may stimulate further active investigation by others.

From a historical perspective, interest in the physiologic responses to exercise has shifted between cardiovascular, respiratory, and electrocardiographic variables. Although the cardiorespiratory variables were considered before the twentieth century, Einthoven [6] in 1908 first observed the increase in ECG voltage of P- and T-waves, as well as in heart rate, as a consequence of the exertion of stair climbing. In 1928 Feil and Siegel [7] observed ST-T changes in association with both spontaneous and exercise-induced angina; they also reported changes in relation to treatment with nitroglycerin. In 1929 Master [8] published his two-step test, using moderate exertion adjusted for sex and body weight, as a technique for the functional evaluation of the cardiovascular system. He later published variations in foot-pounds of energy expenditure with age in both men and women that resemble corresponding differences in functional aerobic capacity [9]. Years later, he added to the procedure ECG recording after exertion and changed the objective of such testing to the detection or diagnosis of coronary insufficiency by means of ST-T changes [10]. This objective has remained the primary concern of physicians for the last three to four decades, especially when follow-up observations by Mattingly [11] and Robb, Marks, and co-workers [12, 13] revealed the predictive value of such abnormal responses for coronary disease.

Meanwhile, others explored the possibility of increasing the diagnostic sensitivity of exercise testing by permitting progressive increments in workloads up to the symptom-limited capacity of asymptomatic, healthy, middle-aged men; this refinement seemed to augment the prevalence of ST depression about two- to threefold in various population samples [14–16]. With the advent of the independent diagnosis of coronary heart disease by coronary arteriography, the clinical value of the ST criterion was seriously questioned: an excessive number of false-positive and false-negative responses were demonstrated in coronary patients, thereby documenting less than optimal diagnostic discrimination [17–20]. The risk of false-positive results has also been pointed out to increase in populations with a low prevalence of disease, and the need to consider both the prior clinical classification

of the individual and the associated responses to exercise has been emphasized [21–23].

## Reasons for and Risks Involved with Exercise Testing

The feasibility and relative safety of multistage treadmill testing of symptom-limited maximal exercise is clearly established in the Seattle community (figure 6–1). The overall clinical experience indicates that such testing supplements the routine history, often helping patients to clarify points of uncertainty or to recall additional, previously forgotten details. It reveals transient changes in the data of physical and ECG examinations that often indicate the presence of heart disease. Such testing also allows differentiation of angina pectoris from various nonspecific chest wall syndromes and anxiety-induced muscle tension states, which usually are not reproduced and which may be alleviated by exercise testing. ECG evidence may be detected regarding exertional or postexertional arrhythmias, ST depression or elevation, and the inability to raise or to sustain systolic pressure because of acute power failure of the left ventricle. (Exercise testing to detect arrhythmias will be commented on only briefly in this chapter because it is discussed at length in chapter 5.) Systolic clicks of mitral valve prolapse, the systolic murmur of papillary muscle dysfunction, and diastolic gallops may be identified.

Once the physician has ascertained the possibility, probability, or certainty of heart disease on the basis of the preliminary history and physical and ECG examinations, he or she should usually supervise the exercise test personally because valuable, noninvasive information is often gained at this time. In general, the presence of a physician is recommended at all tests, but such presence is felt to be mandatory for testing patients with known or suspected heart disease. Thus, exercise testing is properly considered a desirable and informative extension of the initial clinical examination of ambulatory persons with suspected or known heart disease. Equally important, a negative or normal response gives reassurance that even maximal exertion, often to above average-normal performance, does not reveal clinically significant symptoms or signs of

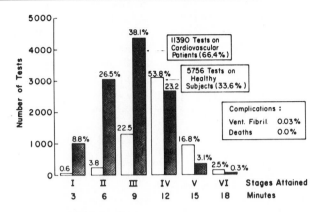

FIGURE 6–1. 17,146 multistage treadmill tests of symptom-limited maximal exercise in fifteen testing facilities (Seattle experience, 6 years, July 1, 1971 to July 1, 1977.)

possible heart disease at this point in the life of an individual concerned about health status.

A significant issue in exercise testing is the risk involved and the attendant responsibilities of the physician. Several concepts have emerged in published reports from large series of testing. A small risk exists of myocardial infarction and ventricular fibrillation, both of which, as in any setting, can lead to death. Rochmis and Blackburn [24], in their national survey of 73 testing laboratories that included 170,000 tests, found 16 deaths reported, or a $\frac{1}{10,000}$ risk, and an approximately $\frac{3}{10,000}$ risk of morbidity. These events were divided equally between maximal and submaximal tests, but a determination of the comparative risk between the two approaches cannot be made because the frequency of use of each method is not known. Although submaximal testing has been said to carry less risk than maximal testing [25, 26], adequate data are not available to prove or disprove that point. A rare instance of unexpected acute myocardial infarction associated with the thermal stress of a hot shower shortly after a maximal exercise test in a normal middle-aged male has been reported; the infarction was followed by cardiac arrest that required ventricular defibrillation and by eventual recovery. Subsequent cardiac catheterization revealed a 90 percent stenosis of the circumflex artery and a small aneurysm [27].

The risk also depends on the test population. Gibbons and associates [28], reporting on 15,-000 maximal tests, of which 83 percent were normal, cited four events (two with myocardial infarction and two with ventricular fibrillation) without death. Three events were in patients with known cardiac disease, yielding the low risk of morbidity of $\frac{1}{12,000}$ of an event in a presumably normal patient.

Certain patients are at greater risk. Myocardial infarction has been reported in testing patients with angina decubitus during Master's test [29], for example, and one of the deaths in the review by Rochmis and Blackburn (24) was in a patient with an unrecognized acute infarction prior to the test. Because of this, it is absolutely essential that a careful history and physical examination with a resting 12-lead ECG be done prior to the test to exclude such conditions.

We have updated our unpublished data since the 1977 report of the Seattle Heart Watch and Exercise Registry experience [30] depicted in figure 6–2. To date, nine cases of ventricular fibrillation have occurred in the approximately 31,000 maximal tests (.03 percent incidence); there were no deaths [Bruce, unreported observations, 1984]. All these cases of ventricular fibrillation occurred in *men* with a *history of coronary heart disease* who had *exertional hypotension* defined as less than a 10 mmHg rise from resting levels or a fall below the normal resting level. (The usual responses of the blood pressure in stage 1 of the Bruce protocol are an increase of 20 mmHg in patients with angina and 30

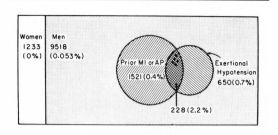

FIGURE 6–2. Relative risk of postexertional ventricular fibrillation in the Seattle population tested (1,233 women and 9,518 men; 10,751 total). Five men experienced ventricular fibrillation (black dots); all five had both exertional hypotension and prior angina pectoris (AP) or myocardial infarction (MI). The overall risk ratio is therefore 5/10,751 (0.047 percent). (From Irving, J.B. and Bruce, R.A. *Am. J. Cardiol.* 39:849, 1977.)

mmHg in normal men.) In this group (see figure 6–2) the relative risk of ventricular fibrillation was 2.2 percent; all such episodes occurred early in recovery from exercise of short duration.

McHenry [31] reported on 12,000 tests in a presumably similar population without noting any episode of ventricular fibrillation. Blood pressures were recorded every minute, with repetition every 15 seconds if a reduction was noted. Tests were terminated if a reduction of 10 mmHg was sustained over two readings. The implication that this approach to the early detection of hypotension may reduce the incidence of ventricular fibrillation is worth consideration, but it should be used with the awareness that pressure recordings may not rise normally in the first minute or two of the test, not until an initially anxious patient with a minor pressure elevation gains confidence with the test protocol.

Thus, the risk of testing is small, and safety can be ensured by carefully following well-accepted guidelines, as outlined in the following exercise testing prerequisites:

1. Select only ambulatory persons without evidence of acute or recent illness.
2. Give preliminary clinical and ECG examinations and classify heart disease.
3. Precede patient orientation and consent with brief demonstration of method.
4. Monitor symptoms and signs: ECG (rhythm) and systolic pressure (each minute).
5. Record duration of exertion, peak heart rate, and systolic pressure.
6. Have emergency facilities and skills immediately available.
7. Provide independent observers, computer processing, or both, of ST responses.

Legal issues of professional liability in testing and informed consent have been reviewed elsewhere [32, 33].

## Who to Test and When

Exercise testing can be used to quantify functional cardiovascular capacity, either individually or in comparison to group norms. It can also be used to determine the diagnosis, prognosis, or both in coronary artery disease, and it is helpful in defining the safety or risk of undertaking certain levels of exertion. Exercise testing is used clinically in three major groups of patients; asymptomatic adults, patients with chest pain of uncertain cause, and patients with known coronary heart disease. It is used for different purposes, however, in each group, and the significance of the information gained differs in each setting.

For an asymptomatic adult, exercise testing is of most value in determining the prognosis or risk and in demonstrating the safety of undertaking a vigorous training program. For the evaluation of atypical chest pain, such testing can be of some diagnostic value. In patients with probable angina or already diagnosed coronary heart disease, testing is of lesser use diagnostically, but it has utility in prognosis, quantification of cardiac capacity, and definition of the safety and advisability of various levels of exertion; the last is especially useful in cardiac rehabilitation programs (see chapter 16). For a discussion of the use of exercise testing in detecting arrhythmias, refer to chapter 5.

DIAGNOSTIC POTENTIAL OF ST RESPONSES
We believe that the *overall* diagnostic potential of ST responses to exercise testing is limited [34]. In spite of the abundance of attention directed to and controversy about this aspect, attempts to justify the diagnostic value of ST responses should be balanced against arguments of its ineffectiveness [35, 36].

Many studies of the sensitivity (i.e., percentage of abnormal responses correctly detected) and specificity (percentage of normal responses correctly identified) of ST depression as a diagnostic sign of exertional myocardial ischemia due to coronary vascular stenosis have been added to the literature in recent years. Koppes and co-workers [1] summarized many of these studies, finding an average sensitivity of 69 percent and a specificity of 90 percent when ischemic ST changes in maximal or near-maximal exercise tests are compared arteriographically. Thus, 31 percent of the patients with anatomic disease are not detected (false-negatives), and 10 percent of normal subjects appear to have ischemic ST depression (false-positives).

Many attempts have been made to preselect patients to improve the diagnostic correlation between the exercise test and coronary anatomy, but three important considerations must not be overlooked. First, ST depression is merely a *functional* sign of an abnormal metabolic supply-demand relationship at the myocardial cell membrane; it does not indicate the cause, anatomic or otherwise, of that abnormality.

In addition to coronary heart disease (which is common in economically developed populations), other causes of ST depression include anemia; hypoxemia due to high altitude or bronchopulmonary disease; binding of hemoglobin with carbon monoxide; myocardial hypertrophy whether idiopathic or secondary to hypertension or valvular heart disease; hypokalemia; treatment with digitalis; or various combinations of these factors. Another mechanism observed by Kasser and Bruce [37] with maximal exercise testing of asymptomatic men may be excessive hemodynamic stress. When performance was compared with that of slightly younger peers without ST depression, the maximal heart rate and systolic pressure, age adjusted by covariance analysis, were higher and the duration of exercise longer in those who exhibited ST depression.

Middle-aged women show false-positive postexertional ST depression more frequently than men [38]. Their hematocrits are lower than those of men, which affects oxygen capacity. Furthermore, invasive hemodynamic observations revealed higher pulmonary and systemic arterial pressures and resistance with higher pressure-rate products in asymptomatic middle-aged women who exhibit ST depression after maximal exercise [39]. Also, evidence of myocardial ischemia associated with angina and ST changes in the presence of normal coronaries have been reported (chapter 4). Linhart and colleagues [40] have argued, however, that in women with normal resting ECGs who are not on medication, the false-positive rate is similar to that in men.

The second issue in the use of ST depression for diagnosis concerns the strong impact that the prevalence of disease in a certain clinical subgroup has upon the significance of normal or abnormal ST changes for that group. The appropriate statistical index is *predictive value* [41], that is, the percentage of patients with a positive test who have disease or, alternatively, the percentage with a negative test who do not have disease. This index is influenced not only by the commonly emphasized sensitivity and specificity of a test, but also by the prevalence of disease in the test population. In low-prevalence groups the predictive value of a positive test can be significantly diminished by a high ratio of false-positive to true-positive results, even at a specificity of 90 percent. Likewise, in high-prevalence groups, the predictive value of a negative test for no disease is diminished by frequent false-negative results. For coronary heart disease, the prevalences in various clinical groups have been determined as follows: approximately 1 percent in asymptomatic males, depending on age; 10 percent in patients with chest pain that probably is not angina; 50 percent in patients with atypical chest pain; and 80 to 90 percent in patients with typical angina [1]. The predictive value or risk of disease with a positive exercise test ("posterior probability") may be compared with the risk established from prevalence data prior to the test ("prior probability") to determine whether there is any added value from the information generated by the test. The higher this increment, the greater the value of doing the test. The closer the posterior (posttest) probability is to unity, the greater its diagnostic power.

This approach has been developed in detail by Rifkin and Hood [21], who used the maximal likelihood ratio of the Bayesian method to document the relative gain in posterior probability over prior probability provided by the use of exercise testing. This study emphasizes the minimal diagnostic gain of exercise testing when the prevalence is very low, as in healthy young adults, because a high proportion of positive responses are false, perhaps as a result of excessive hemodynamic demand at maximal effort relative to a normal coronary supply of oxygenated blood. Likewise, the study documents little gain in diagnostic significance in patients who are carefully selected for angina pectoris, because the prior probability of disease is already very high. In addition, other confounding variables occur in this group that may distort the ST response, especially in patients with prior infarction, cardiac enlargement, marked abnormalities of ventricular contraction, transmural ischemia with ST elevation, or some combination of these disorders. Under such conditions the sensitivity may be lowered due to the excessive proportion of false-negative responses, as will the predictive value of a negative test in excluding coronary disease.

The greatest diagnostic gain occurs in the intermediate region of possible or probable but not definitely established coronary disease if other confounding variables—such as excessive hypertension, hypertrophy, anemia, hypoxemia, unexpected exertional pulmonary hypertension in women, marked hypokalemia, or a combination of such factors—are not operative. In this group, the probability of disease can rise from approximately 50 percent to over 90 percent after a positive exercise test.

The third point regarding the diagnostic value of the ST response is that manipulation of selection and exclusion criteria to try to optimize sensitivity and specificity may not significantly influence the predictive value of exercise testing over clinically achievable ranges. Thus, at the low prevalence seen in asymptomatic adults, a negative test changes the probability that the subject has a normal heart by only 1 percentage point (from 98 to 99 percent), and a positive test, far from being diagnostic, increases the probability of disease only from 2 percent to 10 or 15 percent [41]. The same consideration holds in reverse at the 90 percent prevalence level in patients with typical angina. In neither group is the

ST response to exercise of significant added diagnostic value. Furthermore, even if one could increase the sensitivity from 60 to 95 percent, at 95 percent specificity the posttest probability in the asymptomatic group (1 percent prevalence) would increase only 5 percent, from 10 to 15 percent, far from what could be considered "diagnostic" (i.e., 80 to 90 percent).

Thus, the controversy about the lack of diagnostic utility of exercise testing must be analyzed in statistical terms that relate the use of the test to subpopulations with varying disease prevalences. Even under optimal conditions when specificity and sensitivity might both reach 90 percent, the test still provides significant diagnostic information primarily in that subgroup of patients who have an expected disease prevalence of 30 to 70 percent. On the other hand, exercise testing, both in asymptomatic patients and in certain populations of patients with coronary heart disease, provides considerable *prognostic* information, and as such it can provide a significant dimension to the clinical analysis of risk factors.

PROGNOSTIC VALUE OF ST RESPONSES
Many studies have shown an increased risk of cardiac events and mortality over varying durations of follow-up in asymptomatic people with ischemic ST depression [1, 13], and this represents a risk factor that is independent of the other known risk factors [42]. Erikssen and coworkers [43] studied 2,014 healthy Norwegian men aged 40 to 59 and found 75 had ischemic ST depression of 1.5 mm or more at 0.08 msec from the J-point. Of these, 48 had demonstrable coronary artery disease on arteriography, yielding a predictive value of a positive test of 64 percent. While this value may not be close enough to certainty to be dependable in diagnosis, it clearly identifies a group that is obviously at high risk for coronary events over the next few years, and intervention regarding modifiable risk factors that may be present is warranted. Similar findings have been presented by Froelicher and associates [44].

The inference from the prior statements of the value and safety of exercise testing might be that all ambulatory persons should have at least one exercise test. This, however, is neither possible nor desirable. Accordingly, there is a need for guidelines, and the Seattle Heart Watch studies suggest additional new guidelines. In *asymptomatic, healthy men,* there is no significant prognostic gain over 3.3 years with respect to disease prediction on the basis of maximal exercise testing in about two-fifths of individuals, namely, those who are free from all four commonly accepted risk factors (figure 6–3) [45, 46]. These risk factors include a positive family history for cardiovascular disease, hypertension, hypercholesterolemia, and cigarette smoking. Among the remaining three-fifths of the population with any one or more of such risk factors, the vast majority have a normal exercise test without ST depression, and among them there is no significant increase in the risk of morbidity or mortality from coronary heart disease. Conversely, for the few with one or more risk factors as well as postexertional ischemic ST depression of 1 mm or more, the risk of primary coronary events within 3 years is significantly increased (approximately sevenfold). The interaction of these factors, as determined by sequential evaluation, identifies 3.5 percent of the original sample who warrant careful medical evaluation and follow-

up. Repeated exercise testing at 1- or 2-year intervals in those with risk factors and no ST depression initially also identifies a small fraction who develop ischemia and warrant more attention.

The use of exercise testing in patients with symptoms of typical angina or atypical chest pain has been extensively studied in comparison with findings at coronary angiography. The average sensitivity has been determined to be 69 percent and the specificity 90 percent among population samples with an average disease prevalence of 55 percent. The sensitivity ranged from 43 percent for single-vessel disease to 86 percent for three-vessel disease [1].

The prediction of the location of coronary arterial stenoses on the basis of ST changes during exercise requires a multilead system and has not been generally successful [47]. The *severity* of coronary disease in terms of the number of vessels involved does correlate with ST changes in testing. *In general, the greater the ST depression, the greater the chance of multivessel disease* [36, 48–50]. Among patients with 3 mm or more ST depression, a study by Goldman and associates [51] found 69 percent to have three-vessel disease and 92 percent anterior descending disease. The criterion is not specific, however, in that approximately one-third of patients with 1 to 2.9 mm ST depression also had three-vessel disease and two-thirds had anterior descending involvement. The data are similar for left main coronary artery disease [50].

Several groups [48–50] have found an increased risk of cardiac events over time according to the time of onset of ST changes or the workload level at which they developed; thus, the incidence of subsequent coronary events in patients who had 2 mm ST depression early in the exercise protocol was greatest and was usually indicative of severe disease.

A recent report of a 5- to 10-year follow-up of men without clinical evidence of coronary heart disease who were enrolled in the Seattle Heart Watch reveals the prognostic importance of the preliminary clinical classification before exercise testing in relation to the observation of ST depression with maximal exercise [52]. Among 2,-365 asymptomatic healthy men, 2,184 (92.34 percent) had no evident ST depression and 97.5

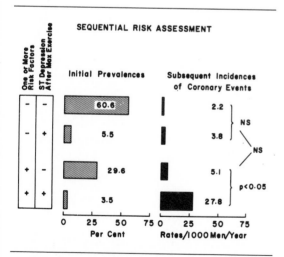

FIGURE 6–3. Relative importance of risk factors and ST depression in 2,760 men initially free of coronary heart disease. Note that significant risk is limited to a small group that has both risk factors and ST depression. (From Bruce, R.A. In McDonald, L. et al. (eds.), *Early Recognition of Coronary Heart Disease.* Amsterdam: Excerpta Medica, 1978.)

percent survived 6 years without a primary coronary heart disease event (figure 6–4A). Of the remaining 181 (7.7 percent) with ischemic ST depression after maximal exercise, only 93.6 percent survived 6 years without a primary coronary heart disease event (p < .001). Among 632 men with hypertension, 560 (88.6 percent) had no ST depression, and 92 percent of those remained free of primary coronary heart disease events for 6 years (figure 6–4B). In contrast, of the 72 (11.4 percent) with ischemic ST depression, only 80 percent remained free of these events for 6 years (p < .05). Among 549 men with atypical chest pain syndromes specifically not angina pectoris, 90.5 percent had no ischemic ST depression after maximal exercise and 95 percent lived over 6 years without primary coronary heart disease events (figure 6–4C). Nevertheless, of 95 percent with ischemic ST depression after maximal exercise, only 85 percent remained free of these events for 6 years (p < .001). The lesser predictive value of ST depression in hypertension, despite its greater prevalence, may reflect the imbalance between myocardial oxygen supply and increased demand as a result of greater mass of cardiac muscle. Prognosis was better in healthy men than in men with atypical chest pain syndromes, whether or not they manifested ST depression.

Inasmuch as patients with atypical chest pain syndromes may make differential diagnosis difficult, it is important to note that the number of conventional risk factors as well as ST depression and functional aerobic impairment are statistically important predictors of risk of primary coronary heart disease events in later years. A low-risk group of patients—41 percent of those patients with atypical chest pain syndromes and without any of these risk variables—has a 97 percent chance of 6-year survival without coronary heart disease events (figure 6–5). An intermediate-risk group (42 percent of such patients) has a corresponding survival rate of 93 percent. In contrast, the high-risk group (17 percent of these patients), with all these risk variables, has a reduced survival rate of 83 percent (p < .001). As for ST depression in these patients, the prognostic sensitivity at 6 years of follow-up is only 73 percent and the specificity is 79 percent.

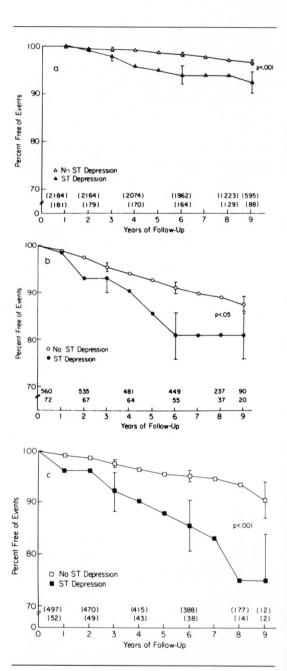

FIGURE 6–4. Life table analysis for percentage of group remaining free of primary coronary heart disease events in (A) asymptomatic men, (B) hypertensive men, and (C) men with atypical chest pain, according to the presence (closed symbols) or absence (open symbols) of ST depression. The difference between asymptomatic men and men with atypical chest pain is apparent in those with and without ST depression, indicating the importance of clinical classification. (From Hossack, K.F., Bruce, R.A., Fisher, L., and Hofer, V. *Int. J. Cardiol.* 3:37, 1983.)

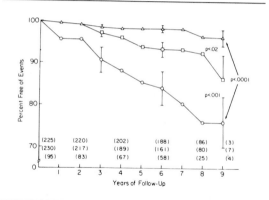

FIGURE 6–5. A life table analysis indicating the difference in percentage remaining free of primary coronary heart disease events in the low-risk (△), medium-risk (○), and high-risk (═) groups in men with atypical chest pain. (From Hossack, K.F., Bruce, R.A., Fisher, L., and Hofer, V. *Int. J. Cardiol.* 3:37, 1983.)

In addition to ST segment depression, ST elevation may occasionally occur during exercise. It is much more common in patients with prior myocardial infarctions [53, 54]. Because the ECG abnormalities are nearly always in the area of the prior infarction and asynergy is usually present, their significance is unclear except that ST segment elevation in leads $V_1$ and/or AVL reliably predicts significant disease of the left anterior descending coronary artery, even when a prior arterior wall infarction has not occurred [55]. Whether these ECG abnormalities indicate that these patients are more susceptible to coronary spasm [56] requires further study.

## OTHER MEASUREMENTS BESIDES ST CHANGES

As has been repeatedly emphasized, exercise testing provides more information than ST changes, and such additional information is now receiving attention. The change in R-wave magnitude from rest to near-maximum exertion is one of these additional measurements. Ellestad and co-workers [57] were the first to point out that the R-wave tends to decrease in normal subjects and to remain the same or increase in coronary patients. In their studies the R-wave increase with exertion in patients with coronary heart disease correlated with the severity of cor-

onary disease and with left ventricular contraction abnormalities. In a study sample that included many patients with false-positive ST segment responses, analyses of the changes in the R-wave, rather than in the ST segment, increased sensitivity from 48 to 63 percent and specificity from 59 to 79 percent [58]. Since the initial report by Ellestad and co-workers, a host of reports have either confirmed (59) or refuted (60) the diagnostic utility of R-wave changes. The mechanism of the R-wave changes has also been challenged. Initially, these changes were attributed to the larger volumes in the transiently ischemic ventricle, but this has not been borne out in studies in which ventricular volumes during exercise were determined [61]. David et al. [62] have suggested instead that changes in intramyocardial conduction may be an important factor in the R-wave amplitude responses to active myocardial ischemia. In addition to the R-wave, ischemia-induced intraventricular conduction disturbances [63] and decreases in Q-wave amplitude [64] have been studied. Both are very uncommon occurrences, but like ST segment elevation in leads 1 and/or AVL, appear specific for significant disease of the left anterior descending coronary artery.

Heart rate and blood pressure changes also carry significance. Ellestad [3] found that a subnormal heart rate response without ST changes carried the same risk as ischemic ST changes and a normal rate response, with an event incidence of about 15 percent per year. Exertional hypotension, as discussed earlier, carries a strong correlation with two- and three-vessel disease and with left main coronary artery lesions. Not surprisingly, therefore, such patients have a poorer prognosis than do patients with normal blood pressure responses [65].

As would be expected, the development of angina during a test changes the prognostic significance over that of ST changes alone. Patients with angina associated with ischemic ST changes on a near-maximal testing protocol had twice the rate of events over a 4-year follow-up as did those with positive ST changes without pain [3]. Also, patients with angina occurring at 4 METS had twice the rate of events as those with angina at 8 to 9 METS of energy expenditure.

The importance of blood pressure, ST

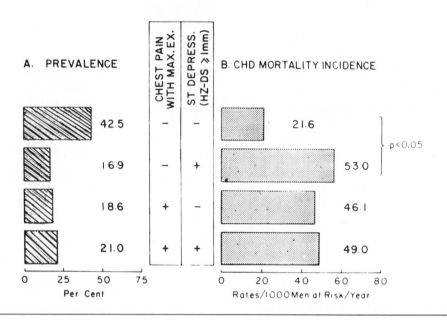

FIGURE 6–6. Risk for death from coronary heart disease (CHD) in relation to ST depression or chest pain with maximal exercise. (From Bruce, R.A. Reprinted, by permission from the *New England Journal of Medicine,* 296:671, 1977.)

changes, the test duration, presence of angina, and other clinical variables has been analyzed in the Seattle Heart Watch data. For ambulatory men *with clinical manifestations of coronary heart disease* on the basis of a typical history of angina pectoris, prior myocardial infarction, or prior cardiac arrest with resuscitation by ventricular defibrillation, the occurrence either of chest pain on exercise testing or of ischemic, horizontal or downsloping ST depression of 1 mm or more after maximal exercise testing is not strongly predictive of future cardiac mortality risks (figure 6–6). Conversely, *cardiomegaly,* as determined by chest roentgenography, combined with the exercise variables of *duration* of maximal exercise and *systolic pressure responses* are indications of disease severity, and such data are important in estimating the prognosis for cardiac mortality (figure 6–7). The purpose of testing in this context is *not* to make a diagnosis of coronary disease that is already clinically evident, but rather to assess the severity of impairment along with the mechanisms limiting left ventricular function and to help obtain guidelines to indicate the *optimal time for invasive studies* for localizing and quantifying the disease that is present.

A recent additional use of exercise testing has been in patients with resolving myocardial infarction prior to discharge from the hospital. Clinical experience indicates that up to 40 to 50 percent of all myocardial infarction patients have no significant complications during their hospitalization and can be safely discharged as early as the seventh day (see chapter 13). A *low-level* multistage exercise test, performed to the level of 2 to 3 METs or to the *first appearance* of symptoms (i.e., the symptom threshold), can be done safely prior to hospital discharge [66]. Since the test is designed to duplicate the activity levels that might be encountered at home during convalescence, it can demonstrate the safety and appropriateness of the anticipated discharge. It also integrates well into programs of early rehabilitation (see chapter 16) by increasing the patient's confidence about returning to an unsupervised home environment and by providing a pulse-rate limit for monitoring activity in the early stages of recovery. Perhaps most impor-

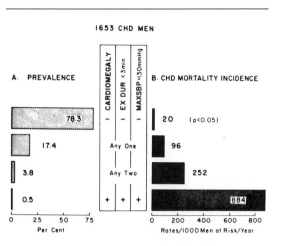

1653 CHD MEN

A. PREVALENCE

CARDIOMEGALY
EX DUR <3min
MAXSBP<130mmHg

B. CHD MORTALITY INCIDENCE

78.3

20 (p<0.05)

17.4     Any One     96

3.8     Any Two     252

0.5     + + +     884

0   25   50   75         0   200   400   600   800
Per Cent          Rates/1000 Men at Risk/Year

FIGURE 6–7. Risk gradient for death from coronary heart disease (CHD) in relation to absence or presence of cardiomegaly or exercise parameters of impaired limits of left ventricular function (exercise duration and maximum systolic blood pressure). Note that 78 percent of patients have lowest risk. (From Bruce, R.A. Reprinted, by permission from the *New Engl. J. of Med.,* 296:671, 1977.)

tantly, information of prognostic (and even therapeutic) value can be acquired, since patients with abnormal responses have a much poorer 1-year survival [66].

A controlled multicenter clinical trial of early cardiac rehabilitation, particularly supervised physical conditioning exercises of 258 randomized patients hospitalized for acute myocardial infarction, revealed unexpected findings [67]. When the same low-level exercise test was used at discharge from the hospital and repeated 3 months later, there were no significant cross-sectional differences in duration of exercises, prevalence of ST displacements, heart rate, or blood pressure responses between exercised and nonexercised control patients at either time. Furthermore, both groups showed equivalent longitudinal improvement after three months of convalescence. This was manifested by a lower resting heart rate and higher systolic and diastolic pressures at rest and submaximal exercise. With symptom-limited exercise testing at 3 months and again at 6 months, there was no further improvement in these variables. As for ECG responses at discharge and at 3 months, presence of arrhythmias (chiefly premature

beats) increased from 20 to 34 percent, whereas prevalence of ST elevation and ST depression decreased from 17 to 5.6 percent and 40 to 27.4 percent, respectively.

## How to Test Exercise Performance and Capacity

### TESTING DEVICES

Whether one uses a series of steps, a stationary bicycle, a treadmill, or a reverse escalator for testing ambulatory persons (or some form of arm work in the case of paraplegics or others), the important physiologic principles are to use a familiar type of exertion that involves large muscle masses and that does not require additional training or skills, to begin with a low workload, to increase the load continuously as a step function every 3 minutes or as a semiramp function at shorter intervals, and to continue until symptom-limited exercise capacity is attained. In about 2 percent of persons, exertion should be stopped before the symptom-limited capacity is achieved because of the sudden manifestation of incapacitation or potentially dangerous signs (see the later section End-Points for Stopping Test).

The relative advantages of various testing devices have been debated. A comparative analysis has been published by the American Heart Association [68, 69]. *Step tests,* such as that designed and popularized by Master, offer the advantages of low cost and portability and use muscular movements that people execute daily. Master's protocol has the advantage of being well studied, so that findings in an individual patient can be related to an epidemiologic data base in terms of the actual presence of coronary disease and the risk of a future coronary event. It suffers, however, in design inasmuch as it substantially overworks the underweight individual and spares the overweight person, even though the number of trips is adjusted for body weight [70]. It also reduces sensitivity by being a submaximal test for all but significantly impaired patients. Disadvantages with step tests also include problems with irregular stepping, tripping, and stumbling; difficulty in obtaining adequate ECG signals during exercise because of motion artifact; and inability to record exercise blood pressures.

The *bicycle ergometer* offers the advantages of relatively low expense compared to treadmills, more stability of the torso to ensure a good ECG signal, as well as easy recording of blood pressures during exercise. Disadvantages include reliance on patient motivation as the sole determinant generating a work output and technical difficulty in maintaining an accurate calibration of the workload unless the Åstrand-type ergometer is used. In addition, the most common limiting symptom is quadriceps pain and weakness rather than the more generalized fatigue that appears on the treadmill test. Furthermore, the systolic pressure response is augmented above that for an equivalent workload during walking [71].

Advantages of a *treadmill* include the use of a familiar type of exercise, a workload that is independent of voluntary factors, and widespread clinical experience. Techniques to reduce ECG signal noise due to movement artifact have been well worked out, but blood pressure recording may be more difficult than on the bicycle, particularly at workloads that require running.

Despite the greater cost of motor-driven treadmills, they represent precision instruments for the differentiation between abnormal and normal functional limits because the workloads are regulated involuntarily, thereby reducing a major variation in observations. This advantage is obtainable, however, only if part of the subject's body weight is not supported by handrails: since the energy requirement for work against gravity is proportioned to the body weight, this advantage will be vitiated if the individual is allowed to support part of his or her body weight by grasping the handrails. The effect of such support can make an average difference in duration of 3.5 minutes—for example, from 14 to 17.5 minutes for active young adults—using the Bruce protocol.

The bicycle ergometer and the treadmill also produce minor physiologic differences [71]. The same persons achieve slightly higher ventilation, oxygen uptake, heart rate, and lactate production, as well as increased cardiac output, when tested on a treadmill. Arterial pressures are higher on a bicycle ergometer at the same

aerobic requirement, even without holding the handlebars (arterial pressure effect is accentuated by a vigorous handgrip). This provides an additional limitation, at least for the cardiac patient, by augmenting the afterload imposed on an ischemic or infarct-scarred left ventricle, as well as accentuating initial regurgitation in a patient with valvular disease. In view of these considerations, the treadmill is preferred for most applications, and with the advent of small and even portable models, it has become the prevailing type of ergometer adopted for routine clinical use, even in office practice, in the United States.

MAXIMAL OXYGEN UPTAKE

The maximal oxygen consumption per minute ($VO_2$ max) per kilogram of body weight at the symptom limit of exercise involving large muscle groups is a reproducible ($r = +0.98$) physiologic limit that represents the maximal aerobic capacity of an individual [72]. In the presence of a normal hematocrit, oxygen dissociation curve, pulmonary function, and neuromuscular and skeletal systems, this capacity is limited by cardiac output and peripheral extraction (as represented by the arterial mixed-venous oxygen difference), and it provides a useful index to each of these variables.

For submaximal work that requires the use of large muscle groups (over 60 percent of body muscle mass), the oxygen uptake increases in direct proportion to the workload up to a maximal limiting value. Beyond this plateau value, increases in workload are not associated with further increments in oxygen consumption, and the body relies on an aerobic glycolysis at this point to supply the extra energy required. Shortly thereafter, exhaustion is reached.

The maximal oxygen uptake thus represents a defined physiologic limit that is relatively uninfluenced by the skill or motivation of an ambulatory person in performing the exercise, and it can be used as a reproducible measure of physiologic fitness [73]. Normal standards have been established, and average values for the maximal oxygen uptake are in the range of 30 to 45 ml/kg/min for the sedentary middle-aged male population [72]; the highest values of 80 to 85 ml/kg/min appear in endurance athletes, such

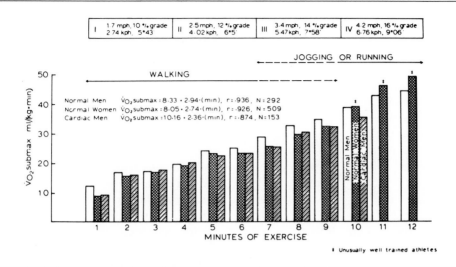

FIGURE 6–8. Variations in oxygen costs (VO₂), weight-adjusted, for middle-aged, healthy men and women with cardiovascular disease. (From Bruce, R.A. et al. Maximal oxygen intake and nomographic assessment of functional aerobic impairment in cardiovascular disease. *Am. Heart J.* 85:546, 1973.)

as Olympic cross-country skiers and runners [74]. Women have values about 15 percent lower than those of males as a result of different body dimensions and composition with respect to fat and muscle. An inexorable decline with age of about 0.9 ml/kg/min occurs each year [75], but weekly activity strenuous enough to produce a training effect on the cardiovascular system can diminish this decline as much as 20 percent [75].

The variations in oxygen cost, weight-adjusted in relation to the variables of sex, age, and habitual physical activity status for a multistage protocol beginning with a requirement of 4 to 5 metabolic units (METs), were published by Bruce and associates [72] in 1973. Several points are noteworthy. First, there is a nearly linear increase in oxygen consumption over time (figure 6–8), in spite of the fact that the workload is changed only every 3 minutes. This allows the oxygen consumption at maximal exertion to be estimated by regression on duration.

Second, using preestablished normal values, the percentage deviation from normal can be calculated using a nomogram (figure 6–9) for any given individual, giving a numerical estimate of the cardiovascular impairment (i.e., the functional aerobic impairment, or FAI). Conversely, one can calculate the equivalent "cardiovascular age" of an individual at which the observed duration would be considered normal. Furthermore, in a way that is incompletely understood, the cardiovascular system grades its response to a workload in proportion to the relative relation of that workload to maximal capacity of the individual. Thus, for different individuals a given workload will require the same oxygen consumption per unit of body weight and cardiac output, but the degree of cardiovascular reserves used to achieve that cardiac output (in terms of heart rate and splanchnic vasoconstriction) will be quite different. The relative cardiovascular stress of a fixed workload varies according to the percentage of the individual's VO₂ max required by the load. This scaling of physiologic changes to exercise as a percentage of the VO₂ max provides the only reasonable basis of comparison for individuals with widely varying capacities [76].

Third, there is as much as a twofold range in maximal oxygen uptake between younger, physically active men and older, sedentary women in middle age. Since the maximal capacity is higher in men than in women, the relative aerobic requirement (i.e., the percentage of the VO₂ max) at any given workload is lower in men than in women (figure 6–10); thus, the relative

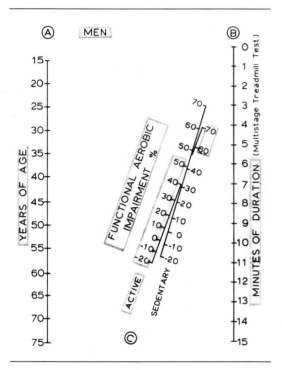

FIGURE 6–9. Nomogram for derivation of functional aerobic impairment (FAI) from age, exercise duration, and prior activity classification. Equivalent normal physiologic age for the same duration of exercise may be derived by extrapolating through zero FAI. (From Bruce, R.A. et al. Maximal oxygen intake and nomographic assessment of functional aerobic impairment in cardiovascular disease *Am. Heart J.* 85:546, 1973.)

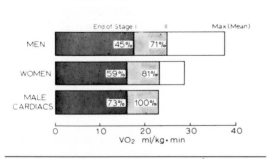

FIGURE 6–10. The same absolute workload represents markedly different cardiovascular stresses relative to the maximal capacity for normal men and women and male cardiac patients. (From Bruce, R.A. et al., Maximal oxygen intake and nomographic assessment of functional aerobic impairment in cardiovascular disease.) *Am. Heart J.* 85:546, 1973.

cardiovascular stress is less. During the final 2 to 3 minutes before maximal oxygen uptake is achieved, the *relative* aerobic requirements are remarkably similar in normal men and women and in men with heart disease (figure 6–11). It must be emphasized, however, that these distinctions cannot be recognized if the test design does not permit symptom-limited exercise capacity to be achieved [77].

Assuming a normal cardiorespiratory capacity and hematocrit, the $VO_2$ depends on the rate of oxygen extraction by working muscle, and it increases as the amount of working muscle increases. Working both legs to maximum on a bicycle generates a $VO_2$ that is 30 percent more than the value obtained using both arms [78], but a maximal value is reached when 60 percent or more of the total body muscle mass is being used, and the addition of arm work to maximum leg work does not significantly increase the $VO_2$ max under most conditions [79, 80].

Studies on $VO_2$ max using various devices have shown that a graded treadmill gives a 15 percent higher result than does an upright bicycle [70, 80] and that the upright bicycle generates the same $VO_2$ max as horizontal running. One study that compared a maximal step test to a treadmill found the $VO_2$ max to be the same in both [83]. Supine bicycle ergometer exercise and swimming generate a 15 percent lower $VO_2$ max than does upright bicycling [83].

Running uphill, as on a treadmill, thus generates the highest $VO_2$ max. Slight differences have been demonstrated in maximal cardiac output, heart rate, and arterial-venous oxygen difference. The responses on the bicycle are about 5 percent lower than on the treadmill, although systolic pressure is increased, representing a slightly different cardiovascular stress [71]. Whether such factors make any difference in the evaluation of cardiovascular performance has not been well established.

TREADMILL PROTOCOLS
Several standardized testing protocols using progressive increments in workloads have become generally accepted for clinical use. Arguments have been put forth for tailoring the design of the test specifically to the capacities of each individual patient, but this approach is used primar-

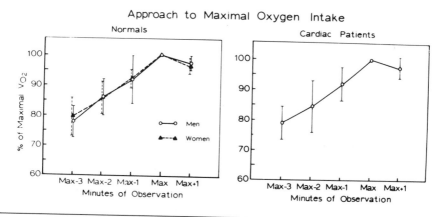

FIGURE 6–11. Relative changes in oxygen uptake (VO$_2$) as the maximum is approached are similar in normal adults as well as in cardiac patients, even though the absolute values differ widely. (From Bruce, R.A., et al. Maximal oxygen intake and nomographic assessment of functional aerobic impairment in cardiovascular disease. *Am. Heart J.* 85:546, 1973.)

ily for research into various aspects of exercise tolerance or the effects of interventions, rather than for clinical determination of exercise capacity and the analysis of a patient's response to exercise.

Pollock and co-workers [85] analyzed four different protocol designs to compare the heart rate responses and oxygen requirements of 51 healthy men: the Åstrand protocol (beginning at a high workload of about 7 to 8 METs), the Ellestad protocol (with three increments in speed before an additional increment in gradient and speed), the Bruce protocol (in which speed and gradient increased every 3 minutes), and the Balke protocol (where the gradient was increased every minute while the speed was held constant at 3.3 miles per hour) (figure 6–12). The first three protocols showed no significant differences in heart rate, blood pressure, or oxygen uptake at maximum. Maximal performance was most rapidly achieved in the Åstrand protocol, but its use is impossible for most cardiac patients because the initial workload is much too high. Likewise, the speed for the Balke protocol may be too fast for many cardiac patients, and the time to reach maximum is prolonged. The average time required to reach maximal effort

ranged from 8 to 20 minutes in the different protocols (figure 6–13). Thus, for clinical purposes, both the Ellestad and Bruce protocols seem appropriate, but the latter is preferred in Seattle because of the more gradual increments in gradient and the extensive documentation of aerobic requirements as well as of normal and abnormal cardiovascular responses in widespread community practice.

REPRODUCIBILITY

The variability of hemodynamic parameters and VO$_2$ max in repeated maximal tests has been demonstrated to be small (on the order of 5 percent) [77]. Often, however, the duration of exercise for second test is increased over the first. Occurring without any change in maximum heart rate, blood pressure, or VO$_2$ max, this increase has been called "habituation" [86, 87].

In patients with angina, Smokler and associates [88] demonstrated that using a subjectively defined end-point of "moderately severe" pain, or 3+ on a 4+ scale, gave similarly reproducible results regarding heart rate and blood pressure maximums, but that the duration of effort that was tolerated increased from a mean of 5.8 minutes to 7.9 minutes with their protocol on the second test. The cause of this habituation response in cardiac patients is presumed to be secondary to increasing familiarity with the procedure, which results in decreased anxiety and sympathetic discharge. In normal subjects, it may be in part a result of a willingness to tolerate

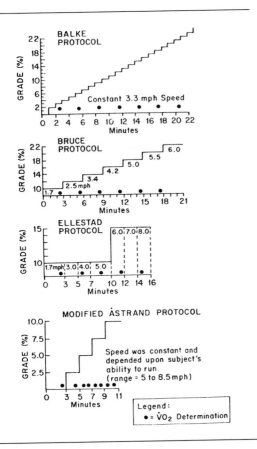

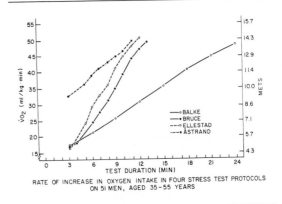

FIGURE 6–13. Maximal oxygen uptake ($VO_2$) is similar for all four protocols, but the time required to attain maximum is prolonged in the Balke design. (From Pollock, M.L. et al. A comparative analysis of four protocols for maximal treadmill stress testing. *Am. Heart J.* 92:39, 1976.)

FIGURE 6–12. Differences in design of treadmill protocols for maximal exercise (see text). (From Pollock, M.L. et al. A comparative analysis of four protocols for maximal treadmill stress testing. *Am. Heart J.* 92:39, 1976.)

increased levels of anaerobic metabolism and possibly an adaptive response leading to increased efficiency.

The reproducibility of an end-point of angina can be modified by the so-called "walk through" phenomenon. This phenomenon has not been commonly observed clinically, but it seems to occur when only moderate workloads are continued for several minutes until a heart load develops and the blood pressure falls slightly as vasodilation develops in the cutaneous circulation. In studies of this phenomenon, two patterns of responses have appeared [89]. In one group a true "walk through" phenomenon occurred when patients developed transient angina at a moderate workload; they then tolerated

it without further difficulty. In these patients, the heart rate and blood pressure declined at the same time as the angina, which reduced the pressure-rate product below the initial level at which the angina appeared. In the other group, patients developed mild angina that they tolerated during continuation of exercise.

Rarely can the psychological factor of expectation play a role, such as in the patient reported by Lown [90]. The patient customarily developed angina with ischemic ST changes on the 44th step of the Master protocol. When the steps had been miscounted (so that his total exertion was less) and he heard the (incorrect) count approaching 44, the patient's typical ischemic changes developed.

Representative coefficients of variation (i.e., standard deviation divided by the mean, expressed in percent) for test response variables are heart rate, 6 percent; pressure-rate product, 10 percent; and duration, 19 percent. The reproducibility of ECG findings varies according to the abnormality. ST segment depression is felt to be reasonably reproducible (see below). Ventricular irritability in coronary patients is poorly reproducible acutely; a second test performed 45 minutes after a first showed a 60 percent reduction in premature ventricular contractions (PVCs) [92]. The design of the protocol used can influence the end-point reproducibility of angina or ischemic ST changes, particularly if the initial workload is near maximal or super-maximal for a given patient by not allowing an opportunity for warm-up and gradual progression to maximum [93].

The long-term (averaging $3 \pm 1$ years) reproducibility of responses to maximal exercise has been evaluated in both healthy subjects and in patients with cardiovascular diseases [94]. The 95 percent confidence intervals for the annual rates of change in duration, exercise heart rate, and systolic pressure responses indicate that only substantial changes in a given individual are likely to be significant. Many patients with coronary heart disease who were considered clinically "unchanged" by their physicians had a substantial improvement that was not recognized prior to symptom-limited testing. Two adaptive changes have been detected in healthy men: one change is a minor (less than 2 percent per year), nonspecific, and statistically insignificant prolongation of exercise duration; the other is a 6.9 percent gain in exercise capacity in those who change from a sedentary to an active status. The prevalence of ST depression remains the same in active men, diminishes in sedentary healthy men or hypertensive men, but increases in coronary heart disease patients (table 6–1). These findings are all consistent with the current understanding that the pressure-rate product correlates well with myocardial oxygen consumption and that in coronary disease, the critical reproducible value during exertion represents the threshold for ischemia and angina.

## FACTORS INFLUENCING RESPONSE TO TREADMILL EXERCISE

A variety of factors have been shown to influence performance on the treadmill, including age, sex, physical training, ambient temperature, circadian rhythms, motivation, previous food intake, anemia, smoking, and prior exercise. Digitalis, $\beta$-adrenergic blockers, and vasodilators are also significant, as are two less obvious factors relevant to the test itself: the subject's holding onto the rails during the test and the rate at which the subject changes pace from walking to jogging or running.

The effects of training on maximal performance are well documented; in normal subjects, these include an increased stroke volume at any level of exertion and, consequently, a lower heart rate [95, 96]. The overall increment in $VO_2$ max ranges from 15 to 25 percent. In patients with coronary heart disease, the primary effect of training is an increased arterial-venous oxygen difference with less marked change in stroke volume [97–99].

Circadian rhythms also exert an effect on exercise performance. A 12 percent difference in $VO_2$ max was reported by Ilmarinen and co-workers [100], with the lowest value being noted at 11 P.M. and the highest at 3 P.M. Maxi-

TABLE 6–1. ECG responses in men with long-term ($3 \pm 1$ yr) unchanged clinical status and same classifications

| Classification of men | Clinical interpretation of ischemic ST depression on last test versus initial test | | | Prevalences | |
|---|---|---|---|---|---|
| | No change (i.e., agreement) (%) | Change + to − (%) | Change − to + (%) | Initial test (%) | Last test (%) |
| Active, healthy | 77.5 | 11.3 | 11.3 | 15.0 | 15.0 |
| Sedentary, healthy | 88.5 | 8.0 | 3.4 | 12.6 | 8.0 |
| Hypertensive | 70.8 | 18.8 | 10.4 | 25.0 | 16.7 |
| Coronary heart disease | 69.1 | 10.8 | 20.1 | 35.6 | 44.8 |
| *Overall* | 75.1 | 12.0 | 9.3 | 24.5 | 28.9 |

From Bruce, R. A. and DeRouen, T. A. In Folinsbee, L. J. (ed.), *Environmental Stress: Individual Human Adaptations.* New York: Academic, 1978.

mum heart rate was lowest at 3 A.M. and was highest at 7 A.M. Crockford and Davies [101] found a similar circadian variation in submaximal heart rates, with the lowest heart rate per load occurring at 4 to 5 A.M. and the highest 4 to 8 P.M. These diurnal variations can affect ST responses, especially in coronary partients. In one study, ST segment displacement on 4 P.M. tests were significantly greater than on 8 A.M. tests [102].

The effect of food prior to exertion was reported by Goldstein and associates [103]. A 1,000-calorie meal taken prior to exertion in 12 patients with angina caused 9 percent of them to have angina at least 1 minute earlier on their protocol; this effect was associated with a resting and submaximal mean heart rate increment of 11 beats/min and a slight increase in systolic pressure. The effect lasted about 1 hour, although in some it continued to be apparent as late as 3 hours after the meal. Similar hemodynamic effects have also been noted in normal subjects. The mechanism for such effects is not clear; possibly, blood is shunted to the splanchnic system for digestion, necessitating a greater cardiac output for any given muscular workload. A similar effect is noted with exertion in high ambient temperatures; in this case, blood is shunted to the skin [104].

As would be expected, significant degrees of anemia also diminish exercise tolerance. Davies and associates [105] showed that a 34 percent reduction in $VO_2$ max occurred with hemoglobin levels under 8g/dl and a 24 percent reduction with levels between 8 and 10g/dl. Reductions in $VO_2$ max at hemoglobin levels above 10g/dl were not significant. Other variables that can influence test duration include the degree of motivation, which can create a 10 to 20 percent difference in work output and duration; this difference results from more utilization of anaerobic metabolism without a change in $VO_2$ max [106]. The choice between running or walking at intermediate speeds also influences exercise duration; subjects who walk through the third or fourth stage of the Bruce protocol continue significantly longer than those who run [107]. This observation is consistent with data that suggest that the mechanical efficiency of movement is greater below approximately 4.75

mph when walking and above 4.75 mph when running [108].

Submaximal testing is equally susceptible to the factors discussed above. The change in response toward greater efficiency with repeated testing may influence submaximal results more than those of maximal testing [109].

## EFFECTS OF DRUGS ON EXERCISE PERFORMANCE

The most commonly used drugs that can alter exercise performance or data and whose effects are well described are the digitalis glycosides, vasodilators, and $\beta$-adrenergic blocking agents (beta-blockers). Other antiarrhythmic and antihypertension drugs have been less well studied.

The effect of *digitalis* on the exercise test was first studied by Liebow and Feil [110] in 1941, who found J-point depression and T-wave modification in 14 adults. The hemodynamic response to exercise is probably not changed significantly in normal subjects with acute digitalization [111, 112], although the blood pressure response to isometric exertion is increased [113]. Sharma and colleagues [114], using 0.01mg/kg ouabain in six patients with angina, found a slight increase in stroke volume and cardiac output, a decrease in left ventricular and diastolic pressure, and an improvement in the relation between stroke work and end-diastolic pressure; others, however, have not duplicated these findings [111].

The major area of clinical concern with digitalis, however, concerns its effect on the exercise ECG. Adair and associates [115] found that 8 of 11 subjects with a normal bicycle exercise tolerance test and a normal resting ECG developed abnormal ST depression during exercise when digitalized acutely; these workers noted that this reaction occurred up to around 80 percent of $VO_2$ max and then resolved. This phenomenon has not been reported elsewhere. Kawai and Hultgren [116] found that 50 percent of normal subjects developed a positive Master's test after acute digitalization. Sketch et al. [117] reported a 24 percent frequency using the treadmill. LeWinter and co-workers [118] found that with digitalization the mean change in ST depression at maximal exertion among cardiac patients was from 2.6 to 3.8 mm.

Although the presence of digitalis, with or without normal repolarization at rest, destroys the significance of ST depression at maximal exertion, nonspecific ST-T wave changes present on the resting ECG in the absence of digitalis may not alter the significance of ST changes with exertion.

The hemodynamic effects of exercise with *chronic beta-blockade* were studied by Reybrouck and associates [119], who demonstrated that in patients not limited by angina, no change occurred in $VO_2$ max; there was a reduction in cardiac output of 14 percent, which was compensated for by an increase in arterial-venous oxygen extraction of 8 percent. Maximum heart rate decreased 33 percent, and there was an increase in stroke volume of 31 percent. Mean blood pressure decreased 14.5 mmHg, and mean pulmonary artery wedge pressure increased 20 percent.

The ST responses to maximal exercise with propranolol, a beta-blocker, were studied by Gianelly and co-workers [120], using 0.15 mg/kg intravenously in 11 patients with angina, all of whom had greater than 1 mm exertional ST depression (mean: 2.3 mm). Acute propranolol therapy changed the mean ST depression for the group from 2.3 to 1.0 mm; two of the 11 patients no longer showed any ST depression, and two showed minimal amounts (0.2 to 0.3 mm). Thus, while digitalis creates a false-positive ST change, propranolol may create a significant number of false-negative tests, which could have significance in the evaluation of coronary disease in patients who are taking the drug for hypertension.

Except for propranolol and related drugs, there are few data regarding the effects of *antihypertension medication* per se on the exercise test. A small study on dose levels of chlorthalidone showed a progressive decrease in exercise blood pressure and pressure-rate product up to a dose level of 100 mg/day; there was also a paradoxical rise of both systolic and diastolic pressures at 200 mg [121]. Although not well studied with treadmill data, antihypertensive drugs may lead to an increased risk of exertional and postexertional hypotension.

The effects of one of the slow-channel *calcium-blocking agents*, namely diltiazem, have been carefully evaluated in a double-blind, triple cross-over, multicenter clinical trial of 57 randomized patients with exercise-induced angina pectoris [122]. Of three dose levels tested— 120, 180, and 240 g/day in four divided doses —the largest dose was most effective. The time for appearance of 1 mm of ST depression was increased from 1.01 to 1.81 minutes ($p < .002$), the time for appearance of angina from 1.17 to 1.81 minutes ($p < .01$), and duration of symptom-limited maximal exercise was extended from 1.05 to 1.87 minutes. At maximal exercise, corresponding roughly with energy requirements of ordinary daily activities, heart rate, diastolic pressure, and the product of heart rate and systolic pressure were significantly reduced by diltiazem, but rate and pressure were unchanged at maximal exercise.

In addition to the use of specific test protocols and our present concepts of reproducibility and modifying variables, major controversial aspects about methods focus on at least three clinically important aspects: (1) end-points for stopping testing, (2) the number and configuration of electrode leads, and (3) the criteria for interpretation of ST changes.

## END-POINTS FOR STOPPING TEST

The preferred end-point is symptom-limited capacity, either for healthy persons or for patients with symptoms. The *threshold* of symptoms is used as an end-point for low-level testing of patients at the time of discharge from hospital, but not when capacity is being determined. *Limiting symptoms*, usually of fatigue and breathlessness, occur when oxygen uptake reaches its peak; if effort is continued, the oxygen uptake reaches a plateau or falls slightly as additional energy is derived from anaerobic glycolysis. If this limit is achieved on a treadmill without partial support of the subject's body weight by use of his or her hands to grip the handrail, it provides a sharply defined end-point with excellent reproducibility, usually within 97 to 103 percent of the observed duration.

*A major source of contention in protocol design has been between maximal and submaximal testing.* The early work by Master popularized a submaximal test, and in some laboratories the feeling persisted that it was safer, although no data substantiate this. A submaximal test cannot measure maximal aerobic capacity, and although a variety of nomograms have been published in attempts to extrapolate to a predicted maximum, there is significant error. In addition, maximal testing has been shown to increase the prevalence of significant ST changes and hence the diagnostic and prognostic yield. Furthermore, the adequacy of a submaximal test is limited in screening for potentially adverse cardiovascular reactions in preparation for an exercise program. The strongest argument, however, against the use of submaximal testing with a fixed protocol for all patients (e.g., testing to an arbitrary heart rate) is that goals set by the protocol may well expect the most seriously impaired patients to perform at maximal or even supramaximal stress; that is, one is actually giving a maximal test to the most impaired patients, while the submaximal test understresses the healthiest persons (figure 6–14).

Others [123] have tried to increase the utility of submaximal testing by setting a heart rate limit of 80 to 90 percent of the age-predicted

maximum heart rate in normal subjects. Research designs using this approach significantly dilute the possible informative value of heart rate or blood pressure changes near or at maximum tolerance, since there is no knowledge of how close to true maximal effort these arbitrary end-points may be in each individual.

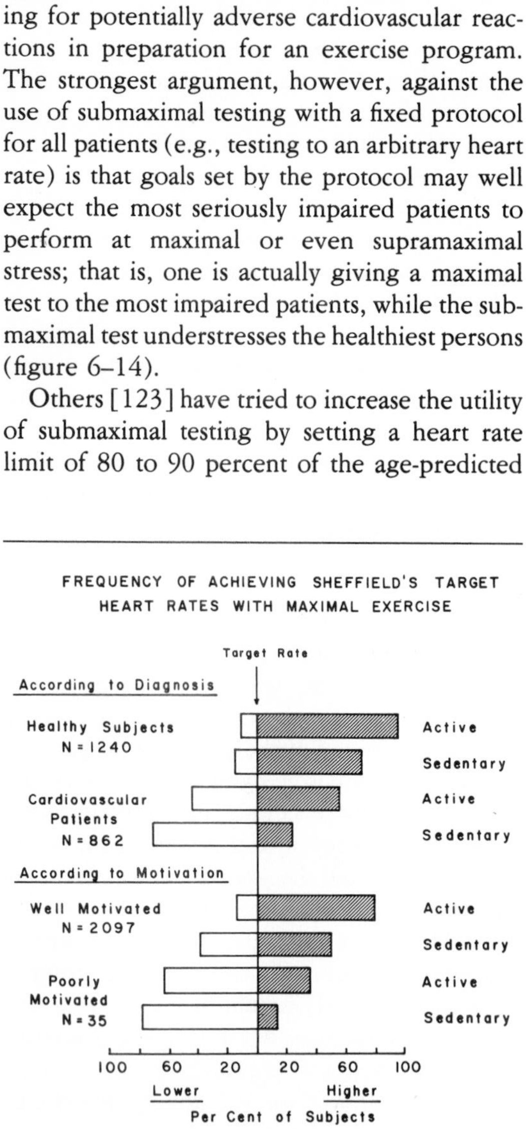

Furthermore, reliance upon target heart rates, such as 90 percent of the age-predicted maximal heart rate for normal persons, is neither physiologic, acceptable, nor necessarily safe. The standard deviation for normal subjects may be 8 to 10 beats/min; thus, the 95 percent confidence intervals are $\pm 16$ to $\pm 20$ beats around the mean [72]. Patients with coronary heart disease have lower maximal rates. In some instances, they are well below the predicted value, especially if the patient has been treated with a beta-blocker. Forcing such patients toward these expected values may occasionally be disastrous or even lethal. Finally, for those investigators who still insist on using such end-points, their own data reveal that the majority of cardiac patients cannot attain these values. Safety might be ensured if the limit is set at 90 percent of the *individual's* maximal heart rate; unfortunately, there is no reliable way to predict this before the first test is performed, and it may change over time.

Testing to symptom-limited capacity has been shown in the Seattle Heart Watch program to be safe and feasible in many different clinical settings in the community. It also correlates well with the accepted physiologic indexes of maximal aerobic capacity, such as a plateau in oxygen consumption, elevated lactate levels, and a respiratory exchange ratio above 1:15.

There are a few mandatory indications for stopping exertion, even in the absence of any symptom. These include the sudden appearance of incapacitating and dangerous signs, such as an ataxic gait (presumably due to inadequate cerebral blood flow); three or more *consecutive* ventricular premature beats, or tachycardia; and exertional hypotension that is defined by a fall in systolic pressure certainly below the *usual* resting level and perhaps by any sustained fall over 10 mmHg. Fortunately, such events are infrequent occurrences (see figure 6–4), but failure to intervene when they occur may precipitate

FREQUENCY OF ACHIEVING SHEFFIELD'S TARGET HEART RATES WITH MAXIMAL EXERCISE

FIGURE 6–14. Variations in proportions of persons who are either unable to attain or able to exceed the arbitrarily recommended target heart rate responses advocated by other investigators (see text). (From Bruce, R.A. et al. *Am. J. Cardiol.* 33:459, 1974.)

injury or even death. Although the wisdom of expecting the achievement of maximal, symptom-limited exercise capacity may be questioned by those unfamiliar with exercise testing, it should be emphasized that there is no safer place to discover the rarely encountered hazards than in a clinical laboratory, with a physician in attendance and with facilities for emergency treatment, including ventricular defibrillation apparatus. Furthermore, it may be more hazardous not to uncover such risks under controlled circumstances than to have an unsuspecting patient encounter them in daily life and incur the risk of unwitnessed sudden cardiac death.

## EXERCISE ECG LEAD SYSTEMS

Areas of technical concern in the detection and faithful delineation of the electrical vectors of the heart include the generation of the signal by the myocardium, transmission through the volume conductor of the torso, possible distortion at the skin-electrode and the electrode-wire junctions, the input impedance of the ECG premplifier, and the frequency-response characteristics of the ECG circuitry.

At the skin-electrode junction, the stratum corneum acts as a significant resistance barrier, attenuating the signal between the body and the electrode. Also, irregular contact can occur between the skin and the electrodes during motion, causing baseline wandering or other artifacts. These may be overcome by the use of lightweight electrodes, which are attached to the skin with adhesive discs after brisk rubbing to remove the stratum corneum in order to lower skin resistance. Others [124, 125] have described an alternative approach that uses relatively stationary parts of the body to achieve continuous recordings.

The amplitude of the signal also depends on the ratio between the resistance of the skin electrodes and the input impedance of the preamplifier; an optimal ratio is less than 1:10 [126]. For an input impedance of 50,000 to 100,000 ohms, the skin resistance should be reduced by rubbing to 5,000 ohms or less, which is usually obtained when erythema develops.

The frequency response of the ECG is a known source of recording error; this error involves the first 25 percent of ventricular repolar-

ization. The recording instrument should have proper frequency responses over a frequency range of 0.05 hertz (Hz) for repolarization events to above 300 Hz for high-frequency depolarization changes. The latter frequency exceeds the range of available direct writers. In 1966 Berson and Pipberger [127] reported a 6 percent error in recording ischemic ST depression with a low-frequency cutoff of 0.1 Hz, but reducing the cutoff to 0.05 Hz obviated the error. The American Heart Association (AHA) subsequently adopted this requirement in their specifications for electrocardiographs [128].

An additional technical modification to reduce recording error was the development of computer averaging of signals [129]. Signal averaging relies on the principle that most noise in the ECG signal is random. The noise can be reduced by the square root of the number of beats sampled, thereby enhancing the actual signal; for example, averaging 100 beats reduces noise to 10 percent of the original level. This method works well for reducing respiratory or muscle movement artifacts as well as 60-Hz interference. Computer averaging and subsequent processing has also allowed a very detailed analysis of specific portions of the ECG signal and precise quantification of changes from the baseline. Bruce and co-workers [130] reported an overall processing error in their computer system of 6 to 11 $\mu$V.

The specific technical issues of ST segment analysis have been well covered recently [131]. The areas of debate concern which lead system to use (i.e., bipolar, 12-lead, or orthogonal XYZ leads), the optimal time during exercise or recovery for discrimination of the ischemic responses, the optimal technique for ST segment and analysis (ST integral, ST slope, or ST index), and the optimal position on the ST segment at which to record depression.

It was well recognized from the use of a 12-lead ECG for post-exercise recordings that the precordial lead $V_5$ most frequently showed the presence of ischemic ST abnormalities. This is a result of the orientation of the ischemic ST vector predominantly toward the right and slightly superior, whether anteriorly or posteriorly tilted. Bipolar lead systems with the positive electrode in the $V_5$ position and the negative electrode on the manubrium ($CM_5$) or at the lower tip of the right scapula ($CB_5$) approximate the axis of the ischemic ST vector. Because they record negative to positive, rather than ground to positive as with the unipolar $V_5$ lead, they record a larger QRS voltage and ST voltage if present; that is, they have a 25 percent higher "lead strength" for any given vector direction. In a few patients (about 10 percent) the ischemic vector is oriented more superiorly and is recorded best in an inferior lead. Frank's [132] orthogonal XYZ leads have also been used, particularly in computerized systems. The X lead is not as parallel to the ischemic vector as in the two bipolar systems mentioned, but the Y lead, although noisy, makes available a vertically oriented recording lead. Use of the Frank lead system requires careful standardization of electrode placement [133].

Blackburn and associates [134] analyzed various lead configurations in detail and found that 90 percent of all abnormal responses were detected by lead $V_5$. Other leads added information as follows: AVF, 4 percent; $V_4$, $V_6$, and 11, 2 percent each; and $V_3$, 1 percent. Phibbs and Buckels [135] found similar results, with lead $V_5$ revealing 80 percent of the abnormal responses, the inferior leads, 13 percent; and $V_6$, 3 percent. A false-negative recording of 15 to 20 percent resulted with the use of any single lead alone. Ascoop [136], after evaluating many lead systems (bipolar, Frank's, and 12-lead) in patients with previously equivocal exercise tests and chest pain suspicious for angina, found the bipolar lead $GM_5$ better than scalar or Frank's leads. Later studies [137] showed the bipolar leads to be equivalent to the Frank system, and Hornsten and Bruce [138] showed the same to be true for the Frank system and $CB_5$. Recently, Simoons and Block [139] have suggested that the Frank system is superior to the bipolar. For routine clinical use, a single bipolar precordial lead from the $V_5$ position to inferior tip of the right scapula, plus a grounding electrode, has usually been satisfactory. For enhancement of arrhythmia detection and the diagnosis of ventricular ectopy, a vertical lead axis is also useful. For research purposes, multiple precordial leads, Frank's XYZ system, or both with computer averaging, analysis, and graphic display of all 12 leads simultaneously (figure 6–15) warrant further exploration, as do vectorcardiograms, polarcardiograms, and spatial trajectories of QRS complexes.

## CRITERIA FOR INTERPRETATION OF ST RESPONSES

It is well established that the higher the workload, the higher the incidence of ischemic responses. A major complaint about the Master test was that the workload was not only variable (depending, for example, on the patient's weight), but it was frequently insufficient to elicit latent ischemia. Ascoop and co-workers [140] found a twofold increase in ischemic responses in maximal treadmill testing over the Master test. Others [141] have found comparable gains. Furthermore, arbitrary discontinuance of a test at 85 percent of normal maximum age-predicted heart rate will fail to elicit up to 54 percent of positive ST changes. Arbitrary discontinuation, even at a 95 percent level, fails to uncover 19 percent of the positive responses seen with a symptom-limited maximum test [141].

The search for deviations from normal that carry the most specific information about cardiac ischemia has stimulated a tremendous volume of literature and, perhaps unfortunately, focused interpretive efforts of exercise results predominantly toward ECG responses and away from other aspects of the overall cardiovascular response.

*T-wave changes* have been evaluated in several laboratories and have been found to be unreliable indicators of ischemia as well as not to influence ST responses [142, 143].

The *repeatability* of ST depression induced by maximal exercise has been analyzed. A study by Blackburn and others [144] revealed marked variability in the visual interpretation of borderline abnormal ST responses both within and among 14 cardiologists who read the records independently and without prescribed or uniform criteria; the prevalence of responses classified as abnormal by individual cardiologists ranged from 5 to 58 percent. When uniform criteria were adopted, agreement increased and the range of prevalence among the readers diminished to 35 to 45 percent.

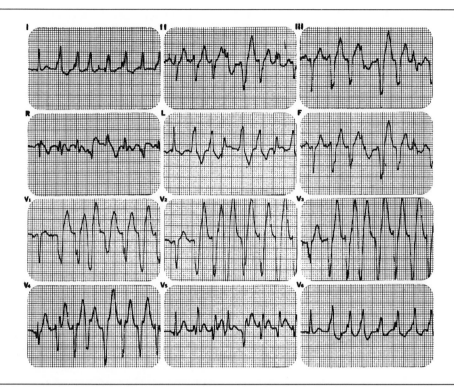

FIGURE 6–15. Advantage of displaying 12 ECG leads simultaneously. The onset of paroxysmal atrial fibrillation with rate-dependent left bundle branch block is recorded and allows easier differentiation from ventricular tachycardia.

Doan and co-workers [145] reported good repeatability in 19 of 20 "positive" men from a group of more than 200 who were studied after an elapsed time of 1 year, and Most and associates [146] reported consistently negative responses in 155 men, consistently positive responses in 10 men, and variable responses in 21 men (11 percent) who were retested again 2 years later.

Trayler [147] evaluated the interpretations of ST responses in 58 asymptomatic men of 24 to 64 years of age (mean age 48.7 years), of whom 16 previously had less than 1 mm depression, 19 exhibited 1 mm of upsloping depression, and 23 showed horizontal or downsloping depression of 1 mm or more. The tracings were read independently by four cardiologists on two separate occasions and analyzed by computer as well. The men were retested exactly 1 week later, plus or minus 1 hour, with specific instructions about

maintaining the same activity and sleeping and eating habits as well as to refrain from smoking. Overall, the ST responses were placed in the same classification by visual interpretations in 69 percent of the second tests, and computer analysis classified them the same in 75 percent of the second tests. Repeatability of clinical or visual interpretation by the different cardiologists ranged from 79 to 91 percent. The highest correlation of several variables defined by computer analysis from measurements obtained one week apart was obtained for $ST_2$ (60 msec from the nadir of R deflection) at 1 and 5 minutes after maximal exercise ($r = +0.94$ and $+0.92$, respectively).

ST segment depression has long been recognized as an indicator of myocardial ischemia, and much effort has been devoted to defining criteria that best separate normal from abnormal responses, either for predicting future coronary events in follow-up or for determining coronary artery stenosis by cardiac catheterization. The three morphologic characteristics studied are the depth of depression, the spatial orientation, and the rate of return to baseline. Isolated J-point depression with the subsequent ST segment returning to baseline with a rapid upslope was described by Sjöstrand [148] as a normal response to tachycardia. Initially, this phenomenon was attributed to the effect of atrial repolarization, but a carefull analysis by Simoons and Hugenholtz [149] demonstrated that the timecourses of J-point depression and P-wave changes during exertion were different, as were the corresponding vector orientations.

The usual criterion for the "ischemic" ST pattern is horizontal or downsloping depression that is either new or superimposed on the nonspecific ST-T wave abnormalities seen on a resting ECG in the absence of digitalis administration [119, 142, 143]. This pattern was associated with the general incidence of coronary events in early studies, but a slowly upsloping pattern has been noted to carry an intermediate risk [12]. "Slow" has been defined as a slope of less than 1 mV/sec or an upsloping depression of 1 mm or more 0.08 second from the J-point [150].

Attempts have also been made to combine the depth of depression and the slope into a single criterion. McHenry and co-workers [151] developed an ST index that adds the depth of depression at $ST_2$ to the slope of the ST segment from 70 to 110 msec after the R-peak. According to this index, above zero is normal, and below zero, abnormal. Sheffield and colleagues [152] analyzed the integrated area between the baseline and the ST segment, and the optimal discriminating value for ischemia was established as $-8$ $\mu V/sec$.

Ascoop and associates [153], in a detailed retrospective evaluation of discriminating criteria among a group of patients with suspected coronary disease and previously equivocal exercise tests, found the direction (not the magnitude) of the ST vector at 80 msec after the J-point to be the optimal criterion. The ST index and the ST integral did not have as much value as criteria in their population. Dower and co-workers [154], using a polarcardiographic technique of mapping vectors in spherical polar coordinates, developed a criterion for an ischemic response to exercise that is based on the product of the spatial magnitude of the vector at the end of the QRS complex (analogous to the open loop of the vectorcardiogram) multiplied by the change

in the spatial angle of the ST vector 75 msec from the midpoint of the integral of the QRS training. This criterion combines a voltage displacement value with the vector direction in space. Notwithstanding the more elaborate computer-based criteria (none of which has shown clear supremacy), the clinical criterion of 1 mm depression, flat or downsloping, and present at 0.08 second after the J-point is commonly accepted. Bruce et al. [155] found, however, that the best statistical discrimination between coronary heart disease patients and normal subjects was obtained by using the criterion of 1.5 mm depression 0.06 second after the J-point occurring 1 minute into recovery after symptom-limited maximal exercise.

To provide a different perspective—namely, that of community practice where many physicians are evaluating ST responses in patients with a variety of clinical manifestations and different degrees of severity of coronary heart disease—the data available from the Seattle Heart Watch may be helpful. These data have been examined in 232 men who received both maximal exercise testing and evaluation by invasive coronary arteriography. The ST responses were classified by visual interpretation by the testing physicians, and in addition, the ECG signals from the same bipolar precordial lead ($CB_5$) were transmitted by telephone from 15 different testing sites to a computer for averaging, analysis, and interpretation. The criterion for significant vascular disease was the presence of at least 70 percent stenosis of one or more arteries. Using the clinical ECG criterion of at least 1 mm of horizontal or downsloping ST depression, the prevalence was 35 percent, the sensitivity 47 percent, and the specificity 81 percent. By computer analysis, using the criterion of $ST_B$ (50 to 69 msec after the nadir of S) equal to or less than $-0.10$ mV (equivalent to 1 mm or more depression), these parameters were 34, 40, and 76 percent, respectively. When the criterion for the same data was changed to less than $-0.20$ mV, the parameters were 15, 17, and 95 percent, respectively. Thus, for comparable criteria, the computer analysis and clinical interpretation exhibited reasonably good agreement. With a more stringent criterion for classification by computer, however, the prevalence and sensitivity were less than one-half of their initial values, but the specificity for exclusion of significant vascular disease was enhanced substantially. This type of appraisal offers the advantages of pooling the experience of several groups of physicians, which may make it more representative of general experience, and of using the same independent and objective assessment of computer measurements to evaluate both the agreement with visual interpretations and the effects of a more stringent criterion.

Another aspect of ST depression is its prognostic value with respect to subsequent mortality from coronary heart disease. Computer analysis is available of the Seattle Heart Watch experience with a 3-year follow-up of 2,766 men, some with and others without clinical manifestations of coronary heart disease initially. At this time, 77 deaths have occurred, and the overall sensitivity for the optimal criterion for computer analysis (namely, less than $-0.15$ mV 1 minute *after* maximal exercise) was 41.6 percent, the specificity 92.4 percent, and the predictive risk ratio 7.7:1. Much higher specificities and predictive risk ratios were obtained for men originally free of clinical manifestations of coronary heart disease.

Finally, despite the attention usually directed toward ST responses, there are three continuous variables that should always be noted on every maximal exercise test: (1) the duration of exertion in seconds using a standardized testing protocol, (2) the heart rate, and (3) the systolic blood pressure observed at maximal exertion. Other observations of importance include the notation of symptoms; the signs on reexamination of the patient after exertion; the blood pressure, which should be recorded at least at each stage; ECG for arrhythmia detection and heart rate; the number of exercise stages; and the duration of testing. Multivariate approaches for interpreting tests with some of these measurements have been proposed [155–160]. It is also important to classify each individual clinically before the exercise test.

## What the Exercise Responses Mean and Why

Interpretation of exercise responses is difficult or impossible without knowledge of expected normal standards in healthy persons of comparable sex, age, and habitual activity status. Whereas data may be appraised in relation to published standards, it is more convenient in the Seattle community to use one of 10 computer terminals linked to dial-up telephone, to enter quickly the preliminary classificatory data and pertinent exercise responses, and then to allow the central computer to make a standard report with quantitative appraisal of key continuous variables. If ST responses are averaged and analyzed on-line next to the treadmill and electrocardiograph, such data may be entered immediately and the results graphed against heart rate responses by the computer terminal program.

When this computer approach is used, body weight is evaluated in proportion to height and reported as relative weight; then "100 percent" represents the average weight for the observed height of normal subjects. Exercise duration is evaluated in terms of *functional aerobic impairment (FAI)*, where "0 percent" represents no impairment or a maximal oxygen uptake of 100 percent of normal for healthy peers, as estimated by regression on the observed duration of exertion (when body weight is not supported by the handrails). Stated differently, the percent of average normal maximal oxygen uptake equals 100 percent minus the FAI percent. *Heart rate impairment* (HRI) represents the percentage deviation between the observed and the age-predicted normal values. Likewise, *left ventricular impairment* (LVI), or the functional limits of this chamber of the heart, represents (in the absence of aortic stenosis) the percentage deviation between the observed and the age-predicted product of heart rate and systolic pressure. These two indexes, representing the chronotropic capacity and the limits of myocardial capacity, separate the cardiac components from the functional aerobic capacity of the entire body. The difference between FAI and LVI, or the *peripheral circulatory impairment* (PCI), is an approximate measure of the noncardiac components; it can vary with peripheral vascular resistance and with physical training.

This systematic method of interpreting exercise responses also reports three prognostic items. The first is the annual mortality rates for white individuals of similar sex and age; these rates are derived from published data of United States Vital Statistics for all deaths from all causes for the entire population. The second is the annual coronary heart disease mortality risk, which is based on the current experience derived from the Seattle Heart Watch in relation to age and clinical classification of heart disease before exercise testing. The third estimates the risk of sudden cardiac death; this estimate is based upon the individual responses to maximal exercise and includes previously identified predictive variables. Thus, with this method, physicians may be provided with an organized report that contains an interpretation of the responses in relation to normal standards and mortality risks.

Contrary to reported practices of other investigators, no attempt is made to define the diagnosis of coronary or any other disease in this report. The functional evaluation may aid the physician who is uncertain about the diagnosis, which in many instances is already apparent from the clinical examination. Of greater importance, this evaluation may suggest whether there is need for invasive arteriographic studies to provide confirmation and quantitation of disease and its anatomic and functional severity.

As noted earlier in this chapter, the combination of findings, rather than any single response, is far more helpful in diagnosis and prognosis. For earlier detection of coronary heart disease in asymptomatic healthy men, the combination of one or more convenient risk factors with ischemic ST depression is associated with a significantly greater mortality risk. Accordingly, the presence of this combination may be more diagnostic of disease and associated with fewer false-positive results, but this is only a hypothesis awaiting further testing.

Similarly, because of the numbers of patients with prior myocardial infarction and contraction abnormalities of the left ventricle, ischemic ST responses, even when associated with pain on testing, have no significant predictive value for sudden cardiac death (SCD). The presence or absence of cardiomegaly, exercise duration more or less than 3 minutes (stage 1), and a systolic pressure at maximal exercise above or below 130 mmHg have major prognostic value for total mortality risk, however [155]. Indeed, the gradient ranges from 20 to 884 per 1,000 men at risk (see figure 6–7). The same variables

are equally important for non-SCD mortality risks. The relation of these predictors to the indications for medical versus surgical treatment of coronary heart disease has also been investigated [160]. The results of this 2,000-man study indicate that such noninvasive predictors, which represent the parameters of left ventricular dimensions and functional limits at maximal exercise, may be clinically useful criteria for determining the optimal time to consider invasive studies and the feasibility of surgical treatment.

Curiously, the occasional appearance of pathognomonic physical signs after maximal exercise may reveal unsuspected diagnostic information. The vigorous but transient pulsations of the jugular veins reveal tricuspid incompetence; a loud second heart sound may reveal pulmonary hypertension; a systolic click may identify mitral valve prolapse; or an ejection murmur may identify clinically important obstructive cardiomyopathy. Likewise, gallops reveal elevated end-diastolic pressure and a noncompliant left ventricle.

## Comparative Value and Cost Effectiveness of Exercise Testing

Several points must be noted in appraising the comparative value and cost effectiveness of exercise testing. First, concerning its value as a technique of patient evaluation, it can be incorporated into the routine clinical examination of patients in office or clinical practice. Second, it can be repeated acutely within a half-hour for immediate evaluation of drug therapy or serially as often as clinically indicated. Third, it can be combined with other procedures, such as myocardial perfusion with thallium (see chapter 8) or invasive research studies of hemodynamic responses that involve measurements of arterial pressures (systemic and pulmonary), arterial-mixed oxygen differences, and cardiac output by the direct Fick principle. As yet, scanning techniques have not been feasible to monitor ejection fraction changes with upright exercise on a treadmill, although this has been achieved with modified bicycle ergometry (chapter 8). Thus, exercise testing is primarily adaptable to clinical practice, yet it provides opportunities for many research applications.

The cost effectiveness of exercise testing varies with the charges imposed, the completeness of data collection, and the adequacy of interpretation, as well as with the relative safety of the test and the value of information generated. The charges for exercise testing are substantially less than those for invasive arteriography and ventriculography, especially if necessary hospitalization costs are considered. The safety of exercise testing is demonstrated by the widespread clinical experience among thousands of patients with coronary heart disease in Seattle, all of whom survived exercise testing; a few, however, did not survive coronary arteriography. Although echocardiography provides anatomic information, unfortunately it cannot easily be combined with treadmill exercise testing to ascertain the changes at the functional limits of the left ventricle. Even invasive hemodynamic studies of exercise responses have been repeated as many as four times over a period of years in the same patients to observe longitudinal changes with the progression of the disease and its treatment. Thus, for moderate cost, little time and inconvenience, and established safety, maximal exercise testing offers valuable clinical information. Looking to the future, the value of such information can be enhanced substantially by the use of a computer terminal to organize reports, interpret measurements, and offer prognostic assessments.

## Conclusions

Exercise testing is a useful supplement to the clinical evaluation of patients with, or suspected of having, coronary heart disease. In a properly supervised setting, the risks of serious complications are extremely small.

The diagnostic potential of the ST response is probably more limited than most physicians realize, especially in asymptomatic populations, but the adverse prognostic implications of marked ST depression are still valid. Other noninvasive measurements besides ST changes are also important in interpreting the exercise test; these include the heart rate response, reduction in blood pressure, development of angina, and duration of the exercise test itself. Functional aerobic capacity can also be evaluated, along with the percentage of normal maximum oxygen uptake and its complement, the functional aerobic impairment (FAI).

The treadmill test has become the prevailing exercise test procedure at present, although bicycle ergometers and step tests are still used by some. Several standardized protocols are available for the treadmill test, and either the Bruce or the Ellestad protocols are recommended. Reproducibility of the treadmill exercise test is generally good. For routine clinical ECG use, a single bipolar precordial lead ($V_5$) is generally satisfactory. Special precautions in interpreting the test results must be taken when the patients are receiving certain cardiac drugs, particularly digitalis (in relation to ST depression) and beta-blockers (in relation to maximal attained heart rate and, perhaps, blood pressure).

Finally, the exercise test appears to be cost effective in relation to invasive procedures, and it may become even more useful when combined with radioisotopic myocardial perfusion studies and noninvasive tests of left ventricular function.

## References

1. Koppes, G., McKiernan, T., Bassan, M., and Froelicher, V.F. Treadmill Exercise Testing, Parts I and II. In *Current Problems in Cardiology.* Chicago: Year Book, 1977.
2. Fortuin, M.J. and Weiss, J.L. Exercise Stress Testing. In A.M. Weissler (ed.), *Review of Contemporary Laboratory Methods. Circulation* 56:699, 1977.
3. Ellestad, M.H. *Stress Testing: Principles and Practice* (2nd ed.). Philadelphia: Davis, 1980.
4. American Heart Association Committee Report. Standards for exercise testing laboratories. *Circulation* 59:412A, 1979.
5. Bruce, R.A., Gey, G.O., Cooper, M.N., Fisher, L.D., and Peterson, D.R. Seattle Heart Watch: Initial clinical, circulatory and electrocardiographic responses to maximal exercise. *Am. J. Cardiol.* 33:459, 1974.
6. Einthoven, W. Weiteres uber das elektrokardiogramm. *Arch. Dtsch. Ges. Physiol.* 172:517, 1908.
7. Feil, H. and Siegel, M.L. Electrocardiographic changes during attacks of angina pectoris. *Am. J. Med. Sci.* 175:255, 1928.
8. Master, A.M. and Oppenheimer, E.T. A simple exercise tolerance test for circulatory efficiency

with standard tables for normal individuals. *Am. J. Med. Sci.* 177:223, 1929.

9. Master, A.M. The two-step test of myocardial infarction. *Am. Heart J.* 10:495, 1935.

10. Master, A.M. and Jaffe, H.L. The electrocardiographic changes after exercise in angina pectoris. *J. Mt. Sinai Hosp.* 7:629, 1941.

11. Mattingly, T.W. The postexercise electrocardiogram: Its value in the diagnosis and prognosis of coronary arterial disease. *Am. J. Cardiol.* 9:-395, 1962.

12. Robb, G.P. and Marks, H.H. Latent coronary artery disease: Determination of its presence and severity by the exercise electrocardiogram. *Am. J. Cardiol.* 13:603, 1964.

13. Entmacher, P.S., Robb, G.P., and Seltzer, F. Detection and prognosis in coronary artery disease. *Cardiac Rehabil.* 4:55, 1973.

14. Doan, A.E., Peterson, D.R., Blackmon, J.R., and Bruce, R.A. Myocardial ischemia after maximal exercise in healthy men. *Am. Heart J.* 69:-11, 1965.

15. Li, Y-B, Ting, N., Chiang, B.N., Alexander, E.R., Bruce, R.A., and Grayson, J.T. Electrocardiographic response to maximal exercise: Treadmill and double Master exercise tests in middle-aged Chinese men. *Am. J. Cardiol.* 20:-541, 1967.

16. Allen, W.H., Aronow, W.S., Goodman, P., and Stinson, P. Five-year follow-up of maximal treadmill stress test in asymptomatic mean and women. *Circulation* 62:522, 1980.

17. Young, S.G. and Froelicher, V.F. Exercise testing: An update. *Mod. Conc. Cardiovasc. Dis.* 52:-25, 1983.

18. Redwood, D.R. and Epstein, S.E. Uses and limitations of stress testing in the evaluation of ischemic heart disease. *Circulation* 46:115, 1972.

19. Borer, J.S., Brensike, J.F., Redwood, D.R., Itscoitz, S.B., Passamani, E.R., Stone, N.J., Richardson, J.M., Levy, R.I., and Epstein, S.E. Limitations of the electrocardiographic response to exercise in predicting coronary-artery disease. *N. Engl. J. Med.* 293:367, 1975.

20. Redwood, D.R., Borer, J.S., and Epstein, S.E. Whither the ST segment during exercise? *Circulation* 54:703, 1976.

21. Rifkin, R.D. and Hood, W.B., Jr. Bayesian analysis of electrocardiographic exercise stress testing. *N. Engl. J. Med.* 297:681, 1977.

22. Hlatky, M., Botvinick, E., and Brundage, B. Diagnostic accuracy of cardiologists compared with probability calculations using Bayes' rule. *Am. J. Cardiol.* 49:1927, 1982.

23. Diamond, G.A., Staniloff, H.M., Forrester, J.S., Pollack, B.H., and Swan, H.J.C. Computer-assisted diagnosis in the noninvasive evaluation of patients with suspected coronary artery disease. *J. Am. Coll. Cardiol.* 1:444, 1983.

24. Rochmis, P. and Blackburn, H. Exercise tests: A survey of procedures, safety, and litigation experience in approximately 170,000 tests. *JAMA* 217:1061, 1971.

25. Bruce, R.A. and McDonough, J.R. Maximal exercise testing in assessing cardiovascular function. *J. S. C. Med. Assoc.* Suppl. 1:26, 1969.

26. Shephard, R.J. Do risks of exercise justify costly caution? *Physician Sports Med.* 2:58, 1977.

27. Bruce, R.A., Hornsten, T.R., and Blackmon, J.R. Myocardial infarction after normal responses to maximal exercise. *Circulation* 38:-552, 1968.

28. Gibbons, L.W., Cooper, K.H., Constant, R.R., Blide, R.W., and Meyer, B. The safety of maximal exercise stress testing in preventive and rehabilitative medicine. *Med. Sci. Sports* 9:74, 1977.

29. Grossman, L.A. and Grossman, M. Myocardial infarction precipitated by Master two-step test. *JAMA* 8:179, 1955.

30. Irving, J.B. and Bruce, R.A. Exertional hypotension and post-exertional ventricular fibrillation in stress testing. *Am. J. Cardiol.* 39:849, 1977.

31. McHenry, P.L. Risks of graded exercise testing. *Am. J. Cardiol.* 39:935, 1977.

32. Ladimer, I. Professional liability in exercise testing for cardiac performance. *Am. J. Cardiol.* 30:-753, 1972.

33. Alexander, J., Holder, A.R., and Wolfson, S. Legal implications of exercise testing. *Cardiovasc. Med.* 3:1137, 1978.

34. Bruce, R.A. Values and limitations of exercise electrocardiography. *Circulation* 50:1, 1974.

35. Goldman, L., Cook, E.F., Mitchell, N., Flatley, M., Sherman, H., Rosati, R., Harrell, F., Lee, K., and Cohn, P.F. Incremental value of the exercise test for diagnosing the presence or absence of coronary artery disease. *Circulation* 66:-945, 1982.

36. Goldschlager, N. Use of the treadmill test in the diagnosis of coronary artery disease in patients with chest pain. *Ann. Int. Med.* 97:383, 1982.

37. Kasser, I.S. and Bruce, R.A. Comparative effects of aging and coronary heart disease on submaximal and maximal exercise. *Circulation* 39:759, 1969.

38. Val, P.G., Chaitman, B.R., Waters, D.D., Gourassa, M.G., Scholl, J.M., Ferguson, R.J., and Wagniart, P. Diagnostic accuracy of exercise ECG lead systems in clinical subsets of women. *Circulation* 65:1465, 1982.

39. Kusumi, F., Bruce, R.A., Ross, M.A., Trimble, S., and Voigt, A.E. Elevated arterial pressure and postexertional ST-segment depression in middle-aged women. *Am. Heart J.* 92:576, 1976.

40. Linhart, J.W., Laws, J.G., and Satinsky, J.D.

Maximum treadmill exercise electrocardiography in female patients. *Circulation* 50:1173, 1974.

41. Vecchio, T.J. Predictive value of a single diagnostic test in unselected populations. *N. Engl. J. Med.* 274:1171, 1966.

42. Blackburn, H.A., Taylor, H.L., and Keys, A. Prognostic significance of the post-exercise electrocardiogram: Risk factors held constant. *Am. J. Cardiol.* 25:85, 1970.

43. Erikssen, J., Rasmussen, K., Forfany, K., and Storstein, O. Exercise ECG and case history in the diagnosis of latent coronary heart disease among presumably healthy middle-aged men. *Eur. J. Cardiol.* 5:463, 1977.

44. Froelicher, V.F., Jr., Yanowitz, F.G., Thompson, A.J., and Lancaster, M.C. The correlation of coronary angiography and the electrocardiographic response to maximal treadmill testing in 76 asymptomatic men. *Circulation* 48:597, 1973.

45. Bruce, R.A., DeRouen, T.A., and Hossack, K.F. Value of maximal exercise tests in risk assessment of primary coronary heart disease events in healthy men: Five years' experience of the Seattle Heart Watch Study. *Am. J. Cardiol.* 46:371, 1980.

46. Bruce, R.A., Hossack, K.F., DeRouen, T.A., and Hofer, V. Enhanced risk assessment for primary coronary heart disease events by maximal exercise testing: 10 years' experience of Seattle Heart Watch. *J. Am. Coll. Cardiol.* 2:565, 1983.

47. Kaplan, M.A., Harris, C.N., Aronow, W.S., Parker, D.P., and Ellestad, M.H. Inability of the submaximal treadmill test to predict the location of coronary disease. *Circulation* 47:250, 1973.

48. Dagenais, G.R., Rouleau, J.R., Christen, A., and Fabia, J. Survival of patients with a strongly positive exercise electrocardiogram. *Circulation* 65:452, 1982.

49. Weiner, D.A., McCabe, C.H., and Ryan, T.J. Prognostic assessment of patients with coronary artery disease by exercise testing. *Am. Heart J.* 105:749, 1983.

50. Schneider, R.M., Seaworth, J.F., Dohrmann, M.L., Lester, R.M., Phillips, H.R., Jr., Bashore, T.M., and Baker, J.T. Anatomic and prognostic implications of an early positive treadmill exercise test. *Am. J. Cardiol.* 50:682, 1982.

51. Goldman, S., Tselos, S., and Cohn, K. Marked depth of ST-segment depression during treadmill exercise testing: Indicator of severe coronary artery disease. *Chest* 69:729, 1976.

52. Hossack, K.F., Bruce, R.A., Fisher, L., and Hofer, V. Prognostic value of risk factors and exercise testing in men with atypical chest pain. *Int. J. Cardiol.* 3:37, 1983.

53. Fox, K.M., Jonathan, A., and Selwyn, A. Significance of exercise induced ST segment elevation in patients with previous myocardial infarction. *Br. Heart J.* 49:15, 1983.

54. Gewirtz, H., Sullivan, M., O'Reilly, G., Winter, S., and Most, A.S. Role of myocardial ischemia in the genesis of stress-induced S-T segment elevation in previous anterior myocardial infarction. *Am. J. Cardiol.* 51:1289, 1983.

55. Dunn, R.F., Freedman, B., Kelly, D.T., Bailey, I.K., and McLaughlin, A. Exercise-induced ST-segment elevation in leads $V_1$ or $aV_L$: A predictor of anterior myocardial ischemia and left anterior descending coronary artery disease. *Circulation* 63:1357, 1981.

56. Specchia, G., DeServi, S., Falcone, C., Angoli, L., Mussini, A., Bramucci, E., Marioni, G.P., Ardissino, D., Salerno, J., and Bobba, P. Significance of exercise-induced ST-segment elevation in patients without myocardial infarction. *Circulation* 63:46, 1981.

57. Bonoris, P., Greenberg, P.S., Castellanet, M., and Ellestad, M.H. Significance of changes in R wave amplitude during treadmill testing: Angiographic correlation. *Am. J. Cardiol.* 41:846, 1978.

58. Bonoris, P.E., Greenberg, P.S., Christison, G.W., Castellanet, M.J., and Ellestad, M.H. Evaluation of R wave amplitude changes versus ST-segment depression in stress testing. *Circulation* 57:904, 1978.

59. Berman, J.A., Wynne, J., Mallis, G., and Cohn, P.F. Improving diagnostic accuracy of the exercise test by combining R-wave changes with duration of ST segment depression in a simplified index. *Am. Heart J.* 105:60, 1983.

60. Fox, K., England, D., Jonathan, A., and Selwyn, A. Inability of exercise-induced R wave changes to predict coronary artery disease. *Am. J. Cardiol.* 49:674, 1982.

61. Deanfield, J.E., Davies, G., Mongiadi, F., Savage, C., Selwyn, A.P., and Fox, K.M. Factors influencing R wave amplitude in patients with ischaemic heart disease. *Br. Heart J.* 49:8, 1983.

62. David, D., Naito, M., Michelson, E., Watanabe, Y., Chen, C.C., Morganroth, J., Shaffenburg, M., and Blenko, T. Intramyocardial conduction: A major determinant of R-wave amplitude during acute mycoardial ischemia. *Circulation* 65:161, 1982.

63. Boran, K.J., Oliveros, R.A., Boucher, C.A., Beckmann, C.H., and Seaworth, J.F. Ischemia-associated intraventricular conduction disturbances during exercise testing as a predictor of proximal left anterior descending coronary artery disease. *Am. J. Cardiol.* 51:1098, 1983.

64. Famularo, M.A., Paliwal, Y., Redd, R., and Ellestad, M.H. Identification of septal ischemia during exercise by Q-wave analysis: Correlation with coronary angiography. *Am. J. Cardiol.* 51:438, 1983.

65. Hammermeister, K.E., DeRouen, T.A., Dodge, H.T., and Zia, M. Prognostic and predictive value of exertional hypotension in suspected coronary heart disease. *Am. J. Cardiol.* 51:1261, 1983.

66. Cohn, P.F. Role of non-invasive cardiac testing after an uncomplicated myocardial infarction. *N. Eng. J. Med.* 309:90, 1983.

67. Sivarajan, E.S., Bruce, R.A., Lindskog, B.D., Almes, M.J., Belanger, L., and Green, B. Treadmill test responses to an early exercise program after myocardial infarction: A randomized study. *Circulation* 65:1420, 1982.

68. The Committee on Exercise. *Exercise Testing and Training of Apparently Healthy Individuals: A Handbook for Physicians.* New York: American Heart Association, 1972.

69. The Committee on Exercise. *Exercise Testing and Training of Individuals with Heart Disease or at High Risk for its Development: A Handbook for Physicians.* New York: American Heart Association, 1975.

70. Rowell, L.B., Taylor, H.L., Simonson, E., and Carlson, W.S. The physiologic fallacy of adjusting for body weight performance of the Master two-step test. *Am. Heart J.* 70:461, 1965.

71. Niederberger, M., Bruce, R.A., Kusumi, F., and Whitkanack, S. Disparities in ventilatory and circulatory responses to bicycle and treadmill exercise. *Br. Heart J.* 36:377, 1974.

72. Bruce, R.A., Kusumi, F., and Hosmer, D. Maximal oxygen intake and nomographic assessment of functional aerobic impairment in cardiovascular disease. *Am. Heart J.* 85:546, 1973.

73. Shephard, R.J., Allen, C., Benade, A.J.S., Davies, C.T.M., dePrampero, P.E., Hedman, R., Merriman, J.E., Myhre, K., and Simmons, R. The maximum oxygen intake: An international reference standard of cardiorespiratory fitness. *Bull. W.H.O.* 38:757, 1968.

74. Dill, D.B. and Montoye, H.J. Man's capacity for consuming oxygen: Comments on an article. *J. Sports Med. Phys. Fitness* 8:245, 1968.

75. Dehn, M.M. and Bruce, R.A. Longitudinal variations in maximal oxygen intake with age and activity. *J. Appl. Physiol.* 33:805, 1972.

76. Rowell, L.B., Blackmon, J.R., and Bruce, R.A. Indocyanine green clearance and estimated hepatic blood flow during mild to maximal exercise in upright man. *J. Clin. Invest.* 43:166, 1964.

77. Froelicher, V.F., Jr., Brammell, H., Davis, G., Noguera, I., Stewart, A., and Lancaster, M.C. A comparison of the reproducibility and physiologic response to three maximal treadmill exercise protocols. *Chest* 65:512, 1974.

78. Astrand, P-O. and Saltin, B. Maximal oxygen uptake and heart rate in various types of muscular activity. *J. Appl. Physiol.* 16:977, 1961.

79. Stenberg, J., Astrand, P-O., Ekblom, B., Royce, J., and Saltin, B. Hemodynamic response to work with different muscle groups, sitting and supine. *J. Appl. Physiol.* 22:61, 1967.

80. Asmussen, E. and Hemmingsen, I. Determination of maximum working capacity at different ages in work with the legs or with the arms. *Scand. J. Clin. Lab. Invest.* 10:67, 1958.

81. Hermansen, L. and Saltin, B. Oxygen uptake during maximal treadmill and bicycle exercise. *J. Appl. Physiol.* 26:31, 1969.

82. Kasch, F.W., Phillips, W.H., Ross, W.D., Carter, J.E.L., and Boyer, J.L. A comparison of maximal oxygen uptake by treadmill and step-test procedures. *J. Appl. Physiol.* 21:1387, 1966.

83. Dixon, R.W., Jr. and Faulkner, J.A. Cardiac outputs during maximum effort running and swimming. *J. Appl. Physiol.* 30:653, 1971.

84. Robinson, B.F. Relation of heart rate and systolic blood pressure to the onset of pain in angina pectoris. *Circulation* 35:1073, 1967.

85. Pollock, M.L., Bohannon, R.L., Cooper, K.H., Ayres, J.J., Ward, A., Purdy, J.G., White, S.R., and Linnerud, A.C. A comparative analysis of four protocols for maximal treadmill stress testing. *Am. Heart J.* 92:39, 1976.

86. Blomqvist, G. and Atkins, J.M. Repeated exercise testing in patients with angina pectoris: Reproducibility and follow-up results. *Circulation* 44 (Suppl. 2):76, 1977.

87. Starling, M.R., Moody, M., Crawford, M.H., Levi, B., and O'Rourke, R.A. Repeat treadmill exercise testing: Variability of results in patients with angina pectoris. *Am. Heart J.* 107:298, 1984.

88. Smokler, P.E., MacAlpin, R.N., Alvaro, A., and Kattus, A.A. Reproducibility of a multi-stage near maximal treadmill test for exercise tolerance in angina pectoris. *Circulation* 48:346, 1973.

89. MacAlpin, R.N. and Kattus, A.A. Adaptation to exercise in agina pectoris. The electrocardiogram during treadmill walking and coronary angiographic findings. *Circulation* 33:183, 1966.

90. Lown, B. Verbal conditioning of angina pectoris during exercise testing. *Am. J. Cardiol.* 40:630, 1977.

91. Hartman, K.E., Nordstrom, L.A., and Gobel, F.L. Effect of placebo on exercise response and nitroglycerin consumption. *Minn. Med.* 12:839, 1976.

92. Sheps, D.S., Ernst, J.C., Briese, F.R., Lopez, L.V., Conde, C.A., Castellanos, A., and Myerburg, R.J. Decreased frequency of exercise-induced ectopic activity in the second of two consecutive treadmill tests *Circulation* 55:892, 1977.

93. Redwood, D.R., Rousing, D.R., Goldstein, R.E., Beiser, G.D., and Epstein, S.E. Impor-

tance of the design of an exercise protocol in the evaluation of patients with angina pectoris. *Circulation* 43:618, 1971.

94. Bruce, R.A. and DeRouen, T.A. Longitudinal Comparisons of Responses to Maximal Exercise. In L.J. Folinsbee (ed.), *Environmental Stress: Individual Human Adaptations.* New York; Academic, 1978.

95. Saltin, B. Physiologic effects of physical conditioning. *Med. Sci. Sports* 7:50, 1969.

96. Hartley, L.H., Grimby, G., Kilbom, A., Nilsson, N.J., Astrand, I., Bjure, J., Ekblom, B., and Saltin, B. Physical training in sedentary middle-aged and older men. III. Cardiac output and gas exchange at submaximal and maximal exercise. *Scand. J. Clin. Lab. Invest.* 24:445, 1969.

97. Detry, J.M.R., Rousseau, M., Vander-Broucke, G., Kusumi, F., Brasseur, L.A., and Bruce, R.A. Increased arteriovenous oxygen difference after physical training in coronary heart disease. *Circulation* 44:109, 1971.

98. Detry, J.M.R., Rousseau, M., and Brasseur, L.A. Early hemodynamic adaptations to physical training in patients with healed myocardial infarction. *Eur. J. Cardiol.* 2:307, 1975.

99. Bruce, R.A., Kusumi, F., and Frederick, R. Differences in cardiac function with prolonged physical training for cardiac rehabilitation. *Am. J. Cardiol.* 40:597, 1977.

100. Ilmarinen, J., Rutenfranz, J., Kylian, H., and Klimt, F. Untersuchung zur Tagesperiodik verschiedener Kreislaufund Atemgrossen bei submaximalen und maximalen Leistungen am Fahrradergometer. *Eur. J. Appl. Physiol.* 34:255, 1975.

101. Crockford, G.W. and Davies, C.T.M. Circadian variations in responses to submaximal exercise on a bicycle ergometer. *J. Physiol.* (Lond.) 201:94, 1969.

102. Joy, M., Pollard, C.M., and Nunan, T.O. Diurnal variation in exercise responses in angina pectoris. *Br. Heart J.* 48:156, 1982.

103. Goldstein, R.E., Redwood, D.R., Rosing, D.R., Beiser, G.D., and Epstein, S.E. Alterations in the circulatory response to exercise following a meal and their relationship to postprandial angina pectoris. *Circulation* 44:90, 1971.

104. Rowell, L.B., Marx, H.J., Bruce, R.A., Conn, R.D., and Kusumi, F. Reductions in cardiac output, central blood volume and stroke volume with thermal stress in normal men during exercise. *J. Clin. Invest.* 45:1801, 1966.

105. Davies, C.T.M., Chukweumeka, A.C., and Van-Haaren, J.P.M. Iron-deficiency anaemia: Its effect on maximum aerobic power and responses to exercise in African males aged 17–40 years. *Clin. Sci.* 44:555, 1973.

106. Wilmore, J.H. Influence of motivation on physi-

107. Cundiff, D. and Schwane, J. Walking vs. jogging in stages III and IV of the Bruce treadmill test. *Med. Sci. Sports* 9:74, 1977.

108. Astrand, P-O. Quantification of exercise capability and evaluation of physical capacity in man. *Prog. Cardiovasc. Dis.* 19:51, 1976.

109. Shephard, R.J. Methodology of exercise tests in healthy subjects and in cardiac patients. *Can. Med. Assoc. J.* 99:354, 1968.

110. Liebow, I.M. and Feil, H. Digitalis and the normal work electrocardiogram. *Am. Heart J.* 22:683, 1941.

111. Niederberger, M., Bruce, R.A., Frederick, R., Kusumi, F., and Marriott, A. Reproduction of maximal exercise performance in patients with angina pectoris despite ouabain treatment. *Circulation* 49:309, 1974.

112. Friesen, W.J. and Cumming, G.R. Effects of digoxin on the oxygen debt and the exercise electrocardiogram in normal subjects. *Can. Med. Assoc. J.* 97:960, 1967.

113. Bruce, R.A., Lind, A.R., Franklin, D., Muir, A.L., Macdonald, H.R., McNicol, G.W., and Donald, K.W. The effects of digoxin on fatiguing static and dynamic exercise in man. *Clin. Sci.* 34:29, 1968.

114. Sharma, B., Majid, P.A., Meeran, M.K., Whitaker, W., and Taylor, S.H. Clinical, electrocardiographic, and hemodynamic effects of digitalis (ouabain) on angina pectoris. *Br. Heart J.* 34:631, 1972.

115. Adair, R.F., Hellerstein, H.K., and White, L.W. Digoxin induced exercise ECG changes in young men: ST-T walk through phenomenon above 80% max heart rate. *Circulation* 46 (Suppl. 2):11, 1972.

116. Kawai, C. and Hultgren, H.N. The effect of digitalis upon the exercise electrocardiogram. *Am. Heart J.* 68:409, 1964.

117. Sketch, M.H., Mooss, A.N., Butler, M.L., Nair, C.K., and Mohiuddin, S.M. Digoxin-induced positive exercise tests: Their clinical and prognostic significance. *Am. J. Cardiol.* 48:655, 1981.

118. LeWinter, M.M., Crawford, M.H., O'Rourke, R.A., and Karliner, J.S. The effects of oral propranolol, digoxin, and combination therapy on the resting and exercise electrocardiogram. *Am. Heart J.* 93:202, 1977.

119. Reybrouck, T., Amery, A., and Billiet, L. Hemodynamic response to graded exercise after chronic beta-adrenergic blockade. *J. Appl. Physiol.* 42:123, 1977.

120. Gianelly, R.E., Treister, B.L., and Harrison, D.C. The effect of propranolol on exercise-induced ischemic S-T segment depression. *Am. J. Cardiol.* 24:161, 1969.

121. Ogilvia, R.I. Cardiovascular response to exercise under increasing doses of chlorthalidone. *Eur. J. Clin. Pharmacol.* 9:339, 1976.

122. Hossack, K.F., Pool, P.E., Steele, P., Crawford, M.H., DeMaria, A.N., Cohen, L.S., and Ports, T.A. Efficacy of diltiazem in angina on effort: A multicenter trial. *Am. J. Cardiol.* 49:567, 1982.

123. Sheffield, L.T. and Roitman, D. Stress testing methodology. *Prog. Cardiovasc. Dis.* 19:33, 1976.

124. Mason, R.E. and Likar, I. A new system of multiple-lead exercise electrocardiography. *Am. Heart J.* 71:196, 1966.

125. Mason, R.E., Likar, I., Biern, R.O., and Ross, R.S. Multiple-lead exercise electrocardiography: Experience in 107 normal subjects and 67 patients with angina pectoris, and comparison with coronary cinearteriography in 84 patients. *Circulation* 36:517, 1967.

126. Blackburn, H. (ed.). *Measurement in Exercise Electrocardiography: The Ernst Simonson Conference.* Springfield, Ill.: Thomas, 1969.

127. Berson, A.S. and Pipberger, H.V. The low-frequency response of electrocardiographs, a frequent source of recording errors. *Am. Heart J.* 71:779, 1966.

128. Committee on Electrocardiography. Recommendations for standardization of leads and of specifications for instruments in electrocardiography and vectorcardiography. American Heart Association. *Circulation* 35:583, 1967.

129. Simoons, M.L., Hugenholtz, P.G., Ascoop, C.A., Distelbrink, C.A., deLand, P.A., and Vinke, R.V.M. Quantitation of exercise electrocardiography. *Circulation* 63:471, 1981.

130. Bruce, R.A., Mazzarella, J.A., Jordan, J.W., Jr., and Green, E. Quantitation of QRS and ST segment responses to exercise. *Am. Heart J.* 71:455, 1966.

131. Chaitman, B.R. and Hanson, J.S. Comparative sensitivity and specificity of exercise electrocardiographic lead systems. *Am. J. Cardiol.* 47:1335, 1981.

132. Frank, E. An accurate, clinically practical system for spatial vectorcardiography. *Circulation* 13:737, 1956.

133. Rautaharju, P.M. Toward standardized VCG systems. (Letter). *Circulation* 55:556, 1977.

134. Blackburn, H., Taylor, H.L., Okamoto, N., Rautaharju, P., Mitchell, PL.L., and Kerkhof, A.C. Standardization of the Exercise Electrocardiogram. A Systematic Comparison of Chest Lead Configurations Employed for Monitoring During Exercise. In M.J. Karvonen and A.J. Barry (eds.), *Physical Activity and the Heart.* Springfield, Ill.: Thomas, 1967.

135. Phibbs, B.P. and Buckels, L.J. Comparative yield of ECG leads in multistage stress testing. *Am. Heart J.* 90:275, 1975.

136. Ascoop, C.A. *ST Forces During Exercise.* Utrecht: Grafisch Bedrijf Schotanus & Jens Utrecht VG, 1974.

137. Distelbrink, C.A., Ascoop, C.A., and deLang, P.A. The diagnostic value of exercise electrocardiograms. *Adv. Cardiol.* 16:529, 1976.

138. Hornsten, T.R. and Bruce, R.A. Computed ST forces of Frank and bipolar exercise electrocardiograms. *Am. Heart J.* 78:346, 1969.

139. Simoons, M.L. and Block, P. Toward the optimal lead system and optimal criteria for exercise electrocardiography. *Am. J. Cardiol.* 47:1366, 1981.

140. Ascoop, C.A., Simoons, M.L., Egmond, W.G., and Bruschke, A.V.G. Exercise test, history, and serum lipid levels in patients with chest pain and normal electrocardiogram at rest: Comparison to findings at coronary arteriography. *Am. Heart J.* 82:609, 1971.

141. Cumming, G.R. Yield of ischemic electrocardiograms in relation to exercise intensity. *Br. Heart J.* 34:919, 1972.

142. Cohn, P.F., Vokonas, P.S., Herman, M.V., and Gorlin, R. Post-exercise electrocardiogram in patients with normal resting electrocardiograms. *Circulation* 43:648, 1971.

143. Surawicz, B. and Saito, S. Exercise testing for detection of myocardial ischemia in patients with abnormal electrocardiograms at rest. *Am. J. Cardiol.* 41:493, 1978.

144. Technical Group on Exercise Electrocardiography. The exercise electrocardiogram: Differences in interpretation. *Am. J. Cardiol.* 21:871, 1968.

145. Doan, A.E., Peterson, D.R., Blackmon, J.R., and Bruce, R.A. Myocardial ischemia after maximal exercise in healthy men: One year follow-up of physically active and inactive men. *Am. J. Cardiol.* 17:9, 1966.

146. Most, A.S., Hornsten, T.R., Hofer, V., and Bruce, R.A. Exercise ST changes in healthy men. *Arch. Intern. Med.* 121:225, 1968.

147. Trayler, R.E. The Reproducibility of the Post-exercise ECG and PCG Indices of Myocardial Ischemia. Ph.D. dissertation. University of Washington, 1977.

148. Sjöstrand, T. The relationship between the heart frequency and the S-T level of the electrocardiogram. *Acta Med. Scand.* 138:201, 1950.

149. Simoons, M.L. and Hugenholtz, P.G. Gradual changes of ECG waveform during and after exercise in normal subjects. *Circulation* 52:570, 1975.

150. Stuart, R.J., Jr. and Ellestad, M.H. Upsloping S-T segments in exercise stress testing: Six-year follow-up study of 438 patients and correlation with 248 angiograms. *Am. J. Cardiol.* 37:19, 1976.

151. McHenry, P.L., Phillips, J.F., and Knoebel, S.B. Correlation of computer quantitated treadmill exercise electrocardiogram with arteriographic location of coronary artery disease. *Am. J. Cardiol.* 30:747, 1972.

152. Sheffield, L.T., Holt, J.H., Lester, F.M., Conroy, D.V., and Reeves, T.J. On-line analysis of the exercise electrocardiogram. *Circulation* 40:935, 1969.

153. Ascoop, C.A., Distelbrink, C.A., deLang, P., and Van Bemmel, J.H. Quantitative comparison of exercise vectorcardiograms and findings at selective coronary arteriography. *J. Electrocardiol.* 7:9, 1974.

154. Dower, G.E., Bruce, R.A., Pool, J., Simmons, M.L., Niederberger, M.W., and Meilink, L.J. Ischemic polarcardiographic changes induced by exercise. A new criterion. *Circulation* 48:725, 1973.

155. Bruce, R.A., DeRouen, T., Peterson, D.R., Irving, J.B., Chinn, N., Blake, B., and Hofer, V. Noninvasive predictors of sudden cardiac death in men with coronary heart disease: Predictive value of maximal stress testing. *Am. J. Cardiol.* 39:833, 1977.

156. Berman, J.L., Wynne, J., and Cohn, P.F. A multivariate approach for interpreting treadmill exercise tests in coronary artery disease. *Circulation* 58:505, 1978.

157. Kansal, S., Roitman, D., Bradley, E.L., Jr., and Sheffield, L.T. Enhanced evaluation of treadmill tests by means of scoring based on multivariate analysis and its clinical application: A study of 608 patients. *Am. J. Cardiol.* 52:1155, 1983.

158. Hollenberg, M., Budge, W.R., Wisenski, J.A., and Gertz, E.W. Treadmill score quantifies electrocardiographic response to exercise and improves test accuracy and reproducibility. *Circulation* 61:275, 1980.

159. Fisher, L.D., Kennedy, J.W., Chaitman, B.R., Ryan, T.J., McCabe, C., Weiner, D., Tristani, F., Schloss, M., and Warner, H.R., Jr. Diagnostic quantification of CASS (Coronary Artery Surgery Study) clinical and exercise test results in determining presence and extent of coronary artery disease: A multivariate approach. *Circulation* 63:987, 1981.

160. Bruce, R.A., DeRouen, T.A., and Hammermeister, K.E. Noninvasive screening criteria for enhanced 4-year survival after aortocoronary bypass surgery. *Circulation* 60:638, 1979.

# 7. ECHOCARDIOGRAPHY

## William E. Lawson
## Claire E. Proctor

Echocardiography has become an increasingly valuable noninvasive procedure in diagnosing the presence of coronary artery disease and assessing its functional consequences. Initially, *M-mode echocardiography* had been useful in demonstrating regional left ventricular dysfunction secondary to ischemic heart disease. However, M-mode echocardiography gives an "ice pick" view of the heart that permits only limited left ventricular regional visualization. The segmental abnormalities typical of coronary artery disease may be missed using M-mode echocardiography and are more readily detected and quantitated using two-dimensional echocardiography. Variations in regional function invalidate assumptions of a normal left ventricular geometry with relatively homogeneous function, thereby making M-mode estimates of global left ventricular function unreliable. In the past, M-mode echocardiography has also shown itself to be useful in the diagnosis of noncoronary chest pain syndromes such as mitral valve prolapse, pericardial disease, and hypertrophic obstructive cardiomyopathy.

The addition of *two-dimensional echocardiography* (cross-sectional echocardiography) has substantially improved the ability to evaluate ischemic heart disease. Direct visualization of the proximal coronary arteries may permit the echocardiographic diagnosis of coronary artery disease in some instances. Standardization of views has permitted localization and quantification of regional and global function in both acute and chronic ischemic heart disease. Many of the complications of myocardial infarction are most easily recognized by two-dimensional echocardiography. Interventional echocardiographic techniques (such as contrast and stress echocardiography) have also become practical, enhancing our ability to detect and localize coronary artery disease.

## M-Mode and Two-Dimensional Techniques

With the patient in the left lateral decubitus position, the echocardiographic exam is begun by moving the M-mode transducer along the left parasternal border until an M-mode sweep can be recorded from the level of the aortic valve to that of the body of the left ventricular cavity (figure 7–1). The end-diastolic left ventricular cavity dimension is measured at the onset of the ECG QRS (and at the level of the tips of the mitral valve) as the vertical distance between the trailing edge of the septal echo and the leading edge of the posterior left ventricular free wall. End-systolic left ventricular dimension is measured at the time of minimal cavity dimension [1]. The ejection fraction and fractional shortening derived from these measurements, however, are unreliable in the presence of regional asynergy. Regional wall thickness changes in the septum and posterior wall may be evaluated by measurements obtained at end-systole and end-diastole. Areas with previous infarction and scarring may be identified by regional thinning, decreased motion, and increased echo density (figure 7–2).

M-mode echocardiography is not satisfactory for directly quantitating the area of left ventricular dysfunction because of variation in the rate of scanning by hand. In addition, the axial chord image provided by M-mode echocardiography

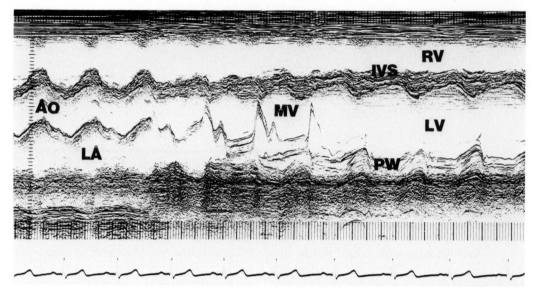

FIGURE 7–1. Normal M-mode echocardiographic sweep from the aortic root to the left ventricular cavity. Ao = aortic root, MV = mitral valve, LA = left atrium, RV = right ventricle, IVS = interventricular septum, PW = posterior wall, LV = left ventricle.

makes it difficult to adequately visualize and correctly spatially orient all the left ventricular segments. The use of cross-sectional echocardiographic techniques has increased the ability to record lateral motion, as well as axial motion, in multiple planes. To evaluate left ventricular regional function, two-dimensional echocardiograms are recorded in several related planes. A parasternal long axis view may be performed that visualizes segments similar to those seen with the standard M-mode echocardiogram sweep, as shown in figure 7–3. Additional parasternal short axis views at the level of the mitral valve, papillary muscle, and apex are commonly recorded as are apical four- and two-chamber views (seen diagramatically in figure 7–4) [2, 3]. Left ventricular segments are identified and graded by the type of wall motion (hyperkinetic, normokinetic, hypokinetic, aki-

netic, or dyskinetic) and by wall thickening (increased, normal, decreased, paradoxical, or no thickening) (table 7–1). Combining the results of this segmental analysis allows a left ventricular wall motion index to be derived:

$$\text{Wall motion index} = \frac{\text{sum of the individual asynergy scores for each segment}}{\text{number of segments}}$$

## Validation

Echocardiography is potentially the ideal method of left ventricular imaging. Using two-

TABLE 7–1. Regional systolic function

| Disorder | Systolic endocardial thickening | Systolic endocardial motion | Asynergy score |
|---|---|---|---|
| Hyperkinesis | +++ | +++, inward | −1 |
| Normal | ++ | ++, inward | 0 |
| Hypokinesis | + | +, inward | +1 |
| Akinesis | 0 | 0 | +2 |
| Dyskinesis | Systolic thinning | Systolic expansion | +3 |

Regional systolic function is assigned an asynergy score based on the systolic function 50 percent or more of the segment (refer to reference 43).

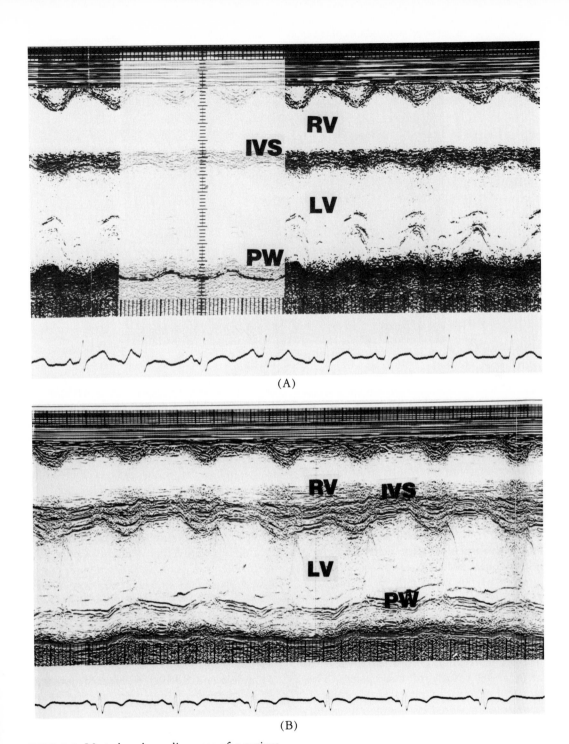

FIGURE 7–2. M-mode echocardiograms of a patient
with an (A) anteroseptal infarction and one with a
(B) inferoposterior infarction. IVS = interventricular
septum, PW = posterior wall, LV = left ventricle,
RV = right ventricle.

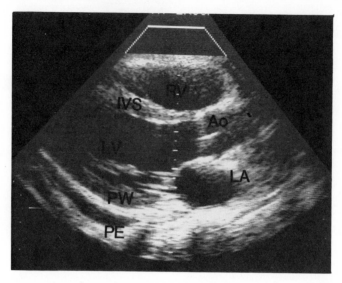

FIGURE 7–3. Two-dimensional echocardiographic parasternal long axis view of a patient with a pericardial effusion. LV = left ventricle, LA = left atrium, Ao = aortic root, IVS = interventricular septum, PW = posterior wall, PE = pericardial effusion.

dimensional echocardiography, the left ventricle can be imaged in multiple planes in a tomographic fashion, potentially allowing examination of all left ventricular segments. Left ventricular wall motion as determined by two-dimensional echocardiography has compared favorably with the results of biplane left ventriculography in several studies. For example, Kisslo and co-workers [4] compared phased array two-dimensional echocardiography obtained in 105 consecutive patients with standard biplane left ventriculography. Echocardiograms judged adequate for analysis were obtained in 82 percent of the potentially comparable regions. A region-by-region comparison of wall motion assessed by the two methods yielded agreement 90 percent of the time. In those regions where the two methods gave different evaluations of wall motion, an attempt was made to identify the reason for discrepancy. Two-dimensional echocardiography errors in identifying wall motion were most commonly attributable to one of three problems: (1) inadequate visualization of an area previously thought to be adequately visualized; (2) problems with technique whereby spatial orientation was incorrect or tangential imaging caused left ventricular distortion; or (3) observer errors. It was recommended that at least 50 percent of a particular segment be adequately visualized throughout the cardiac cycle to reliably evaluate asynergy. A major problem of two-dimensional echocardiog-

raphy was the significant number of patients and wall segments that could not be evaluated due to poor visualization. With ventriculography there were no problems with adequate visualization. Ventriculographic errors occurred mainly as a result of the superimposition of normally and abnormally contracting segments. Other potential problems in using biplane left ventriculography as a standard with which to compare two-dimensional echocardiography include the following: (1) the regions compared may not be similar, and (2) the use of radiopaque contrast affects vascular tone and cardiac function, potentially affecting global and regional function.

Pandian and Kerber [5] have demonstrated, using sonomicrometers, the ability of two-dimensional echocardiography to detect transient regional ischemia in open-chest dogs. The sonomicrometers were oriented side by side to yield segment length changes and in an endocardial-epicardial orientation to give changes in wall thickness. During normal systolic function, wall thickening and segment length shortening was seen with both methods. During ischemia, paradoxical systolic thinning and segment length bulging were also appreciated with both methods. There were quantitative differences in the

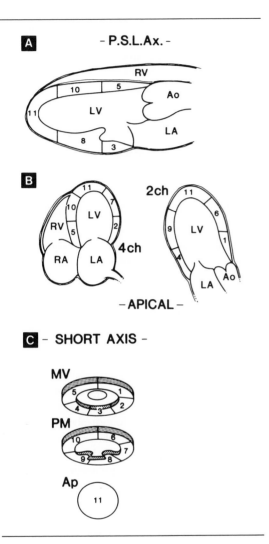

FIGURE 7–4. Diagram of standard left ventricular two-dimensional echocardiographic views. (A) parasternal long axis (P.S.L.Ax). (B) apical 4- and 2-chamber (ch) views, (C) parasternal short axis at levels of mitral valve, papillary muscles and apex. Numbered segments include anterior left ventricular free wall (LVFW) base (1) and mid (6); lateral LVFW base (2) and mid (7); posterior LVFW base (3) and mid (8); inferior LVFW base (4) and mid (9); interventricular septum base (5) and mid (10); apex (Ap) (11). RV = right ventricle; LV = left ventricle; RA = right atrium; LA = left atrium; Ao = aorta.

degree of thickening or thinning seen with the two methods, but qualitatively they were in complete agreement.

Weiss and colleagues [6] have assessed the accuracy of two-dimensional echocardiography in detecting, localizing, and quantitating myocardial injury in man by correlation with postmortem studies. All transmural myocardial infarctions were identified as hypokinetic, akinetic, or dyskinetic in the majority of cases (79 percent). Abnormal wall motion segments were seen, however, in 46 percent of the areas deemed normal at postmortem. Most (82 percent) of these latter segments were hypokinetic, and many (66 percent) were adjacent to areas of scarring. These results suggest that evaluation of wall motion abnormalities using two-dimensional echocardiography is sensitive in the detection of myocardial infarction, but overestimates the extent and localization of myocardial injury.

## Technical Problems

Present limitations in the use of two-dimensional echocardiography in patients with coronary artery disease are related to a number of factors. A major limitation of the technique is that images that are completely adequate for analysis can be obtained in only about 70 to 80 percent of patients because of factors such as body habitus and lung disease. Technical problems in performing the echocardiographic examination may also be reflected in oblique or tangential endocardial imaging, inadequate segment visualization, and incorrect segment identification. If not recognized, these problems will cause errors in the assessment of regional function.

While wall thickening analysis may be more accurate than wall motion analysis in defining and quantifying regional dysfunction secondary to coronary artery disease, analysis is limited by the ability of two-dimensional echocardiography to visualize adequately endocardial and epicardial borders throughout the cardiac cycle. New automated edge detection algorithms and microprocessors may soon make quantitative assessment of both regional wall motion and thickening easier to perform [7–9]. Wall thickening changes may be especially helpful in evaluating regional function in conditions that may have associated wall motion abnormalities such as atrial septal defect, valvular heart disease, mitral valve prolapse, cardiomyopathy, interventricular conduction defects, and volume overload states.

Using two-dimensional echocardiography, lateral relationships can be appreciated and quantitated that would not be possible with M-mode echocardiography. The ability to visualize lateral cardiac structures has improved the ability to reproducibly spatially orient the sampling plane and thus correctly identify left ventricular segments and their function. Cross-sectional echocardiography has also proved to be of assistance in verifying placement of the M-mode chord relative to surrounding structures. Inherent cardiac motion may affect analysis of regional motion, but floating axis systems have not been shown to be clearly superior to fixed frames of reference in correcting this problem [10]. Using M-mode echocardiography, this effect is most noticeable where the posterior wall usually shows greater systolic inward motion than the interventricular septum, in part because of the anterior motion of the normal heart during systole. As smaller areas of the left ventricle are examined, however, problems with cardiac motion and rotation throughout the cardiac and respiratory cycles may become more noticeable. The internal landmarks used to identify regions do not permit precise segment localization (i.e., the papillary muscle heads may be visualized over a 1 to 2 cm range in the short axis projection). This may result in a small but unquantifiable and irreducible source of error, since the same exact region is not examined throughout the cardiac cycle.

Another problem limiting the accuracy of regional analysis is the significant heterogeneity of function that has been shown to be present in normal hearts [11, 12]. However, while segments with decreased thickening and hypokinesis may be present both in normal patients and in those with ischemic heart disease, the more severe abnormalities of systolic wall thinning and dyskinesis appear specific for ischemia or infarction.

Calculation of global left ventricular function is currently time consuming and often inaccurate despite the availability of modeling equations, which have been shown to potentially yield an excellent correlation with angiography. This is partly due to frequent difficulties in adequately visualizing all the left ventricular segments and in standardizing and reproducing the apical two-dimensional echocardiography views in particular. Improvements in automatic edge detection and computer processing may significantly improve the accuracy and facility with which such calculations can be made. The use of multiple two-dimensional echocardiography planes to reconstruct a three-dimensional model [14] may be possible with advances in computer technology. This would hopefully limit current spatial orientation problems.

## Direct Visualization of Coronary Arteries

Symptomatic left main coronary artery disease is known to be associated with high mortality, despite medical therapy, and remains a clear-cut indication for coronary artery bypass graft surgery [15, 16]. Invasive coronary angiography has been widely employed as the only modality capable of defining coronary anatomy and diagnosing this lethal lesion. By contrast, single-, double-, and triple-vessel coronary artery disease in patients with good left ventricular function and stable exertional angina have been shown to have comparable mortality with either medical or surgical therapy [17]. Since the first report by Weyman and co-workers [18] in 1976 of left main coronary artery visualization, interest has focused on the ability of echocardiography to detect left main disease.

Weyman and co-workers, using a parasternal short axis approach, were able to identify the normal left main coronary artery as two parallel linear echoes separated by an echo-free space [18]. Each of their three patients with angiographically confirmed left main coronary artery disease was identified by luminal narowing on echocardiography.

Echocardiographic examination of the coronary arteries is difficult because the coronary arteries are small and in motion throughout the cardiac cycle (figure 7–5). Left main coronary artery visualization requires review of many individual frames in several cardiac cycles. Using the short axis orientation, the aortic root, pulmonary artery, and superior margin of the left ventricle have been used for orientation, and the failure to visualize these structures by echocardiogram limits the ability to detect left main coro-

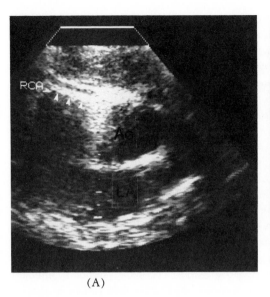

(A)

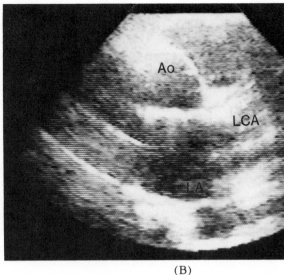

(B)

FIGURE 7-5. Two-dimensional echocardiographic visualization of right (**A**) and left (**B**) coronary arteries from a parasternal short axis position. LCA = left coronary artery, RCA= right coronary artery, Ao= aoric root, LA = left atrium.

nary artery disease. Because other linear echoes may be seen in the vicinity of the left main coronary artery, continuity of the echoes with the aortic root and the left main coronary artery ostia must be demonstrated. Left main coronary artery disease may be visualized as a localized luminal narrowing on the echocardiogram with proximal and distal patency. Because the left main coronary artery may not run a linear course that permits visualization of the left main coronary artery from ostium to bifurcation, small adjustments of transducer angulation may be required to visualize the left main coronary artery throughout its course. This makes analysis more difficult. High-intensity, localized, irregular intraluminal echoes from the left main coronary artery have also been reported as useful in detecting disease. Examining the left main coronary artery from an apical orientation as described by Chen and his co-workers [19] has also increased the ability to image the left main coronary artery and thus identify left main coronary artery disease.

To date, results of studies examining the ability of echocardiography to detect left main coronary artery disease have been promising. In the study by Chen and his colleagues involving 73 patients [19], the left main coronary artery was adequately visualized in 52 patients (71 percent). Of the 16 patients with left main coronary disease by angiography, 12 were correctly identified by echocardiography. Of the patients without left main coronary artery disease, three patients were falsely identified as having left main coronary artery disease. Echocardiographic analysis showed a sensitivity of 75 percent and specificity of 91 percent for detection of left main coronary artery disease in those patients in whom adequate left main visualization was possible.

A recent study by Block and Popp [20] showed similar results with the left main coronary artery adequately visualized in 37 of 50 patients (74 percent). Four of the five patients with left main coronary artery disease were correctly identified, a sensitivity of 80 percent. Of the 32 patients with left main disease, six were incorrectly identified, yielding a specificity of 81 percent.

Recent technical advances promise to increase the practicality of echocardiography for the detection of left main coronary artery disease. A study by Rink and his co-workers [21] made use of a strobe freeze-frame feature to extract and continuously display a portion of the cardiac cycle when the left main coronary artery was visible. Digital gray scale analysis enhanced the ability to detect high-intensity echoes in the left main coronary artery. In their prospective study of 31 patients, the three with left main coronary artery disease were correctly identified, for a sensitivity of 100 percent. There was only one false-positive, for a specificity of 96 percent.

Friedman and his colleagues [22] have recently described a method utilizing a modified antilog curve to enhance strong echoes and suppress weak ones. In their study, images of the left main coronary artery adequate for analysis were obtained in 30 of 37 patients (80 percent). The 16 patients with left main coronary artery disease were all correctly identified, for a sensitivity of 100 percent. There was one false-positive, yielding a specificity of 93 percent.

The direct visualization of the left main coronary artery by echocardiography is an extremely promising area. In patients with stable angina and good left ventricular function, concern about left main coronary artery disease is still a major reason for cardiac catheterization and coronary angiography. Echocardiographic identification of left main coronary artery disease may in the future offer a cost-effective and noninvasive means of screening such patients for left main coronary artery disease. Only when abnormalities were found would follow-up angiography and bypass surgery be necessary. Other coronary artery segments—including the left main bifurcation, the proximal left anterior descending and left circumflex coronary arteries, and the proximal right coronary artery—have been visualized with limited success, but are an area of future clinical promise. One of the current major limitations in coronary artery imaging is that echocardiographic examinations adequate for analysis can be performed in only 70 to 80 percent of the at-risk population. Further improvements in visualization and image processing offer promise in improving the ability of two-dimensional echocardiography to diagnose left main coronary artery disease.

## Evaluating Regional and Global Left Ventricular Function

Within seconds of the onset of transmural ischemia, regional contractility and wall motion

are affected. As we have discussed, direct visualization of the proximal coronary arteries is sometimes possible with two-dimensional echocardiography, but most of the time the presence of significant coronary artery disease must be inferred from the presence of segmental wall motion and thickening abnormalities.

### ANIMAL MODELS

Using sonomicrometers to evaluate myocardial thickening, Gallagher and his co-workers [23] demonstrated in open-chest dogs the effect of various degrees of left circumflex coronary artery stenosis produced by an hydraulic cuff occluder. Regional myocardial blood flow was assessed by radioactive microspheres. They found that progressive coronary stenosis affected *subendocardial* blood flow first and most significantly. Moderate and severe hypokinesis was produced without a significant decrease in mean transmural blood flow, but with a significant reduction in perfusion of the inner half of the myocardium. Akinesis occurred with a 42 percent reduction in transmural blood flow, but with no significant changes in *subepicardial* perfusion. Dyskinesis was seen with a 58 percent reduction in transmural blood flow; there was also significant reduction in perfusion of the subepicardial and subendocardial layers (i.e., transmural ischemia). These findings suggest that progressive reductions in coronary artery blood flow over a wide range produced graded reductions in wall thickening and eventual paradoxical systolic thinning. Systolic thinning was associated with a significant transmural reduction in blood flow.

A study by Lieberman and his colleagues [24] examined wall motion and thickening as indicators of myocardial infarction in dogs 48 hours after snare coronary artery occlusion. Using two-dimensional echocardiography in open-chest anesthetized dogs, they found wall motion abnormalities to be less precise than thickening in separating infarct, peri-infarct, and distal normal areas. Myocardial infarction affecting > 20 percent of the transmural wall thickness produced systolic thinning, which did not increase in degree with increases in the transmural extent of the infarction. For myocardial infarctions affecting less than 20 percent of the transmural wall thickness, a graded effect was demonstrable, with smaller infarcts causing less of a decrease in systolic thickening than larger ones. This study is important in showing that infarction produces wall motion and thickening abnormalities, both of which can be detected by two-dimensional echocardiography. Wall thickening appeared more precise as an indicator of myocardial infarction. The threshold phenomenon that they described by which infarctions involving > 20 percent of the wall thickness produce similar systolic thinning is a possible reason for consistent overestimation of acute myocardial infarction size by echo. While two-dimensional echocardiography could give an accurate estimate of functional infarct size, the inability to grade the transmural extent of infarction could cause overestimation of actual pathological infarct size. Certain complications of transmural myocardial infarction, such as infarct expansion or myocardial rupture, would be overpredicted because of mixing of subendocardial and transmural infarctions.

Nieminen and his associates [25] examined serial changes in regional function in dogs with acute myocardial infarctions produced by coronary artery ligation. Closed-chest echocardiograms were performed at 2, 24, and 48 hours postinfarct to assess regional wall thickening and compared with the infarct size determined at 48 hours. The echo-predicted infarct size at 2 hours, arrived at by summing the areas of segments showing systolic thinning or failure to thicken, was much larger than the infarct size seen at 48 hours. Significant reductions were found in the echo-predicted infarct size at 24 and 48 hours, with the 48-hour observations still overestimating but most accuractely predicting actual infarct size.

The study by Nieminen and co-workers showed that in dogs, evaluation of regional function will overestimate eventual infarct size in the early postinfarction period. Regional function evaluation became increasingly accurate at 24 hours and 48 hours postmyocardial infarction. The tendency of two-dimensional echocardiography to overestimate infarct size early in the course of an acute myocardial infarction, and the spontaneous resolution of regional dysfunction with time, must obviously be considered when two-dimensional echocardiography is used to follow the course of a myocardial infarction or to evaluate the efficacy of early interventions to limit infarct size. Improved regional function in these dogs may have been due to the functional recovery of jeopardized myocardium in the peri-infarction border zone. Similar at-risk areas in humans with coronary artery disease that may show reversible dysfunction include areas with jeopardized collaterals and areas that are supplied by a significantly stenotic coronary artery.

By contrast with the previous study, Gibbons and co-workers [26, 27] did not find significant changes in abnormal wall motion in echocardiograms performed at 30 minutes, 48 hours, and 1 week postinfarction in closed-chest dogs. A further follow-up by echocardiography showed the abnormal wall motion significantly decreased at 3 weeks, with a further significant reduction at 6 weeks (with wall motion abnormalities virtually absent in four of the eight dogs). Simultaneous blood flow changes measured with radioactive microspheres were suggestive of scar contraction. This study demonstrates that wall motion abnormalities as indicators of chronic ischemia (especially old myocardial infarction) may diminish with time as the area of infarction develops scar tissue and then contracts.

In another study of clinical interest, Blumenthal and his associates [28] used two-dimensional echocardiography to evaluate late regional function in dogs with medically salvaged myocardium 1 week postsnare coronary artery occlusion. The area of infarction was minimal, with an average necrosis of 2.2 percent of the left ventricle. Despite the minimal amount of infarction, thickening abnormalities were demonstrable in salvaged areas adjacent to the center of the occluded bed. These functional abnormalities were present despite normal regional blood flow and no histologic evidence of infarction. Whether the functional dysfunction was due to persistent biochemical abnormalities resulting in "stunned" myocardium or to "tethering" by adjacent ischemic segments was unclear. This study demonstrates that two-dimensional echocardiography may overestimate infarct size, including as abnormal those peri-infarction areas with normal blood flow and histology. It also sounds a cautionary note in the use of two-dimensional echocardiography to assess success after interventions designed to produce myocardial salvage in acute myocardial infarction. Thus, despite histologic salvage, functional abnormalities can persist at 1 week in the dog model.

During acute myocardial infarction, areas with abnormal regional function and a potentially similar two-dimensional echocardiography appearance include areas of infarction and ischemia and bordering zones. Contrast two-dimensional echocardiography has attracted interest because it may allow another "independent" assessment of regional flow and function.

Sakamaki and colleagues [29] showed that contrast two-dimensional echocardiography could provide information regarding regional myocardial perfusion, identifying the area at "risk" for myocardial infarction. Using a saline-renografin contrast solution with monastral blue dye to evaluate regional perfusion in closed-chest dogs, they demonstrated that the under-perfused zones could be identified on two-dimensional echocardiography as perfusion defects. The actual size of infarction, as identified by triphenyltetrazolium-chloride, was slightly overestimated. Similarly, Tei and co-workers [30] demonstrated that the underperfused zones correlated well with regional asynergy and that the use of a saline-renografin contrast solution was associated only with minor and transient hemodynamic and ECG changes.

By contrast, Armstrong and co-workers [31, 32], using two-dimensional echocardiography with gelatin-encapsulated microbubbles and a hydrogen peroxide contrast solution in open-chest dogs, demonstrated that contrast two-dimensional echocardiography was more accurate than abnormal wall motion and/or thickening in identifying and quantitating areas of reduced perfusion or infarction.

An exciting alternative approach to identifying areas with reduced perfusion by contrast two-dimensional echocardiography is based on computer analysis of the rate of regional contrast washout. In closed-chest dogs, using an agitated saline-renografin contrast solution, Maurer and Tei and colleagues [33, 34] were able to demonstrate that the greater the degree of experimen-

tal stenosis the more prolonged the contrast disappearance rate. A significant prolongation in the contrast washout index was even seen with 50 percent coronary artery stenosis.

This technique promises, by allowing quantitation of regional coronary blood flow, to be helpful in assessing both the presence and severity of coronary artery disease. It may also prove helpful in identifying ischemic but potentially salvageable areas, and in assessing the efficacy of interventions aimed at improving regional coronary blood flow. Areas of "stunned" myocardium—with normal perfusion but regional dysfunction—may also be identified by this technique.

Myocardial viability may also be demonstrable by interventions that cause reversibility of regional dysfunction. Sakamaki and co-workers [35] have used two-dimensional echocardiography in conjunction with post extrasystolic potentiation to demonstrate functional reserve. They found that when segmental necrosis was greater than 60 percent, no postextrasystolic potentiation occurred. Normal and ischemic regions and areas with less than 40 percent segmental necrosis demonstrated a postextrasystolic increase in wall thickening and systolic fractional area change. Comparable results, in distinguishing potentially viable from necrotic myocardium in dogs, were demonstrated using IV nitroglycerin by Shimoura and colleagues [36]. If these interventions fulfill their potential in patients with coronary artery disease, they will be extremely helpful in therapeutic decision making by allowing differentiation of reversible ischemia from infarction. Introduction of the ventricular premature beat may be achieved in humans with the use of the external cardiac stimulator, as demonstrated by Cohn and colleagues in their M-mode echocardiographic studies [37], to be discussed in the next section.

CLINICAL STUDIES

In humans, the ability of echocardiography to detect transient myocardial ischemia has been demonstrated in patients with Prinzmetal's angina. Distante and colleagues [38] studied 29 episodes of Prinzmetal's angina in a group of 12 patients using M-mode echocardiography. During the 29 spontaneous episodes, 18 M-mode echocardiograms showed an average 76 percent reduction in wall motion and 88 percent reduction in wall thickening in the affected area (septum or posterior wall). M-mode echocardiography performed at the time of resolution of the ST-T wave abnormalities revealed transient supernormal function in the previously affected area. When 11 episodes of Prinzmetal's angina were induced by ergonovine, regional dysfunction was found to precede angina or significant ST-T abnormalities.

Because regional wall motion abnormalities are a sensitive indicator of myocardial ischemia and infarction, two-dimensional echocardiography has been tested as a potential screening procedure in patients with acute chest pain syndromes. Horowitz and associates [39] examined 80 consecutive patients presenting with suspected first myocardial infarctions. Two-dimensional echocardiograms adequate for analysis were obtained in 81 percent of the study patients. Of these patients, 33 were eventually diagnosed as having an acute myocardial infarction, while a myocardial infarction was ruled out in the remaining 32. Regional wall motion abnormalities were detectable in all 19 of the patients with a transmural infarction and in 12 of the 14 patients with a subendocardial infarct. By contrast, the initial ECG was nondiagnostic in 55 percent of the 33 patients eventually diagnosed as having an acute myocardial infarction. There were five patients with regional wall motion abnormalities in whom a myocardial infarction was ruled out. Cardiac catheterization in three of these patients revealed coronary artery disease in all three. All 10 of the patients developing complications from their infarcts had transmural infarctions that were detected by echocardiography.

A study by Heger and co-workers [40] also demonstrated the ability of two-dimensional echocardiograms to identify and localize wall motion abnormalities in acute myocardial infarction. Two-dimensional echocardiograms were performed in 44 patients with acute myocardial infarctions, of which 37 echocardiograms (84 percent) were adequate for analysis. The two-dimensional echocardiograms revealed areas of asynergy in all patients studied; the area most commonly affected was the apex. Correlation

with ECG revealed asynergy of posterior segments in 19 out of 20 patients with inferior wall myocardial infarctions, asynergy of anterior segments in all of the 14 patients with anterior wall myocardial infarctions, and asynergy of anterior and posterior segments in all of the three patients with combined anterior and inferior myocardial infarctions. Four patients died, and postmortem examination revealed evidence of myocardial infarction in 21 of the 22 areas with asynergy by two-dimensional echocardiography.

An interesting study by Brad Stamm and co-workers [41] examined the extent of asynergy in acute myocardial infarction with single- and multivessel coronary artery disease. As a baseline for comparison, 51 patients with recent myocardial infarction and single-vessel coronary artery disease were evaluated by two-dimensional echocardiography to establish usual and maximal zones of asynergy for each coronary artery. Two-dimensional echocardiograms were subsequently performed in a group of 30 patients with acute myocardial infarctions and single- or multivessel disease, and regional wall motion abnormalities were compared. Remote asynergy (asynergy outside the maximal zone previously established for one-vessel disease) was present in 17 of the 22 (77 percent) patients with multivessel disease. Of the five multivessel disease patients without remote asynergy, four had only a 70 percent lesion in a second coronary artery. No remote asynergy was seen in the anterior myocardial infarction patients with one-vessel disease. By comparison, regional compensatory hyperkinesis was seen in four of the eight patients (50 percent) with one-vessel disease, but in only one of the 22 patients (45 percent) with multivessel disease. A follow-up echocardiogram performed in the early convalescent course demonstrated improvement in asynergy in two of the six patients (33 percent) with one-vessel disease and in 10 of the 13 multivessel disease patients (79 percent).

These findings suggest that remote asynergy in acute myocardial infarctions is common and is strongly suggestive of multivessel disease. Possible mechanisms for this "ischemia at a distance" include (1) jeopardized collaterals and/or (2) increased functional demands on an area supplied by a stenotic coronary artery. Compensatory hyperkinesis, as might be expected, was seen much more frequently in one-vessel disease. Resolution of asynergy was seen in both single- and multivessel groups, but with a higher frequency in the multivessel-disease patients. This would suggest that the greater the extent of coronary artery disease in the patient with acute myocardial infarction, the greater the likelihood that two-dimensional echocardiography wall motion analysis will overestimate infarct size.

Another clinical application of interest is the use of two-dimensional echocardiography to evaluate ST-T wave abnormalities in areas distant to the acute myocardial infarction. As reported by Camara and his associates [42], two-dimensional echocardiography can be used to evaluate remote asynergy of the left ventricle. The absence of remote asynergy implies that the ECG changes are truly "reciprocal" and not due to distant ischemia or infarction. Thus, using two-dimensional echocardiography to determine whether distant wall areas are at risk of infarction is a potentially useful procedure in guiding therapeutic decisions in the patient with an acute myocardial infarction.

The leading cause of in-hospital mortality in the patient with an acute myocardial infarction is pump failure. As we have discussed, two-dimensional echocardiography overestimates actual pathological infarct size when performed during an acute myocardial infarction, because it identifies wall motion abnormalities in peri-infarction segments, as well as in ischemic but uninfarcted areas. Despite this tendency, however, the degree of functional impairment can be related to the extent and severity of regional dysfunction. Several clinical studies using wall motion indexes, based on a summation of the function of individual segments, have shown the ability of two-dimensional echocardiography to grade pump dysfunction, identify patients with multivessel disease, and predict hemodynamic deterioration, reinfarction, and death [43–46].

The extent and severity of left-vessel dysfunction is the most important single prognosticator of morbidity and mortality in the postmyocardial infarction patient. Nishimura and his co-workers [47] demonstrated the ability of predischarge echocardiograms to identify a group of convalescent myocardial infarction patients at higher risk of morbidity and mortality in the first year post-infarction. Based on a wall motion score index, 88 percent of the patients with more extensive and severe regional abnormalities had a postdischarge course complicated by severe congestive heart failure, severe angina, death, or reinfarction. By contrast, only 9 percent of the patients with limited regional abnormalities developed complications.

During ischemia and infarction, changes in chemical composition occur that alter ultrasound attenuation and may prove to be detectable by backscatter analysis. Changes such as tissue edema secondary to acute ischemia or injury, and increasing collagen content postinfarction, if detectable, could be clinically useful. Rasmussen and co-workers [48], in a classic article using M-mode echocardiography, demonstrated that echocardiography is a sensitive and specific method for detecting myocardial scar tissue. Areas of myocardial scar tissue were characteristically thinned, echo dense, and demonstrated decreased wall motion and thickening. Further work on ultrasound myocardial tissue characterization may make possible the identification of the more subtle changes seen with acute ischemia and infarction.

Cohn and co-workers [37] have shown that postextrasystolic potentiation can be used to differentiate ischemic from infarcted areas with M-mode echocardiography. Postextrasystolic potentiation that demonstrates contractile reserve can be used to identify areas of reversible ischemia for possible revascularization.

## Evaluating the Complications of Ischemic Heart Disease

Echocardiography has been extremely successful in recognizing some of the complications of ischemic heart disease. Differentiating infarct expansion from infarct extension or reinfarction is a common clinical problem in the early postmyocardial infarction patient. Both extension and expansion may be associated with chest pain and ECG changes, and both may result in clinical congestive heart failure and increased mortality. Extension is seen more commonly with nontransmural myocardial infarctions than with transmural myocardial infarctions and may usu-

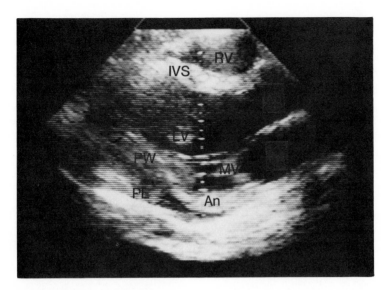

FIGURE 7–6. Two-dimensional echocardiographic pa-rasternal long axis view of a patient with a post-erobasal left ventricular aneurysm and pericardial effusion. An = aneurysm, PE = pericardial effusion, LV = left ventricle, LA = left atrium, Ao = aortic root, MV = mitral valve, IVS = interventricular sep-tum, PW = posterior wall, RV = right ventricle.

ally be recognized by additional segmental dys-function on two-dimensional echocardiography. Expansion is associated with transmural infarc-tions. Eaton, Erlebacher, and colleagues [49, 50] have shown early expansion to be character-ized echocardiographically by regional thinning and segmental dilation. This leads to chronic, generalized left ventricular dilation and func-tional limitation.

Left ventricular aneurysms are another com-mon complication of myocardial infarctions and probably occur in about 15 percent of survivors, with the most common location being anteroapi-cal. Aneurysms are frequently unrecognized on physical examination, chest x-ray, and serial ECGs, though clinically they are associated with congestive heart failure, angina, arrhythmias, and thrombi. Aneurysms are recognized on the echocardiograms as a well-demarcated bulge present in both diastole and systole, with thinned, akinetic or dyskinetic walls (figure 7–6). Using biplane ventriculography as the "gold standard," Visser and co-workers [51], in a study of 386 patients with 111 angiographic aneurysms, showed a two-dimensional sensitiv-ity of 93 percent and a specificity of 94 percent in detecting aneurysms.

Many investigators have demonstrated the utility of two-dimensional echocardiography in detecting left ventricular mural thrombi (figure 7–7). Ezekowitz and colleagues [52] demon-strated comparable sensitivities of two-dimen-sional echocardiography and indium-111 plate-let imaging. The mechanisms of detection are different; two-dimensional echocardiography re-lies on thrombus size, motion, and location, while indium imaging relies on thrombus activ-ity. Thus, the two techniques are complemen-tary. Used separately, indium scanning showed a sensitivity of 71 percent versus 77 percent for two-dimensional echocardiography. When the two techniques were used conjointly, all thrombi were detected. Echocardiography has been shown to be superior in sensitivity and spe-cificity to single-plane left ventriculography for diagnosis of thrombi by Takamoto and co-work-ers [53]. The same workers also showed that chronic anticoagulation significantly decreased the incidence of left ventricular thrombi.

Besides identifying patients with postinfarc-tion thrombi who are at high risk for systemic embolization, two-dimensional echocardiogra-phy has been used to follow the natural history of untreated versus anticoagulated patients with thrombi. A study by Weinreich and associates [54] demonstrated that chronic anticoagulation significantly decreased the incidence of throm-

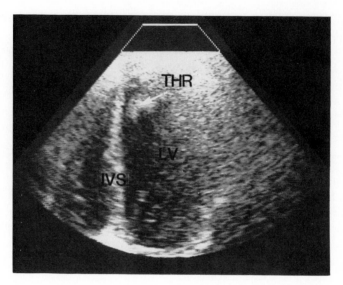

FIGURE 7-7. Apical four-chamber two-dimensional echocardiographic view showing an apical left ventricular mural thrombus in a patient with an anteroapical infarction. LV = left ventricle, IVS = interventricular septum, RV = right ventricle, THR = thrombus.

boembolism in patients with anteroapical infarcts and left ventricular thrombi. Of interest is that all embolic events in untreated patients occurred within 4 months of the acute myocardial infarction, despite persistent thrombi being demonstrable in 17 of the 28 patients (61 percent) on follow-up echo study. While most patients with untreated postinfarction thrombi appear to embolize within 4 months, if at all, it will be interesting to see whether the group of patients who have benefited from chronic anticoagulation show sustained benefit after discontinuation of anticoagulation.

Rupture of the left ventricle postinfarction is an infrequent but life threatening complication. Ventricular septal defects resulting from infarction may vary in size, shape, and number. While large defects in the muscular septum may be readily detectable by direct echocardiographic visualization, small, multiple, or linear defects may be missed. Drobac and co-workers [55] demonstrated that right heart contrast echocardiography is a rapid, sensitive method of detecting ventricular septal defects. Even without being directly visualized, the ventricular septal defects may be appreciated by an area of absent contrast in the right ventricle or by the presence of contrast appearing in the left ventricle. While sensitive for the presence of a ventricular septal defect, size of the defect could not be accurately predicted based on the size of the contrast defect.

Rupture of the left ventricular free wall is usually rapidly fatal from massive hemopericardium and resulting cardiac tamponade. Occasionally, free wall rupture may occur with clotted blood being retained by the fibrous pericardium, resulting in the formation of a pseudoaneurysm. Unlike true aneurysms, fatal delayed spontaneous rupture of a pseudoaneurysm is common if the pseudoaneurysm is not recognized and repaired. Catherwood and colleagues [56] demonstrated that echocardiography can identify pseudoaneurysms and distinguish them from true aneurysms. Features characteristic of pseudoaneurysms included (1) sudden endocardial discontinuity at the entrance of the pseudoaneurysm, (2) a saccular or globular pseudoaneurysm configuration, and (3) a narrow orifice neck relative to the body of the pseudoaneurysm.

Papillary muscle dysfunction is often first clinically detected in the myocardial infarction patient as the development of a new mitral regurgitation murmur accompanying congestive heart failure. Differentiation from heart failure due to extensive infarction is important because the congestive heart failure resulting from mitral regurgitation secondary to papillary muscle dysfunction is surgically correctable. With functional papillary muscle dysfunction the associated myocardium may be ischemic, infarcted, and scarred or ruptured. Mintz et al. [57] and Godley et al. [58] have shown that papillary muscle dysfunction is most commonly associated with echocardiographic evidence of ischemia/infarction (inferoposterior wall motion abnormalities) at the bases of the papillary muscles. With actual rupture of one or more papillary muscle heads the echocardiogram shows evidence of a flail mitral leaflet. Papillary muscle ischemia and scarring may be manifest on the echocardiogram as apical retraction of a mitral valve leaflet. Retraction of a leaflet prevents appropriate systolic coaptation, resulting in mitral regurgitation.

The right ventricle is often involved in left ventricular inferior wall infarctions, though right ventricular infarction is rarely predominant hemodynamically. Clinically, when the right ventricular infarction predominates, hemodynamically common features are an elevated central venous pressure, clear lungs, and hypotension—features that may also be seen with pericardial constriction or tamponade. The use of two-dimensional echocardiography can usually readily distinguish these conditions. The two-dimensional echocardiographic characterization of global and regional right ventricular size and function is difficult, however, because the normal right ventricular "banana" shape is difficult to characterize geometrically and measure reproducibly. Recent reports by Kaul et al. [59] and Panidis et al. [60] have shown that two-dimensional echocardiography can yield comparable results to radionuclide angiography in assessing global right ventricular ejection fraction, as well as demonstrating that right ventricular ejection fraction is commonly depressed with inferior wall myocardial infarctions.

Regional right ventricular function has been studied by Lopez-Sendon et al. [61], and Jugdutt et al. [62]. Regional right ventricular asynergy was commonly associated with inferoposterior left ventricular infarctions. The most commonly affected portion of the right ventricle was also inferoposterior. Analysis of patients with hemodynamically predominant right ventricular infarctions revealed echocardiographic evidence of biventricular dysfunction, but with the extent of the right ventricular wall motion abnormalities exceeding that of the left ventricular wall motion abnormalities. Other echocardiographic features of right ventricular infarcts included right ventricular dilation, paradoxical septal motion, and right ventricular thrombi.

About half of all patients who have had a transmural myocardial infarction develop a localized pericarditis. About 15 percent develop a more diffuse serofibrinous pericarditis. While the pericardial effusion associated with a myocardial infarction may be large, clinical tamponade is rare. Echocardiography is useful in detecting, localizing, and grossly quantitating pericardial effusions (see figure 7-3). In the patient with cardiomegaly on chest x-ray, echocardiography may be particularly useful in differentiating chamber dilation from pericardial effusion. Characteristic echocardiographic features of pericardial effusions include (1) separation of the visceral and the parietal pericardium throughout the cardiac cycle by a relatively echo-free space, (2) decreased motion of the parietal pericardium, and (3) swinging of the entire heart with large effusions.

## Stress Testing and Other Interventions

Since myocardial ischemia rapidly causes regional ventricular dysfunction, the use of two-dimensional echocardiography could potentially increase both the sensitivity and specificity of stress testing in detecting exercise-induced ischemia. The major problems with dynamic exercise have been recording technically adequate studies with correct spatial orientation, particularly during upright treadmill exercises. Both ventricular pacing [63] and cold pressor tests [64] have been used in conjunction with two-dimensional echocardiography and promise to be useful in patients incapable of dynamic exercise. For the patient capable of exercise, both bicycle and treadmill tests have been used to produce myocardial ischemia.

Using supine bicycle exercise, Morganroth and co-workers [65] were frequently able to demonstrate wall motion abnormalities during exercise. The rate of false-negative studies, however, was 52 percent. Subcostal imaging during upright bicycle exercise by Ginzton and his colleagues [66] was used successfully to produce diagnostic quality studies in 39 of his 41 patients (95 percent), both at rest and with exercise. The regional wall motion abnormalities detected by this technique were shown to correlate well with first-pass radionuclide angiography.

Crawford and associates [67] were able to obtain biapical two-dimensional echocardiography suitable for regional analysis at rest and during upright bicycle exercise in 72 percent of 25 patients with coronary artery disease. They found the technique useful in assessing the global left ventricular response to exercise and in evaluating the therapeutic effects of nitroglycerin.

Because regional wall motion abnormalities produced by exercise do not immediately resolve, several groups have studied the accuracy of two-dimensional echocardiography in detecting wall motion abnormalities when performed immediately after treadmill exercise.

In a study by Scott Robertson and associates [68], two-dimensional echocardiography was performed at rest and immediately after the treadmill test in 30 patients with known or suspected coronary artery disease. Echocardiograms suitable for analysis were obtained in 92 percent. In the group of 11 patients suspected of having coronary artery disease, two-dimensional echocardiography identified resting wall motion abnormalities after exercise in all seven patients shown to have coronary artery disease on subsequent catheterizations. Of 14 patients with known coronary artery disease prior to catheterization, two-dimensional echocardiography identified resting wall motion abnormalities in all 14 and new wall motion abnormalities after exercise in 10; furthermore, two-dimensional echocardiography substantially increased the sensitivity of the exercise test for detection of myocardial ischemia from 10 out of 21 to 17 out of 21. Regional analysis of wall motion also proved useful in predicting the distribution of coronary artery obstructions. Corresponding wall motion abnormalities correctly identified 12 of 14 patients as having right coronary artery disease, 14 of 17 patients as having left anterior descending coronary artery disease, and 2 of 7 patients as having circumflex coronary artery

disease. All eight patients with one-vessel coronary artery disease were correctly identified, compared to only five of nine patients with two-vessel disease. These findings suggest that two-dimensional echocardiography performed immediately after treadmill exercise significantly enhances the sensitivity of stress testing for myocardial ischemia. It may also be useful in identifying specific coronary arteries with significant occlusions.

Exercise radionuclide ventriculography is the standard method of assessing global and regional left ventricle function during exercise. Limacher and his co-workers [69] compared the results of post-treadmill two-dimensional echocardiography with standard exercise radionuclide ventriculography in patients with and without angiographic coronary artery disease. Compared to the group of patients with normal coronary arteries in whom mean global echocardiographic ejection fraction rose from 66 to 73 percent, the mean global echocardiographic ejection fraction of the coronary artery patients fell from 56 to 53 percent. Using an abnormal global ejection fraction response to exercise, or the development of regional dyssynergy, as indicators of left ventricular ischemia, 51 of 56 patients (91 percent) with coronary artery disease were detected. Exercise radionuclide ventriculography and two-dimensional echocardiography were then compared in a group of 41 patients of which 24 had coronary artery disease. As compared to radionuclide ventriculography, two-dimensional echocardiography showed an overall sensitivity of 92 percent versus 71 percent for radionuclide ventriculography in detecting coronary artery disease patients. The relative specificities were 88 percent for two-dimensional echocardiography and 82 percent for radionuclide ventriculography. Both modalities showed increased sensitivity with a greater extent of coronary artery disease. The degree of exercise-induced global dysfunction detected by two-dimensional echocardiography correlated well with the number of arteries with disease. Also, the regional wall motion abnormalities detected in patients with coronary artery disease after exercise were predictive of significant coronary artery disease in the coronary artery supplying that segment. This study suggests that posttreadmill two-dimensional echocardiography compares favorably with standard exercise radionuclide ventriculography in detecting coronary artery disease. Besides improving the sensitivity and specificity of stress testing, it offers information regarding the extent and location of coronary artery disease that may have therapeutic value.

Taking advantage of the fact that regional myocardial ischemia decreases global ejection fraction and changes left ventricle geometry toward a more globular configuration, Berberich and co-workers [70] demonstrated that simple M-mode echocardiography immediately posttreadmill could be used to detect coronary artery disease. Using the criteria of a normal decrease in end-systolic dimension ($\geq 3$mm) and a normal increase in fractional shortening ($\geq 5$ percent), M-mode echocardiography showed a 94 percent sensitivity for the detection of patients with coronary artery disease, the only false-negatives being in patients with single-vessel coronary artery disease.

## Hemodynamic Information

Most echocardiographic hemodynamic information is inferential, being based on calculations to determine left ventricular size and function. An exciting development has been the use of Doppler echocardiography to provide a clinically useful noninvasive cardiac output. The Doppler shift produced by moving blood cells in the ascending aorta enables the calculation of an instantaneous mean blood flow velocity. Integrating the blood flow velocity over the cross-sectional area of the ascending aorta during a cardiac cycle yields the stroke volume and when multiplied by the heart rate, the cardiac output. The cardiac outputs obtained by this technique have been shown to correlate well with those obtained by thermodilution [71, 72].

A method for estimating left ventricular filling pressures using M-mode echocardiography in patients in normal sinus rhythm, attractive in its simplicity, has been described by Askenazi and co-workers [73]. Using the ratio of the time intervals obtained from mitral valve closure (MVC) to the onset of the QRS and from aortic valve closure (AVC) to the maximal early diastolic opening of the anterior mitral valve leaflet (E), an excellent correlation was demonstrated with pulmonary capillary wedge pressure (PCW). The derived regression equation predicts that

$$PCW \text{ (mmHg)} = 36.6 \frac{[(Q-MVC)]}{(AVC-E)} - 2.0,$$

with a standard error of 2.7 mmHg.

## Cardiac Surgery

Echocardiography has found multiple uses in the patient undergoing coronary artery bypass surgery. Preoperatively, echocardiography is commonly used to evaluate global and regional left ventricular function. Intraoperatively, echocardiography, as demonstrated by Sahn and colleagues [74], may be useful in imaging the coronary arteries. While coronary angiography is clearly the "gold standard," in selected cases echocardiographic imaging is useful in confirming intraoperatively the location and severity of coronary lesions to optimize graft placement. This may be particularly true in vessels that have been inadequately angiographically visualized because of technical difficulties or high-grade proximal disease. While this study demonstrated that intraoperative imaging with a $9MH_z$ transducer provided a close correlation with angiographic results, a newly available $13MH_z$ transducer (the size of a crayon) may further enhance results.

Postoperatively, echocardiography has been used to evaluate changes in global and regional left ventricular function. Both radionuclide ventriculography and echocardiography have often demonstrated postoperative deterioration in septal function and enhanced lateral wall function as assessed by wall motion changes. An interesting study by Force and co-workers [75] suggests that the commonly seen wall motion abnormalities are due to postoperative changes in cardiac motion. Using the usual fixed frame of reference for analysis in patients who had uncomplicated coronary artery bypass graft surgery, there was a clear-cut deterioration in septal wall motion and improvement in lateral wall motion with no change in global ejection fraction.

However, septal thickening, by echocardiography, remained unchanged. When a floating axis frame of reference was used, which corrected for translational effects of cardiac motion, lateral and septal wall motion was unchanged from preoperative values. This study suggests that changes in cardiac motion commonly occur after coronary bypass surgery and may lead to errors in the assessment of regional function. Either regional thickening or wall motion assessment by a floating axis frame of reference may be used to correctly assess regional function.

Pericardial effusions are demonstrable in as many as 50 to 85 percent of patients postbypass surgery. Weitzman and colleagues [76], using M-mode echocardiography, found pericardial effusions in 85 percent of 112 postbypass graft patients, with virtually all being visualized by the fifth postoperative day. Most effusions became gradually smaller and more echo dense before resolving by 30 days postoperatively. Complications due to pericardial effusions were shown to be extremely rare and not dependent on effusion size.

## Conclusions

Echocardiography has become an indispensable tool in the diagnosis and management of ischemic heart disease and its complications. Current applications range from the direct visualization of proximal coronary artery disease to evaluation of the affects of coronary artery disease on regional and global left ventricular function. Echocardiography overestimates the actual pathologic area of acute infarction or ischemic "area at risk," but is useful in evaluating left ventricular functional impairment and identifying the complications of myocardial infarctions. Used in conjunction with stress testing, echocardiography adds to the sensitivity and specificity for detecting coronary artery disease and, by identifying regional wall motion abnormalities, may identify specific coronary arteries as having significant disease.

## References

1. *Recommendations of the American Society of Echocardiography Regarding Quantitation in M-Mode Echocardiography.* Report of the American Society of Echocardiography, Indianapolis, Indiana, March 7, 1978.
2. Henry, W.L., DeMaria, A., Gramiak, R., King, D.L., Kisslo, J.A., Popp, R.L., Sahn, D.J., Schiller, N.B., Tajik, A., Teichholz, L.E., and Weyman, A.E. *Report of the American Society of Echocardiography Committee on Nomenclature and Standards in Two-Dimensional Echocardiography,* June 1980.
3. Henry, W.L., DeMaria, A., Feigenbaum, H., Kerber, R., Kisslo, J., Weyman, A.E., Nanda, N., Popp, R.L., Sahn, D., Schiller, N.B., and Tajik, A.J. *Report of the American Society of Echocardiography Committee on Nomenclature and Standards: Identification of Myocardial Wall Segments,* November 1982.
4. Kisslo, J.A., Robertson, D., Gilbert, B.W., von-Ramm, O., and Behar, V.S. A comparison of real-time, two-dimensional echocardiography and cineangiography in detecting left ventricular asynergy. *Circulation* 55:134, 1977.
5. Pandian, N.G. and Kerber, R.E. Two-dimensional echocardiography in experimental coronary stenosis. I. Sensitivity and specificity in detecting transient myocardial dyskinesis: Comparison with sonomicrometers. *Circulation* 66:597, 1982.
6. Weiss, J.L., Bulkley, B.H., Hutchins, G.M., and Mason, S.J. Two-dimensional echocardiographic recognition of myocardial injury in man: Comparison with postmortem studies. *Circulation* 63:401, 1981.
7. Buda, A.J., Delp, E.J., Meyer, C.R., Jenkins, J.M., Smith, D.N., Bookstein, F.L., and Pitt, B. Automatic computer processing of digital 2-dimensional echocardiograms. *Am. J. Cardiol.* 52:384, 1983.
8. Henschke, C.I., Risser, T.A., Sandor, T., Hanlon, W.B., Neumann, A., and Wynne, J. Quantitative computer-assisted analysis of left ventricular thickening and motion by 2-dimensional echocardiography in acute myocardial infarction. *Am. J. Cardiol.* 52:960, 1983.
9. Zwehl, W., Levy, R., Garcia, E., Haendchen, R.V., Childs, W., Corday, S.R., Meerbaum, S., and Corday, E. Validation of a computerized edge detection algorithm for quantitative two-dimensional echocardiography. *Circulation* 68:1127, 1983.
10. Moynihan, P.F., Parisi, A.F., and Feldman, C.L. Quantitative detection of regional left ventricular contraction abnormalities by two-dimensional echocardiography. I. Analysis of methods. *Circulation* 63:752, 1981.
11. Pandian, N.G., Skorton, D.J., Collins, S.M., Falsetti, H.L., Burke, E.R., and Kerber, R.E. Heterogeneity of left ventricular segmental wall thickening and excursion in 2-dimensional echocardiograms of normal human subjects. *Am. J. Cardiol.* 51:1667, 1983.

12. Haendchen, R.V., Wyatt, H.L., Maurer, G., Zwehl, W., Bear, M., Meerbaum, S., and Corday, E. Quantitation of regional cardiac function by two-dimensional echocardiography. I. Patterns of contraction in the normal left ventricle. *Circulation* 67:1234, 1983.

13. Weyman, A.E. *Cross-Sectional Echocardiography.* Philadelphia: Lea & Febiger, 1982.

14. Nixon, J.V., Saffer, S.I., Lipscomb, K., and Blomqvist, C.G. Three-dimensional echoventriculography. *Am. Heart J.* 106:435, 1983.

15. Takaro, T., Hultgren, H.N., Detre, K.M., and Peduzzi, P. The Veterans Administration cooperative study of stable angina: Current status. *Circulation* 65(suppl. II):60, 1982.

16. European Coronary Surgery Study Group. Prospective randomized study of coronary artery bypass surgery in stable angina pectoris: A progress report on survival. *Circulation* 65(suppl. II):67, 1982.

17. CASS Principal Investigators and Their Associates. Myocardial infarction and mortality in the coronary artery surgery study (CASS) randomized trial. *N. Engl. J. Med.* 310:750, 1984.

18. Weyman, A.E., Feigenbaum, H., Dillon, J.C., Johnston, K.W., and Eggleton, R.C. Noninvasive visualization of the left main coronary artery by cross-sectional echocardiography. *Circulation* 54:169, 1976.

19. Chen, C.C., Morganroth, J., Ogawa, S., and Mardelli, T.J. Detecting left main coronary artery disease by apical, cross-sectional echocardiography. *Circulation* 62:288, 1980.

20. Block, P.J. and Popp, R.L. Two-dimensional echocardiographic assessment of left main coronary artery disease in man (abstract). *Circulation* 68(Suppl. II):1463, 1983.

21. Rink, L.D., Feigenbaum, H., Godley, R.W., Weyman, A.E., Dillon, J.C., Phillips, J.F., and Marshall, J.E. Echocardiographic detection of left main coronary artery obstruction. *Circulation* 65:719, 1982.

22. Friedman, M.J., Sahn, D.J., Goldman, S., Eisner, D.R., Gittinger, N.C., Lederman, F.L., Puckette, C.M., and Tiemann, J.J. High predictive accuracy for detection of left main coronary artery disease by antilog signal processing of two-dimensional echocardiographic images. *Am. Heart J.* 103:194, 1982.

23. Gallagher, K.P., Kumada, T., Koziol, J.A., McKown, M.D., Kemper, W.C., and Ross, J., Jr. Significance of regional wall thickening abnormalities relative to transmural myocardial perfusion in anesthetized dogs. *Circulation* 62:1266, 1980.

24. Lieberman, A.N., Weiss, J.L., Jugdutt, B.I., Becker, L.C., Bulkley, B.H., Garrison, J.G., Hutchins, G.M., Kallman, C.A., and Weisfeldt, M.L. Two-dimensional echocardiography and infarct size: Relationship of regional wall motion and thickening to the extent of myocardial infarction in the dog. *Circulation* 63:739, 1981.

25. Nieminen, M., Parisi, A.F., O'Boyle, J.E., Folland, E.D., Khuri, S., and Kloner, R.A. Serial evaluation of myocardial thickening and thinning in acute experimental infarction: Identification and quantification using two-dimensional echocardiography. *Circulation* 66:174, 1982.

26. Gibbons, E.F., Franklin, T.D., Hogan, R.D., Nolting, M., and Weyman, A.E. Correlation of myocardial infarct scar contraction with resolution of regional dysfunction in the canine left ventricle *Circulation:* 68(Suppl. III):282, 1983 (abstract).

27. Gibbons, E.F., Franklin, T.D., Hogan, R.D., Nolting, M., and Weyman, A.E. The course of resolution of regional dysfunction in the chronic infarct. Experimental cross-sectional echocardiographic studies *Circulation* 68(Suppl. III):109, 1983 (abstract).

28. Blumenthal, D.S., Becker, L.C., Bulkley, B.H., Hutchins, G.M., Weisfeldt, M.L., and Weiss, J.L. Impaired function of salvaged myocardium: Two-dimensional echocardiographic quantification of regional wall thickening in the open-chest dog. *Circulation* 67:225, 1983.

29. Sakamaki, T., Tei, C., Meerbaum, S., Shimoura, K., Kondo, S., Fishbein, M.C., Y-Rit, J., Shah, P.M., and Corday, E. Verification of myocardial contrast two-dimensional echocardiographic assessment of perfusion defects in ischemic myocardium. *J. Am. Coll. Cardiol.* 3:34, 1984.

30. Tei, C., Sakamaki, T., Shah, P.M., Meerbaum, S., Shimoura, K., Kondo, S., and Corday, E. Myocardial contrast echocardiography: A reproducible technique of myocardial opacification for identifying regional perfusion deficits. *Circulation* 67:585, 1983.

31. Armstrong, W.F., Mueller, T.M., Kinney, E.L., Tickner, E.G., Dillon, J.C., and Feigenbaum, H. Assessment of myocardial perfusion abnormalities with contrast-enhanced two-dimensional echocardiography. *Circulation* 66:166, 1982.

32. Armstrong, W.F., West, S.R., Mueller, T.M., Dillon, J.C., and Feigenbaum, H. Assessment of location and size of myocardial infarction with contrast-enhanced echocardiography. *J. Am. Coll. Cardiol.* 2:63, 1983.

33. Maurer, G., Ong, K., Haendchen, R., Torres, M., Tei, C., Wood, F., Meerbaum, S., Shad, P., and Corday, E. Myocardial contrast two-dimensional echocardiography: Comparison of contrast disappearance rates in normal and underperfused myocardium. *Circulation* 69:418, 1984.

34. Tei, C., Kondo, S., Meerbaum, S., Ong, K., Maurer, G., Wood, F., Sakamaki, T., Shimoura, K., Corday, E., and Shah, P.M. Correlation of myocardial echo contrast disappearance rate

("washout") and severity of experimental coronary stenosis. *J. Am. Coll. Cardiol.* 3:39, 1984.

35. Sakamaki, T., Corday, E., Meerbaum, S., Torres, M.A.R., Fishbein, M.C., Y-Rit, J., and Aosaki, N. Relation between myocardial injury and postextrasystolic potentiation of regional function measured by two-dimensional echocardiography. *J. Am. Coll. Cardiol.* 2:52, 1983.

36. Shimoura, K., Meerbaum, S., Sakamaki, T., Kondo, S., Fishbein, M.C., Y-Rit, J., Tei, C., Shah, P.M., and Corday, E. Relation between functional response to nitroglycerin and extent of myocardial necrosis in dogs: Mapping of the left ventricle by 2-dimensional echocardiography. *Am. J. Cardiol.* 52:177, 1983.

37. Cohn, P.F., Angoff, G.H., and Sloss, L.J. Noninvasively induced postextrasystolic potentiation of ischemic and infarcted myocardium in patients with coronary artery disease. *Am. Heart J.* 97:187, 1979.

38. Distante, A., Rovasi, D., Picano, E., Moscarelli, Palombo, C., E., Morales, M.A., Michelassi, C., and L'Abbate, A. Transient changes in left ventricular mechanics during attacks of Prinzmetal's angina: An M-mode echocardiographic study. *Am. Heart J.* 107:465, 1984.

39. Horowitz, R.S., Morganroth, J., Parrotto, C., Chen, C.C., Sofer, J., and Pauletto, F.J. Immediate diagnosis of acute myocardial infarction by two-dimensional echocardiography. *Circulation* 65:323, 1982.

40. Heger, J.J., Weyman, A.E., Wann, L.S., Rogers, E.W., Dillon, J.C., and Feigenbaum, H. Cross-sectional echocardiographic analysis of the extent of left ventricular asynergy in acute myocardial infarction. *Circulation* 61:1113, 1980.

41. Stamm, R.B., Gibson, R.S., Bishop, H.L., Carabello, B.A., Beller, G.A., and Martin, R.P. Echocardiographic detection of infarct-localized asynergy and remote asynergy during acute myocardial infarction: Correlation with the extent of angiographic coronary disease. *Circulation* 67:233, 1983.

42. Camara, E.J.N., Chandra, N., Ouyang, P., Gottlieb, S.H., and Shapiro, E.P. Reciprocal ST change in acute myocardial infarction: Assessment by electrocardiography and echocardiography. *J. Am. Coll. Cardiol.* 2:251, 1983.

43. Gibson, R.S., Bishop, H.L., Stamm, R.B., Crampton, R.S., Beller, G.A., and Martin, R.P. Value of early two-dimensional echocardiography in patients with acute myocardial infarction. *Am. J. Cardiol.* 49:1110, 1982.

44. Horowitz, R.S. and Morganroth, J. Immediate detection of early high-risk patients with acute myocardial infarction using two-dimensional echocardiographic evaluation of left ventricular regional wall motion abnormalities. *Am. Heart J.* 103:814, 1982.

45. Abrams, D.S., Starling, M.R., Crawford, M.H., and O'Rourke, R.A. Value of noninvasive techniques for predicting early complications in patients with clinical Class II acute myocardial infarction. *J. Am. Coll. Cardiol.* 2:818, 1983.

46. Heger, J.J., Weyman, A.E., Wann, L.S., Dillon, J.C., and Feigenbaum, H. Cross-sectional echocardiography in acute myocardial infarction: Detection and localization of regional left ventricular asynergy. *Circulation* 60:531, 1979.

47. Nishimura, R.A., Reeder, G.S., Miller, F.A., Jr., Ilstrup, D.M., Shub, C., Seward, J.B., and Tajik, A.J. Prognostic value of predischarge 2-dimensional echocardiogram after acute myocardial infarction. *Am. J. Cardiol.* 53:429, 1984.

48. Rasmussen, S., Corya, B.C., Feigenbaum, H., and Knoebel, S.B. Detection of myocardial scar tissue by M-mode echocardiography. *Circulation* 57:230, 1978.

49. Eaton, L.W., Weiss, J.L., Bulkley, B.H., Garrison, J.B., and Weisfeldt, M.L. Regional cardiac dilatation after acute myocardial infarction: Recognition by two-dimensional echocardiography. *N. Engl. J. Med.* 300:57, 1979.

50. Erlebacher, J.A., Weiss, J.L., Eaton, L.W., Kallman, C., Weisfeldt, M.L., and Bulkley, B.H. Late effects of acute infarct dilation on heart size: A two-dimensional echocardiographic study. *Am. J. Cardiol.* 49:1120, 1982.

51. Visser, C.A., Kan, G., David, G.K., Lie, K.I., and Durrer, D. Echocardiographic-cineangiographic correlation in detecting left ventricular aneurysm: A prospective study of 422 patients. *Am. J. Cardiol.* 50:337, 1982.

52. Ezekowitz, M.D., Wilson, D.A., Smith, E.O., Burow, R.D., Harrison, L.H., Jr., Parker, D.E., Elkins, R.C., Peyton, M., and Taylor, F.B. Comparison of indium-111 platelet scintigraphy and two-dimensional echocardiography in the diagnosis of left ventricular thrombi. *N. Engl. J. Med.* 306:1509, 1982.

53. Takamoto, T., Kim, D., Urie, P.M., Guthaner, D.F., Gordon, H.J., Keren, A., Popp, R.L. Comparative recognition of left ventricular thrombi by echocardiography and cineangiography (abstract). *J. Am. Coll. Cardiol.* 3:614, 1984.

54. Weinreich, D.J., Burke, J.F., and Pauletto, F.J. Serial echocardiographic evaluation of mural thrombi. *J. Am. Coll. Cardiol.* 3:614, 1984 (abstract).

55. Drobac, M., Gilbert, B., Howard, R., Baigrie, R., and Rokowski, H. Ventricular septal defect after myocardial infarction: Diagnosis by two-dimensional contrast echocardiography. *Circulation* 67:335, 1983.

56. Catherwood, E., Mintz, G.S., Kotler, M.N., Parry, W.R., and Segal, B.L. Two-dimensional echocardiographic recognition of left ventricular pseudoaneurysm. *Circulation* 62:294, 1980.

57. Mintz, G.S., Victor, M.F., Kotler, M.N., Pary, W.R., and Segal, B.L. Two-dimensional echocardiographic identification of surgically correctable complications of acute myocardial infarction. *Circulation* 64:91, 1981.

58. Godley, R.W., Wann, L.S., Rogers, E.W., Feigenbaum, H., and Weyman, A.E. Incomplete mitral leaflet closure in patients with papillary muscle dysfunction. *Circulation* 63:565, 1981.

59. Kaul, S., Tei, C., Hopkins, J.M., and Shah, P.M. Assessment of right ventricular function using two-dimensional echocardiography. *Am. Heart J.* 107:526, 1984.

60. Panidis, I.P., Ren, J-F., Kotler, M.N., Mintz, G., Iskandrian, A., Ross, J., and Kane, S. Two-dimensional echocardiographic estimation of right ventricular ejection fraction in patients with coronary artery disease. *J. Am. Coll. Cardiol.* 2:911, 1983.

61. Lopez-Sendon, J., Garcia-Fernandez, M.A., Coma-Canella, I., Yanguela, M.M., and Banuelos, F. Segmental right ventricular function after acute myocardial infarction: Two dimensional echocardiographic study in 63 patients. *Am. J. Cardiol.* 51:390, 1983.

62. Jugdutt, B.I., Sussex, B.A., Sivaram, C.A., and Rossall, R.E. Right ventricular infarction: Two-dimensional echocardiographic evaluation. *Am. Heart J.* 107:505, 1984.

63. Kondo, S., Meerbaum, S., Sakamaki, T., Shimoura, K., Tei, C., Shah, P.M., and Corday, E. Diagnosis of coronary stenosis by two-dimensional echographic study of dysfunction of ventricular segments during and immediately after pacing. *J. Am. Coll. Cardiol.* 2:689, 1983.

64. Gondi, B. and Nanda, N.C. Cold pressor test during two-dimensional echocardiography: Usefulness in detection of patients with coronary disease. *Am. Heart J.* 107:278, 1984.

65. Morganroth, J., Chen, C.C., David, D., Sawin, H.S., Naito, M., Parrotto, C., and Meixell, L. Exercise cross-sectional echocardiographic diagnosis of coronary artery disease. *Am. J. Cardiol.* 47:20, 1981.

66. Ginzton, L.E., Conant, R., Brizendine, M., Lee, F., Mena, I., and Laks, M.M. Exercise subcostal two-dimensional echocardiography: A new method of segmental wall motion analysis. *Am. J. Cardiol.* 53:805, 1984.

67. Crawford, M.H., Amon, K.W., and Vance, W.S. Exercise 2-dimensional echocardiography: Quantitation of left ventricular performance in patients with severe angina pectoris. *Am. J. Cardiol.* 51:1, 1983.

68. Robertson, W.S., Feigenbaum, H., Armstrong, W.F., Dillon, J.C., O'Donnell, J., and McHenry, P.W. Exercise echocardiography: A clinically practical addition in the evaluation of coronary artery disease. *J. Am. Coll. Cardiol.* 2:1085, 1983.

69. Limacher, M.C., Quinones, M.A., Poliner, L.R., Nelson, J.G., Winters, W.L., Jr., and Waggoner, A.D. Detection of coronary artery disease with exercise two-dimensional echocardiography: Description of a clinically applicable method and comparison with radionuclide ventriculography. *Circulation* 67:1211, 1983.

70. Berberich, S.N., Zager, J.R.S., Plotnick, G.D., and Fisher, M.L. A practical approach to exercise echocardiography: Immediate postexercise echocardiography. *J. Am. Coll. Cardiol.* 3:284, 1984.

71. Chandraratna, P.A., Nanna, M., McKay, C., Nimalasuriya, A., Swinney, R., Elkayam, U., and Rahimtoola, S.H. Determination of cardiac output by transcutaneous continuous-wave ultrasonic Doppler computer. *Am. J. Cardiol.* 53:234, 1984.

72. Huntsman, L.L., Stewart, D.K., Barnes, S.R., Franklin, S.B., Colocousis, J.S., and Hessel, E.A. Noninvasive Doppler determination of cardiac output in man: Clinical validation. *Circulation* 67:593, 1983.

73. Askenazi, J., Koenigsberg, D.I., Ziegler, J.H., and Lesch, M. Echocardiographic estimates of pulmonary artery wedge pressure. *N. Engl. J. Med.* 305:1566, 1981.

74. Sahn, D.J., Barratt-Boyes, B.G., Graham, K., Kerr, A., Roche, A., Hill, D., Brandt, P.W.T., Copeland, J.G., Mammana, R., Temkin, L.P., and Glenn, W. Ultrasonic imaging of the coronary arteries in open-chest humans: Evaluation of coronary atherosclerotic lesions during cardiac surgery. *Circulation* 66:1034, 1982.

75. Force, T., Bloomfield, P., O'Boyle, J.E., Pietro, D.A., Dunlap, R.W., Khuri, S.F., and Parisi, A.F. Quantitative two-dimensional echocardiographic analysis of motion and thickening of the interventricular septum after cardiac surgery. *Circulation* 68:1013, 1983.

76. Weitzman, L.B., Tinker, W.P., Kronzon, I., Cohen, M.L., Glassman, E., and Spencer, F.C. The incidence and natural history of pericardial effusion after cardiac surgery—an echocardiographic study. *Circulation* 69:506, 1984.

# 8. NUCLEAR CARDIOLOGY

Robert Soufer

Barry L. Zaret

Nuclear cardiology had its beginning in 1927, when Blumgart and Weiss described the technique for measuring circulation time in man using injected radioactive radon and modified Wilson cloud chambers as radiation detectors [1]. In 1949 Prinzmetal and Corday first described the radiocardiogram. However, it was not until the late 1960s and early 1970s that a host of new technologies suitable for assessing coronary disease were developed and described. These included equilibrium radionuclide angiocardiography, first-pass radionuclide angiocardiography, myocardial perfusion scintigraphy (first with potassium-43 and rubidium-81 and now with thallium-201), and infarct avid scintigraphy. These techniques provided a means for assessing global and regional ventricular function, myocardial perfusion, and viability. Studies could be performed not only at rest but under conditions of exercise or other physiologic and pharmacologic stress.

The efforts of many investigators in the 1970s centered on the refinement of these techniques and the definition of their relative sensitivity and specificity for the diagnosis of coronary artery disease. In the 1980s work has begun to focus on other clinical issues, namely, functional and prognostic stratification of patients with known coronary disease, both stable and unstable. Further technical advances have propelled nuclear cardiology into a new era, with increased dependence upon advanced computer techniques. This orientation has led to new approaches, such as quantification of image defects and advanced-image processing, quantification of regional wall motion, definition of diastolic function parameters based upon the filling characteristics of the generated volume curve, absolute chamber volume calculations, definition of intracellular radioactive tracer washout kinetics as a parameter of ischemia, single-photon emission computed tomography (SPECT), and studies of myocardial metabolism involving both positron and single-photon instrumentation. In addition to computer advances, new advances in imaging instrumentation have occurred, including rotating detector systems for SPECT, "digital" cameras for high-count rate, first-pass radionuclide angiocardiograms and small portable imaging probes and miniaturized detectors for monitoring of cardiac function. In general, techniques now have been incorporated into clinical practice and are used in ambulatory as well as acutely ill patients.

The purpose of this chapter is to deal with techniques currently employed clinically in nuclear cardiologic assessment of coronary artery disease. Techniques will be described briefly, their attributes and limitations defined, and their clinical relevance placed in current perspective.

## Radionuclide Studies of Cardiac Performance

### EQUILIBRIUM (GATED BLOOD POOL) RADIONUCLIDE ANGIOCARDIOGRAPHY

Equilibrium radionuclide angiocardiography (ERNA) provides relevant functional data following the stable labeling of the entire intravascular blood pool. The whole cardiac cycle is sampled repetitively, and sampling is synchronized with electrocardiographic events. The data are continuously summed from repetitive cardiac cycles until sufficient count density is obtained to allow for meaningful analysis [2–4]. The most reliable data are obtained in the presence of stable cardiac performance, minimal patient motion, and a constant concentration of intravascular radioactivity. The appropriate number of frames per cardiac cycle (i.e., framing interval) must be chosen to allow adequate temporal resolution for a given heart rate. That is, the faster the heart rate the shorter the framing interval. This, however, must be balanced against sufficient duration of data acquisition for adequate count density and statistical accuracy.

An optimal blood pool label is necessary for good definition of cardiac structures, adequate edge definition, and precise delineation of defined regions of interest. Frequently, this is the most relevant technical aspect of this particular study. Basically, three techniques are employed for red blood cell labeling: in vivo, in vitro, and modified in vivo [5, 6]. The modified in vivo technique is currently recommended. With this approach, stannous pyrophosphate is injected intravenously into the patient, as is performed in the conventional in vivo technique. However, labeling of the patient's red blood cells occurs in a closed heparinized syringe—extension tube system attached to the patient by a needle. This technique minimizes the presence of free intravascular pertechnetate and consequently improves target-to-background ratios and the entire quality of the study. Again, it is worth emphasizing that adequate labeling of the patient's blood pool is often the crucial aspect of a technically adequate study. A poor red blood cell label will interfere with adequate image interpretation and will definitely hinder attempts at precise quantification of image data.

To ensure adequate visual assessment of the cardiac chambers and the great vessels, imaging at rest should be performed in at least three and preferably four views. The anteroposterior view gives information regarding the anterobasal, anterolateral, and apical portions of the left ventricle as well as visualization of the right ventricular apex. The left anterior oblique gives the best separation of both ventricles and displays the septum, inferoapical and lateral portions of the

left ventricle, as well as a portion of the right ventricle (this should be done in the "best septal" orientation, which optimally separates the ventricles; this generally occurs from 35 to 55 degrees). The left lateral position displays the apical, inferior, and posterior basal portion of the left ventricle. A recommended fourth view is the left posterior oblique; this gives better angulation of the left ventricle and allows assessment of the posterobasal wall and gives confirmatory data about the inferior wall in a select but significant number of patients (figure 8–1). The addition of the left lateral and left posterior oblique views is useful in defining the presence of aneurysms of the posterobasal and anteroapical segments, which are not routinely seen on either the anterior or left anterior oblique views. At least one of these two views is necessary. Which of the two will provide optimal anatomic definition and technical data is difficult to predict in advance.

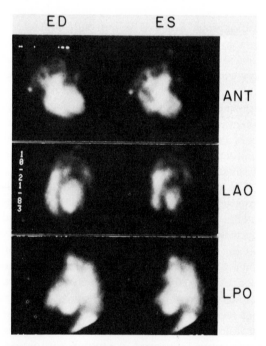

FIGURE 8–1. Equilibrium radionuclide angiocardiogram obtained in a patient with a posterobasal aneurysm. End-diastolic images are shown on the left, and systolic images on the right. The upper panels represent anterior view images; middle panel, left anterior oblique view; and lower panel, left posterior oblique view. Note the presence of a significant aneurysm that is seen only in the left posterior oblique view.

Visual interpretation is best performed from an endless loop cine display rather than from static images. The factors to consider in visual interpretation are size, synchrony, and symmetry of contraction. An initial qualitative assessment of global performance should be reached before analysis of regional wall motion. Relevant regional data may also be obtained using standard visual analysis. In our laboratory, we divide the left ventricle into 11 segments analyzed from three or four views. Each segment is graded using a 5-point scale, from 3 being normal to $-1$ being dyskinetic. Using this system, a normal left ventricle would have a score of 33.

The evaluation of the septum is difficult on a purely visual basis. Although edge motion occurs with the long axis of the heart, systolic thickening of the septum in the 45-degree LAO position is the best way to characterize septal wall motion. This is facilitated by the fact that both sides of the interventricular septum are visualized. When the septum (basal, apical, or both) moves paradoxically, it moves toward the right ventricle in systole. This finding does not necessarily imply septal infarction or ischemia. Paradoxical motion of the septum is a common finding after cardiac surgery, conduction defects, or right ventricular dilatation (especially volume overload).

Quantitative measurements of global left ventricular function generally are obtained in the left anterior oblique view, since in this view count-based measures will have minimal contribution from right ventricle activity. Left ventricular regions of interest using either manually derived or automated approaches are both accurate and reliable [7–10]. Within this region of interest, background activity not arising from the left ventricle must be accounted for. This background activity is corrected for in all count-based calculations. A left ventricular time-activity curve is generated, which is comparable to the left ventricular volume curve (figure 8–2). Many noninvasive parameters, such as ejection fraction, ejection rate, peak filling rate, and relative or absolute left ventricular volume, are derived from this curve. Although ejection fraction is influenced significantly by loading conditions, it still remains an important clinically relevant index of ventricular global pump function. In addition, if ventricular volumes and blood pressure are measured, then other contractile indices such as systolic pressure–volume relationships can also be assessed.

Additional quantitative measurements may also be derived. Absolute ventricular volume can be calculated nongeometrically from the total number of counts in the ventricular region of interest and the mean depth of the ventricle relative to the detector surface. After accounting for the framing interval and the blood radioactivity concentration during the study, absolute volumes may be measured by a simple calculation using the linear attenuation coefficient for technetium-99m in soft tissue. This is also based upon the fact that at equilibrium, counts are directly proportional to volume [11–13].

The ratio of right to left ventricular stroke counts may be used to derive a measure of valvular regurgitation. This is based upon the assumption that the stroke volumes of the right and left ventricles are equal in the absence of intracardiac shunting or regurgitation. The pitfalls of this regurgitant index approach involve the need for precise validation within each laboratory, difficulty in differentiating mild degrees of regurgitation from normals, and problems with specificity in the presence of left ventricular dysfunction [14].

The accurate and reproducible quantitative assessment of regional function is of fundamental importance. The quantitative analysis of regional wall motion may be determined by computer-generated chords, hemaxes, radii, and contours [15]; regional count-based ejection fractions [16, 17]; ejection fraction or stroke volume functional images [18, 19]; and Fourier phase and amplitude images and histograms [20, 21]. Count-based techniques are performed only in the left anterior oblique view. Geometric methods such as radial shortening, etc., may be performed in any view. The critical issue in the technique involves appropriate edge detection. Application of new computer approaches such as artificial intelligence offers great promise in this area [22]. The Fourier fitting technique is also useful when the temporal sequence of mechanical events is an issue, as in conduction disturb-

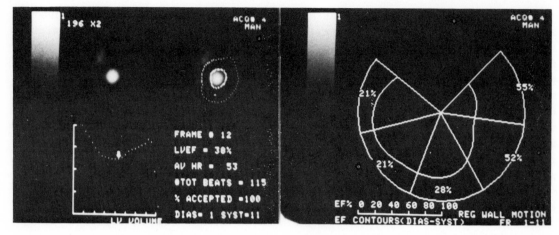

FIGURE 8–2. Global and regional ejection fraction measurements obtained in a patient following an anteroseptal myocardial infarction. Global ejection fraction data are shown on the left, regional ejection fraction data obtained from five distinct regions are shown on the right. Note that there is a significant decrease in the regional ejection fractions recorded from the 2 anteroseptal and apical regions as compared to the lateral regions of the ventricle as seen in the left anterior oblique view. This study points out the importance of obtaining appropriate regional data in coronary artery disease.

ances or in certain types of asynchrony that can be encountered in coronary disease.

## NONIMAGING NUCLEAR PROBE

A recent modification of the traditional equilibrium blood pool technique, the nonimaging nuclear probe, allows assessment of global left ventricular function using a collimated nonimaging nuclear probe and microprocessor [23–25]. The logistic advantages involve portability and decreased cost. The technical advantages are its higher sensitivity and temporal resolution, which enable accurate measurement of the diastolic portion of the time activity curve. However, this instrument is limited to global left ventricular performance and does not provide assessment of regional left or right ventricular function.

The time activity curve is displayed on a beat-to-beat basis, facilitating immediate analysis of the effect of various interventions. However a volume curve summing the gated cardiac cycles for 30 to 120 seconds may also be obtained (figure 8–3). This high temporal resolution volume curve is analagous to that obtained with equilibrium radionuclide angiocardiography. The monitoring of beat-to-beat LV performance is advantageous in several circumstances. These include assessment of the hemodynamic consequences of rhythm disturbances [26], assessment of left ventricular stiffness in patients with heart failure and normal systolic function [27], definition of ventricular function during rapidly changing reflex events [28], and beat-to-beat pressure-volume relationships [29].

## FIRST-PASS RADIONUCLIDE ANGIOCARDIOGRAPHY

First-pass radionuclide angiocardiography (FPRNA) differs from ERNA in that there is temporal and anatomic segregation of radioactivity within each of the cardiac chambers. This results from the sampling of radioactivity only during the first-pass, or transit, state, in contrast to ERNA where the radioactivity is in equilibrium throughout the blood pool. The FPRNA technique allows rapid sequential assessment of both right and left ventricular performance from the same study [30].

Each measurement or study requires a separate injection of a radiopharmaceutical. Technetium-99m radiopharmaceuticals generally are used. It is possible that gold-195m, which has an extremely short half-life and is generator produced, could replace technetium-99m for first-transit studies [31, 32]. This would allow performance of repetitive studies with low background and low radiation burden.

Since data are derived from a few cardiac cycles, the scintillation camera must provide ade-

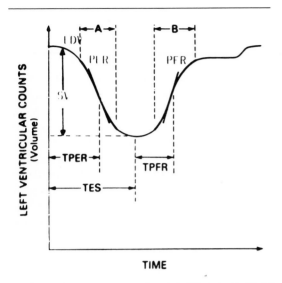

FIGURE 8–3. Diagram of a relative ventricular volume curve generated from nuclear data. The systolic ejection phrase is indicated by A and the diastolic filling phase by B. A variety of measurements can be obtained from this volume curve as indicated in this illustration. EDV = end-diastolic volume, SV = stroke volume, PER = peak ejection rate, TPER = time to peak ejection rate, TES = time to end-systole, PFR = peak filling rate, TPFR = time to peak filling rate.

quate temporal and spatial resolution with adequate count density. Thus, it is critical to have appropriate instrumentation for first-pass studies. Presently, the multicrystal scintillation camera and newly developed "digital" cameras permit such rapid acquisition and allow accumulation of high count rates. A "gated" FPRNA may be obtained using the conventional gamma cameras and radiopharmaceuticals; it is employed currently to evaluate right ventricular function.

Analysis of the FPRNA involves visual assessment of the morphology of the cardiac blood pool and great vessels and determination of the overall flow pattern. The concepts used in calculating ejection fraction are similar to those employed in equilibrium blood pool imaging. Through data processing, low count rate data are summed, images constructed, and ventricular and background regions of interest are assigned [30]. Time-activity curves are generated and representative ventricular volume curves

are derived. It is important to keep in mind that radioactivity is analyzed sequentially and only at the time it is in the chamber being assessed. Statistical reliability dictates summation of four to five cardiac cycles for the calculation of ejection fraction. In addition, images may be viewed in a cine continuous loop manner to visualize better structural and functional abnormalities. Additional indices such as cardiac output, stroke volume, pulmonary transit time, and shunts may also be determined.

COMPARISON OF THE FIRST-PASS AND EQUILIBRIUM TECHNIQUES
Because of the limitations and attributes of each technique, the clinician should decide which study will provide the most useful information in each of the varying clinical situations that radionuclide-derived functional data would be of value. This decision will depend to a major extent upon the equipment available, quality of the laboratory, and the experience and training of the laboratory personnel. Ejection fraction measurements are not always equivalent in the same patient when the two techniques are compared [33]. With ERNA, a single radionuclide injection provides simultaneous and continuous evaluation of the cardiac chambers. In addition, regional wall motion can be assessed in multiple views in a near simultaneous fashion. Therefore, pharmacologic and physiologic interventions may be evaluated serially over several hours, and if necessary, studies may be obtained in multiple views. With the FPRNA each new evaluation requires a separate injection of radionuclide. On the other hand, multiple sequential FPRNA studies are limited in number if technetium-99m is employed. This problem may be obviated if the short-lived generator-produced gold-195m becomes commercially available [31, 32]. At present this radionuclide is available only for experimental studies. In terms of regional wall motion analysis, the equilibrium method probably allows more detailed assessment of cardiac structures in multiple views. First-pass radionuclide angiocardiography provides sequential chamber assessment without superimposition from other structures, but the data are of lower count density and hence pos-

sess less statistical reliability. Time for data acquisition by the first-pass technique is less than 1 minute versus 2 to 10 minutes per view with equilibrium imaging. Therefore, when analysis of rapid physiologic events is an issue, FPRNA is preferable.

Although exercise ventricular performance can be evaluated with either technique, the rapid data acquisition of the first-pass technique minimizes time for patient motion, thus making that technique more suitable for upright exercise, when control of patient motion is more difficult. The latter form of exercise certainly is preferable in heart failure and ventilatory-impaired patients and generally is more comfortable for most patients. Exercise equilibrium studies generally are limited to supine or semisupine exercise. In this position loading conditions of the ventricles are altered, which may alter the observed ventricular performance characteristics. The high count density offered by ERNA, which facilitates analysis of regional wall motion, must be balanced with the problems involved with superimposition of great vessels and other cardiac chambers, which can at times confound both qualitative interpretation and quantitative analysis.

Currently in our laboratory, FPRNA is the preferred technique for the evaluation of right ventricular function, intracardiac shunts, and exercise performance.

### EXERCISE VENTRICULAR FUNCTION STUDIES

Exercise ventricular function studies may be performed using either ERNA or FPRNA techniques [34–37]. The exercise protocols will vary slightly, depending on the technique employed. As previously mentioned, equilibrium studies may be performed for several hours after a single injection. Therefore, if exercise is to be done with ERNA, a routine resting equilibrium study is recommended before exercise. This can be used to evaluate chamber size, configuration, and wall motion in multiple views. Equilibrium studies generally are performed in the supine or semisupine position with a bicycle ergometer and the patient's legs outstretched and at the same level as the torso. Exercise is begun at a workload of 150 to 200 kilopond-meters/min

and increased by 150 to 200 kilopond-meters/-min until symptom limited. Imaging is performed and data accumulated from the last 2 minutes of each 3-minute exercise stage. An endless loop cine display is developed for analysis of wall motion. A left ventricular time-activity curve is derived, from which ejection fraction and other functional parameters are calculated. Only one view is recorded per exercise protocol. The "best septal" LAO view is preferred for separation of right and left ventricles in order to obtain an accurate count-based nongeometric ventricular volume curve for functional analysis. Unfortunately, this view allows assessment only of the posterolateral, inferolateral, apical, and septal segments of the left ventricle and is probably least suitable for conventional wall motion analysis. It has been suggested that if detailed analysis of regional wall motion is to be performed with ERNA, then two distinct periods of exercise are necessary, with each obtained in a different orientation [38].

The alternative approach to exercise ERNA studies is exercise FPRNA. A resting study is performed initially; the subsequent graded exercise protocol is similar to the one previously described for the equilibrium study. However, in this instance exercise generally is performed in the upright position. The ability of FPRNA to be performed routinely in the upright position during exercise should provide accurate physiologic data that can be related more directly to routine daily activities. In the supine position, loading conditions are altered in a manner that is distinct from upright exercise. This can have a profound impact on the observed results, particularly in the presence of significant cardiovascular disease or heart failure. In addition, upright FPRNA exercise studies can be performed in positions other than the LAO. Because there is no ventricular chamber overlap with the FPRNA, studies are usually obtained in the RAO or anterior positions. Both regional wall motion and global function can be assessed in these views. Thus, problems attendant to relatively lower counting statistics of the FPRNA data may be more than compensated for by the ability to assess wall motion in positions more favorable for appropriate anatomic definition and analysis.

## CLINICAL UTILITY IN THE DIAGNOSIS OF CORONARY ARTERY DISEASE

It is generally believed that exercise radionuclide angiocardiography can augment diagnostic accuracy for detection of coronary artery disease over that achieved with exercise electrocardiography alone. However, criteria on which a positive or negative test are based clearly hinge upon the definition of the normal left ventricular response to exercise. These normal responses are based upon data acquired in populations with a low pretest likelihood of coronary artery disease using Bayesian analysis [39, 40], as well as those "proven" at the time of coronary angiography to be free of significant disease.

The most widely used definition of normal ventricular response to exercise is an absolute increase in at least 5 ejection fraction units (5 percent) without development of concomitant regional wall motion abnormalities [34, 41]. This definition carries an average sensitivity of 87 percent [42] and a specificity of 93 percent. However, Rosanski et al. [43] recently reported a decline of the specificity of exercise ERNA, when a more recent series from the same laboratory was compared to the initial group of normals studied in that laboratory when the technique was first being developed and implemented. This difference was attributed to differences in the selection of the normal populations during the two time periods. In the initial period, normals were derived from those with low likelihood of disease, frequently "supernormal" volunteers, laboratory personnel, etc. In the later period, "normals" were derived from those studied in the catheterization laboratory and determined to have no major anatomic lesions. The second group had a higher pretest probability of disease. A posttest referral bias also contributed to this decline in specificity, since all patients with a positive ERNA were referred for catheterization. Alternatively, identification of patients with abnormal exercise responses and angiographically normal coronary arteries, rather than unmasking a tendency toward false-positive responses, may be providing a means of defining heretofore unrecognized preclinical myocardial disease states or supply-demand imbalances that require new definitions and classifications [44].

For certain patient subsets the criterion of a normal exercise increment of at least 5 percent may not be suitable. Included in this group are patients with exaggerated sympathetic tone and resting left ventricular ejection fractions greater than 70 to 75 percent. In this population a normal response is best defined by no fall in ejection fraction with stress. Furthermore, in comparison with other "normals," female patients do not augment ejection fraction to the same degree [45]. Patients more than 60 years of age with no clinical evidence of coronary artery disease also frequently have abnormal exercise responses [46]. It is important to keep in mind that if one is to maximize the specificity of stress radionuclide angiocardiography, then patients with conditions associated with left ventricular dysfunction and poor left ventricular reserve must be excluded. These conditions include hypertrophic cardiomyopathy [47], doxorubicin cardiotoxicity [48], dilated cardiomyopathy, radiation-induced myocardial fibrosis [49], and valvular disease, to mention but a few [50–53]. In our experience, hypertension alone is not associated with an abnormal LV response [54].

A recent study observed that standard visual analysis of coronary angiograms is inaccurate as a measure of the physiologic significance of coronary stenosis. In this study the measurement of the percentage of stenosis from coronary angiograms was not significantly correlated ($r = -0.25$) with the reactive hyperemic response as measured with the Doppler technique intraoperatively [55]. Traditionally, the percentage of coronary luminal narrowing on coronary angiogram is the "gold standard" against which all comparisons are made concerning sensitivity and specificity of radionuclide studies. However, a positive exercise ventricular function study in the presence of a vascular distribution with only an apparent 40 to 50 percent stenosis may still be quite significant physiologically. It is worthwhile to remain aware of the fact that the gold standard for assessing the diagnostic accuracy of noninvasive studies frequently might have its own highly significant intrinsic limitations.

Three factors, when present, appear to maximize the sensitivity of exercise ventricular performance studies. These factors include exercise to a heart rate or double-product end-point appropriate for age and sex, the presence of left main or triple-vessel coronary stenosis, and the presence of exercise-induced electrocardiographic evidence of ischemia [56–59].

For certain patients who cannot perform dynamic exercise, other forms of stress that alter ventricular function have been proposed as diagnostic alternatives. These include atrial pacing, cold pressor stimulation, and isometric handgrip. These interventions differ in the mechanism(s) by which they alter left ventricular performance. The physiologic alterations may range from altered loading conditions to imbalance of regional oxygen-supply ratios. It is important to keep in mind that the response to isometric handgrip must include analysis of regional performance. This is due to the fact that global left ventricular ejection fraction falls routinely in normals as well as in patients with coronary artery disease in response to this intervention, rendering the analysis of global function totally nonspecific. However, abnormalities in regional wall motion may occur more specifically in response to handgrip in patients with coronary artery disease [60]. Although regional dysfunction in response to handgrip has been reported to be 90 percent sensitive in patients with coronary artery disease, another direct comparison of handgrip and dynamic exercise suggests that dynamic exercise results in a significantly higher sensitivity and specificity for the diagnosis of coronary artery disease [61]. Several years ago, based upon preliminary results, the cold pressor test also was felt to be a suitable diagnostic study. However, it has been demonstrated subsequently by several laboratories that the diagnostic accuracy of the cold pressor test is limited by the overlap of responses observed in normals and in patients with coronary artery disease [62, 63]. Currently, this test is not considered to be clinically useful.

Atrial pacing ventricular function studies have been shown to have reasonable sensitivity and specificity. However, the technique requires placement of a temporary pacing catheter, thereby altering the noninvasive nature of the study and complicating its logistics.

In an effort to expand the diagnostic detection of patients with coronary artery disease, indices of diastolic function derived from radionuclide angiocardiography recently have been studied at rest. If found to be suitable, this could obviate the need for concomitant exercise in certain instances. Using ERNA, peak filling rate and time to peak filling rate are obtained from the diastolic portion of the left ventricular volume curve. Peak filling rate is the maximal rate of change in counts occurring within early- to mid-diastole, normalized to end-diastolic volume. Time to peak filling rate is the time from end-systole (minimal number of counts) to peak filling rate (see figure 8–3). These are the major noninvasive radionuclide parameters presently employed to reflect noninvasive estimates of diastolic function. Their actual relationship to more detailed parameters of diastolic function involving compliance indices, pressure-volume relations, and relaxation remains to be defined.

Recently, a group of patients with normal resting left ventricular ejection fraction and coronary artery disease were evaluated at rest. The peak filling rate was abnormal (PFR $\leq$ 2.5 EDV/sec) in 85 percent of these patients [64]. The combination of time to peak filling rate and peak filling rate identified 90 percent of patients with coronary artery disease. These findings occurred in the absence of myocardial infarction and clinically evident myocardial ischemia. In addition, these parameters appear to be capable of dynamic change and consequently may be used to follow therapy. Successful coronary angioplasty [65] and antianginal therapy with calcium channel blockers [66] have been shown to reverse these abnormal diastolic parameters. It should be emphasized that acquisition of these diastolic parameters from the radionuclide relative volume curve requires augmented computer memory capability, high temporal resolution, forward/backward construction of the volume curve, and careful beat length windowing in order to obtain accurate diastolic data. This is clearly not the case with systolic function. The reason for this difference involves the fact that the systolic portion of the cardiac cycle is relatively fixed in duration, whereas modest changes in cycle length can impact significantly on the more variable diastolic portion of the cycle. Because of its high sensitivity and temporal resolution, the portable nuclear probe obviates some of these complex computational requirements and provides these same measures of diastolic left ventricular performance.

## Myocardial Perfusion Scintigraphy

Thallium-201 ($^{201}$T1) myocardial perfusion imaging is an important clinical tool in the diagnosis and categorization of patients with coronary artery disease. In addition, uses involving definition of extent and functional significance of known disease make this technique quite valuable in certain clinical situations.

The delivery of $^{201}$T1 (a potassium analog) to the myocardial cell is a function of both regional blood flow and the fraction of the locally delivered tracer that is extracted by the myocardial cell. The defects in $^{201}$T1 images are predominantly due to regional abnormalities of flow distribution. Although there are drugs such as digitalis [67, 68] that may alter extraction of $^{201}$T1 by the myocardial cell, their contribution to the ultimate image analysis is probably quite small, albeit not yet totally defined. There are qualitative differences in the manner in which myocardium subjected to coronary disease will handle thallium-201 injected at peak exercise and thereafter. Myocardium that is scarred from previous infarction will behave differently from myocardium that is ischemic. The myocardium receives approximately 4 percent of the cardiac output. Thus, approximately 4 percent of the injected intravenous dose is initially delivered and accumulated in the left ventricle. The radionuclide is extracted efficiently by the myocardium (88 percent).

When a segment of the myocardium is ischemic, the input-output ratio of thallium is such that a defect is seen in early images. However, approximately 2 to 4 hours later, equilibrium is reached between the release and input of $^{201}$T1 on a cellular level. This may result in resolution of the previous defect. This phenomenon of redistribution discriminates between areas that are ischemic (reversible) from areas that are infarcted (irreversible). When compared to the early postexercise image defects, the irreversible "cold spots" at redistribution time 2 to 4 hours postexercise appear the same. This indicates myocardial scar, although in certain instances

redistribution may be quite a slow process and a repeat image 24 hours later is necessary to demonstrate at least a degree of reversibility.

Multistage treadmill exercise testing according to the Bruce protocol is commonly used in association with imaging. The sensitivity of this technique in the detection of coronary artery disease and definition of its extent is influenced by the amount of exercise performed and the increase in myocardial oxygen requirement achieved. Therefore, the sensitivity of this technique in the detection of coronary artery disease in patients receiving adequate doses of propranolol would be expected to be reduced. Three cc of saline containing 2 mCi of $^{201}$T1 is injected intravenously 60 to 120 seconds prior to termination of exercise. Thereafter imaging should be done within 10 minutes. Imaging is performed in three views, at approximately 10 minutes per view. The views employed are the anterior, 45 degrees left anterior oblique (LAO), and left lateral or steep LAO views. A heavy meal or exercise should be avoided between the initial and delayed images because it may alter redistribution kinetics. An alternative to exercise involves use of persantine as a pharmacologic means of increasing coronary flow and demonstrating heterogeneity of vascular responsiveness in the presence of coronary stenosis.

Despite the advent of computer processing of the images, visual interpretation of the unprocessed images is still commonly employed. Qualitative interpretation of planar $^{201}$T1 images requires experience. The observer must acquire the ability to discriminate between perfusion defects due to ischemia and/or infarction from apparent abnormalities that are more appropriately attributed to soft tissue attenuation and normal variation [69, 70]. Soft tissue attenuation of myocardial $^{201}$T1 uptake frequently is due to large breasts and overlap of the diaphram in the left lateral supine position. Breast artifacts may be obviated by elevation of the breasts with tape on both initial and redistribution studies. Apparent inferior defects due to diaphragmatic attenuation may be minimized by performing left lateral views in the right decubutis position [71]. Additionally, narrow defects with sharp borders seen at the apex frequently are due to normal thinning of the myocardium where the two ventricles are bordered. The latter is termed "an apical variant" and can be seen in up to 20 percent of normals [72]. The normal study shows an even distribution of radioactivity throughout the left ventricular myocardial mass (figure 8–4). At rest, because of its larger muscle mass, the left ventricle is the only cardiac chamber routinely visualized in normals. Visualization of the right ventricular myocardium at rest is associated with either right ventricular hypertrophy [73, 74] or acute increase in right ventricular blood flow or afterload, as can be seen in acute pulmonary embolism. However, right ventricular uptake is commonly seen in exercise images and is attributable to increased right ventricular blood flow.

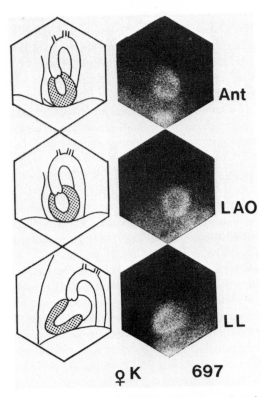

FIGURE 8–4. Normal thallium-201 planar imaging obtained in the anterior (Ant, upper panel), anterior oblique (LAO, middle panel), and left lateral (LL, lower panel). Diagrammatic representations of the myocardial distribution is shown to the left of each image. Note the homogeneous myocardial uptake and central clear space representing the ventricular cavity. (From Wackers, et al. *Clin. Nucl. Med.* 2:64, 1977. Reproduced with permission.)

The one extracardiac finding of diagnostic importance is the finding of increased $^{201}$Tl uptake in the lungs on exercise images. This finding is attributable to reversible exercise-induced left ventricular dysfunction. Left ventricular failure at the time of exercise is suggested by a lung-to-myocardium ratio greater than 0.5. Generally, however, the finding is readily evident from simple inspection of the images. Increased pulmonary uptake is indicative of ischemic-related left ventricular dysfunction when associated with a focal perfusion defect [75, 76].

In terms of qualitative image analysis, myocardial perfusion defects are considered as reversible, partially reversible, or irreversible. The reversible abnormality is associated with defects on the initial image (either exercise, dipyrimadole, or rest) that are no longer evident on a delayed follow-up redistribution image 2 to 4 hours later. This occurs in patients with physiologically significant coronary artery disease but no myocardial infarction. An irreversible (persistent) abnormality is seen in patients who have previous infarction and associated myocardial scarring. This defect is seen equally well on the initial and redistribution images. These defects correlate with irreversible resting regional wall motion abnormalities in the same region [77–79]. On occasion there are persistent defects at 4 hours that fill in at 24 hours. These defects represent prolonged severe ischemia with slow washout [80]. Clearly, an individual patient may have reversible and irreversible defects in separate segments of myocardium. In addition, both patterns (reversible and irreversible) may be evident in the same myocardial segment. This is indicative of a component of residual ischemia despite the presence of established scar and is consistent with the pathological finding of frequent admixture of viable myocardium and scar in infarct zones.

When a perfusion defect is detected, it should be observed in the same myocardial segment on more than one view (figure 8–5). Since perfusion defects can be correlated with the geographical location of specific vascular beds, the qualitative assessment of $^{201}$Tl images may provide information on the extent of

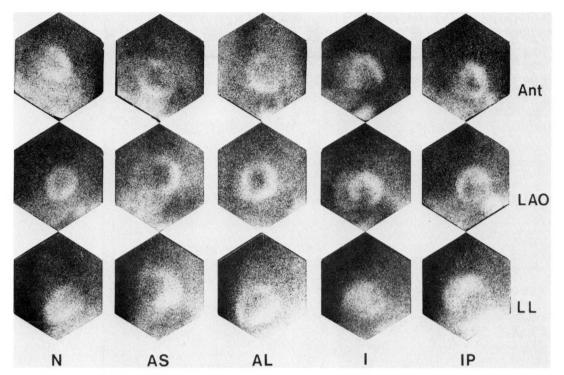

Ant

LAO

LL

N          AS          AL          I          IP

FIGURE 8-5. Thallium-201 uptake patterns seen in various locations of myocardial infarction. Images are displayed in the anterior (Ant), left anterior oblique (LAO), and left lateral (LL) views. Studies are shown for normal (N), anteroseptal infarction (AS), anterior lateral infarction (AL), inferior infarction (I), inferoposterior infarction (IP). Note the perfusion defects in each view corresponding to the zones of infarction. (From Wackers et al. *Clin. Nucl. Med.* 2:64, 1977. Reproduced with permission.)

coronary artery disease. Defects in the septum seen on the 45 degree LAO are attributed to stenosis of the left anterior descending coronary artery proximal to the first septal perforator. Other stenosis of the left anterior descending may appear as a defect of the anterior wall or apex observed in the anterior steep LAO or lateral views. Stenosis of the right coronary artery will appear as a defect in the inferior wall seen on the anterior and left lateral views. Circumflex disease usually appears as a perfusion defect in the posterolateral region as viewed on the 45 degree LAO view. However, it must be emphasized that these patterns can vary substantially, based primarily upon normal variation in coronary anatomy and vascular distributions.

QUANTITATIVE THALLIUM-201 ANALYSIS
Planar $^{201}$Tl imaging displays relative differences in perfusion between vascular beds. As a consequence, frequently only the most severe abnormality may be detected qualitatively. A balanced reduction in perfusion in patients with diffuse disease could result in the absence of visually identifiable focal defects despite extremely severe disease. Fortunately, this occurs relatively infrequently. Underestimation of the extent of disease may also occur in unbalanced multivessel disease. Hypoperfused mycardial segments may appear relatively normal on the same image in *comparison* with the most severely hypoperfused segments. For these reasons attempts have been made to develop new techniques that would allow quantitative assessment of $^{201}$Tl visual image data such that ischemia could be detected in multiple vascular beds. The principles of $^{201}$Tl myocardial kinetics are applicable to quantitative analysis of image data. Specifically, not only is the initial uptake of $^{201}$Tl reduced in myocardial segments that are hypoperfused, but the washout of $^{201}$Tl from these regions is slower as well. Indeed, abnormal washout characteristics may be the only manifes-

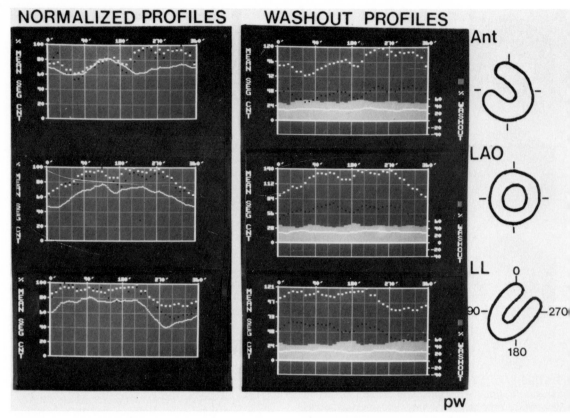

FIGURE 8–6. Thallium-201 kinetic washout profiles from a rest and exercise study obtained in a normal individual. Profiles are obtained in the three views demonstrated. Each data point represents thallium-201 quantitative data from a 10 degree segment. The white dots are the data obtained immediately following exercise; the black dots, the data obtained on a redistribution study; and the white curve indicates the lower limit of normal. The data here are clearly normal. (Illustration courtesy of Dr. Frans J. Wackers.)

tation of regional ischemia. Thus, quantified regional washout of thallium over 2 to 4 hours following injection can be obtained and compared directly to data generated in normals. This technique allows definition of ischemic responses in a nonrelative manner, based upon absolute numbers generated regionally and compared to a previously defined normal range.

Images are obtained in three views (45 degrees LAO, ANT, left lateral, or steep LAO), immediately postinjection and 2 to 4 hours later. Special attention must be given to obtaining identical reproduction of the initial imaging views during the subsequent delayed study. If this is not done, major errors in analysis may occur. This is the principal technical concern in the performance of the study. Computer processing involves bilinear interpolative background subtraction to compensate for tissue crosstalk. The images are smoothed, generally using a 9-point standard algorithm. Myocardial activity may be profiled in a circumferential or linear manner, assessing average or maximal activity at each point. The activity for each segment of the myocardium is determined shortly after injection and at redistribution. The value termed "washout" is the difference in the amount of activity following exercise (or other stress) and redistribution, divided by the activity at exercise. Data frequently are expressed as profile curves with direct comparison made to normal values (figures 8–6 and 8–7). In direct comparison with visual planar imaging, quantitative analysis improves the ability to localize individual coronary artery stenosis and therefore to define the extent of disease. When all vascular

# NORMALIZED PROFILES    WASHOUT PROFILES

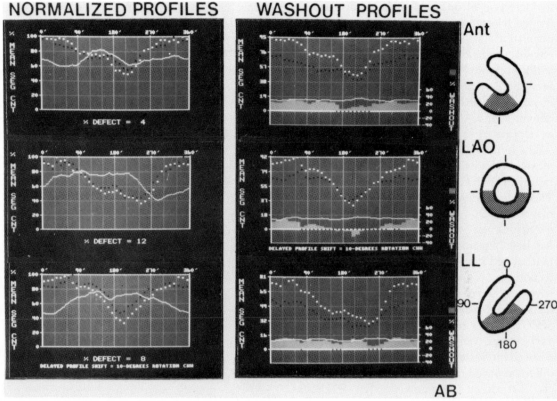

FIGURE 8–7. Abnormal washout from a quantitative thallium-201 kinetic study in a patient with abnormal uptake and washout in the inferior and apical portions of the ventricle. The format is the same as in figure 8–6. (Data courtesy of Dr. Frans J. Wackers.)

beds were evaluated individually, visual analysis was found to have a sensitivity of 52 percent (56 percent for left anterior descending, 34 percent for left circumflex, and 65 percent for right coronary artery) versus 79 percent with qualitative analysis (80 percent, 63 percent, 94 percent, respectively) [81, 82].

This technique is of value in providing improved objectivity in image analysis. However, of greater value is the increased ability to define decreased perfusion in segments that are visually normal on qualitative planar images. This allows more complete definition of the extent of disease even if sensitivity with respect to overall disease detection is not augmented. Quantitative analysis also showed improved sensitivity when compared to visual analysis in instances when vessels were graded as being moderately diseased on angiography (50 to 70 percent stenosis). Quan-

titative analysis in this particular subset had a sensitivity of 70 percent versus 35 percent with planar imaging [81]. The major concern with this technique (as with any new computer approach) is that sensitivity will be improved at the expense of specificity. This does not appear to be the case in initial reports. However, further data are necessary to establish this point.

## SINGLE-PHOTON EMISSION COMPUTED TOMOGRAPHY

The overlap of myocardial segments on routine planar $^{201}$Tl images may obscure visual detection of small and/or multiple defects and also can lead to errors in quantitative analysis. The avoidance of regional overlap, at least theoretically, should lead to improved detection of zones of ischemic myocardium as well as definition of subendocardial processes. Such thinking has provided the focus for recent developmental work in the area of single-photon emission computed tomography (SPECT). Work in the field still is in a very early stage. Several groups have demonstrated what appears to be good results for detection of infarcted or ischemic zones in limited selected experimental models or patient populations [83–86]. In general, [201]T1, with its physical limitation of relatively low photon flux and low energy, is not an optimal radionuclide for SPECT studies. The full potential of the technique will probably not be realized until a technetium-99m flow-related radiopharmaceutical is developed.

The tomographic technique as currently employed can provide myocardial images in frontal, saggital, and transaxial sections (figure 8–8). These views are obtained by a camera detector that rotates on a gantry acquiring counts at frequent intervals over 180 degrees. This approach has been reported to have a sensitivity of 96 percent and specificity of 89 percent for the detection of coronary artery disease [83]. The inherent relative attributes and limitations of qualitative analysis versus quantification in SPECT studies remain to be defined. Preliminary studies comparing 7 pinhole tomography and conventional imaging show no significant differences with regard to sensitivity and specificity of coronary artery detection [87–89]. Controversy still exists concerning the best method of acquisition (i.e., rotating camera(s) versus circumference stationary detectors, etc.). A physiologic concern with the tomographic approach involves the prolonged acquisition time of 22 minutes. This may allow redistribution to commence during summed acquisition and therefore affect the accuracy of reconstructed data. However, despite concerns, the results obtained with this technique thus far are sufficiently encouraging to warrant further study.

## THALLIUM-201 SCINTIGRAPHY FOR DIAGNOSIS AND ASSESSMENT OF SEVERITY OF CORONARY ARTERY DISEASE

The diagnostic clinical utility of stress [201]T1 scintigraphy is obviously dependent upon its relative sensitivity and specificity. However, sensitivity and specificity may vary with the anticipated prevalence of coronary artery disease in the population studied. In many of the reported studies analyzing the clinical utility of stress-redistribution [201]T1 scintigraphy, the prevalence of coronary artery disease in the populations under evaluation was high. On the basis of the cur-

rently reported literature, qualitative planar [201]T1 scintigraphy has a sensitivity of approximately 80 percent and a specificity of 90 percent [42, 90] for detecting angiographically documented coronary disease. The caveat concerning the reliability of a coronary angiographic "gold standard," as discussed earlier in this chapter, is equally applicable here.

Application of these sensitivity and specificity figures to an individual patient is benefited by a Bayesian approach. When the pretest probability of coronary artery disease in the patient is either too low (i.e., < 30 percent) or high (i.e., > 70 percent), the posttest probability of coronary artery disease based on either a positive or negative test would not be significantly altered. Thus, based on the relative sensitivity and specificity of the test, there are clearly patient populations and individual patients who, from a *diagnostic* standpoint, would *not* benefit from the procedure. It must be emphasized that here the relevant issue is only diagnosis and not the extent of disease or its physiologic significance. In the latter two instances, thallium-201 scintigraphy data may be quite helpful, irrespective of Bayesian considerations.

In contrast, in a population with a pretest probability of disease in the range of 30 to 70 percent a positive test increases the posttest probability to approximately 90 percent, and a negative test decreases the probability to 10 percent. Diamond and Forrester [91] have reviewed literature reports involving 28,948 patients in order to define the prevalence of suspected coronary artery disease in various populations based upon clinical symptoms, age, and sex. The prevalence of disease in a symptomatic population was as follows: typical angina (89 percent), atypical angina (50 percent), nonangina (16 percent). In any patient, based upon probability analysis, the pretest likelihood

FIGURE 8–8. Single-photon emission-computed tomography images obtained with thallium-201 in a patient with significant coronary artery disease. (A) A transverse section in which the upper images, obtained at exercise, demonstrate a clear-cut perfusion defect in all cuts, with substantial redistribution readily evident. (B) A longitudinal section in which the same format is employed and reversible ischemia is also apparent in this different tomographic plane.

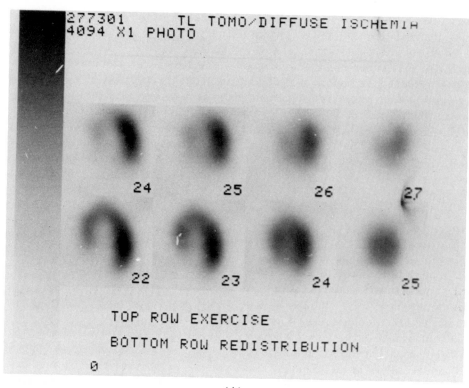

(A)

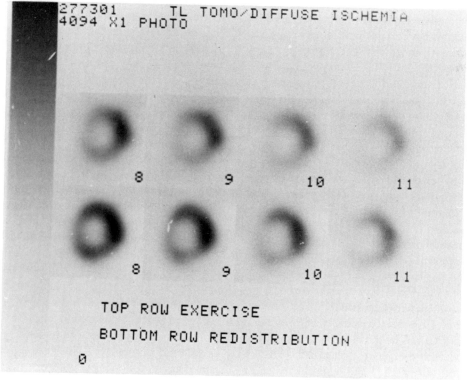

(B)

of coronary disease ranges from 1 percent (35-year-old asymptomatic female) to 94 percent (65-year-old male with typical angina). This approach should be utilized in terms of both triage of patients referred for laboratory evaluation and interpretation of the results of scintigraphic examinations.

Certain limitations of treadmill electrocardiography may be overcome by [201]Tl scintigraphy, thereby accounting in part for its current clinical utilization. Resting abnormalities on an ECG (i.e., left bundle branch block, left ventricular hypertrophy, digoxin) render ST segment changes nondiagnostic during and following exercise. The [201]Tl images in these instances may still reveal perfusion abnormalities. However, it must be realized that [201]Tl scintigraphy also may be associated with false-positive results in the setting of either LBBB and LVH [92]. Furthermore, perfusion defects may be visualized when inadequate exercise fails to elicit ischemic ST depression. However, in this instance the anticipated sensitivity of the technique also will be reduced. In general, [201]Tl scintigraphy also will add to the overall specificity of data obtained from conventional studies.

The defined extent of coronary artery disease in any patient has certain implications concerning subsequent morbidity and mortality. Current concepts would indicate that patients with multivessel disease and left main stenosis are at a higher risk than those with single-vessel disease. Classification of patients into these two categories based upon [201]Tl scintigraphy would appear to have clinical significance. Four studies evaluating the ability of [201]Tl scintigraphy to predict the extent of coronary artery disease have been pooled and reviewed by Berman et al. [81]. A total of 338 patients were available for evaluation. Left anterior descending stenosis was accurately predicted in 174 of 234 patients (74 percent sensitivity). The specificity for evaluating this particular vascular bed in 80 normals was 90 percent. Prediction of right coronary artery stenosis carried a sensitivity of 69 percent (124 out of 199) and a specificity of 86 percent (101 out of 117). The left circumflex system was associated with the poorest sensitivity (38 percent, or 60 out of 157) and a specificity of 91 percent.

Because of the high specificities involved in analysis of each of the vascular beds, defects in multiple vascular beds strongly suggest multivessel disease. In addition, quantitative analysis increases the sensitivity of [201]Tl in the detection of each of the previously mentioned vascular beds [82]. This latter observation clearly requires further study.

Rigo et al. [93] have described a pattern associated with left main stenosis involving perfusion defects in the anterior, septal, and lateral vascular distributions. Although the pattern is highly sensitive (92 percent), this pattern may be seen with double- or triple-vessel disease, accounting for its low specificity (15 percent). The absence of this pattern speaks against the presence of left main disease.

## RADIONUCLIDE ASSESSMENT AND PROGNOSIS

Recent studies suggest that certain abnormal patterns in radionuclide assessment appear to have strong prognostic value by predicting subsequent coronary events in patients with coronary artery disease and/or previous infarction. Questions relating to risk of future infarction and mortality are being addressed. Studies may be considered in two broad categories: those that identify anatomic and pathophysiologic subsets believed to be at high risk, and those that more directly address the role of the individual radionuclide evaluation in defining prognosis. When compared to exercise treadmill testing in patients postinfarction, exercise [201]Tl scintigraphy improves sensitivity (92 percent versus 72 percent) for detection of multivessel disease, a recognized high-risk subset [94]. With respect to extent and localization of infarction, electrocardiographic abnormalities do not correlate as well as [201]Tl imaging does with anatomic pathological localization of infarct site [95]. The extent of infarction as determined by both creatine kinase kinetics [96–98] and pathologic studies [99–101] generally has correlated with the size of the [201]Tl perfusion defect. In one study recurrent angina, reinfarction, and sudden death were more likely to occur in patients with large as opposed to small [201]Tl perfusion defects obtained at rest following acute myocardial infarction [102]. In this study a late follow-up (average 9 months) revealed a 92 percent mortality rate in those patients with large perfusion defects. In some of the patients coming to necropsy, the visual perfusion defect was larger than the observed extent of infarction on pathologic examination [101]. This allows speculation that $^{201}$T1 perfusion defects at rest early after infarction are defining zones of infarction as well as related ischemia, thereby providing an estimate of the total risk region.

Using radionuclide evaluation of ventricular function, several studies have evaluated the impact of assessment upon prognosis in myocardial infarction [103–105]. One report noted that in a population of 56 patients with first myocardial infarction, 11 patients had left ventricular ejection fraction less than or equal to 30 percent. Six (total mortality for the entire group was 7 out of 56) of these patients died during this initial period of hospitalization. Interestingly, pump dysfunction was not evident by clinical examination in 5 of these 6 patients [106].

Becker et al. recently reported prognostic results in a group of patients evaluated postinfarction with resting $^{201}$T1 scintigraphy and ERNA. $^{201}$T1 imaging within the first 15 hours of the onset of symptoms was useful in predicting mortality in patients with acute myocardial infarction. Scintigrams were scored using an objective computer-based technique. Perfusion defects were graded based on a profile curve compared to standards developed from the study of normals. A defect score of 7 or greater identified a high-risk subgroup with a 6-month mortality of 64 percent. This was in direct comparison to patients with defect scores less than 7 who experienced a mortality of only 8 percent. Similarly, patients with ejection fraction <35 percent within the peri-infarction period had a 60 percent 6-month mortality versus one of 11 percent in patients with an ejection fraction >35 percent. The highest risk was in the subset of patients with both high-risk radionuclide findings in whom the 6-month mortality was 83 percent [107].

In the recent study of the Multicenter Postinfarction Research Group, 888 patients were studied with 24-hour Holter monitoring and radionuclide ejection fraction measurement before discharge. Four risk factors were identified

as independent predictors of survival after myocardial infarction: LVEF <40 percent, ventricular ectopy of greater than or equal to 10 beats per hour, advanced New York Heart Association class before discharge, and rales in the upper two-thirds of the lung fields during the coronary care unit course. In this study all four factors were independent predictors. However, LVEF was demonstrated to be an extremely powerful predictor of subsequent mortality (figure 8–9) The presence of a predischarge ejection fraction <40 percent presented a 2.4-fold increased risk of cardiac death in 12 to 36 months postinfarction when compared with patients with ejection fraction >40 percent [105]. In contrast to the positive prognostic value of ejection fraction, one recent study indicated that in patients with pulmonary edema in the early phase of infarction, the ejection fraction did not impact on prediction of survival [108]. The key factor appeared to be the presence of pulmonary edema alone, whether related to transient ischemia or loss of a substantial amount of myocardium. The recent study of Meizlich et al. would indicate that regional wall motion analysis also is of importance [109]. In this study a group of 53

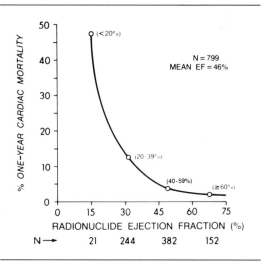

FIGURE 8–9. The relationship of four categories of left ventricular ejection fraction to survival following myocardial infarction. Reproduced from the Multicenter Post infarction Research Group, N. Eng. J Med. 309:331, 1983. Reprinted with permission of the *New England Journal of Medicine*.

patients with an initial transmural anterior infaction were studied serially with multiview ERNA. Patients were divided into those with and without functional aneurysm formation development during the course of hospitalization. The two groups had comparable ejection fraction (27 versus 31 percent, pNS); however, those with aneurysm development had a 61 percent one-year mortality as compared to 9 percent in those with large infaction but no aneurysm (p < 0.01). Thus, ejection fraction is not the entire answer to prognostic stratification, inasmuch as regional left ventricular functional analysis must also be considered.

In addition to resting function assessment, investigators also have demonstrated the predictive value of the left ventricular response to exercise [110]. For example, Corbett et al. [111], using failure to improve ejection fraction by greater than 5 percent, reported that the sensitivity for a poor outcome in 6 months is 95 percent (versus 54 percent with standard treadmill exercise) and the specificity is 96 percent (versus 58 percent).

Use of dipyridamole-$^{201}$T1 scintigraphy following infarction also has been shown to have prognostic import [112]. In a study of 51 patients recovering from acute myocardial infarction, 12 patients died or had reinfarction on a mean follow-up of 19 months. Eleven of these 12 patients had manifested redistribution in the predischarge dipyridamole $^{201}$T1 study. In addition, 24 of these 51 patients required readmission for management of angina. Twenty-two of these 24 also showed redistribution on the dipyridamole-$^{201}$T1 study. In this preliminary study, dipyridamole-$^{201}$T1 scintigraphy proved to be a more sensitive indicator of subsequent cardiac events than submaximal stress electrocardiography.

## Approach to the Patient with Coronary Artery Disease

It is relevant to question how radionuclide studies can best be integrated into the systematic, rational evaluation and care of patients with coronary artery disease. Clearly, the utility of the tests employed will be dependent upon several factors, including the expertise of the laboratory in which the studies are performed, the patient

population(s) to be evaluated, and the demonstrated intrinsic "value" of the individual study in the clinical circumstance evaluated. In the following sections we suggest several approaches to coronary patients, employing the radionuclide procedures described in this chapter. It should be emphasized that at the present the issues discussed are not resolved and will require further prospective evaluation.

SUSPECTED CORONARY ARTERY DISEASE
In the patient with suspected coronary artery disease, the initial diagnostic procedure should probably still be the routine maximal stress electrocardiographic study. In appropriately defined patient subpopulations this safe and relatively inexpensive test may provide the necessary diagnostic information. In certain clinical circumstances, however, the exercise electrocardiogram will be predictably nondiagnostic. To mention but a few; situations involving inadequate workload, abnormal baseline ECG, or nonspecific drug effects as are seen with digitalis will present this problem. If the stress electrocardiogram is expected to be nondiagnostic, then an exercise radionuclide method should be the initial evaluative procedure. Otherwise, if the initial exercise study is nondiagnostic or provides inconsistent clinical data, then and exercise radionuclide study also should be undertaken. As stated earlier in this chapter, which of the two exercise-stress radionuclide studies is to be undertaken will be in part dependent upon local skills and experiences. Based upon our current understanding of the techniques, there clearly are circumstances when one of the two will be preferable. If one gives equivocal or nondiagnostic data, then the alternative should be considered. A positive result should lead to appropriate diagnostic categorization. The magnitude of abnormality can lead to appropriate functional stratification and, in the case of markedly positive abnormal results, could lead to more invasive evaluation and/or intensive pharmacologic or surgical therapy.

KNOWN CORONARY ARTERY DISEASE
In patients with known coronary disease, studies would be undertaken to attempt functional categorization. In this instance the questions asked

surround (1) definition of patients into high- and low-risk strata that might mandate specific approaches, i.e. left main disease; and (2) monitoring and assessing the efficacy of therapy. In this latter instance, studies might be regularly performed to follow the results of bypass surgery or angioplasty (exercise studies) or assess acute pharmacologic effect in intensive care unit environment with instruments such as the nuclear probe. The specific nuclear study employed, and whether it would be obtained at rest or with stress, will clearly vary with the clinical circumstance and the clinical questions to be answered.

## POST MYOCARDIAL INFARCTION

Patients sustaining an acute infarction define a distinct subset that has been studied more intensively than others. Based upon current knowledge it would seem reasonable for patients sustaining an acute infarction to have a complete multiview left ventricular function study prior to discharge. This would provide important data concerning ejection fraction and wall motion and would be a first step in prognostic categorization. Patients also should have had a stress study prior to discharge. Current data would suggest that an exercise radionuclide study (probably $^{201}$Tl scintigraphy rather than ventricular function) will provide additional relevant data beyond the exercise ECG. Alternatively, one could argue that a conventional modified exercise test could be employed prior to discharge and, if normal, could be supplemented by a maximal exercise study with radionuclides in several weeks. If the initial study was abnormal, then further testing might not be indicated. Clearly, in these settings, the results of nuclear studies could provide appropriate branch points in clinical decision making concerning the need for angiography and/or further intervention.

## Technetium-99m Stannous Pyrophosphate Infarct-Avid Scintigraphy

Technetium-99m stannous pyrophosphate infarct-avid scintigraphy was one of the first procedures proposed for the radionuclide study of coronary artery disease. Demonstration of the zone of infarction as a "hot spot" of increased radionuclide accumulation triggered the imagination of investigators interested in radionuclide imaging of cardiovascular disease. Following the publication of a plethora of papers dealing with this subject, it became apparent that frequently the clinical indication for the performance of such studies is limited. Indeed, frequently there are easier and less expensive manners of diagnosing acute myocardial infarction. Nevertheless, in certain clinical instances the diagnosis of infarction is difficult. In such instances, for clinical purposes, infarct-avid imaging can play an important diagnostic role. Such clinical circumstances include (1) patients with electrocardiograms such as left bundle branch block that make it difficult to define the presence of acute infarction, (2) those presenting several days after onset of infarction such that conventional diagnostic electrocardiographic or enzymatic modalities for detecting infarction are no longer applicable, (3) those in whom infarction or necrosis may develop in the perioperative cardiovascular surgical setting. In such instances infarct-avid imaging can play an important clinical role. In addition, utilization of the technique to define infarct size may be of clinical as well as investigational value. This has achieved increasing importance with the development of thrombolytic therapy for the treatment of the evolving infarct. In this setting, particularly if thrombolytic therapy is to be administered intracoronary, technetium-99m pyrophosphate may be administered directly through the coronary artery, thereby altering its conventional kinetics and leading to the definition of zones of necrosis within the early hours of infarction.

The exact mechanism of myocardial uptake of this radiopharmaceutical is still somewhat controversial. Current evidence suggests that the mechanism involves complexing of the radiopharmaceutical with intracellular calcium within the infarcted segment. There is probably also complexing with macromolecules present in the infarct zone [112–114].

Images are generally evaluated visually on a scale of 0 to 4+, based on the intensity of accumulation: 0 = no activity, 1+ = minimal activity, 2+ = myocardial activity not as intense as that of the sternum, 3+ = myocardial activity as intense as the sternum, and 4+ = myocardial activity more intense than the sternum. In addition, uptake is graded as being either "diffuse" or "focal" [115]. When a 2+ focal or greater pattern is used as a criterion for a positive study, the sensitivity for detection of transmural myocardial infarction is greater than 80 percent. However, using the same criteria for subendocardial infarction, the sensitivity is only between 30 and 45 percent [116–118]. The specificity of the technique is dependent upon the patient population evaluated. A number of conditions will lead to abnormal cardiac accumulation of technetium-99m pyrophosphate. These include a previous infarction [119, 120] or aneurysm [121–123], unstable angina [124–130], cardiomyopathy [124], cardioversion [127, 131, 132], valvular calcification [133–135], pericarditis [136], and trauma [137, 138]. In addition, it must be noted that when administered intravenously, maximal uptake in the zone of infarction occurs 24 to 72 hours after the onset [139, 140]. Therefore, under routine circumstances the ability of this imaging technique to detect infarction will be limited by time constraints. However, if the issue of diagnosis is removed, this time constraint will not affect the ability to size infarction and use the data derived therefrom in prognostic stratification of patients.

## Imaging of Cardiac Metabolism

One of the earliest reports of cardiac imaging in general involved the attempt by Evans et al. [141] to employ iodinated oleic acid to image myocardial infarction. Since that study a broad experience has occurred with respect to myocardial metabolic imaging. This has generally taken two major lines of investigation: positron emission–computed tomography and single-photon radioiodinated fatty acid imaging. To date, these studies remain primarily experimental and therefore will be reviewed only briefly. Studies have been performed in experimental animals as well as in man. Positron studies have involved the use of carbon-11 palmitic acid to study fatty acid uptake and washout as well as fluorodeoxyglucose to study glucose metabolism [142, 143]. The positron studies currently require onsite cy-

clotron facilities for preparation of radioactive tracers. These studies have demonstrated decreased fatty acid accumulation following ischemia or infarction and altered metabolic washout rates. Furthermore, in acute infarction and ischemia there has been increased uptake of radioactive glucose, indicating a shift in metabolism within the myocardium favoring this less efficient metabolic pathway (figure 8–10) [142–147].

Single-photon radioiodinated free fatty acid studies have involved the use of iodine-123 as the radioactive label with a number of fatty acids employed as the radioactive metabolic substrate [148–151]. Problems have arisen from interpreting the data of washout curves regionally, because the release of iodine from the fatty acid leading to a high level of nonmetabolic background can confound metabolic kinetic analysis [152]. Currently, attempts are being made to derive new fatty acid tracers that will not be subject to the same kinetic and theortical difficulties occurring with the current radioiodinated tracers.

In general, these compounds, both positron and nonpositron emitters, present a great potential for future studies. Use of such tracers will allow definition of the metabolic integrity of various regions of myocardium, even in the presence of altered perfusion or function. Clearly, this general class of studies represents the next stratum of nuclear cardiologic investigation.

## Studies During Thrombolysis and Reperfusion

All of the studies discussed in this chapter have potential application to the evaluation of the reperfused myocardium following thrombolytic therapy. Preliminary studies already have been reported involving ventricular function, perfusion and infarct-avid scintigraphy, and metabolic scintigraphy. Studies involving ventricular functional analysis clearly must focus not only on global ventricular function, but also regional assessment. This has been emphasized in previous studies involving contrast angiography as well as radionuclide studies [153]. Clearly, within the context of noninvasive evaluation, radionuclide ventricular function studies should play an important role. Evaluation of perfusion as well as

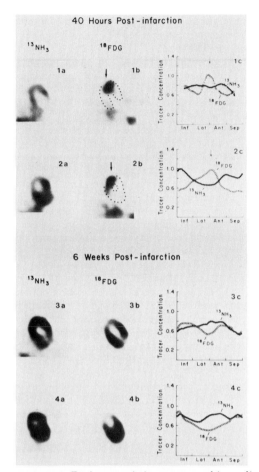

40 Hours Post-infarction

6 Weeks Post-infarction

FIGURE 8–10. Positron emission tomographic studies obtained with fluorodeoxyglucose (FDG) representing glucose metabolism, and ammonia representing perfusion. Images in the upper panel were obtained 40 hours following infarction, those in the lower panel obtained 6 weeks after infarction. Note the area of increased uptake of glucose present in images 1b and 2b, indicating increased uptake of glucose resulting from an altered metabolic pathway. At 6 weeks postinfarction this is no longer apparent. Quantitative analysis to the right confirms the visual impression. (From Marshall et al. Identification of and differentiation of resting myocardial ischemia and infarction in man with position-computed tomography,[18] F-labeled fluorodeoxyglucose and M-13 ammonia. *Circulation* 67:766, 1983. Reprinted by permission of the American Heart Association, Inc.)

viability and metabolic performance should likewise be quite important. Studies in this area are currently under active investigation (see Chapter 9), and detailed explication awaits further reports in this field.

*References*

1. Blumgart, H.C. and Weiss, S. Studies on the velocity of blood flow: VII. The pulmonary circulation time in normal resting individuals. *J. Clin. Invest.* 4:399, 1927.
2. Burow, R.D., Strauss, H.W., Singleton, R., Pond, M., Rehn, T., Bailey, I.K., Griffith, L.C., Nickoloff, E., and Pitt, B. Analysis of left ventricular function from multiple gated acquisition cardiac blood pool imaging: Comparison to contrast angiography. *Circulation* 56:1024, 1977.
3. Green, M.V., Ostrow, H.G., Douglas, M.A., Myers, R.W., Scott, R.N., Bailey, J.J., and Johnston, G.S. High temporal resolution ECG-gated scintigraphic angiocardiography. *J. Nucl. Med.* 16:95, 1975.
4. Strauss, H.W., Zaret, B.L., Hurley, P.J., Natarajan, T.K., and Pitt B. A scintiphotographic method for measuring left ventricular ejection fraction in man without cardiac catheterization. *Am. J. Cardiol.* 28:575, 1971.
5. Pavel, D.G., Zimmer, A.M., and Patterson, V.N. In vivo labeling of red blood cells with Tc-99m: A new approach to blood pool visualization. *J. Nucl. Med.* 18:305, 1977.
6. Callahan, R.J., Froelich, J.W., McKusick, K.A., Leppo, J., and Strauss, H.W. A modified method for the in vivo labeling of red blood cells with Tc-99m: Concise communication. *J. Nucl. Med.* 23:315, 1982.
7. Bourguignon, M.H., Douglass, K.H., Links, J.M., and Wagner, H.N., Jr. Fully automated data acquisition, processing, and display in equilibrium radioventriculography. *Eur. J. Nucl. Med.* 6:343, 1981.
8. Chang, W., Henkin, R.E., Hale, D.J., and Hall, D. Methods for detection of left ventricular edges. *Semin. Nucl. Med.* 10:39, 1980.
9. Turner, D.A., Von Gehren, P.L., Ruggie, N.T., Hauser R.G., Denes, P., Ali, A., Messer, J.V., Fordham, E.W., and Groch, M.S. Noninvasive identification of initial site of abnormal ventricular activation by least-square phase analysis of radionuclide cineangiograms. *Circulation* 65:1511, 1982.
10. Wackers, F.J., Berger, H.J., Johnstone, D.E., Goldman, L., Reduto, L.A., Langou, R.A., Gottschalk, A., and Zaret, B.L. Multiple gated cardiac blood pool imaging for left ventricular ejection fraction: Validation of the technique and assessment of variability. *Am. J. Cardiol.* 43:1159, 1979.
11. Dehmer, G.J., Lewis, S.E., Hillis, L.D., Twie, S., DiFalkoff, M., Parkey, R.W., and Willerson, J.T. Nongeometric determination of left ventricular volumes from equilibrium blood pool scans. *Am. J. Cardiol.* 45:293, 1980.
12. Links, J.M., Becker, L.C., Shindledecker, J.G., Guzman, P., Burow, R.D., Nickoloff, E.L., Al-

derson, P.O., and Wagner, H.N. Measurement of absolute left ventricular volume from gated blood pool studies. *Circulation* 65:82, 1982.

13. Slutsky, R., Karliner, J., Ricci, D., Kaiser, R.P., Fisterer, M., Gordon, D., Peterson, K., and Ashburn, W. Ventricular volumes by gated equilibrium radionuclide angiography: A new method. *Circulation* 60:556, 1979.

14. Lam, W., Pavel, D., Byrom, E., Sheikh, A., Best, D., and Rosen, K. Radionuclide regurgitant index: Value and limitations. *Am. J. Cardiol.* 47:292, 1981.

15. Alpert, N.M., Strauss, H.W., Tarolli, E.J., and Chesler, D.A. Determination of ventricular borders by adaptive filtering. *J. Nucl. Med.* 21(6):P47, 1980 (abstract).

16. Maddox, E.E., Wynne, J., Uren, R., Parker, J.A., Idoine, J., Neill, J.M., Cohn, P.F., and Holman, B.L. Regional ejection fraction: A quantitative radionuclide index of regional left ventricular performance. *Circulation* 59:1001, 1979.

17. Papapietro, S.E., Yester, M.V., Logic, J.R., Tauxe, W.N., Mantle, J.A., Rogers, W.J., Russell, R.O., Jr., and Rackley, C.E. Method for quantitative analysis of regional left ventricular function with first pass and gated blood pool scintigraphy. *Am. J. Cardiol.* 47:618, 1981.

18. Adam, W.E., Tarkowska, A., Bitter, F., Stauch, M., and Geffer, H. Equilibrium (gated) radionuclide ventriculography. *Cardiovasc. Radiol.* 2:161, 1979.

19. Maddox, E.E., Holman, B.L., Wynne, J., Idoine, J., Parker, J.A., Uren, R., Neill, J.M., and Cohn, P.F. Ejection fraction image: A noninvasive index of regional left ventricular wall motion. *Am. J. Cardiol.* 41:1230, 1978.

20. Ratib, O., Henze, E., Schön, H., and Schelbert, H.R. Phase analysis of radionuclide ventriculograms for the detection of coronary artery disease. *Am. Heart J.* 104:1, 1982.

21. Vos, P.H., Vossepoel, A.M., and Pauwels, E.K.J. Quantitative assessment of wall motion in multiple-gated studies using temporal fourier analysis. *J. Nucl. Med.* 24:388, 1983.

22. Duncan, J.S. Intelligent detection of left ventricular boundaries in gated nuclear medicine image sequences. Presented: Proceedings of the 7th International Conference on Pattern Recognition, Montreal, Quebec, Canada, July 30–August 2, 1984. In press.

23. Bacharach, S.L., Green, M.V., Borer, J.S., Ostrow, H.G., Redwood, D.R., and Johnston, G.S. ECG-gated scintillation probe measurement of left ventricular function. *J. Nucl. Med.* 18:1176, 1977.

24. Berger, H.J., Davies, R.A., Batsford, W.P., Hoffer, P.B., Gottschalk, A., and Zaret, B.L. Beat-to-beat left ventricular performance as-

sessed from the equilibrium cardiac blood pool using a computerized nuclear probe. *Circulation* 63:133, 1981.

25. Wagner, H.N., Jr, Wake, R., Nickoloff, E., and Natarajan, T.K. The nuclear stethoscope: A simple device for generation of left ventricular volume curves. *Am. J. Cardiol.* 38:747, 1976.

26. Schneider, J., Berger, H.J., Sands, M., Lachman, A., and Zaret, B.L. Beat to beat left ventricular performance in atrial fibrillation: Radionuclide assessment with the computerized nuclear probe. *Am. J. Cardiol.* 51:1189, 1983.

27. Soufer, R., Wohlgelernter, D., Vita, N.A., Amuchestegui, M., Sotsman, D., Berger, H.J., and Zaret, B.L. Intact systolic left ventricular function in congestive heart failure: Clinical description and mechanistic considerations. *Am. J. Cardiol.,* in press, 1985.

28. Giles, R.W., Berger, H.J., Barash, P.G., Tarabadkar, S., Marx, P.G., Hammond, G.L., Geha, A.S., Laks, H., and Zaret, B.L. Continuous monitoring of left ventricular performance with the computerized nuclear probe during laryngoscopy and intubation prior to coronary artery bypass surgery. *Am. J. Cardiol.* 50:735, 1982.

29. Berger, H.J., Byrd, W., Giles, R., Orphanoudakis, S., and Zaret, B.L. Beat-to-beat left ventricular pressure-volume relationships assessed from the equilibrium cardiac blood pool using a computerized nonimaging nuclear probe. In *Computers in Cardiology.* New York, IEEE Computer Society, 1982, pp. 55–60.

30. Berger, H.J., Matthay, R.A., Pytlik, L.M., Gottschalk, A., and Zaret, B.L. First-pass radionuclide assessment of right and left ventricular performance in patients with cardiac and pulmonary disease. *Semin. Nucl. Med.* 9:275, 1979.

31. Wackers, F.J., Giles, R.W., Hoffer, P.B., Lange, R.C., Berger, H.J., and Zaret, B.L. Gold-195m, a new generator-produced short-lived radionuclide for sequential assessment of ventricular performance by first-pass radionuclide angiocardiography. *Am. J. Cardiol.* 50:89, 1982.

32. Wackers, F.J., Stein, R., Pytlik, L., Plankey, M.W., Lange, R., Hoffer, P.B., Sands, M.J., Zaret, B.L., and Berger, H.J. Gold-195m for serial first pass radionuclide angiocardiography during upright exercise in patients with coronary artery disease. *J. Am. Coll. Cardiol.* 2:497, 1983.

33. Kaul, S., Boucher, C.A., Okada, R.D., Newell, J.B., Strauss, H.W., and Pohost, G.M. Sources of variability in the radionuclide angiographic assessment of ejection fraction: A comparison of first-pass and gated equilibrium techniques. *Am. J. Cardiol.* 53:823, 1984.

34. Berger, H.J., Reduto, L.A., Johnstone, D.E., Borkowski, H., Sands, M., Cohen, L., Langou,

R., Gottschalk, A., and Zaret, B.L. Global and regional left ventricular response to bicycle exercise in coronary artery disease: Assessment by quantitative radionuclide angiocardiography. *Am. J. Med.* 66:13, 1979.

35. Borer, J.S., Bacharach, S.L., Green, M.V., Kent, K.M., Epstein, S.E., and Johnston, G.S. Real-time radionuclide cineangiography in the noninvasive evaluation of global and regional left ventricular function at rest and during exercise in patients with coronary artery disease. *N. Engl. J. Med.* 296:839, 1977.

36. Caldwell, J.H., Hamilton, G.W., Sorensen, S.G., Ritchie, J.L., Williams, D.L., and Kennedy, J.W. The detection of coronary artery disease with radionuclide techniques: A comparison of rest-exercise thallium imaging and ejection fraction response. *Circulation* 61:610, 1980.

37. Rerych, S.K., Scholz, P.M., Newman, G.E., Sabiston, D.C., Jr., and Jones, R.H. Cardiac function at rest and during exercise in normals and in patients with coronary heart disease: Evaluation by radionuclide angiocardiography. *Ann. Surg.* 187:449, 1978.

38. Borer, J.S., Bacharach, S.L., Green, M.V., Kent, K.M., Epstein, S.E., and Johnston, G.S. Real time radionuclide cineangiography in the noninvasive evaluation of global and regional left ventricular function at rest and during exercise in patients with coronary artery disease. *N. Engl. J. Med.* 296:839, 1977.

39. Kent, K.M., Borer, J.S., Green, M.V., Bacharach, S.L., McIntosh, C.L., Conkle, D.M., and Epstein, S.E. Effects of coronary artery bypass on global and regional left ventricular function during exercise. *N. Engl. J. Med.* 298:1434, 1978.

40. Poliner, L.R., Dehmer, G.J., Lewis, S.E., Parkey, R.W., Blomquist, C.G., and Willerson, J.T. Left ventricular performance in normal subjects: A comparison of the responses to exercise in the upright and supine positions. *Circulation* 62:528, 1980.

41. Brady, T.J., Lo, K., Thrall, J.H., Walton, J.A., Brymer, J.F., and Pitt, B. Exercise radionuclide ejection fraction: Correlation with exercise contrast ventriculography. *Radiology* 132:703, 1979.

42. Okada, R.D., Boucher, C.A., Strauss, H.W., and Pohost, G.M. Exercise radionuclide imaging approaches to coronary artery disease. *Am. J. Cardiol.* 46:1188, 1980.

43. Rosanski, A., Diamond, G.A., Berman, D., Forrester, J.S., Morris, D., and Swan, H.J.C. The declining specificity of exercise radionuclide ventriculography. *N. Engl. J. Med.* 309:518, 1983.

44. Berger, H.J., Sands, M.J., Davies, R.A., Wack-

ers, F.T., Alexander, J., Lachman, A.S., Williams, B.W., and Zaret, B.L. Exercise left ventricular performance in patients with chest pain, ischemic-appearing exercise electrocardiograms, and angiographically normal coronary arteries. *Ann. Intern. Med.* 94:186, 1981.

45. Gibbons, R.H., Lee, J.L., Cobb, F.R., and Jones, R.H. Ejection fraction response to exercise in patients with chest pain and normal coronary arteriograms. *Circulation* 64:952, 1981.

46. Port, S., Cobb, R.R., Coleman, R.E., and Jones, R.H. Effect of age on the response of the left ventricular ejection fraction to exercise. *N. Engl. J. Med.* 303:1133, 1980.

47. Borer, J.S., Bacharach, S.L., Green, M.V., Kent, K.M., Maron, B.J., Rosing, D.R., Seides, S.F., and Epstein, S.E. Obstructive vs. nonobstructive symmetric septal hypertrophy: Differences in left ventricular function with exercise. *Am. J. Cardiol.* 41:379, 1978 (abstract).

48. Gottdiener, J.S., Mathisen, D.J., and Borer, J.S. Doxorubicin cardiotoxicity: Assessment of late left ventricular dysfunction by radionuclide cineangiography. *Ann. Int. Med.* 94:430, 1981.

49. Gottdiener, J.S., Katia, M.J., Borer, J.S., Bacharach, S.L., and Green, M.V. Late cardiac effects of therapeutic mediastinal irradiation. *N. Engl. J. Med.* 308:569, 1980.

50. Borer, J.S., Bacharach, S.L., Green, M.V., Kent, K.M., Rosing, D.R., Seides, S.F., McIntosh, C.L., Conkle, D., Morrow, A.G., and Epstein, S.E. Left ventricular function in aortic stenosis: Response to exercise and effects of operation. *Am. J. Cardiol.* 41:382, 1978 (abstract).

51. Borer, J.S., Bacharach, S.L., Green, M.V., Kent, K.M., Henry, W.L., Rosing, D.R., Seides, S.F., Johnston, G.S., and Epstein, S.E. Exercise induced left ventricular dysfunction in symptomatic and asymptomatic patients with aortic regurgitation: Assessment with radionuclide cineangiography. *Am. J. Cardiol.* 42:351, 1978.

52. Borer, J.S., Gottdiener, J.S., Rosing, D.R., Kent, K.M., Bacharach, S.L., Green, M.V., and Epstein, S.E. Left ventricular function in mitral regurgitation: Determination during exercise. *Circulation* 60:II-38, 1979 (abstract).

53. Gottdiener, J.S., Borer, J.S., Bacharach, S.L., Green, M.V., and Epstein, S.E. Left ventricular function in mitral valve prolapse: Assessment with radionuclide cineangiography. *Am. J. Cardiol.* 47:7, 1981.

54. Francis, C.K., Cleman, M., Berger, H.J., Davies, R.A., Giles, R.W., Black, H.R., Zito, R.A., and Zaret, B.L. Left ventricular systolic performance during upright bicycle exercise in patients with essential hypertension. *Am. J. Med.* 75:40, 1983.

55. White, C.W., Wright, C.B., Doty, D.B.,

Hiratza, L.F., Eastham, C.L., Harrison, D.G., and Marcus, M.L. Does visual interpretation of the coronary arteriogram predict the physiologic importance of a coronary stenosis? *N. Engl. J. Med.* 310:819, 1984.

56. Borer, J.S., Kent, K.M., Bacharach, S.L., et al. Sensitivity, specificity, and predictive accuracy of radionuclide cineangiography during exercise in patients with coronary artery disease; comparison with exercise electrocardiography. *Circulation* 60:572, 1979.

57. Jones, R.H., McEwan, P., Newman, G., Port, S., Rerych, S.K., Scholz, P.M., Upton, M.T., Peter, C.A., Austin, E.H., Leong, K., Gibbons, R.J., Cobb, F.R., and Sabiston, D.C., Jr. The accuracy of diagnosis of coronary artery disease by radionuclide measurements of left ventricular function during rest and exercise. *Circulation* 64:586, 1981.

58. Newman, G.F., Rerych, S.K., Upton, M.T., Sabiston, D.C., Jr., and Jones, R.H. Comparison of electrocardiographic and left ventricular functional changes during exercise. *Circulation* 62:1204, 1980.

59. Gibbons, R.J., Lee, K.L., Cobb, F.C., Coleman, E., and Jones, R.H. Ejection fraction response to exercise in patients with chest pain, coronary artery disease, and normal resting ventricular function. *Circulation* 66:643, 1982.

60. Bodenheimer, M.M., Banka, V.S., Fooshee, C.M., Gillespie, J.A., and Helfant, R.H. Detection of coronary heart disease using radionuclide determined regional ejection fraction at rest and during handgrip exercise: Correlation with coronary arteriography. *Circulation* 58:640, 1978.

61. Benge, W., Litchfield, R.L., and Marcus, M.L. Exercise capacity in patients with severe left ventricular dysfunction. *Circulation* 61:955, 1980.

62. Giles, R., Marx, P., Commerford, P., Zaret, B.L., and Berger, H.J. Rapid sequential changes in left ventricular function during cold pressor and isometric handgrip: Relationship to blood pressure and mechanistic implications. *Am. J. Cardiol.* 49:1002, 1982 (abstract).

63. Jordan, L.J., Borer, J.S., Zullo, M., Hayes, D., Kubo, S., Moses, J.W., and Carter, J. Exercise versus cold temperature stimulation during radionuclide cineangiography: Diagnostic accuracy in coronary artery disease. *Am. J. Cardiol.* 51:1091, 1983.

64. Bonow, R.O., Bacharach, S.L., Green, M.V., Kent, K.M., Rosing, D.R., Lipson, L.C., Leon, M.B., and Epstein, S.E. Impaired left ventricular diastolic filling in patients with coronary artery disease: Assessment with radionuclide angiography. *Circulation* 64:315, 1981.

65. Bonow, R.O., Kent, K.M., Rosing, D.R. Lipson, L.C., Bacharach, S.L., Green, M.V., and Epstein, S.E. Improved left ventricular diastolic filling in patients with coronary artery disease after percutaneous transluminal coronary angioplasty. *Circulation* 66:1159, 1982.

66. Bonow, R.O., Leon, M.B., Rosing, D.R., Kent, K.M., Lipson, L.C., Bacharach, S.L., Green, M.V., and Epstein, S.E. Effects of verapamil and propranolol on left ventricular systolic function and diastolic filling in patients with coronary artery disease: Radionuclide angiographic studies at rest and during exercise. *Circulation* 65:1337, 1981.

67. Pohost, G.M., Alpert, N.M., Ingwall, J.S., and Strauss, H.W. Thallium redistribution: Mechanisms and clinical utility. *Sem. Nuc. Med.* 10:70, 1980.

68. Gehring, P.J. and Hammond, P.B. The interrelationship between thallium and potassium in animals. *J. Pharacol. Exp. Ther.* 155:187, 1967.

69. Botvinick, E.H., Dunn, R.F., Hattner, R.S., and Massie, B.M. The consideration of factors affecting diagnostic accuracy of thallium-201 myocardial perfusion scintigraphy in detecting coronary artery disease. *Sem. Nuc. Med.* 10:157, 1980.

70. Dunn, R.F., Wolff, L. Wagner, S., and Botvinick, E.H. Inconsistent pattern of thallium defects: A clue to the false positive perfusion scintigram. *Am. J. Cardiol.* 48:224, 1981.

71. Johnstone, D.E., Wackers, F.J., Berger, H.J., Hoffer, P.B., Kelley, M.J., Gottschalk, A., and Zaret, B.L. Effect of patient positioning on left lateral thallium-201 myocardial images. *J. Nucl. Med.* 20:183, 1979.

72. Cook, D.J., Bailey, I., Strauss, H.W., Rouleau, J., Wagner, H.N., Jr., and Pitt, B. Thallium-201 for myocardial imaging: Appearance of the normal heart. *J. Nucl. Med.* 17:583, 1976.

73. Stevens, R.M., Baird, M.G., Fuhrman, C.F., Rouleau, J., Summer, W.P., Strauss, H.W., and Pitt, B. Detection of right ventricular hypertrophy by thallium-201 myocardial perfusion imaging. *Circulation* 52:II-243, 1975 (abstract).

74. Wackers, F.J., Klay, J.W., Laks, H., Schnitzer, J., Zaret, B.L., and Geha, A.S. Pathophysiologic correlates of right ventricular thallium-201 uptake in a canine model. *Circulation* 64:1256, 1981.

75. Gibson, R.S., Watson, D.O., Carabello, B.A., Holt, N.D., and Beller, G.A. Clinical implication of increased lung uptake of thallium-201 during exercise scintigraphy 2 weeks after myocardial infarction. *Am. J. Cardiol.* 49:1586, 1982.

76. Boucher, C.A., Zir, L.M., Beller, G.A., Okada, R.D., McKusick, K.A., Strauss, H.W., and Pohost, G.M. Increased pulmonary uptake of thallium-201 during exercise myocardial imaging:

Clinical hemodynamic and angiographic implications with patients with coronary artery disease. *Am. J. Cardiol.* 46:189, 1980.

77. Rozanski, A., Berman, D.S., Gray, R., Levy, R., Raymond, R.N., Maddahi, J., Pantaleo, N., Waxman, A.D., Swan, H.J.C., and Matloff, J. Use of thallium-201 redistribution scintigraphy in the preoperative differentiation of reversible and nonreversible myocardial asynergy. *Circulation* 64:936, 1981.

78. Jengo, J.A., Freeman, R., Brizendine, M., and Mena, I. Detection of coronary artery disease: Comparison of exercise stressed radionuclide angiocardiography and thallium stress perfusion scanning. *Am. J. Cardiol.* 45:535, 1980.

79. Kirshenbaum, H.D., Okada, R.D., Boucher, C.A., Kushner, F.G., Strauss, H.W., and Pohost, G.M. Relationship of thallium-201 myocardial perfusion to regional and global left ventricular function with exercise. *Am. Heart. J.* 101:734, 1981.

80. Blood, D.K., McCarthy, D.M., Sciacca, R.R., and Cannon, P.J. Comparison of single-dose and double-dose thallium-201 myocardial perfusion scintigraphy for the detection of coronary artery disease and prior myocardial infarction. *Circulation* 58:777, 1978.

81. Berman, D.S., Garcia, E.V., and Maddahi, J. Thallium-201 Myocardial Scintigraphy in the Detection and Evaluation of Coronary Artery Disease. In D.S. Berman and D.T. Mason (eds), *Clinical Nuclear Cardiology.* New York: Grune & Stratton, 1981, pp. 86–93.

82. Maddahi, J., Garcia, E.V., Berman, D.S., Waxman, A., Swan, H.J.C., and Forrester, J. Improved noninvasive assessment of coronary artery disease by quantitative analysis of regional stress myocardial distribution and washout of thallium-201. *Circulation* 64:924, 1981.

83. Tamaki, N., Mukai, T., Ishii, Y., Yonekura, Y., Kambara, H., Kawai, C., and Torizuka, K. Clinical evaluation of thallium-201 emission myocardial tomography using a rotating gamma camera: Comparison with 7 pinhole tomography. *J. Nucl. Med.* 22:849, 1981.

84. Tamaki, S., Nakajima, H., Murakami, T., Yui, Y., Kambara, H., Kadota, K., Yoshida, A., Kawai, C., Tamaki, N., Mukai, T., Ishii, Y., and Torizuka, K. Estimation of infarct size by myocardial emission computed tomography with thallium-201 and its relation to creatine kinase-MB release after myocardial infarction in man. *Circulation* 66:994, 1982.

85. Ritchie, J.L., Williams, D.L., Harp, G., Stratton, J.L., and Caldwell, J.H. Transaxial tomography with thallium-201 for detecting remote myocardial infarction: Comparison with planar imaging. *Am. J. Cardiol.* 50:1236, 1982.

86. Roesler, H., Hess, T., Weiss, M., Noelpp, U.,

Mueller, G., Hoeflin, F., and Kinser, J. Tomoscintigraphic assessment of myocardial metabolic heterogeneity. *J. Nucl. Med.* 24:285, 1983.

87. Berman, D.S., Staniloff, H., Freeman, M., Garcia, E., Pantaleo, N., Maddahi, J., Waxman, A., Forrester, J., and Swan, H.J.C. Thallium-201 stress myocardial scintigraphy: Comparison of multiple pinhole tomography with planar imaging in the assessment of patients undergoing coronary arteriography. *Am. J. Cardiol.* 45:481, 1980 (abstract).

88. Green, A., Alderson, P., and Berman, D., A multicenter comparison of standard and 7 pinhole tomographic myocardial perfusion imaging: RVC analysis of quantitative visual interpretation. *J. Nucl. Med.* 21:70, 1980.

89. Berman, D., Garcia, E. Maddahi, J., Freeman, M., Pantaleo, N., Waxman, A., and Forrester, J. Quantitative analysis of thallium-201 distribution and washout for comparison of multiple pinhole tomography with planar imaging. *Circulation* 62:II-103, 1980 (abstract).

90. Massie, B.M., Botvinick, E.H., and Brundage, B.H. Correlation of thallium-201 scintigrams with coronary anatomy: Factors affecting region by region sensitivity. *Am. J. Cardiol.* 44:616, 1979.

91. Diamond, G.A. and Forrester, J.S. Analysis of probability as an aid in the clinical diagnosis of coronary artery disease. *N. Engl. J. Med.* 300:1350, 1979.

92. Hirzel, H.O., Senn, M., Nuesch, K., Buettner, C., Pfeiffer, A., Hess, O.M., and Krayenbuehl, H.P. Thallium-201 scintigraphy in complete left bundle branch block. *Am. J. Cardiol.* 53:764, 1984.

93. Rigo, P., Bailey, I.K., Griffith, L.S.C., Pitt, B., Burow, R.D., Wagner, H.N., and Becker, L.C. Value and limitations of segmental analysis of stress thallium myocardial imaging for localization of coronary artery disease. *Circulation* 61:973, 1980.

94. Dunn, R. Freedman, B., Bailey, I.K., Uren, R., and Kelly, D.T. Noninvasive prediction of multivessel disease after myocardial infarction. *Circulation* 62:726, 1980.

95. Wackers, F.J., Becker, A.E., Samson, G., Sokole, E.B., van der Schoot, J.B., Vet, H.J., Lie, K.I., Durrer, D., and Wellens, H. Location and size of acute transmural myocardial infarction estimated from thallium-201 scintiscans: A clinicopathological study. *Circulation* 56:72, 1977.

96. DiCola, V.C., Downing, S.F., Donabedian, R.K., and Zaret, B.L. Pathophysiological correlates of thallium-201 myocardial uptake in experimental infarction. *Cardiovas. Res.* 11:141, 1977.

97. Henning, H., Schelbert, H.R., Righetti, A.,

Ashburn, W.L., and O'Rourke, R.A. Dual myocardial imaging with technetium-99m pyrophosphate and thallium-201 for detecting, localizing and sizing acute myocardial infarction. *Am. J. Cardiol.* 40:147, 1977.

98. Mueller, H.S., Fletcher, J.W., and Ayres, S.M. 201-thallium image and creatine kinase MB infarct size: Evaluation of variable treatment responses. *Circulation* 60:II-163, 1979.

99. Buja, L.M., Parkey, R.W., Stokely, E.M., Bonte, F.J., and Willerson, J.T. Pathophysiology of technetium-99m stannous pyrophosphate and thallium-201 scintigraphy of acute anterior myocardial infarcts in dogs. *J. Clin. Invest.* 57:1508, 1976.

100. Schuster, E.H., Bulkely, B.H., Jugdutt, B.I., Burow, R., Clulow, J., and Becker, L.C. Assessment of extent of myocardial infarction by computer analysis of thallium-201 scintigrams (TS). *Circulation* 60:II-134, 1979.

101. Bulkley, B.H., Silverman, K., Weisfeldt, M.L., Burow, R.D., Pond, M., and Becker, L.C. Pathologic basis of thallium-201 scintigraphic defects in patients with fatal myocardial injury. *Circulation* 60:785, 1979.

102. Silverman, K.J., Becker, L.C., Bulkley, B.H., Burow, R.D., Mellits, E.D., Kallman, C.H., and Weisfeldt, M.L. Value of early thallium-201 scintigraphy for predicting mortality in patients with acute myocardial infarction. *Circulation* 61:996, 1980.

103. Schulze, R.A., Jr., Strauss, H.W., and Pitt, B. Sudden death in the year following myocardial infarction: Relation to ventricular premature contractions in the late hospital phase and left ventricular ejection fraction. *Am. J. Med.* 62:192, 1977.

104. Shah, P.K., Pichler, M., Berman, D.S., Singh, B.N. and Swan, H.J.C. Left ventricular ejection fraction determined by radionuclide ventriculography in early stages of first transmural myocardial infarction: Relation to short-term prognosis. *Am. J. Cardiol.* 45:542, 1980.

105. The Multicenter Postinfarction Research Group. Risk stratification and survival after myocardial infarction. *N. Engl. J. Med.* 309:331, 1983.

106. Berman, D.S., Garcia, E.V., and Maddhi, J. Thallium-201 Myocardial Scintigraphy in the Detection and Evaluation of Coronary Artery Disease. In D.S. Berman and D.T. Mason (eds), *Clinical Nuclear Cardiology.* New York: Grune & Stratton, 1981, pp. 270–272.

107. Becker, L.D., Silverman, K.J., Bulkely, B.H. Kallman, C.H., Mellits, E.D., and Weisfeldt, M.D. Comparison of early thallium-201 scintigraphy and gated blood pool imaging for predicting mortality in patients with acute myocardial infarction. *Circulation* 67:6, 1983.

108. Warnowicz, M.A., Parker, H., and Cheitlin, M.D. Prognosis of patients with acute pulmonary edema and normal ejection fraction after acute myocardial infarction. *Circulation* 67:330, 1983.

109. Meizlish, J., Berger, H.J., Plankey, R.T., Errico, D., Levy, W., and Zaret, B.L. Functional left ventricular aneurysm formation following acute anterior transmural myocardial infarction: Incidence, natural history and prognostic implications. *New Engl. J. Med.* 311:1001, 1984.

110. Pryor, D.B., Harrell, F.E., Jr., Lee, K.L., Rosati, R.A., Coleman, E., Cobb, F.R., Califf, R.M., and Jones, R.H. Prognostic indicators from radionuclide angiography in medically treated patients with coronary artery disease. *Am. J. Cardiol.* 53:18, 1984.

111. Corbett, J.R., Dehmer, G.J., Lewis, S.E., Woodward, W., Henderson, E., Parkey, R.W., Blomquist, C.G., and Willerson, J.T. The prognostic value of submaximal exercise testing with radionuclide ventriculography before hospital discharge in patients with recent myocardial infarction. *Circulation* 64:535, 1981.

112. Leppo, J.A., O'Brien, J., Rothendler, J.A., Getchell, J.D., and Lee, V.W. Dipyridamole-thallium-201 scintigraphy in the prediction of future cardiac events after acute myocardial infarction. *N. Engl. J. Med.* 310:1014, 1984.

113. Buja, L.M., Tofe, A.J., Kulkarni, P.V., Mukherjee, A., Parkey, R.W., Francis, M.D., Bonte, F.J., and Willerson, J.T. Sites and mechanisms of localization of technetium-99m phosphorus radiopharmaceuticals in acute myocardial infarcts and other issues. *J. Clin. Invest.* 60:724, 1977.

114. Poliner, L.R., Buja, L.M., Parkey, R.W., Bonte, F.J., and Willerson, J.T. Clinicopathologic findings in 52 patients studied by technetium-99m stannous pyrophosphate myocardial scintigraphy. *Circulation* 59:257, 1979.

115. Willerson, J.T., Parkey, R.W., Buja, L.M., and Bonte, F.J. Detection of Acute Myocardial Infarcts Using Myocardial Scintigraphic Techniques. In R.W. Parkey, F.J. Bonte, L.M. Buja, et al. (eds), *Clinical Nuclear Cardiology.* New York: Appleton-Century-Crofts, 1979, p. 141.

116. Willerson, J.T., Parkey, R.W., Bonte, F.J., Meyer, S.L., and Stokely, E.M. Acute subendocardial infarction in patients: Its detection by technetium-99m stannous pyrophosphate scintigrams. *Circulation* 51:436, 1975.

117. Massie, B.M., Botvinick, E.H., Werner, J.A., Chatterjee, K., and Parmley, W.W. Myocardial scintigraphy with technetium-99m stannous pyrophosphate: An insensitive test for nontransmural myocardial infarction. *Am. J. Cardiol.* 43:186, 1979.

118. Lyons, K.P., Olson, H.G., and Aronow, W.S.

Pyrophosphate myocardial imaging. *Semin. Nucl. Med.* 10:168, 1980.

119. Olson, H.G., Lyons, K.P., Aronow, W.S., Brown, W.T., and Greenfield, R.S. Follow-up technetium-99m stannous pyrophosphate myocardial scintigrams after acute myocardial infarction. *Circulation* 56:181, 1977.

120. Malin, F.R., Rollow, F.D., and Gertz, E.W. Sequential myocardial scintigraphy with technetium-99m stannous pyrophosphate following myocardial infarction. *J. Nucl. Med.* 19:1111, 1978.

121. Ahmad, M., Dubid, J.P., Verdon, T.A., Jr, and Martin, R.H. Technetium-99m stannous pyrophosphate myocardial imaging in patients with and without left ventricular aneurysm. *Circulation* 53:833, 1976.

122. Crowley, M.J., Mantle, J.A., Rogers, W.J., Russell, R.O., Jr., Rackley, C.E., and Logic, J.R. Technetium-99m stannous pyrophosphate myocardial scintigraphy: Reliability and limitations in assessment of acute myocardial infarction. *Circulation* 56:192, 1977.

123. Curry, R.C. and Jackmon, W.M. Persistently positive Tc-pyrophosphate myocardial scintigram in patients with a left ventricular aneurysm. *Clin. Nucl. Med.* 1:91, 1976.

124. Perez, L.A., Hayt, D.B., and Freeman, L.M. Localization of myocardial disorders other than infarction with 99m-Tc-labelled phosphate agents. *J. Nucl. Med.* 17:241, 1976.

125. Donsky, M.S., Curry, G.C., Parkey, R.W., Meyer, S.L., Bonte, F.J., Platt, M.R., and Willerson, J.T. Unstable angina pectoris: Clinical, angiographic, and myocardial scintigraphic observations. *Br. Heart. J.* 38:257, 1976.

126. Abdulla, A.M., Canedo, M.I., Cortez, B.C., McGinnis, K.D., and Wilhelm, S.K. Detection of unstable angina by 99m-technetium pyrophostphate myocardial scintigraphy. *Chest* 69:-168, 1976.

127. Prasquier, R. Taradash, M.R., Botvinick, E.H., Shames, D.M., and Parmley, W.W. The specificity of the diffuse pattern of cardiac uptake in myocardial infarction imaging with technetium-99m stannous pyrophosphate. *Circulation* 55:-61, 1977.

128. Ahmad, M., Dubiel, J.P., Logan, K.W., Verdon, T.A., and Martin, R.H. Limited clinical diagnostic specificity of technetium-99m stannous pyrophosphate myocardial imaging in acute myocardial infarction. *Am. J. Cardiol.* 39:-50, 1977.

129. Jaffe, A.S., Klein, M.S., Patel, B.R., Siegel, B.A., and Roberts, R. Abnormal technetium-99m pyrophosphate images in unstable angina: Ischemia versus infarction? *Am. J. Cardiol.* 44:-1035, 1979.

130. Holman, B.L., Lesch, M., and Alpert, J.S. Myo-

cardial scintigraphy with technetium-99m pyrophosphate during the early phase of acute infarction. *Am. J. Cardiol.* 41:39, 1978.

131. Pugh, B.R., Buja, L.M., Parkey, R.W., Poliner, L.R., Stokely, E.M., Bonte, F.J., and Willerson, J.T. Cardioversion and "false positive" technetium-99m stannous pyrophosphate myocardial scintigraphy. *Circulation* 54:399, 1976.

132. Davidson, R., Spies, S.M., Przybylek, J., Hai, H., and Lesch, M. Technetium-99m stannous pyrophosphate myocardial scintigraphy after cardiopulmonary resuscitation with cardioversion. *Circulation* 60:292, 1979.

133. Klein, M.S., Weiss, A.N., Roberts, R., and Coleman, R.E. Technetium-99m stannous pyrophosphate scintigrams in normal subjects, patients with exercise-induced ischemia and patients with a calcified valve. *Am. J. Cardiol.* 39:360, 1977.

134. Epstein, E.A., Solar, M., and Levin, E.J. Demonstration of long-standing metastatic soft tissue calcification by 99m Tc-diphosphate. *A.J.R.* 128:145, 1977.

135. Righetti, A., O'Rourke, R.A., Schelbert, H., Henning, H., Hardarson, T., Daily, P.O., Ashburn, W., and Ross, J. Usefulness of preoperative and postoperative Tc-99m (Sn) pyroscans in patients with ischemic and valvular heart disease. *Am. J. Cardiol.* 39:43, 1977.

136. Lyons, K.P. Olson, H.G., Brown, W.T., Aronow, W.S., and Kuperus, J. Persistence of an abnormal pattern on Tc-99m pyrophosphate myocardial scintigraphy of acute myocardial infarction. *Clin. Nucl. Med.* 1:253, 1976.

137. Chiu, C.L., Roelofs, J.D., Go, R.T., Doty, D.B., Rose, E.F., and Christie, J.H. Coronary angiographic and scintigraphic findings in experimental cardiac contusion. *Radiology* 116:679, 1975.

138. Go, R.T., Doty, D.B., and Chiu, C.L. A new method of diagnosing myocardial contusion in man by radionuclide imaging. *Radiology* 116:-107, 1975.

139. Rossman, D.J., Strauss, H.W., Siegel, M.E., and Pitt, B. Accumulation of 99m Tc-glucoheptonate in acutely infarcted myocardium. *J. Nucl. Med.* 16:875, 1975.

140. Alonso, D.R., Jacobstein, J.G., Cipriano, P.R., Roberts, A.J., Alonson, M.L., and Kline, S.A. Early quantification of experimental myocardial infarction with technetium-99m glucoheptonate: Scintigraphic and anatomic studies. *Am. J. Cardiol.* 42:251, 1978.

141. Evans, J.R., Phil, D., Gunton, R.W., Baker, R.G., Beanlands, D.S., and Spears, J.C. Use of radioiodinated fatty acid for photoscans of the heart. *Circ. Res.* 16:1, 1965.

142. Marshall, R.C., Tillisch, J.H., Phelps, M.E., Huang, S.C. Carson, R., Henze, E., and Schelbert, H.R. Identification of and differentiation

of resting myocardial ischemia and infarction in man with positron computed tomography, [18]F-labeled fluorodeoxyglucose and N-13 ammonia. *Circulation* 67:766, 1983.

143. Bergmann, S.R., Lerch, R.A., Fox, K.A., Ludbrook, P.A., Welch, M.J., Ter-Pogossian, M.M., and Sobel, B.E. Temporal dependence of beneficial effects of coronary thrombolysis characterized by positron tomography. *Am. J. Med.* 73:573, 1982.

144. Ter-Pogossian, M.M., Klein, M.S., Markham, J. Roberts, R., and Sobel, B.E. Regional assessment of myocardial metabolic integrity in vivo by positron-emission tomography with C-11 labeled palmitate. *Circulation* 61:242, 1980.

145. Lerch, R.A., Ambos, H.D., Bergmann, S.R., Welch, M.J., Ter-Pogossian, M.M., and Sobel B.E. Localization of viable, ischemic myocardium by positron emission tomography with C-11 palmitate. *Circulation* 64:689, 1981.

146. Lerch, R.A., Bergmann, S.R., Ambos, H.D., Welch, M.J. Ter-Pogossian, M.M., and Sobel, B.E. Effect of flow-independent reduction of metabolism on regional mycardial clearance of C-11 palmitate. *Circulation* 65:731, 1982.

147. Ratib, O., Phelphs, M.E., Huang, S-C, Henze, E., Selin, C.E., and Scheblert, H.R. Positron tomography with deoxyglucose for estimating local myocardial glucose metabolism. *J. Nucl. Med.* 23:577, 1982.

148. Wall, E.E., Hollander, W. den, Westera, G., Majid, P.A., and Roos, J.P. Dynamic myocardial scintigraphy with I-123 labeled free fatty acids in patients with myocardial infarction. *Eur. J. Nucl. Med.* 6:383, 1981a.

149. Wall, E.E., Heidendal, G.A.K., Hollander, W. den, Westera G., and Roos, J.P. Metabolic myocardial imaging with I-123 labeled hetadecanoic acid in patients with angina pectoris. *Eur. J. Nucl. Med.* 6:391, 1981c.

150. Hoeck, A., Freundlieb, C., Vyska, K., Loesse, B., Erbel, R., and Feinendegen, L.E. Myocardial imaging and metabolic studies with [17-I-123] idoheptadecanoic acid in patients with idiopathic congestive cardiomyopathy. *J. Nucl. Med.* 24:22, 1983.

151. Wall, E.E., Westera, G., Hollander, W. den, Visser, F.C., Roos, J.P., and Heidendal, G.A.K. The effect of pindolol on myocardial uptake of free fatty acids in the dog. *Curr. Ther. Res.* 33:591, 1983.

152. Visser, F.C., Eenige, J. van, Wall, E.E., and Roos, J.P. The mechanism of the elimination rate of 123I-heptadecanoic acid from the myocardium. *J. Am. Coll. Cardiol.* 3:476, 1984 (abstract).

153. Sheehan, F.H., Mathey, D.G., Schofer, J., Krebber, H-J, and Dodge, H.T. Effect of interventions in salvaging left ventricular function in acute myocardial infarction: A study of intracoronary streptokinase. *Am. J. Cardiol.* 52:431, 1983.

# 9. CARDIAC CATHETERIZATION AND CORONARY ARTERIOGRAPHY

Peter F. Cohn

Sheldon Goldberg

The first recognized catheterization procedure was performed 50 years ago in Germany, when Werner Forssmann, using fluoroscopy to guide him, advanced a catheter through his own left antecubital vein and into his right atrium [1]. Although Forssmann did not actively pursue his remarkable achievements, others did. Particularly noteworthy are the physiologic investigations of the right heart in the 1940s by Cournand et al. [2] and by Dexter et al. [3]. In 1950, Zimmerman and colleagues [4] helped popularize retrograde left heart catheterization; this procedure was greatly advanced by the development of a percutaneous technique for introducing catheters into the vascular system by Seldinger in 1953 [5]. Early attempts at visualization of the coronary arteries in humans were nonselective: a bolus of radiopaque contrast material was injected into the ascending aorta just above the aortic valve [6]. A variety of such nonselective methods were employed in the 1950s and early 1960s [7], but these were rapidly replaced by the selective technique developed by Sones et al. [8]. Subsequently, Ricketts and Abrams [9], Wilson and co-workers [10], and Judkins [11] modified the percutaneous technique for this purpose. Today, several methods are available for selectively visualizing the coronary arteries.

Although the standard clinical procedures described in chapter 4 (history, physical examination, electrocardiography, and routine laboratory tests) and the special noninvasive procedures described in chapters 5 through 8 (multistage exercise tests, echocardiograms, and myocardial perfusion studies) all have an important place in the evaluation of patients with known or suspected coronary artery disease, there is little disagreement that it is the cardiac catheterization procedure—and particularly the selective coronary arteriogram—that is the "gold standard." With this procedure, the in vivo morphologic characteristics of the coronary arteries can be demonstrated, and there is a reasonable degree of accuracy when compared to postmortem studies [12, 13]. Narrowing of the large coronary arteries by as little as 20 percent can be appreciated, and critical stenosis of 75 percent or more of the cross-sectional area is almost always accurately shown. There are obviously gray zones in which the significance of a given lesion is in question, but when the arteriogram is combined with hemodynamic measurements and left ventriculography, a comprehensive anatomic and physiologic profile can often be obtained for the individual who is being evaluated for coronary artery disease.

This chapter will discuss the indications and contraindications for "diagnostic" cardiac catheterization and coronary arteriography *in patients suspected of having coronary artery disease,* the various physiologic and angiographic methods for evaluating patients in the catheterization laboratory, and the complications of the procedure. The newer "therapeutic" types of cardiac catheterization (angioplasty and thrombolytic therapy administered via the intracoronary route) will also be considered. *Areas of controversy* include the diagnostic and therapeutic indications themselves, the composition of the catheterization team, the use of Sones' versus Judkins' technique, the role of angled projections, the diagnostic potential of digital subtraction ventriculography versus standard ventriculography, and the advantages of out-patient coronary arteriography.

## Indications for "Diagnostic" Cardiac Catheterization

There is a popular misconception that cardiac catheterization and coronary arteriography are performed only as prelude to coronary artery bypass surgery. While some physicians may espouse this policy, most do not accept it, and the rationale for the procedure encompasses a wide range of categories [14, 15]. In some instances, the nature of the patient's chest pain syndrome may suggest coronary artery disease, but more precise data are needed because of uncertainties about the cause of the syndrome. Alternatively, the patient may be asymptomatic but may have a markedly abnormal electrocardiogram (ECG) at rest or after exercise. The patient, his physician, his employer, or his insurance company may be concerned about the possibility of silent coronary artery disease. In patients in whom the diagnosis is more certain but the appropriate therapeutic approach must be determined, cardiac catheterization and coronary arteriography may be useful in defining the sites of obstruction within the coronary tree, the patency of vein grafts, the severity of a concomitant stenotic or regurgitant valvular lesion, the size and operability of a ventricular aneurysm, and so on.

Not all physicians agree on the indications for cardiac catheterization and coronary arteriography; furthermore, any individual physician's list of indications is constantly changing. With this in mind, rather than centering this discussion of the various points of view on broad indications, we will use a more specific approach based on whether or not the patient's predominant symptom is *chest pain*. Listed below are indications for cardiac catheterization and coronary arteriography in patients being evaluated for possible coronary artery disease:

A. Patients in whom chest pain is the predominant symptom
  1. Chronic chest pain
     a. Severe angina pectoris
     b. Angina that is not severe
     c. Atypical chest pain
  2. Unstable angina pectoris
  3. Prinzmetal's angina
  4. Preoperative evaluation of valvular heart disease
  5. Evaluation of recurrent angina following bypass surgery
  6. Suspected anomalies of the coronary circulation
B. Patients in whom chest pain is absent or is not the predominant symptom
  1. Asymptomatic individuals with abnormal ECGs
  2. Asymptomatic individuals with normal ECGs
  3. Persistent heart failure or shock following a myocardial infarction
  4. Unexplained ventricular failure as the predominant symptom
  5. Preoperative evaluation of valvular heart disease
  6. Intractable ventricular arrhythmias or history of cardiac arrest not associated with recent myocardial infarction
  7. Suspected congenital anomalies of the coronary circulation
  8. Evaluation of the coronary circulation following bypass surgery.

WHEN CHEST PAIN IS THE PREDOMINANT SYMPTOM

*Chronic Chest Pain.*

SEVERE ANGINA PECTORIS. This type of patient is typified by the middle-aged male with multiple risk factors who has had classic, severe angina pectoris for several years. In spite of an aggressive medical approach—including the administration of nitroglycerin and long-acting nitrates, effective β-adrenergic blockade, and the use of calcium antagonists—the patient still experiences symptoms that make his life-style unacceptable to him. Obviously, the definition of "unacceptable life-style" is not a rigid one; a 45-year-old carpenter, for example, may have a different definition from that of a 65-year-old retired executive. In the former situation, catheterization *is* a prelude to surgery or angioplasty since the effectiveness of direct revascularization procedures in improving *symptoms* is well established (see chapters 12 and 14).

Thus, patients experiencing angina pectoris that does not respond adequately to a maximal medical program are commonly recommended for cardiac catheterization and selective coronary arteriography. The catheterization should be planned to assess ventricular function, as well as precisely define the site and severity of the obstructive lesions in the coronary arterial tree. Using the information derived from the catheterization, patients can be divided into low-risk and high-risk groups on the basis of left ventricular function and the caliber of the distal vessels.

ANGINA PECTORIS THAT IS NOT SEVERE. In contrast to the group of patients with severe angina (in whom the objective of the catheterization is to define suitability for operation to obtain symptomatic relief), catheterization in these patients may be either for prognostic reasons or for assessing possible surgery or angioplasty.

As discussed in chapter 12, the demonstration of either no disease or only single-vessel disease presages a better prognosis than does that of more advanced disease. In a certain number of patients, however, left main stem stenosis will be found. This lesion, which most often coexists with severe proximal disease in the rest of the coronary tree, is unusually lethal; in three multicenter studies from the United States and Europe, the average yearly mortality in nonoperated patients averaged 10 percent [16].

Many physicians use the exercise test as an important screening tool in this kind of patient in order to detect critical left main arterial stenosis or a left main "equivalent" (i.e., severe narrowing of both the proximal left anterior descending and the circumflex trunks). On the ECG, ST depression of 2 mm or more, especially at a moderate level of exercise and when combined with hypotension, is very suggestive of left main artery disease or its "equivalent" in symptomatic patients [17]. It is on the basis of this kind of exercise response that patients with less that severe angina are often recommended for coronary arteriography. In those who turn out to have left main coronary artery lesions, surgery may be recommended at some centers, regardless of the degree of angina. When triple-vessel or double-vessel disease is found, the decision is less clear (again, see chapters 12 and 14).

What of those patients with less than severe angina who do not have very markedly positive exercise tests? The proponents of early catheterization in such patients base their arguments on the previously cited importance of the prognostic data obtained from catheterization, even while realizing that there is less likelihood of finding severe disease in this type of patient. Opponents argue that the reduced likelihood of severe disease does not warrant subjecting the patient to an invasive procedure with known risks. Not surprisingly, therefore, in this group of patients with chronic but not severe angina there is considerable controversy regarding the need for cardiac catherterization and coronary arteriography.

ATYPICAL CHEST PAIN. Among the groups of patients with both severe and less than severe angina pectoris, discussed in the previous sections (as well as in the group with unstable angina to be discussed in the subsequent section) is a small subset of patients with normal coronary arteriograms. By contrast, although some patients with coronary artery disease may have less than classical angina, *it is probably more common for patients with atypical presentations to have normal coronary arteriograms.* It is sometimes difficult to identify such patients by standard clinical procedures, because (as discussed in chapter 4) some of these patients can have ECG abnormalities that are indistinguishable from those of patients with documented coronary disease and because exercise testing may also yield equivocal results. The lives of such patients are punctuated by frequent visits to emergency rooms and admissions to intensive care units. The response to medical management is variable. It is important to identify this type of patient, because the prognosis is good and reassurance is warranted [18]. A normal coronary arteriogram provides the physician and patient with invaluable information that may prevent unnecessary disruption of the patient's life-style and vocational opportunities.

Before recommending patients with atypical

chest pain for cardiac catheterization and coronary arteriography, every attempt should be made to treat their complaints fully. In many cases, however, there comes a time when after 3, 6, or 9 months of unsuccessful therapy, physicians may have increasing doubt that coronary artery disease is present in some patients who initially were thought to have the disease based on the noninvasive workup. On the other hand, there may be increasing concern that other patients initially thought not to have the disease might actually be on the way to a myocardial infarction.

Both the threshold of decision for each physician and the number of patients with this kind of problem that each physician will encounter will obviously vary. Nonetheless, there is general consensus that such patients are suitable candidates for catheterization if it will help their management, either medically or psychologically, although the approach to a given patient and circumstance may vary from physician to physician.

*Unstable Angina Pectoris.* Unstable angina pectoris is discussed in detail in chapter 12. This classification includes patients with stable angina and a recent spontaneous increase in severity, patients with rest angina, as well as patients with angina of recent onset with progressive increase in severity. In many instances, chest pain episodes are often accompanied by marked ST-T wave changes, pallor, nausea, and diaphoresis, and there is poor response to nitrate administration. At present, there is no evidence that *routinely* treating unstable angina as an acute surgical emergency provides any real benefits. However, angiography in such patients is often uneventful even if they are in the evolutionary phase of an acute myocardial infarction.

A common approach to managing such patients is to treat the patient with aggressive medical management and to study the patient with cardiac catheterization on an urgent basis; the timing of the procedure varies from hospital to hospital. In those who are refractory to medical management (e.g., a patient who continues to have severe pain in spite of adequate doses of nitrates, beta-blockers, and calcium antagonists), intravenous nitroglycerin or the intra-aortic balloon counterpulsation device can be employed, followed by angiography and emergency surgery. This has reduced the risk of catheterization in these patients at many institutions to levels usually observed for stable angina. It should be noted that some institutions are able to study most patients with unstable angina at no apparent risk *without* the need for the balloon device.

There is general agreement that patients with unstable angina are suitable candidates for cardiac catheterization and coronary arteriography. This consensus is most evident in the "increasing severity" and "rest pain" categories of unstable angina, but less evident in the "new-onset" category.

*Prinzmetal's Angina.* This special form of angina pectoris occurs at rest and is associated with striking ECG changes, especially transient ST elevations. This syndrome can also be associated with a high incidence of early myocardial infarction, ventricular arrhythmias, and sudden death. Catheterization is primarily indicated in such patients to differentiate anatomic patterns, since patients with Prinzmetal's angina may have coronary arterial spasm *with or without* fixed obstructive disease. If the vessels appear normal and no spontaneous spasm is demonstrated, then a provocative maneuver, such as the use of ergonovine to stimulate spasm, may be utilized to confirm the diagnosis [19]. Techniques for this type of testing are discussed later in the chapter. The recognition of this form of Prinzmetal's angina has important therapeutic implications because the prognosis may be somewhat better than in coronary atherosclerosis [20]. If a patient has spasm without fixed lesions, surgery is not recommended. There is a general agreement that cardiac catheterization and coronary arteriography are indicated with this clinical syndrome.

*Preoperative Evaluation of Valvular Heart Disease.* In patients with clinically severe valvular heart disease and angina pectoris in whom valvular surgery is contemplated, there is a consensus that coronary arteriography is indicated preoperatively. In some types of valvular heart disease (particularly aortic stenosis and regurgitation), angina may be a consequence of either the valvular disease, the coronary disease, or both. The ECG often is not helpful, showing left ventricular hypertrophy and nonspecific ST-T wave abnormalities. Changes in the exercise ECG are difficult to interpret, and coronary arteriography affords the only means to assess the cause of the anginal syndrome in such patients. In patients with mitral valve disease, angina is much more likely to be due to concomitant coronary artery disease. If obstructive lesions are demonstrated on the coronary arteriogram, bypass surgery is usually performed in conjunction with valvular surgery.

Coronary artery disease may be the cause of anginal pain in valvular heart disease in two other situations: the mitral valve prolapse (Barlow's) syndrome and idiopathic hypertrophic subaortic stenosis (the latter, of course, is not strictly a "valvular" disorder). Such patients do not usually require surgical correction of the valvular abnormality, but when angina is present the possibility of coronary artery disease must be evaluated. In some circumstances (i.e., severe chest pain), it is important to know the state of the coronary circulation *regardless* of the severity of the valvular condition.

Although most catheterization laboratories perform the entire study (including hemodynamic and angiographic evaluation) at one sitting, it is important to stress that if the patient with valvular heart disease seems unduly uncomfortable or fatigued or if the procedure has been unusually prolonged, then a separate study on a different day to assess the coronary arteries is justified.

*Evaluation of the Patient with Recurrent Angina Following Bypass Surgery.* Patients who have undergone revascularization procedures and who have recurrent severe angina may have symptoms due to any of the following causes: (1) incomplete revascularization; that is, the number of grafts placed was less than the number of vessels with severe stenosis; (2) graft closure; or (3) progression of disease in the native circulation distal to a graft or in a nonoperated vessel. Coronary arteriography offers the best way of determining the explanation for such symptoms, and it serves as a basis for recommending appropriate therapy.

*Suspected Anomalies of the Coronary Circulation.* Chest pain may be the predominant symptom in coronary anomalies, especially with respect to the origin of the left coronary artery from the pulmonary artery. This disorder can be suspected clinically when the patient is under 40 years of age, has a history of prior myocardial infarction, and has a continuous audible murmur. When the continuous murmur is not present, the patient may be diagnosed as having premature coronary artery disease, and the true nature of the disorder will be realized only at catheterization. The reader is referred to chapter 18 for a more complete discussion of congenital anomalies.

WHEN CHEST PAIN IS ABSENT OR IS NOT THE PREDOMINANT SYMPTOM

*Asymptomatic Individuals with Abnormal ECGs.* Individuals with abnormalities of their resting ECGs (such as conduction disturbances, arrhythmias, and QRS or T-wave abnormalities) may be recommended for cardiac catheterization and coronary arteriography for a variety of reasons. Insurance companies will not grant some of these individuals policies without objective evidence that they are free of disease. Persons in certain occupations that involve public safety (e.g., airline pilots, bus drivers, and the like) may require similar verification. In many instances, the need for the catheterization procedure can be greatly minimized or even eliminated if a battery of low-risk, noninvasive studies (such as echocardiography, Holter monitoring, radioisotope perfusion studies, and multistage exercise tests) can be performed when indicated and are normal. If one or more of these studies are abnormal, however, cardiac catheterization may become necessary.

A markedly abnormal exercise test, with 2 mm or more ST segment depression or malignant arrhythmias in the first or second stage, is one such result that, to many physicians, justifies catheterization. This view is based on the known correlation between strikingly positive tests and multivessel coronary disease in symptomatic subjects, as well as on data in small numbers of asymptomatic subjects [21]. Because the diagnostic value of a less positive exercise test is uncertain in asymptomatic individuals, however, a stronger case can be made for recommending cardiac catheterization and coronary arteriography if one or more coronary risk factors are also present.

Patients with a *prior myocardial infarction,* but without symptoms at present and with a negative exercise test, may occasionally be referred for coronary arteriography to ascertain the state of their coronary anatomy for prognostic purposes. A small number will have no coronary artery disease or will have disease limited to a single vessel system. Many cardiologists would be reluctant to study such patients unless other factors were present: young age (less than 45), several coronary risk factors, undue concern by the patient or family, and so on. If the exercise test is positive—even in the absence of symptoms—the "need to know" is stronger, since substantial portions of viable myocardium may be in jeopardy because of a high-grade coronary lesion.

To summarize, while the indications for cardiac catheterization are becoming more liberal in asymptomatic patients with abnormal ECGs, the decision still depends in large part on the needs of the particular patient and the physician's approach to the problem.

*Asymptomatic Individuals with Normal ECGs.* Cardiac catheterization and coronary arteriography are occasionally performed in young adults with familial hyperlipidemia, but only as part of specific research protocols.

*Persistent Heart Failure or Shock Following a Myocardial Infarction.* In patients who sustain rupture of the interventricular septum or rupture of a papillary muscle following a myocardial infarction, catheterization and angiography should be considered as soon as it is possible to do so. This often requires therapy with appropriate drugs, fluid repletion, and intra-aortic balloon counterpulsation. In patients in shock, however, immediate surgery may be indicated (chapters 13 and 14).

Patients suspected of having ventricular aneurysm with chronic and intractable failure are also prime candidates for cardiac catheterization procedures. Left ventriculography (preferably biplane) can accurately delineate the extent of the aneurysm and help in the assessment of con-

tractility in the nonaneurysmal portions of the ventricle. Coronary arteriography may reveal that a viable area of myocardium is served by a severely compromised coronary artery so that, in addition to aneurysmectomy, coronary artery bypass grafting should be considered.

*Unexplained Ventricular Failure as the Predominant Symptom.* Cardiac catheterization and coronary arteriography should be used to distinguish ischemic cardiomyopathy due to coronary disease from valvular, pericardial, congenital, or other primary myocardial diseases. Appropriate therapy depends upon accurate diagnosis. Since surgical treatment of all but primary myocardial disease (short of cardiac transplantation) is possible, it is important to detect these other treatable disorders before irreparable myocardial damage results. Sometimes, standard clinical procedures combined with low-risk, noninvasive tests (such as M-mode or two-dimensional echocardiography and radionuclide studies to detect shunts, abnormal ventricular function, or both) may provide enough data. In other cases, the results of such procedures are equivocal, and cardiac catheterization is then recommended.

*Preoperative Evaluation of Patients with Valvular Heart Disease.* In patients in whom the valvular lesion is severe enough to warrant heart surgery, many physicians feel coronary arteriography should be routinely performed even if chest pain is *not* a major symptom. In some cases, significant coronary artery disease will be found —the percentage varies from one series to another, as the literature on aortic valve disease attests [22, 23]—and in such circumstances, "prophylactic" myocardial revascularization may be recommended to assist the patient through the perioperative period. Whether it helps is unclear, but if bypass surgery can be performed without adding appreciable risk to the valvular surgery, a reasonable case can be made for such an approach.

*Intractable Ventricular Arrhythmias or History of Resuscitation from Cardiac Arrest.* Occasionally, a patient is encountered in whom the major or only manifestation of myocardial ischemia is malignant ventricular arrhythmias that are unresponsive to therapy with antiarrhythmic agents. In this small group, cardiac catheterization and coronary arteriography are recommended if all attempts at medical management fail, since there are increasing numbers of surgical procedures reported that suggest ventricular aneurysm resection being effective in abolishing the arrhythmia. These operations are discussed in chapter 15, as are the electrophysiological testing procedures that are often used to localize the involved area in the ventricle.

Patients resuscitated from cardiac arrest that was not associated with recent myocardial infarction have a high recurrence rate of ventricular fibrillation, and a substantial proportion have coronary arterial anatomy that is suitable for bypass surgery. Because of the dire prognosis, cardiac catheterization and coronary arteriography are justifiable in such patients. Again, electrophysiological testing is often recommended as well.

*Suspected Congenital Anomalies of the Coronary Circulation.* In certain anomalies of the coronary circulation, heart failure, rather than angina, is the predominant symptom. In a young adult with a continuous murmur, for example, a congenital coronary arteriovenous fistula may be suspected and subsequently demonstrated at catheterization. The reader is again referred to chapter 18 for more detailed discussion.

*Evaluation of the Coronary Circulation Following Bypass Surgery.* Following bypass surgery, patients may be angina-free because of perioperative infarctions (although some may develop heart failure), while others who are completely asymptomatic may be subsequently shown to have closed grafts. For these reasons, periodic recatheterization for angina-free patients with bypass grafts is often recommended. In some institutions, the patients are admitted under a special research protocol, since the knowledge derived from the study is probably of more benefit to medical science than it is in influencing therapy in asymptomatic patients.

CONTRAINDICATIONS
Cardiac catheterization and coronary arteriography are considered to be contraindicated if they cannot be performed by an adequately trained team of physicians and support personnel in a well-equipped laboratory with a large caseload and a good safety record, as defined by appropriate agencies [24]. Consistently excellent studies are required to spare the patient the double jeopardy of reexaminations or, even worse, an inaccurate diagnosis.

Medical contraindications include fever, mental incompetence (this may require legal advice in certain situations if the family is in favor of the procedure), and overt or latent cardiac electrical instability (latent situations include digitalis toxicity or hypokalemia and other electrolyte-pH disturbances). Bleeding diatheses may present particular problems; when there is a potential problem due to warfarin or heparin therapy, they can be temporarily reversed. A history of previous reaction to the contrast agent may suggest pretreatment with antihistamines and steroids for 3 days if the procedures are essential. With severe congestive heart failure, excessive contrast agent can precipitate acute pulmonary edema, and the procedure must be tailored to yield maximal information at minimal risk. The same is true in patients who are being maintained by renal dialysis. *Elective* cardiac catheterization procedures are usually not performed within 3 to 6 weeks of a myocardial infarction, although investigational and clinical studies have been done safely earlier in the postinfarction period. Of course, "therapeutic" catheterization with antithrombolytic agents is performed within hours of the event, as discussed later in the chapter.

Finally, there is the problem of the patient suffering from a noncardiac disorder that is either clearly terminal or not correctable and so severely impairs another organ system (e.g., the liver, lungs, or brain) that there is little chance that cardiac surgery would be offered in any event. In such circumstances, the risk of the catheterization procedure will outweigh any information obtained from it. This situation is confronted most frequently in the setting of unstable angina, where the pros and cons of revascularization surgery must be evaluated *individually.* It should be emphasized that in patients in whom the outlook is otherwise reasonable for the short term (e.g., those with metastatic but treatable malignancies), cardiac catheterization and cardiac surgery should not be automatically excluded from such considerations because the *quality of life* of the patient may be significantly improved.

## Techniques of Diagnostic Cardiac Catheterization

To perform cardiac catheterization and coronary arteriography in a safe and successful manner, an experienced, cohesive team is required. In most centers, the physicians are only cardiologists; in some hospitals, the cardiologists perform hemodynamic measurements at one sitting, and radiologists perform angiographic procedures on another day. As recommended by the latest report of the Inter-society Commission for Heart Disease Resources [24], a cardiac catheterization team should ideally consist of (1) at least one physician skilled in the performance of coronary arteriography and all aspects of catheterization, with the optimal arrangement being one with *both* a cardiologist and radiologist on the team; (2) radiologic and recording technicians; and (3) experienced nursing personnel. In addition, safe, reliable equipment for blood-pressure and ECG monitoring should be used, as well as appropriate camera and image-intensification equipment. These facilities are described in detail in the above-mentioned report of the Inter-society Commission.

RECOMMENDED GENERAL PRINCIPLES
The procedure should be explained to the patient by the cardiac catheterization team on the day before it takes place. Hopefully, the patient's physician will have already done this as well. Written consent must be obtained, and the patient should be frankly advised as to the relative risks and benefits of the proposed study. Less educated patients require more time to have the procedure explained [25]. Whenever possible, the patient's family should also be informed of the possible risks in the hospital where the procedure will be done. Table 9–1 describes the average risks nationwide, but it is the *specific* catheterization laboratory's complication rate that is of most importance to the patient.

*Patients should never be coerced into undergoing this uncomfortable and potentially dangerous procedure.* Specific guidelines are as follows:

1. The patient should be fasting but not dehydrated.

2. Oral premedication with sedatives (usually antihistamines such as diphenhydramine, 50 mg), tranquilizers (e.g., diazepam, 5 to 10 mg), or both may be helpful 30 to 60 minutes prior to the procedure. Antibiotics need not be routinely administered prophylactically, although in patients with valvular or congenital heart diseases, some laboratories prefer to do so. (The use of atropine and nitroglycerin will be commented on during the discussion of specific coronary arteriographic procedures.) Unless the patient requires digitalis for control of ventricular rate when atrial fibrillation is present, the morning dose can be omitted. Potent diuretics should similarly be omitted. Nitrates should be continued if the patient is having angina while in the hospital. Beta-blockers and calcium antagonists may also be continued in such circumstances, but if withheld, they should immediately be restarted after the procedure.

3. All patients should have an intravenous line established *before* the start of the procedure.

4. There should be ECG monitoring, and pressure monitoring via an intra-arterial catheter. The ventriculographic and coronary catheter is attached to a manifold system that allows for (1) continuous pressure monitoring through the coronary or ventricular catheter, (2) filling with contrast medium for injection, and (3) flushing of the catheter with a heparinized saline solution.

5. Before each study, a protocol should be posted in the laboratory so that the information sought in a particular study is understood by all participants. One recommended order of procedure is to obtain physiologic data before any contrast agent is used. Ventriculography is performed next and *prior* to coronary arteriography, since all contrast agents have a direct myocardial depressant effect and prior multiple coronary injections can "artifactually" depress left ventricular function. An alternative order for the procedure is to obtain the *most* critical information first, namely, the coronary arteriogram. This alternative is especially preferred in severely ill patients.

TABLE 9–1. Complications of coronary arteriography

| Complication | Incidence (No. patients = 89,079) | | |
|---|---|---|---|
| | Overall (%) | Brachial (%) | Femoral (%) |
| Death | 0.14 | 0.12 | 0.16 |
| Myocardial infarction | 0.18 | 0.15 | 0.20 |
| Ventricular fibrillation | 0.76 | 0.70 | 0.82 |
| Thrombosis | 0.67 | 1.13 | 0.20 |
| Hemorrhage | 0.09 | 0.05 | 0.14 |
| Pseudoaneurysm | 0.04 | 0.04 | 0.05 |
| Cerebral embolus | 0.09 | 0.08 | 0.09 |
| Contrast reaction | 1.08 | 1.17 | 1.00 |

Adapted from Adams, D.F. and Abrams, H.L. *Circulation* 52 (Suppl. 4):27, 1975.

6. Systemic heparinization is recommended with both Sones's and Judkins's techniques (5,-000 units IV).

7. The coronary arteries are visualized in multiple views. For the left coronary artery, the left anterior oblique, anteroposterior, and right anterior oblique views should be used routinely. If doubt exists concerning the left anterior descending coronary artery, a left lateral projection is often helpful. The proximal trunks of the left circumflex and left anterior descending arteries are nicely separated using hemiaxial views with a left anterior oblique rotation and cranial-caudal angulation [26, 27]. Figure 9–1 displays examples of some of these projections when C- or U-arms are not available. For the right coronary artery, the right anterior oblique and left anterior oblique views usually suffice.

8. Specific factors related to the contrast agent are worthy of special mention. The use of meglumine diatrizoate has markedly reduced the frequency of asystole and ventricular fibrillation, but untoward effects of injection of contrast medium into the coronary tree still occur, such as hypotension, bradycardia, and T-wave changes on the ECG. These are generally transient. Usually, injection of the right coronary artery produces T-wave inversions in lead II, while left coronary injection produces T-wave peaking. *Before* the study, the patient must be instructed how to cough deeply a few times when requested. The catheterization team always waits for the ECG changes and hypotension to resolve before proceeding with the next injection. ECG changes are physiologic and do not indicate myocardial hypoxia. The amount varies of contrast agent necessary to visualize adequately the coronary arteries; in general, the rapid injection of 7 or 8 ml will allow visualization of the left coronary artery, while 3 to 5 ml will allow visualization of the right. The person injecting the solutions through the manifold should watch the television monitor during the injection required.

9. Postcatheterization care includes vessel repair and application of dressings and seeing the patient several hours later for signs of bleeding, loss of peripheral pulses, inadequate fluid intake, and so forth.

PHYSIOLOGIC MEASUREMENTS

Physiologic measurements are most accurate when performed prior to any contrast studies, although in most patients the effects of contrast agents are transient. Any of the standard catheters (e.g., the NIH, Eppendorf, or Lehman) may be inserted via the brachial artery, or a percutaneous "pigtail" may be inserted via the femoral artery. Resting left ventricular end-diastolic pressure is routinely obtained; its normal value is considered to be 12 mmHg or less in most laboratories and less than 15 mmHg in others. Right heart catheterization is often performed, as well. The normal value for right atrial mean pressure is usually considered to be 5 mmHg or less; for right ventricular end-diastolic pressure, 7 mmHg or less; for mean pulmonary artery pressure, 20 mmHg or less; and for mean pulmonary capillary wedge pressure, 10 mmHg or less. The values may vary slightly from laboratory to laboratory. Systemic arteriovenous oxygen differences are obtained by simultaneously

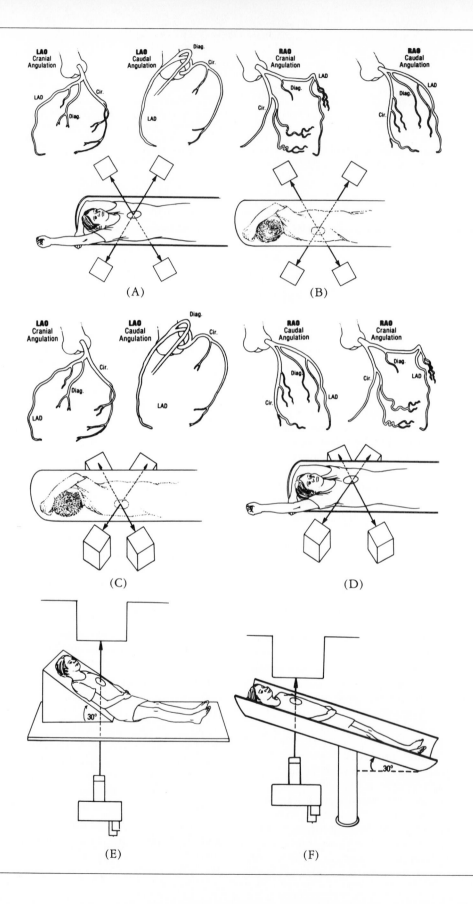

sampling from a peripheral artery and a pulmonary artery. When these data are combined with those for oxygen consumption—measured directly or obtained from tables based on linear regression equations [28]—a "forward" cardiac output (and index) is obtained. This is normally 3.0 liter/min/m² or greater, although some laboratories use 2.8 or even 2.5 liter/min/m² as the lower limit of the normal range because of the varying effects of the premedications administered.

The additional data gained from right heart catheterization can be particularly useful in patients with symptoms of congestive heart failure. In addition, complete right and left heart catheterizations in such patients facilitate testing of potentially beneficial pharmacologic agents (such as preload- and afterload-reducing drugs). Before-and-after measurements of pressure and output aid in the selection of those agents that have the most potential for inducing clinical improvement in individual patients, based on the salutary hemodynamic effects observed during the catheterization procedure.

If more sophisticated measurements are to be obtained (isovolumic indices, ventricular function curves during pacing, and the like), they should probably be performed at this point rather than after the angiographic procedures (with the exception of simultaneous pressure-volume determinations). For an excellent discussion of catheterization laboratory measurement of myocardial muscle mechanics, the reader is referred to the review by Karliner and associates [29].

Other physiologic studies (see below) may have to be performed *after* the angiographic procedures because of questions raised about the angiographic findings. Thus, in patients in whom there is a questionable relation between symptoms and coronary anatomy, additional objective measurements to assess the presence of myocardial ischemia are valuable. In the case of a patient, for example, in whom the coronary arteriogram shows a lesion of questionable importance in the left anterior descending artery (i.e., 50 to 75 percent stenosis), atrial pacing at rapid rates may be employed with simultaneous determination of the arterial and coronary sinus lactate levels. A completely negative result (i.e., net lactate extraction with rapid pacing) would suggest that the lesion in question is not hemodynamically significant and would, therefore, deter one from operation.

In addition to metabolic studies, techniques measuring regional myocardial blood flow (when available) may provide useful complementary information in assessing the hemodynamic significance of coronary arterial lesions. In the catheterization laboratory, these include the intracoronary injection of xenon-133 or microspheres (see chapter 2).

LEFT VENTRICULOGRAPHY
Left ventriculography is a standard part of the evaluation of patients with suspected coronary disease, and as noted earlier, it is usually performed prior to coronary injection. After the ventriculographic catheter is placed into a "quiet" position in which the catheter does not evoke undue irritability (e.g., just beneath the mitral valve leaflets), the catheter is connected to a volume injector and is cleared with a small amount of contrast agent under fluoroscopic control. This maneuver ensures that the tip of the catheter is free in the ventricular cavity. If there is catheter entrapment, transient "stain-

FIGURE 9–1. Variety of projections available for performing coronary arteriography. (**A, B**) Techniques for cranial and caudal angulation using a fixed, vertical x-ray source in the left anterior oblique (LAO) and right anterior oblique (RAO) positions. (**C, D**) Techniques used when the fixed x-ray source is horizontal to the patient. Panel C shows the LAO position, and panel D, the RAO position. The patient must be rotated along his axis into the desired obliquity. The x-ray beam (depicted as an arrow pointing to cranial or caudal imaging systems, respectively) may originate in front of or behind the patient's chest. The diagrams of the coronary arteriograms (above the imaging systems) have been rotated into the conventional LAO and RAO viewing positions. (**E, F**) Techniques for cranial angulation projection, using angulation of the patient or table rather than the x-ray system. In panel E, the patient is elevated 30 degrees, and in panel F, the table is elevated. The x-ray source is beneath the table and the cine camera overhead, but this arrangement could also be reversed without changing the angulation. (From Sos, T.A. and Baltaxe, H.A. Cranial and caudial angulation for coronary angiography revisited. *Circulation* 56:119, 1977. Reproduced by permission of the American Heart Association, Inc.)

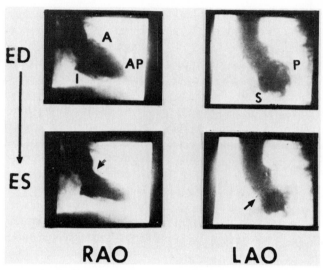

ing" of the myocardium can be readily detected.

When the operator is satisfied with the catheter position, a test injection is delivered at a preselected rate and time (e.g., 12 ml/sec for 1 second). The purpose of this test injection is to ensure adequate ventricular filling without causing undue irritability. Reducing the injection rate will often reduce ventricular irritability, but it may result in decreased opacification. If less than satisfactory results are obtained with this injection, then the catheter is repositioned. When the catheter position is satisfactory, the ventriculogram is performed in either the 30-degree right anterior oblique projection alone or combined with a 60-degree left anterior oblique projection (figure 9–2). (Posteroanterior and lateral projections are preferred in some laboratories for all studies, whereas other laboratories use them only for certain congenital lesions or idiopathic hypertrophic subaortic stenosis.) The standard program for left ventricular injection in our laboratory is to inject at a rate of 10 to 18 ml/sec for 3 to 4 seconds, depending on the left ventricular size, the resting left ventricular end-diastolic pressure, and ventricular irritability. Ventriculography is usually recorded on 35 mm cine film, but it can also be performed with either 16 mm cine film or large size x-ray film.

*Measurement of Left Ventricular Function.*
Ventriculography identifies aneurysms, ventricular clot, and mitral regurgitation in addition to providing quantitative data derived from the outlines of the silhouette in different places of

FIGURE 9–2. Cine left ventriculogram in simultaneous right anterior oblique (RAO) and left anterior oblique (LAO) projections. The RAO projections at end-diastole (ED) and end-systole (ES) are useful in demonstrating movement of the anterior (A), apical (AP), and inferior (I) surfaces of the left ventricle, while in the LAO projection movement of the septal (S) and posterolateral (P) surfaces can be visualized. In this patient, the sinuses of Valsalva above the aortic valve and the origin of the coronary arteries are also opacified with contrast agent. (Arrows depict the location of the aortic valve.)

contraction. Using the area-length method for determining ventricular volume, the following useful clinical measurements can be obtained: end-diastolic volume, end-systolic volume, and angiographic stroke volume (i.e., the difference between end-diastolic and end-systolic volumes). The ejection fraction can then be calculated as the ratio of stroke volume to end-diastolic volume. The area-length method assumes that the left ventricle can be represented by a prolate ellipsoid with a major diameter and two minor diameters.

As discussed at length by Rackley [30], there are formulas available (based on the initial studies of Dodge and associates) for both single-plane and biplane volume determinations. Thus,

$$V = \frac{4}{3\pi} \left(\frac{L}{2}\right) \left(\frac{D_a}{2}\right) \left(\frac{D_b}{2}\right),$$

where $V$ = volume (ml), $L$ = longest length measured directly (cm), and $D_a$ and $D_b$ =

minor axes (cm) in either the right or left anterior oblique projections (or, as some prefer, the anteroposterior and lateral projections). Probably the most widely used version is that employing *only* the right anterior oblique projection, for which the "short" single-plane formula can then be written:

$$V = 0.524D^2L.$$

In using this formula, one assumes that the length of the minor axis in the left anterior oblique projection is similar to that in the right anterior oblique (D); hence, the latter value is squared. (If the single plane used is the anteroposterior projection, then one again assumes that the minor axis in that projection is similar to that of the lateral projection, and the length of the anteroposterior minor axis is squared.) An illustration of the lengths L and D in the right anterior oblique projection is provided in figure 9–3. Because of the irregular contour of the left ventricle in many patients with coronary artery disease, a preferred method of calculating volume is to use a *calculated* minor axis rather than a directly measured one. Thus $D = 4A/\pi L$, where A is the area of the silhouette and L is again the length.

For all formulas, suitable correction factors for x-ray beam distortion and image magnification are necessary. Filming a grid of known dimensions at the level of the patient's heart can often provide the basis for such correction factors. In addition, regression equations should be established in each laboratory (based on casts of autopsied hearts) to correct the calculated volume to "true" volume [31].

Normal values for end-diastolic volume in adults range from 70 to 95ml/m², end-systolic volume ranges from 24 to 36ml/m², and the lower limit of the normal range for the ejection fraction is 0.50 to 0.60, depending on the series [30]. These values are greater than two standard deviations from the norm ($0.67\pm0.08$ in one series and $0.67\pm0.03$ in another).

Other useful measurements obtained from these silhouettes include the average rate of circumferential fiber shortening, or mean $V_{cf}$, and the mean normalized ejection rate [29]. Because wall thickness can be measured, left ventricular mass and stress can also be calculated [30].

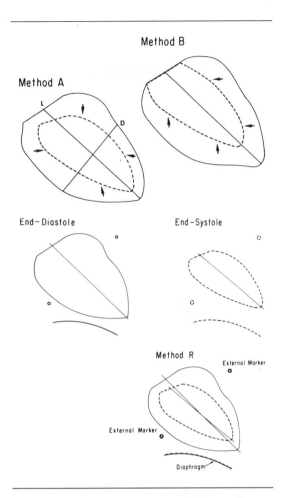

FIGURE 9–3. Graphic illustration of three reference methods for determining left ventricular volumes and wall motion disorders in the right anterior oblique projection. The end-diastolic silhouette is shown by a solid line, and the end-systolic silhouette, by interrupted lines. The long axis (L) and the minor axis that is perpendicular to it (D) are also depicted. Method A assumes all parts of the left ventricle contract toward the appropriate geometric center, and method B assumes the entire left ventricle contracts symmetrically toward the base of the heart. In method R (based on fixed reference points), the end-systolic silhouette is superimposed on the end-diastolic silhouette using two external markers (lead-impregnated letters taped to the image intensifier) and the diaphragm as reference points. The long axis is drawn in both silhouettes, and the angle subtended determines the degree of movement about the long axis. Although method R takes into account any possible movement of the patient, the diaphragm and the long axis (which the other methods do not), methods A and B nonetheless remain the most widely used techniques at the present time. (From Chaitman, B.R., et al. *Circulation* 48:1043, 1973. Reprinted by permission of the American Heart Association, Inc.)

Segmental contraction abnormalities (see chapter 2) may be quantitated with a variety of approaches: hemiaxial shortening, "area" ejection fractions, or percentage of asynergic segments [30]. Several methods for superimposing the ventricular silhouettes have been suggested and are illustrated in figure 9–3. These can be done by hand or by a semiautomated, computerized image-processing system [32].

The ventriculogram helps guide the coronary examination even when it only provides a qualitative judgment based on the tape playback. A ventriculogram showing inferior akinesis, for example, will alert the angiographer to the probability of severe right coronary artery disease. In general, there is excellent correlation between the presence of an akinetic segment and a totally occluded major coronary artery that is not visualized by collateralization. The subject of left ventricular dysfunction in coronary artery disease is discussed in detail in chapter 2.

*When to Perform Biplane Ventriculography.* Biplane projections are most useful in patients who have had prior myocardial infarctions, since these patients have a higher frequency of wall motion abnormalities than do patients without infarction [33]. When the diagnosis of a prior myocardial infarction is not certain, other clues (e.g., cardiomegaly, congestive heart failure, or even third heart sounds) alert the catheterization team to the likelihood of wall motion abnormalities and the need for the most comprehensive type of ventriculgraphic study. To limit the total amount of contrast agent and to avoid depression of function due to the first injection of contrast agent, the biplane study should be simultaneous rather than sequential. Most laboratories use the right and left anterior oblique views; others prefer anteroposterior and lateral views. Ventricular volumes are similar [34]. There is a good correlation between single-plane and biplane studies in the *absence* of asynergy, but not a good a correlation when asynergy is present [33]. Biplane ventriculography is also preferred (but not essential) when pressure-volume relations (e.g., compliance) are analyzed [30]. With the development of image intensifier–x-ray tube configurations with triaxial motion capability (C or U arms), there has been increasing interest in

obtaining axial or angulated views of the left ventriculogram instead of the conventional biplane projections. For example, the caudocranial left anterior oblique view has allowed more accurate assessment of the precise degree and extent of asynergy, left ventricular aneurysms, and septal defects [35].

*Intervention Ventriculography.* Intervention ventriculography (also known as two-stage or dynamic ventriculography) consists of two basic types. In the first type, the resting ventriculogram is normal, and the coronary arteriogram shows a lesion of questionable hemodynamic significance. Latent ventricular dysfunction may be uncovered by means of an intervention that can induce myocardial ischemia (e.g., atrial pacing or dynamic or static exercise). If myocardial ischemia ensues, the second "stress" ventriculogram will demonstrate new segmental wall motion abnormalities and often a decrease in overall left ventricular performance as well. If the ventriculogram remains normal despite the intervention, the coronary lesion is assumed to be nonsignificant. Complementary procedures, such as lactate determinations and myocardial perfusion studies, are also helpful in determining the significance of equivocal lesions (see Chapter 2).

The second type of intervention ventriculogram serves a different purpose: to test the contractile reserve (segmental or global) of apparently depressed myocardium. This cannot be assessed by routine ventriculography. A patient with equivocal evidence of a prior myocardial infarction, for example, may have a 95 percent stenosis of the left anterior descending coronary artery, and ventriculography may show anterior wall hypokinesis with an overall ejection fraction of 0.40. To determine whether this area is merely ischemic or totally fibrotic, intervention ventriculography may be performed using either inotropic stimulation (e.g., catecholamine infusion or postextrasystolic potentiation) or agents, such as nitroglycerin, that unload the ventricle.

In the former technique, 1-epinephrine is infused, a second ventriculogram is performed [36], and contraction patterns are compared (figure 9–4). Alternatively, a ventricular premature contraction is induced either by manipula-

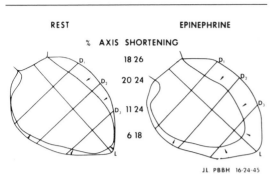

FIGURE 9–4. End-diastolic and end-systolic silhouettes of a patient with coronary artery disease, showing improvement in wall motion on administration of 1-epinephrine as determined by the increase in the percentage of axis shortening. $D_1$, $D_2$, and $D_3$ = minor axes, L = long axis. (From Horn, H.R. et al. Augmentation of left ventricular contraction pattern in coronary artery disease by an inotropic catecholamine: The epinephrine ventriculogram. *Circulation* 49:1063, 1974. Reprinted by permission of the American Heart Association, Inc.)

tion of a right heart catheter during left ventriculography or by use of an R-wave-triggered pacemaker, and the ejection fraction and contraction patterns in the postventricular premature contraction beat are compared with those of a normal beat [37] (see also chapter 2, figure 2–12).

In the latter technique, a second ventriculogram is performed several minutes after 0.3 or 0.4 mg of nitroglycerin is administered sublingually and asynergy is reversed [38] (see figure 2–13). A good correlation has been reported with both techniques between the reversal of asynergy using nitroglycerin and the return to normal contraction of the same myocardial segments after bypass surgery (38) (figure 2–12).

Each technique has advantages in demonstrating contractile reserve. Catecholamines and ventricular premature beats are true inotropic stimuli, and the latter require only a single ventriculogram. On the other hand, the ventricular premature contraction may not always be successfully induced. Nitroglycerin is an easily used drug whose actions are consistent, although the mechanism of action is not that of an inotropic stimulus. Therefore, either the inotropic agent or nitroglycerin technique is acceptable.

*Intravenous Digital Left Ventriculography.* Recent advances in computer technology have resulted in the ability to convert angiographic images directly into a digital format in real time. An image of insufficient resolution can be enhanced by the process of rapid digitization and subtraction of background. This has permitted the obtaining of high-quality ventriculography with either intravenous [39] or diluted intraventricular [40] injections of iodinated contrast material. The former technique eliminates the risks involved with direct left heart catheterization, while the latter technique reduces considerably the hemodynamic alterations seen with conventional intraventricular doses of iodinated contrast agents. Digital subtracting ventriculography can also be performed both at rest and after atrial pacing to assess segmental wall motion abnormalities [41]. These wall motion abnormalities can often be quantitated in a more precise manner than with conventional ventriculographic techniques. The diagnostic potential of this technique is obviously enormous. It has the ability to retain the contrast ventriculogram as the "gold standard" while reducing its risks (when contrast agent is injected intravenously) to nearly that of two-dimensional echocardiography or radioisotopic ventriculography.

## CORONARY ARTERIOGRAPHY

*Direct Brachial (Sones) Technique.* After direct exposure of the right brachial artery, a small arteriotomy is made and the Sones catheter is introduced into the artery. The catheter is made of woven Dacron; it is 100 cm long and 7 or 8 French in diameter, tapering to 5.5 French. There are two to four side holes and an end hole. The catheter is then connected to the manifold, and it is advanced from the brachial artery to the central aorta using both fluoroscopic and pressure control. If a tortuous subclavian artery is encountered, then maneuvers such as having the patient take a deep breath, shrug the shoulders, and turn the head to the left are tried while the catheter is advanced. The use of a guide wire is often helpful. The catheter should *never* be forced if it meets resistance, because dissection of the subclavian artery or central aorta may ensue. Pressure damping and lack of free blood return through the catheter should alert the operator to this possibility.

With the catheter in the central aorta, systemic heparin is administered along with 0.4 or 0.6 mg of atropine IV and 0.3 mg sublingual nitroglycerin—though some prefer to give nitroglycerin later [42]. With the patient in the left anterior oblique position, the catheter is advanced to the left sinus of Valsalva and a J-loop is made (figure 9–5A). By moving the catheter up and down with the loop, the left ostium is engaged. Having the patient take a deep breath is often helpful when one is engaging the left ostium. When this is done, the tip of the Sones catheter appears to be stationary. A test injection is made to ensure that the ostium has been properly engaged, and one then proceeds with arteriography in multiple views. If one has reason to suspect a critical stenosis of the left main coronary artery, then a forceful, nonselective injection into the left sinus of Valsalva is a useful maneuver. If pressure damping occurs while the catheter is in the coronary orifice, it should be immediately removed.

When the operator is satisfied that the left system has been adequately visualized, the catheter is removed from the left ostium while maintaining a gentle loop and applying clockwise torque. It is manipulated toward the right sinus of Valsalva until the right coronary artery is engaged (figure 9–5B). If damping occurs, the catheter is removed and the coronary ostium is again approached. Occasionally, selective catheterization of the conus artery occurs. This is often accompanied by pressure damping, and again, if damping occurs, the catheter should be removed from the orifice of the artery. Advantages of the Sones' approach are that the entire coronary examination is performed with one catheter, and although the Sones' technique is more difficult to master than the percutaneous approach, the skill is eventually acquired with sufficient supervised training. The technique is especially useful in patients with severe peripheral vascular disease, bleeding diatheses, or severe aortic regurgitation.

*Percutaneous Femoral (Judkins') Technique.*
This technique requires direct puncture of the femoral artery with a Seldinger needle; after vigorous blood return is demonstrated, a Teflon-coated guide wire is advanced. The needle is then removed, the guide wire is wiped with a wet sponge, a sheath is introduced and the wire removed; the "pigtail" catheter "loaded" with a J-wire is then advanced into the aorta. Systemic heparin is then administered. The catheter is connected to the manifold and is then advanced into the left ventricle.

After ventriculography is performed, the Judkins catheter is introduced over the guide wire. The catheters used in this technique are preformed to engage selectively either the left or the right coronary ostium. These catheters are 100 cm in length and may be either 7 French or 8 French in diameter, tapering to 5 French. There is an end hole and no side holes. Several different sizes are available. The number 4 is an average catheter; the 5, a large one; and 6, the largest one. These sizes do not reflect French size, but rather the distance between the primary and secondary curves for normal, slightly dilated, and dilated aortas, respectively. The left catheter is usually introduced first and is gently advanced around

(A)

(B)

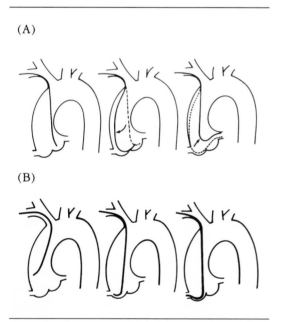

FIGURE 9–5. Selective catheterization (**A**) of the left coronary artery and (**B**) of the right coronary artery by Sones' technique. See text for description. (From Conti, C.R. Coronary arteriography. *Circulation* 55:-227, 1977. Reprinted by permission of the American Heart Association, Inc.)

the aortic arch so as not to "snap" into the left coronary ostium (figure 9–6A). The ease with which the Judkins' catheters engage the respective ostia is the chief hazard in their use. Proper care should be exercised in introducing the catheters into the coronary ostia. The preformed curve of the left catheter makes catheterization of the left ostium quite simple, requiring little manipulation. Again, damping of pressure through the catheter should be cause for immediate removal of the catheter from the ostium.

After completion of left coronary arteriography, the catheter is withdrawn to the level of the diaphragm, the guide wire is reintroduced, and the left coronary catheter is removed and replaced with the right Judkins' catheter. Some manipulation is required here. After the catheter is around the aortic arch, it is advanced to a level about 2 cm above the right sinus of Valsalva, and clockwise torque is then slowly applied until the tip of the catheter "dives" to the right and into the right ostium (figure 9–6B).

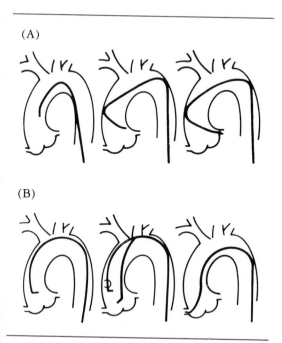

(A)

(B)

FIGURE 9–6. Selective catheterization (A) of the left coronary artery and (B) of the right coronary artery by Judkins' technique. See text for description. (From Conti, C.R. Coronary arteriography. Circulation 55:-227, 1977. Reprinted by permission of the American Heart Association, Inc.)

The advantage of this approach is its ease, but it cannot be used in the presence of severe iliofemoral disease.

*Other Techniques.* The Amplatz technique represents a modification of Judkins' technique, and it also uses a percutaneous femoral approach. The major difference is in the shape of the preformed catheter used. The Amplatz catheters are particularly useful for injecting saphenous vein bypass grafts.

Preformed catheters are also available for use by means of brachial cutdowns. Several groups have reported their experience with such catheters [43], and their results seem to indicate an advantage with the use of these catheters when the conventional Sones approach is unsuccessful and the catheterization team does not wish to employ the femoral route. The Amplatz preformed catheter is also well suited for coronary arteriography via the brachial approach, although it was not designed for that purpose. The flexible tip is useful in navigating tortuous arterial systems, and the preshaped curve facilitates engagement of the coronary ostia.

In occasional patients, neither the brachial nor the femoral approach can be used, and the rarely used transaxillary approach is sometimes helpful [44].

*Provocation of Spasm.* Coronary artery spasm may occasionally be detected on routine coronary arteriography in patients with Prinzmetal's angina if the patient experiences a typical anginal attack at a time when angiography can quickly be performed. Since this is fortuitous, the use of spasm-provoking agents, particularly the ergonovine preparations, has been proposed. Ergonovine testing is not without potentially serious complications, and certain precautions should therefore be taken. First, the procedure should be performed *after* the coronary artery is completely defined. Second, the initial ergonovine doses should probably be either 0.0125 mg or 0.025 mg, but in no instances more than 0.05 mg. Signs of progressive ischemia should be carefully sought even if the vessel narrowing appears to be "pharmacological," i.e., diffuse narrowing up to 30 percent of the vessel diameter. After a wait of 5 to 10 min-

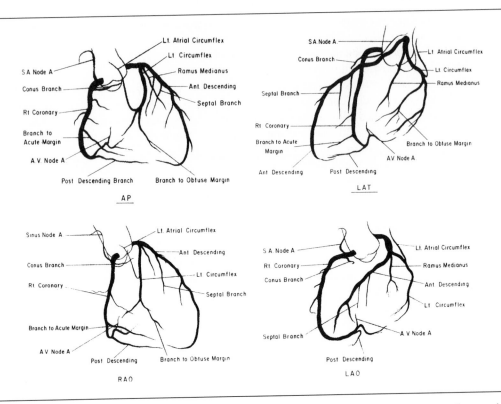

FIGURE 9–7. Normal coronary arteriogram in four standard views: anteroposterior (AP), lateral (LAT), right anterior oblique (RAO), and left anterior oblique (LAO). (From Abrams, H. and Adams, D.F. Reprinted, by permission of the *New England Journal of Medicine,* 281:1277, 1969.)

utes, a second dose may be given. Total doses should probably not exceed 0.2 mg. The spasm is usually relieved with sublingual or intravenous nitroglycerin (see figure 2–9), but intracoronary nitroglycerin must be available for refractory cases [45].

*Interpretation of the Study.* The experienced angiographer evaluates the coronary tree (figure 9–7) from several points of view: Is the anatomy normal? If irregularities are present in the lumen, how severe are they?

According to current convention and based on animal experiments, lesions involving less than 50 percent of the luminal diameter (corresponding to about 75 percent of the cross-sectional area) are generally considered not to be hemodynamically significant, those of 75 percent or more reduction in luminal diameter are considered significant, and the 50 to 75 percent range is a "gray zone." However, reliance on this visual "gold standard" has recently been challenged by White et al. [47] in a series of studies utilizing coronary flow velocity measurements obtained with a Doppler technique during coronary bypass surgery. They concluded that the physiologic effects of many coronary obstructions cannot be determined accurately by conventional angiographic techniques.

Examples of coronary artery stenoses are shown in figures 9–8, 9–9, and 9–10. Whenever possible, the stenosis is measured by comparing it to the vessel width before the stenosis. Because of the eccentric nature of atherosclerotic plaques, the greatest degree of stenosis in any projection is considered as most important. If there is any question of a possibly significant lesion in the proximal left coronary system, angled projections should be employed (see figure 9–1). The location of the lesion is important and should be recorded (i.e., proximal, midvessel, or distal).

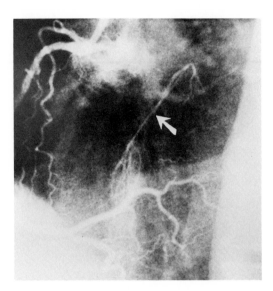

FIGURE 9-8. Angiogram of the right coronary artery (RCA) in the left anterior oblique view. The RCA has several areas of minimal luminal narrowing. There is extensive collateralization to a totally occluded left anterior descending artery (arrow) via septal branches of the posterior descending branch of the RCA.

For doing this schematically, coded reporting systems are available [48] (figure 9-11), as well as more flexible computer-assisted programs [49]. Collateralization should also be noted (examples are depicted in figures 9-8 and 9-9), as well as muscular "bridges." Normally, the coronary arteries lie free on the epicardial surface of the heart, and although the significance of these short muscular "bridges" across sections of the coronary arteries is unclear, ischemic symptoms have been attributed to them [50].

Some laboratories prefer to report their findings in terms of significant disease (usually more than 75 percent reduction of the luminal diameter) of one, two, or three vessels. In reality, these are vessel *systems*. The left anterior descending artery's diagonal branch may, for example, be severely diseased while the main left anterior descending is spared, but the system is still considered diseased. Other groups "score" the degree of stenosis and report their results as a numerical value (table 9-2); either technique is acceptable.

Misinterpretation may be due to an inadequate number of projections, pulsatile or superselective injections, ectopic origins of vessels, spasm, or total occlusion. Pepine and co-workers [51] have also pointed out that the *length* of the diseased segment, as well as of the reduced diameter, can alter the angiographer's assessment of the degree of narrowing at sites of

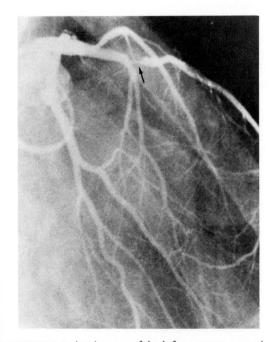

FIGURE 9-9. Angiogram of the left coronary artery in the right anterior oblique view. An almost total occlusion of the proximal left anterior descending artery is present (arrow). Extensive collateralization within the left coronary system is visible.

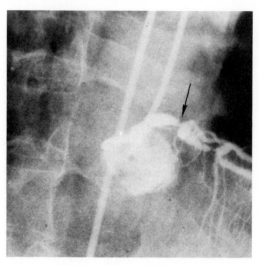

FIGURE 9–10. Angiogram of the left coronary artery (LCA) in a sit-up view. High-grade lesions of the main LCA (arrow) and left anterior descending (LAD) arteries are present (the circumflex artery is completely occluded). The lesion in the LAD was not clearly visualized on the standard projections.

experimentally fixed lumen reduction. The presence of additional narrowings in sequence can also alter the assessment.

Several studies have addressed themselves to problems of variability within and among observers [52–54], and it is recommended that the final report be the *consensus* of at least two experienced angiographers, preferably a cardiologist and a radiologist. At the present time, visual inspection of the arteriogram is still the standard method of assessment of the severity of coronary atherosclerosis. New methods have been developed, however, that combine the arteriogram with digital computation for more precise analysis of a diseased coronary arterial segment [55, 56]. What degree of future acceptance these

techniques will be accorded in most hospitals is uncertain.

Finally, there is the question raised earlier in the chapter regarding the accuracy of the coronary angiogram in relation to autopsied specimens or experimental arterial lesions. Although several studies have shown generally good correlation with autopsied specimens [12, 13], they have also reported a tendency for the arteriogram to *underestimate* the coronary artery lesion

TABLE 9–2. Examples of a coronary artery scoring system

| Score for vessel in question | Degree of reduction in luminal diameter |
| --- | --- |
| 0 | None |
| 1 | <25% |
| 2 | 25–50% |
| 3 | 50–70% |
| 4 | 70–90% |
| 5 | 90–99% |
| 6 | Total occlusion with distal vessel adequately visualized by collaterals |
| 7 | Total occlusion with distal vessel visualized but too poorly to interpret |
| 8 | Total occlusion with distal vessels not visualized |

Adapted from Conti, C.R. *Circulation* 55:227, 1977.

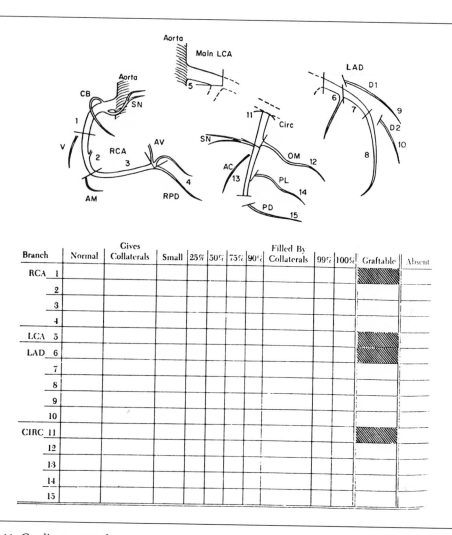

| Branch | Normal | Gives Collaterals | Small | 25% | 50% | 75% | 90% | Filled By Collaterals | 99% | 100% | Graftable | Absent |
|--------|--------|-------------------|-------|-----|-----|-----|-----|-----------------------|-----|------|-----------|--------|
| RCA 1  |        |                   |       |     |     |     |     |                       |     |      |           |        |
| 2      |        |                   |       |     |     |     |     |                       |     |      |           |        |
| 3      |        |                   |       |     |     |     |     |                       |     |      |           |        |
| 4      |        |                   |       |     |     |     |     |                       |     |      |           |        |
| LCA 5  |        |                   |       |     |     |     |     |                       |     |      |           |        |
| LAD 6  |        |                   |       |     |     |     |     |                       |     |      |           |        |
| 7      |        |                   |       |     |     |     |     |                       |     |      |           |        |
| 8      |        |                   |       |     |     |     |     |                       |     |      |           |        |
| 9      |        |                   |       |     |     |     |     |                       |     |      |           |        |
| 10     |        |                   |       |     |     |     |     |                       |     |      |           |        |
| CIRC 11|        |                   |       |     |     |     |     |                       |     |      |           |        |
| 12     |        |                   |       |     |     |     |     |                       |     |      |           |        |
| 13     |        |                   |       |     |     |     |     |                       |     |      |           |        |
| 14     |        |                   |       |     |     |     |     |                       |     |      |           |        |
| 15     |        |                   |       |     |     |     |     |                       |     |      |           |        |

FIGURE 9–11. Grading system for coronary arteriograms recommended by the American Heart Association. The right coronary artery (RCA) and its branches are shown in the left panel. The main left coronary artery (LCA) is shown at the top, and the two major branches of the LCA—the left circumflex artery (Circ) and the left anterior descending artery (LAD)—are in the middle and right panels, respectively. The numbering system refers to the area of the vessel (between the cross lines) that is being evaluated. (From American Heart Association Committee Report. A reporting system on patients evaluated for coronary artery disease. *Circulation* 51:5, 1975. Reprinted by permission of the American Heart Association, Inc.)

(figure 9–12). Cinically, this is preferable to overestimation. However, when arteriographic and direct measurements were recently compared in a dog model, the accuracy of the arteriogram was again generally good, but now there was a tendency to *overestimate* the lesions that directly reduced cross-sectional area 85 percent or more [57]. In another study, Pepine and associates [51] also found that there was a tendency to overestimate the degree of narrowing in short segments but not in longer ones. These latter studies have clinical implications, since the decision to refer a patient for surgery is often based on the degree of narrowing seen on the arteriogram. If the arteriogram underestimates the lesion rather than overestimates it, there is less chance that vessels with lesions that are not hemodynamically significant will be operated on. On the other hand, if the arteriogram overestimates the lesion, then it is possible that noncritical lesions will be bypassed and that a higher graft closure rate might ensue. These studies again em-

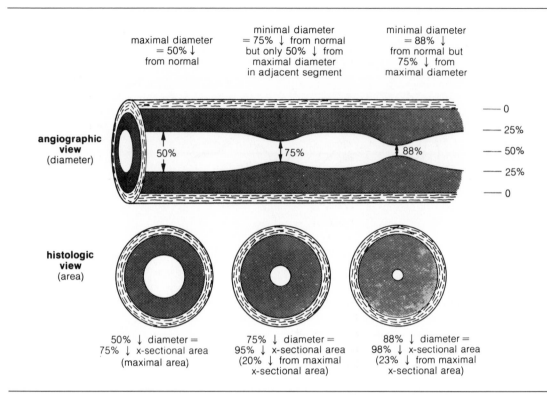

FIGURE 9–12. Reasons for discrepancies between angiographic and histologic findings in stenotic lesions. A 50 percent reduction in diameter seen on angiogram is actually a 75 percent narrowing on histologic cross section. Similarly, an angiographic reading of 75 percent becomes 95 percent on cross section. Moreover, on angiography, narrowing is measured only in relation to the diameter of the adjacent arterial segment, whereas histologic cross sections permit accurate measurements of plaque formation by comparison with the original vessel wall instead of with the adjacent site, which may also be narrowed but to a lesser degree. Other problems include eccentricity of the lesions, especially when viewed in limited angiographic projections. (From Roberts, W.C. *Cardiovasc. Med.* 2:29, 1977.)

phasize the need for a consensus in interpretation of the films, which hopefully will minimize some of such problems as much as possible.

In conclusion, mention should be made of a new experimental technique that might one day supplant the coronary arteriogram: in vivo coronary angioscopy using a 1.8 mm fiber-optic scope and replacement of blood with optically clear fluids [58].

## Complications of Diagnostic Cardiac Catheterization

The incidence of complications during coronary arteriography has, in the past, been related to the technique utilized [59]. The femoral approach in the early years of its use, and especially in those institutions with low case loads, had a dramatically greater complication rate than did the brachial approach. With increased utilization of the femoral approach and coincident with (although not necessarily because of) the use of systemic heparinization for the femoral approach, the risks of death, myocardial infarction, and cerebral embolism became similar for the two procedures when the same centers were reanalyzed [60].

While a recent multicenter study by Davis and co-workers [61] did reveal increased risks utilizing the *brachial* procedure, the most recent large-scale study (involving 53,581 cardiac catheterizations) found no difference between the two techniques [62]. Most deaths occurred in patients with far-advanced disease. This emphasizes the relation of the *experience* of the cardiac catheterization and coronary arteriography team to the risk a patient encounters in that laboratory. It appears at present, then, that whatever technique is utilized by a particular laboratory can be practiced safely provided enough procedures are done each year in that laboratory.

While it has been difficult to document, it seems almost certain that the risk of the procedure increases with time and complexity. What is very clear is that the examination of the coronary arteries adds significantly to the rest of the procedure and that catheterization of infants is similarly associated with a high complication rate.

During coronary arteriography, the most serious complications—namely, death, myocardial infarction, or cerebral embolism—are the result of thrombi that are formed on the tip of the catheter, atheromas that are displaced by the tip of the catheter, or atheromas that are displaced by the introduction of too much contrast agent, especially when the catheter is not lying free within the lumen of the vessel ostium. Studies utilizing scanning electron microscopy have indicated that internal and external surface irregularities play a major role in the initiation of thrombosis in and on intravascular catheters. This seems particularly true of catheters made of polyurethane [66]. Systemic heparinization has been reported to decrease the frequency of thromboembolic complications when the femoral approach is employed, but it does not eliminate them entirely [64]. Since such complications cannot be completely eliminated, however, systemic heparinization should not be considered as a substitute for careful technique. The importance of an experienced laboratory rather than the technique chosen is emphasized by detailed analysis of one of the large surveys cited [60]. On the basis of the responses from 178 institutions in that study that performed 89,079 examinations over 2 years, the mortality within 24 hours of the procedure was .14 percent overall, .12 percent for the brachial technique, and .16 percent for the femoral technique. Laboratories performing 100 or fewer procedures per year had a .29 percent mortality rate (.30 percent brachial and .25 percent femoral), whereas those doing 400 or more cases per year ex-

perienced a .07 percent mortality (.06 percent brachial and .10 percent femoral). Myocardial infarction occurred in .18 percent (.15 percent brachial and .20 percent femoral), and the thromboembolic complication rate was .75 percent (1.2 percent brachial and 0.29 percent femoral). Table 9–1 lists the major complications and incidence rates.

While end-points like death or stroke are relatively clear-cut, the diagnosis of a myocardial infarction may be difficult to make after catheterization, because frequently ST-T changes occur on the ECG and cardiac enzymes can be elevated, especially when premedication is administered intramuscularly. The development of techniques for measuring creatine phosphokinase (CPK) isoenzymes has made this diagnosis much easier, and normal MB-CPK isoenzyme activity effectively rules out the diagnosis of a myocardial infarction [65]. A full-blown infarction may be prevented if the clot obstructing the vessel can be lysed using a guide-wire and/or streptokinase [66]. Thrombolytic therapy is discussed at length in the next section.

Finally, the issue of out-patient coronary cardiac catheterization must be considered when complications are discussed. The proponents of this program reported a complication rate comparable to that of hospitalized patients in one report of over 5,000 consecutive catheterizations [67]. Economic savings and increased bed utilization are also stressed, but many cardiologists are still reluctant to undertake such a program, even in selected patients. Whether this view will change in the future remains to be seen.

## *"Therapeutic" Cardiac Catheterization Procedures*

### TRANSLUMINAL CORONARY ANGIOPLASTY

Since its inception by Gruentzig in 1977 [68], transluminal dilatation of coronary stenoses has become an important therapeutic advance in the treatment of coronary atherosclerosis. The past seven years have witnessed dramatic improvements in equipment design and techniques of angioplasty, and the original criteria for patient selection have been expanded accordingly. This section will describe criteria for patient selection, procedure technique, and results of coronary angioplasty.

*Patient Selection.* The profile of the ideal candidate for transluminal coronary angioplasty is a patient with recent-onset angina who is found on coronary angiography to have a single, proximal, concentric stenosis in a major epicardial coronary artery. In addition, objective evidence for transient myocardial ischemia as documented by stress testing or spontaneous electrocardiographic changes should be present. Importantly, patients should be candidates for coronary artery bypass graft surgery, and the angioplasty procedure should be performed with "surgical standby." Recent refinements in equipment and technique have expanded substantially the number of patients who are candidates for the procedure, and at appropriate experienced centers, higher risk subgroups—i.e., patients with more distal stenoses and eccentric and/or calcified lesions—can be offered the option of transluminal coronary angioplasty. In addition, patients with multivessel disease, prior coronary bypass surgery, and evolving myocardial infarction have been successfully treated with this approach [68–72].

*Technique.* Initially, transluminal coronary angioplasty was carried out via a fixed guide wire catheter system (figure 9–13). These early catheters were double lumen 4 French devices. One lumen was used for pressure monitoring through a distal port as well as contrast injections, while the second lumen connected to the balloon itself. A nonmovable, flexible, straight or J-tipped guide wire was fastened to the distal end of the dilatation catheter.

A most important advance has been the introduction of an angioplasty system that consists of a dilatation catheter through which a soft, steerable guide wire can be passed and moved independently of the dilatation catheter (figure 9–14). The use of this system permits safer passage through tight, eccentric stenoses or even totally occluded coronary arteries [73]. In addition, pressure monitoring through the guiding catheter, seated in the ostium of the coronary artery to be dilated, and the distal port of the dilation catheter permit measurement of the gradient across the stenosis before and after balloon inflation.

Guiding catheters come in a variety of shapes and are either 8 or 9 French (figure 9–15). Once the guiding catheter is properly seated in the coronary ostium, diagnostic angiograms may be performed. Guidelines are as follows: Inject intracoronary nitroglycerin, approximately 200 ug, into the coronary ostium to be dilated. This, in addition to pretreatment with nifedipine, usually 20 mg sublingual, assures coronary vasodilation and decreases the tendency to develop coronary spasm during subselective coronary catheter manipulation. Adequate anticoagulation is critical, and heparin, 10,000 units, is administered prior to insertion of the dilating cath-

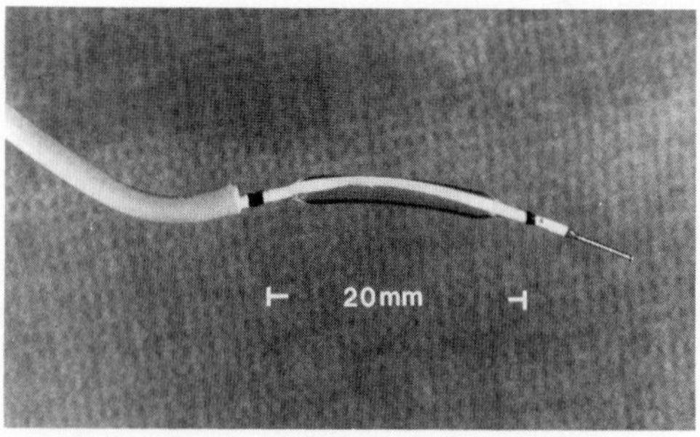

FIGURE 9–13. Early design fixed guide wire–balloon dilatation catheter system used in guiding catheter. (From Greenspon, A. and Goldberg, S. *Cardiovascular Clinics* 13/1:265, 1983.)

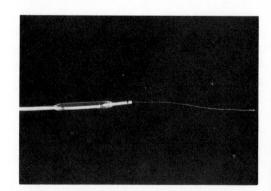

FIGURE 9–14. The newer guide wire–dilatation catheter system. The guide wire itself can be maneuvered independent of the dilatation catheter, and different guide wires may be used during the procedure.

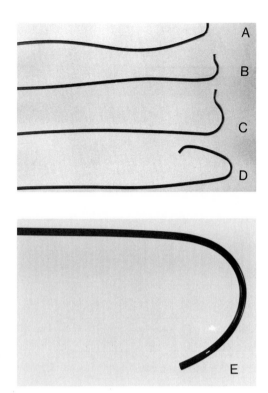

FIGURE 9–15. Variety of guiding catheters using Judkins and Amplatz end hole configurations for transfemoral angioplasty, and the Stertzer catheter with side holes for brachial transluminal coronary angioplasty.

eter. Frequent monitoring of the anticoagulation status by means of the activated coagulation time using a hemochron [R] prevents thrombotic complications. Proper seating of the guiding catheter relative to the coronary ostium is a critical step in the angioplasty procedure. It is not satisfactory just to have an adequate dye injection into the coronary artery; rather the operator must be satisfied that the geometric orientation of the guiding catheter will permit safe passage of the guide wire dilatation system into the ostium of the coronary artery and through the stenosis to be dilated. Special care is taken to prevent "wedging" of the guiding catheter in the coronary ostium with reduction of coronary blood flow and subsequent myocardial ischemia. Certain guiding catheter configurations will also help the operator in subsequent passage of certain stenoses. For example, the Amplatz configuration is particularly helpful in approaching left

circumflex coronary lesions. In some instances modification of the approach may become important; some feel, for example, that use of the brachial approach is helpful in dilating right coronary artery and bypass graft stenoses. Consideration of the geometric configuration of the coronary ostium relative to the aorta, the portion of the coronary artery segment proximal to the stenosis, and the distal coronary anatomy are all features taken into account before selection of the appropriate components of the guide catheter–dilitation system. Realizing the various problems that may be encountered during the dilatation procedure prior to undertaking catheter selection is important in maximizing success rate. Other noteworthy factors include careful scrutiny of the region of the stenosis, with reference to bends, calcification, side branch vessels, degree of eccentricity, and the severity of the stenosis itself.

After the operator is satisfied with the guiding catheter position and the pressure tracings from the guiding catheter, it is time to insert the dilating catheter guide wire system. A variety of dilating catheters are available with different balloon sizes. They usually vary in size from 2.0 to 4.0 mm in inflated diameter (figure 9–14) and are usually 25 mm in length. Metallic markers indicate the position of the balloon segment during fluoroscopy. The "deflated profile" of the balloon-dilating catheters also differs depending on the manufacturer. A variety of guide wires are available (figure 9–16), each with different characteristics and trade-offs. The United States Catheter and Instrument (USCI) wire, for example, is .016 inches in diameter, is highly radiopaque, and steerable. It is somewhat stiffer than the Advanced Catheter System, (ACS) .018 inch "floppy" wire, which is much less radiopaque except for the distal 3cm; however, the floppiness of the ACS wire is especially useful in crossing tight, eccentric stenosis or finding a path through totally occluded coronary arteries. The latter also has very little chance of causing disection; the trade-off of using this "floppy" wire, of course, is that it is much less steerable. In addition, pressure measurements with this wire in place are not easily obtainable, and once a stenosis is crossed an exchange should be made for another wire (the pressure, dye, torque [PDT]

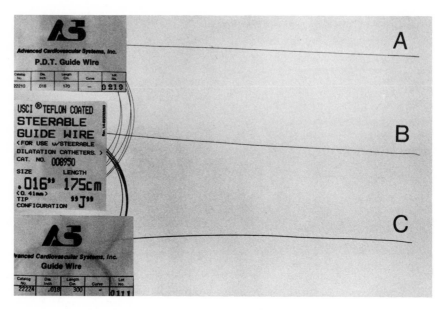

FIGURE 9–16. Movable guide wires. (A) The ACS PDT wire. (B) The USCI steerable guide wire. (C) The ACS "floppy" guide wire. Each has advantages and trade-offs (see text).

of ACS, or the steerable USCI) to obtain coronary pressure. A 300 cm "floppy" exchange wire is particularly useful in the circumstance of having to use more than one dilating balloon catheter to achieve a satisfactory dilatation. For example, in the case of a very tight stenosis present in a large coronary artery, it may be necessary to first perform dilatation with a 2.0 or 2.5 mm balloon, then exchange this for a 3.0 mm balloon to achieve the desired result. Remaining across the stenosis with the 300 cm guide wire obviates the need to recross the lesion.

Advancement of the dilitation catheter–guide wire system should be done with a 5 to 6 cm length of wire protruding beyond the distal tip of the dilating catheter. Having the guide wire extend just beyond the dilating catheter is not advisable because it increases the risk of dissection. The operator or operators need to carefully coordinate the movement of the guide wire, the dilating catheter, and the position of the guiding catheter. Fluoroscopic views that are the best for crossing the stenosis should be preselected. The use of a rapidly movable image intensifier or, better yet, biplane imaging capability is needed for optimal performance of the procedure.

Once the guide wire is steered away from side branches and through the stenosis, the wire is passed to the distal coronary artery. Careful attention is paid to the way in which the guide

wire rests in the distal vessel—the operator should avoid kinking of the guide wire or its entry into small side branches. The balloon segment of the dilatation catheter is positioned into the stenosis itself. The use of the guiding catheter and/or dilating catheter for test injections of dye during the positioning of the guide wire and the balloon catheter, with confirmation of proper position in several views, is necessary. Without these, it is easy, for example, to mistakenly enter a septal or diagonal branch of the left anterior descending artery when the stenosis is in the anterior descending artery itself. Once the guide wire–dilating catheter is well positioned, the gradient across the stenosis can be measured (figure 9–17) with certain guide wire–catheter combinations and balloon inflation can take place. The use of a hand-held device is preferred but the mounted gun devices are acceptable as well. Begin with gradual inflation while constantly watching the shape of the balloon. Look specifically for the "dog bone" effect (Figure 9–18, 9–19, 9–20) present when the dilating balloon engages the stenoses at lower inflation pressures. Careful checking of the "dog bone" helps assure proper positioning of the balloon

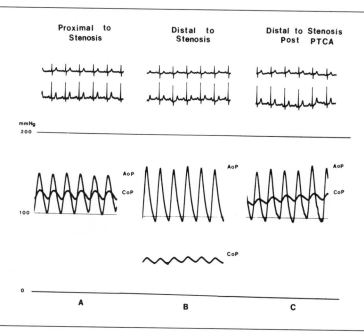

FIGURE 9–17. Measurements of the pressure gradient across a severe left anterior descending stenosis. (A) Simultaneous guiding catheter and dilating catheter measurements with the dilating catheter positioned proximal to the stenosis. (B) The pressure drop across the lesion is recorded after the dilating catheter has passed through the stenosis before balloon dilatation. (C) The simultaneous aortic and distal coronary pressure after balloon dilatation, showing abolition of the pressure gradient across the stenosis. (From Greenspon, A. and Goldberg, S. *Cardiovascular Clinics* 13/1:265, 1983.)

relative to the stenosis. With gradually increasing inflation pressure the "dog bone" disappears and the pressure at which this occurs is a guide to the softness or resistance of the lesion. Longer inflations at higher pressures (up to 11 atmospheres) may be performed if necessary. Generally, the first inflation is done for 10–20 sec with constant arterial pressure and electrocardiogram monitoring, with close scrutiny for the development of chest pain or ST segment elevation. After the "dog bone" has disappeared, deflate the balloon and recheck the gradient and angiographic flow. Inflations are repeated with gradually increasing inflation pressure until a satisfactory hemodynamic and angiographic result occurs (see figure 9–18, 9–19, 9–20). A final gradient less than 15 mm Hg is desirable. The

guide wire is left across the stenosis and in the distal vessel for about 30 minutes following the final balloon inflation, and during this time period any change in the magnitude of the gradient should be checked for. A fall in distal coronary pressure recorded through the tip of the dilatation catheter in the 30 minutes following the last inflation may signal coronary dissection. If this occurs, repeat the dye injection and, if appropriate, reinflate the balloon with a long, low-pressure inflation in an attempt to "tack down" the dissection. Another cause for a drop in distal coronary pressure may be the development of coronary spasm, which can be treated by intracoronary nitroglycerin injection. Balloon inflation is repeated until there is no further gain in distal coronary pressure and the angiographic result appears satisfactory. Attempt to increase the inflation time to 45 to 90 seconds or longer, if feasible, as preliminary evidence suggests that longer inflations may increase the primary success rate and perhaps reduce the restenosis rate. If all appears well after the 30-minute period, remove the guide wire–dilatation balloon catheter system and repeat the coronary angiograms in multiple views. Typically, a certain amount of "haziness" is present in the area of dilatation; occasionally small dissections are clinically visi-

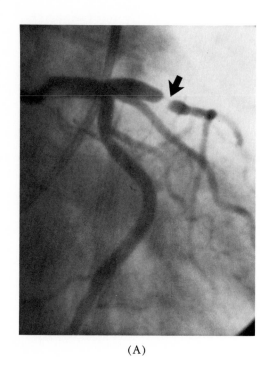

(A)

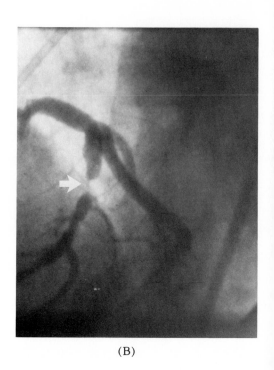

(B)

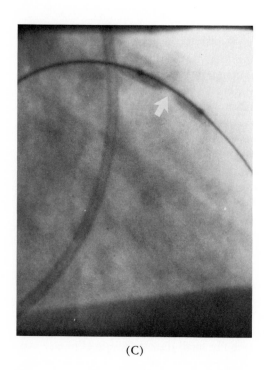

(C)

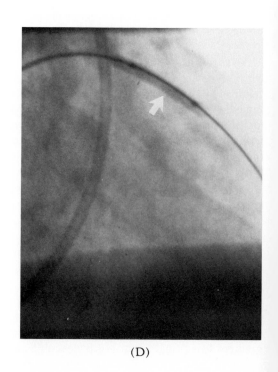

(D)

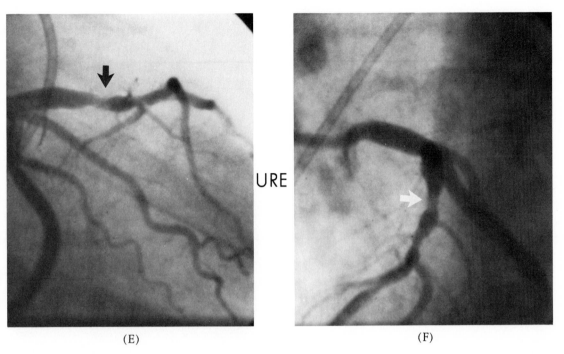

(E)          (F)

FIGURE 9–18. Dilatation of a left anterior descending stenosis using a steerable system consisting of an ACS 3.0mm balloon catheter and USCI guiding catheter and USCI steerable guide wire. (A) A 99 percent left anterior descending stenosis seen in the right anterior oblique view in a patient with unstable angina. (B) The severe stenosis visualized in the left anterior oblique cranial view. (C) The steerable wire is well positioned at the apex; the appearance of the balloon at 2 atmospheres inflation pressure showing the classic "dog bone" effect. (D) Appearance of the balloon at 4 atmospheres showing loss of the "dog bone" effect, indicating dilatation of the stenosis. (E) The left anterior descending coronary artery after dilatation in the right anterior oblique view. Note the hazy appearance in the area of the stenosis. The final gradient was 7 mmHg and the patient's symptoms were relieved. Post-angioplasty stress thallium testing was normal. (F) Post-dilatation left anterior oblique cranial view.

ble. In certain instances there is perhaps a suboptimal or ambiguous result. In this latter circumstance the hemodynamic measurements made across the coronary stenosis assume critical, clinical significance. Coronary dissection that causes abrupt vessel closure usually does so in the first 30 minutes after the last balloon inflation. Any patient who develops an increasing stenosis gradient along with electrocardiographic and/or clinical evidence of myocardial ischemia should be immediately taken for bypass surgery.

Once dilatation is successfully accomplished, the patient is returned to the coronary care unit for 24 hours. Maintain patients on aspirin and persantine indefinitely and nifedipine and nitrates for 6 months. Stress electrocardiography is repeated in the 2-week period following successful angioplasty, and repeat coronary angiography 6 months after angioplasty or sooner if in-

dicated. Restenosis, when it occurs, usually does so in the first 3 to 6 months.

*Results and Future Directions of Angioplasty.*
In 1979 the National Heart Lung and Blood Institute (NHLBI) established a voluntary registry to assess the efficacy of transluminal coronary angioplasty. In the most recent report the results of 3,079 patients undergoing the procedure were analyzed [74]. Briefly, the findings may be summarized as follows. The patients were predominately male (77 percent) with a mean age of 53.5 years. Twenty-six percent of patients were in Canadian Heart Class 4, 37 percent were in Class 3, 28 percent in Class 2, 4 percent in Class 1, and 5 percent had no symptoms. Seventy-three percent of patients had single-vessel disease, 25 percent had multivessel disease, and 2 percent had left main coronary artery disease.

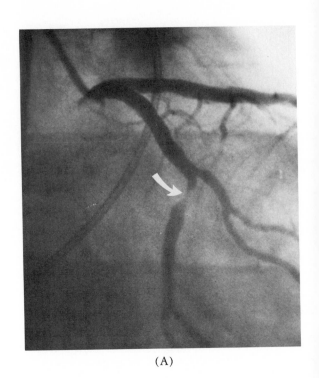

(A)

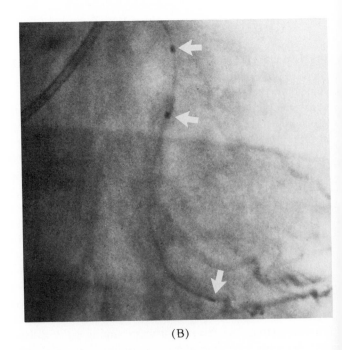

(B)

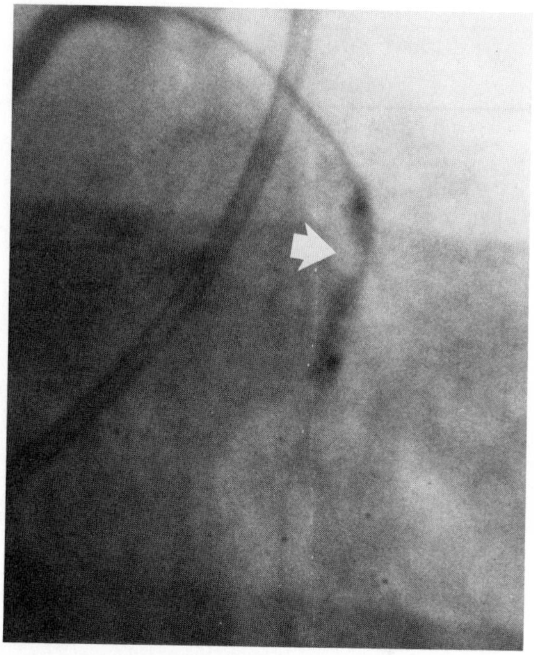

(C)

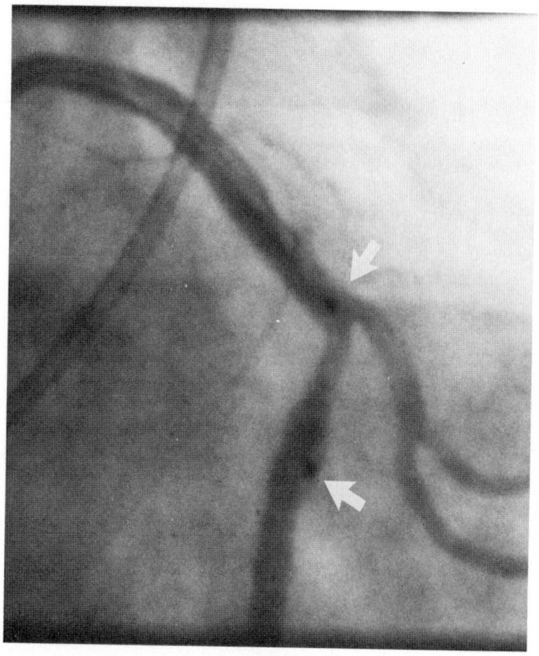

(D)

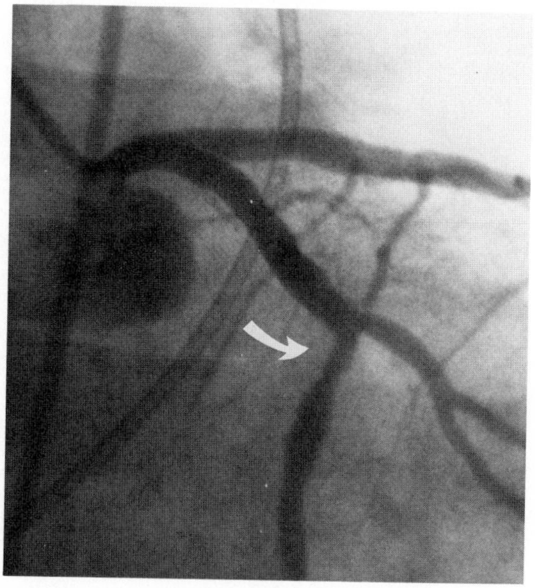

(E)

FIGURE 9–19. Dilatation of a left circumflex (LCFx) stenosis using a moveable guide wire-dilatation system. **(A)** Right anterior oblique view of a 90 percent, LCFx stenosis. **(B)** An ACS "floppy" guide wire is positioned in the distal LCFx marginal branch. **(C)** Inflation of ACS balloon showing the typical "dog bone" effect. **(D)** Repeat guiding catheter injection with the dilating system in place. **(E)** Repeat coronary injection showing final result reduction of the 90 percent stenosis to a luminal irregularity.

The left anterior descending artery was attempted in 64 percent, the circumflex in 6 percent, the right coronary artery in 25 percent, and the left main coronary artery in 1 percent. Four percent had saphenous vein bypass grafts attempted. The angiographic success rate was somewhat higher in males than in females (68 percent versus 63 percent), and the overall complication rate was 19 percent in males and 27 percent in females. In-hospital deaths occurred in 0.7 percent of men and 1.8 percent of women. The major complications included coronary dissection/occlusion/spasm, which occurred in 10.4 percent; myocardial infarction occurred in 5.5 percent, ventricular tachycardia or fibrillation occurred in 2.3 percent, and prolonged angina in 6.7 percent. Longer term follow-up of 1 year following angioplasty was assessed in 1,397 patients. At the end of 1 year, 72 percent of patients with a primary successful result did not require repeat angioplasty or bypass, and 12 percent required repeat dilatation. Therefore, 84 percent of patients with a primary successful result could be managed by angioplasty alone at the end of one year.

It must be stated emphatically that these results represent "early" angioplasty prior to the widespread availability of the newer guide wire–

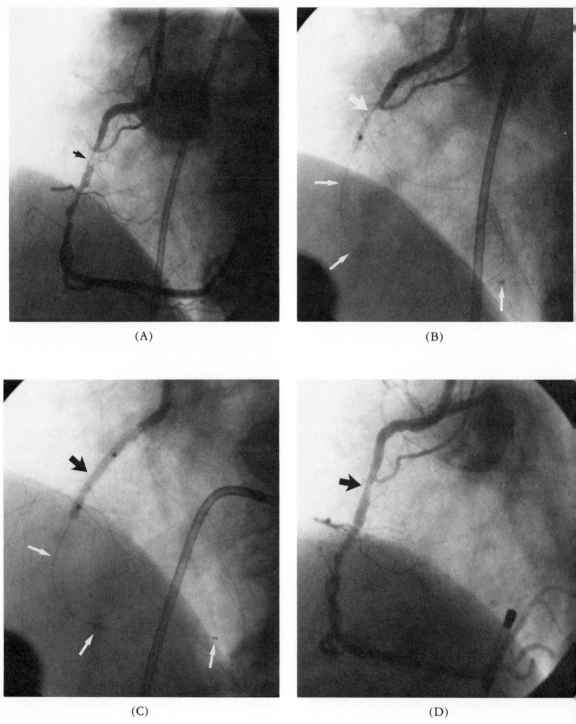

(A)  (B)

(C)  (D)

FIGURE 9–20. Dilatation of a right coronary artery (RCA) stenosis in a patient with variant angina. (A) Baseline view of the RCA lesion in left anterior oblique view. (B) The "floppy" guide wire is well positioned in the distal RCA and the balloon is engaging the stenosis. (C) Inflation of the balloon in the stenosis. (D) Repeat RCA angiogram showing the final result.

dilatation catheter systems. Experienced operators using state-of-the-art equipment are approaching a 90 percent primary success rate, although the restenosis rates remain substantial (15 to 33 percent). It is hoped that with further experience and development of safer catheter systems, along with improvements in imaging, transluminal coronary angioplasty will have even more of an impact.

## THROMBOLYTIC THERAPY FOR EVOLVING MYOCARDIAL INFARCTION

Acute transmural myocardial infarction is associated with total occlusion of the infarct-related artery in approximately 90 percent of patients studied within 6 hours of symptom onset [75] (figure 9–21). Since evolving myocardial infarction is a dynamic ongoing process that takes hours to complete, attempts have been made to salvage myocardium at risk of necrosis by arterial recanalization using thrombolytic drugs [76–78]. These agents have been administered by the intravenous [79] as well as introcoronary routes. The overall success rate of vessel reopening has been higher with the intracoronary route: approximately 75 to 85 percent with intracoronary administration versus

approximately 50–70 percent with intravenous administration.

There has been much speculation regarding the efficacy of thrombolytic agents on myocardial cell salvage, with some studies showing some improvement in left ventricular function [76–80], and others showing no discernible effect [81]. For example, Rentrop et al. [76] found that in 14 patients left ventricular ejection fraction was $50.5 \pm 12$ percent before versus $54.6 \pm 9$ percent immediately after intracoronary thrombolysis (p < 0.05). Similarly, Mathey et al. [78] observed an increase in left ventricular ejection fraction from $37 \pm 5$ percent to $47 \pm 4$ percent (p < 0.05) predischarge in 11 patients in whom intracoronary streptokinase therapy was successful. Anderson et al. [80] performed a controlled randomized trial in which 50 patients with acute myocardial infarction were assigned to receive either intracoronary streptokinase therapy or standard therapy. Intracoronary streptokinase treatment was associated with improved wall motion on echocardiogram, improved radionuclide ejection fraction, and improved electrocardiographic indices as compared to standard treatment. By contrast Khaja et al. [81] found no statistical difference in their randomized trial of intracoronary streptokinase verses placebo with respect to left ventricular function, angiographic ejection fraction, and serial radionuclide ejection fraction. Even so, short-term mortality seems to be significantly reduced in patients who have undergone successful vessel recanalization via intracoronary thrombolysis. In the Western Washington randomized trial, Kennedy et al. [82] enrolled 250 patients with acute evolving transmural myocardial infarction in a multicenter study. The overall 30-day mortality was 3.7 percent in the intracoronary streptokinase group versus 11.2 percent in the control group (p < 0.02).

*Technique of Intracoronary Thrombolysis.* Once the diagnosis of acute transmural myocardial infarction is made on the basis of history and electrocardiographic criteria and the appropriate enzyme and laboratory studies have been obtained, thrombolysis is performed using the following guidelines. First, sheaths are placed in both the femoral vein and artery in preparation for the

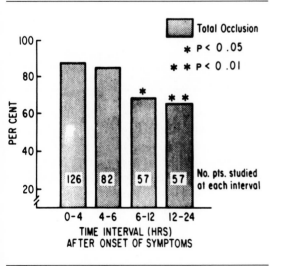

FIGURE 9–21. Relative incidence of total coronary occlusion during the early hours of acute transmural myocardial infarction. (From DeWood, et al. Reprinted, by permission of the *New England Journal of Medicine,* 303:897, 1980.)

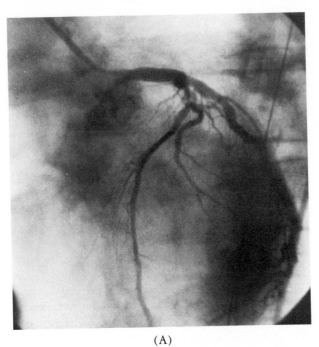

(A)

FIGURE 9–22. (A) Left anterior oblique angiogram of left coronary artery during acute anteroseptal myocardial infarction. There is total occlusion of the left anterior descending coronary artery (LAD). (B) Electrocardiographic tracings before administration of intracoronary streptokinase (upper panel). There is marked ST elevation. During streptokinase administration (middle panel) accelerated idioventricular rhythm develops. Repeat angiogram (see panel C) with appearance of AIVR showed successful reflow of LAD. Later during procedure, ST segment elevation has resolved (lower panel). (C) Repeat angiogram within seconds of onset of AIVR, showing recanalized LAD. (From Goldberg, S. et al., Am. Heart J. 105:-26, 1983. Reproduced with permission.)

cardiac catheterization. This permits later safe removal of catheters, leaving sheaths in place while the patient is anticoagulated with streptokinase. A pacing catheter (for example, a Zucker catheter) is used as the right heart catheter. This is of particular importance during coronary recanalization, as bradycardia is likely to develop during coronary thrombolysis, especially when the right coronary artery is the affected vessel. Following right heart pressure measurements (often the key to the diagnosis of right ventricular infarction), left ventricular function and wall motion are assessed—either by contrast ventriculography and/or noninvasive techniques. The unaffected coronary is visualized next, with special reference to collaterial flow to the affected artery. Following this, the infarct-related artery is visualized. In most instances this will show thrombotic total occlusion of the vessel with typical late staining of thrombus. Nitroglycerin 200 to 300 ug is injected into the affected coronary artery prior to the administration of thrombolytic agents. A 2.5 French subselective Ganz infusion catheter is placed through the diagnostic guiding catheter just proximal to the occluded arterial segment, and streptokinase is infused through this at a rate of 4,000 IU/minute. Continuously monitor the electrocardiogram, since specific dysrhythmias

occur, usually precisely at the time of successful restoration of antegrade coronary flow [83, 84]. The arrhythmias most often noted are accelerated idioventricular rhythm (AIVR) with reperfusion of all myocardial zones (figure 9–22); reflex sinus bradycardia and hypotension occur during right coronary artery recanalization. Usually no specific therapy is required for AIVR. When this arrhythmia does occur, there is some mild drop in arterial pressure due to the loss of the atrial transport mechanism. If necessary, pharmacologic overdrive with atropine is useful. The development of sinus bradycardia and hypotension often requires temporary pacing and volume expansion. These rhythm changes and reflexes are transitory.

BASELINE

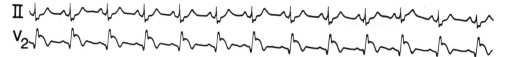

II

$V_2$

IMMEDIATE REPERFUSION

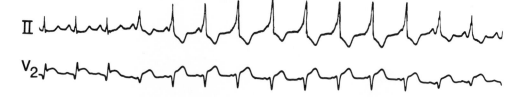

II

$V_2$

50 MIN. POST REPERFUSION

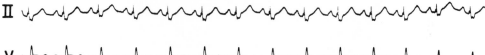

II

$V_2$

(B)

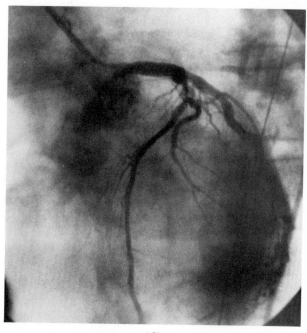

(C)

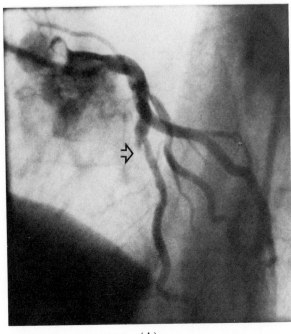

(A)

FIGURE 9–23. (A) Baseline left coronary angiogram in a 52-year-old man with acute anterior myocardial infarction. There is total occlusion of the left anterior descending artery. (B) A 2.5 French Ganz subselective catheter is placed in the LAD artery. (C) Repeat coronary angiogram after successful clot lysis-pain and ST segment elevation have subsided. (D) Three days following thrombolysis, the patient was taken back for angioplasty of the residual 95 percent LAD stenosis, the inflated dilatation balloon in the stenosis. Note the "dog bone" effect on the balloon. A USCI steerable guide wire is in place. (E) Angiographic result after angio-plasty. There has been marked improvement in the lesion. Final gradient was 0 mmHg.

Contrast injections are repeated approximately every 10 minutes or if rhythm disturbances occur. Vessel opening usually occurs in under 30 minutes when the subselective route is utilized. Continue infusion of streptokinase at least until there is angiographic evidence of complete clot dissolution. The average dose of streptokinase in our laboratory has been approximately 250,000 IU. Doses as high as 500,-000 IU have been given for effective clot dissolution. In addition to rhythm disturbances, monitor pain pattern and ST segment changes. In successful cases, ST segment elevation usually subsides in approximately the first hour following coronary reflow.

Intracoronary streptokinase restores coronary flow in the majority of cases, but postthrombolytic management is controversial since reocclusion rates are considerable [85]. In the majority of patients, after clot dissolution has occurred a fixed high-grade stenosis remains at the site of prior total thrombotic occlusion. In order to lessen the tendency for rethrombosis, coronary angioplasty and/or coronary bypass surgery have been advocated [86–88] in selected cases. Both procedures have been performed with very acceptable complication and mortality rates. Some investigators have advocated angio-

plasty during the initial procedure. Others prefer doing a two-step procedure; in the interim, left ventricular recovery can be assessed by electrocardiographic and noninvasive echocardiographic and ventriculographic end-points. If there is evidence of viable myocardium at risk, proceed with coronary angioplasty or bypass surgery, depending on coronary anatomy (figure 9–23).

*Future Directions.* The development of more selective thrombolytic agents [89] with rapid action and less systemic effect is underway. In addition, an aggressive approach to catheterization of a high-risk subgroup of patients with "preinfarction" angina may become more widespread,

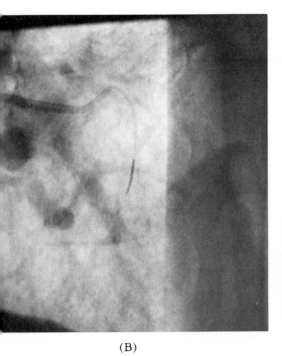

(B)

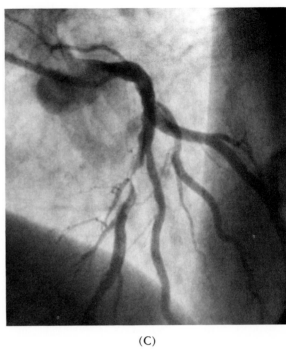

(C)

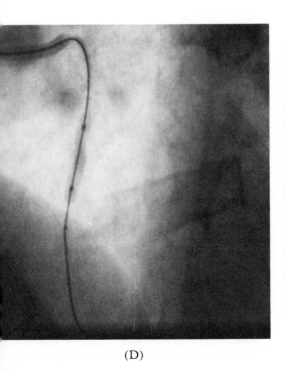

(D)

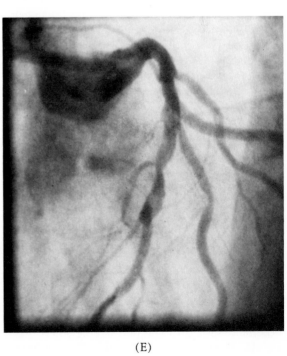

(E)

255

i.e., for those patients with recurrent ST segment elevation especially if they have evidence of a recent subendocardial infarction. These patients are often refractory to maximal medical therapy and frequently have high-grade stenosis with nonocclusive intracoronary thrombi [90]. Intervention in this high-risk subgroup affords the best possibility for myocardial salvage.

## Conclusions

Cardiac catheterization (including coronary arteriography and left ventriculography) provides useful data concerning coronary anatomy, ventricular function, and prognosis in patients requiring this procedure. In experienced hands, it is a safe technique, yielding critical information currently unobtainable by noninvasive methods. In particular, a large group of patients exists for whom the information provided by the catheterization examination can be used to tailor surgical therapy for relief of debilitating symptoms.

The indications for cardiac catheterization are undergoing change and becoming more liberal, most notably in the patient group with chronic but not severe angina in whom the procedure is performed with the idea of recommending surgery to prolong life span. There is far from unanimous opinion, however, regarding this category of patient. The consensus for the use of catheterization seems strongest in patients with severe chronic angina, unstable angina, valvular heart disease with angina, Prinzmetal's angina, persistent heart failure or shock postinfarction, and angina following bypass surgery. There is *less* agreement regarding patients with ventricular arrhythmias or unexplained ventricular failure and in the diagnostic category of atypical chest pain syndromes of uncertain cause. There is *least* agreement in the category of asymptomatic patients, especially those individuals who have had an uncomplicated myocardial infarction.

The makeup of the catheterization team differs from hospital to hospital, but whether the team consists of cardiologists or cardiologists plus radiologists, the physician with the most skill and experience should actually perform the procedure.

The advantages of the Sones and Judkins techniques seems to be a trade-off, and both procedures are employed at most hospitals. Angled projections are especially valuable in some cases and should become part of the angiographer's expertise. Adjunctive procedures—such as resting and intervention ventriculography and physiologic, metabolic, and blood flow studies—are often helpful components of a complete examination. The biplane left ventriculogram is most valuable when asynergy is suspected clinically and when contractile reserve must be evaluated either with nitroglycerin or on the basis of ventricular premature beats. Either intervention technique is acceptable. Digital subtraction ventriculography appears to be a major advance in our ability to image the left ventricle without direct catheterization. Therapeutic procedures are important new aspects of cardiac catheterization: thrombolytic therapy for the early hours of acute infarction and angioplasty for severe stenoses in suitable patients.

As with cardiac surgery, the cardiac catheterization procedure should be performed only in centers that perform an adequate number of cases per year in order to minimize risk and maximize the yield of useful data. Out-patient procedures probably should still be considered as experimental, though this may change with more widespread acceptance.

## References

1. Forssmann, W. Die Sondierung des rechten Herzens. *Klin. Wochenschr.* 8:2085, 1929.
2. Cournand, A.F., Riley, R.L., Breen, E.S., Baldwin, E. de F., and Richard, D.W., Jr. Measurement of cardiac output in man using the technique of catheterization of the right auricle or ventricle. *J. Clin. Invest.* 24:106, 1945.
3. Dexter, L., Haynes, F.W., Burwell, C.S., Eppinger, E.C., Sagerson, R.P., and Evans, J.M. Studies of congenital heart disease. II. The pressure and oxygen content of blood in the right auricle, right ventricle, and pulmonary artery in control patients, with observations on the oxygen saturation and source of pulmonary "capillary" blood. *J. Clin. Invest.* 26:554, 1947.
4. Zimmerman, H.A., Scott, R.W., and Becker, N.D. Catheterization of the left side of the heart in man. *Circulation* 1:357, 1950.
5. Seldinger, S.I. Catheter replacement of the needle in percutaneous arteriography: A new technique. *Acta Radiol.* 39:368, 1953.

6. Radner, S. Attempt at roentgenologic visualization of coronary blood vessels in man. *Acta Radiol.* 26:492, 1945.

7. Bellman, S., Frank, H.A., Lambert, P.B., Littman, D., and Williams, J.A. Coronary arteriography. I. Differential opacification of the aortic stream by catheters of special design—experimental development. *N. Engl. J. Med.* 262:325, 1960.

8. Sones, F.M. and Shirey, E.K. Cine coronary arteriography. *Mod. Concepts Cardiovasc. Dis.* 31:735, 1962.

9. Ricketts, J.H. and Abrams, H.L. Percutaneous selective coronary cine arteriography. *JAMA* 181:620, 1962.

10. Amplatz, K., Formanek, G., Stanger, P., and Wilson, W. Mechanics of selective coronary artery catheterization via femoral approach. *Radiology* 89:1040, 1967.

11. Judkins, M.P. Selective coronary arteriography. I. A percutaneous transfemoral technic. *Radiology* 89:815, 1967.

12. Kemp, H.G., Evans, H., Elliot, W.C., and Gorlin, R. Diagnostic accuracy of selective coronary cinearteriography. *Circulation* 36:526, 1967.

13. Vlodaver, Z., Frech, R., VanTassel, R.A., and Edwards, J.E. Correlation of the antemortem coronary arteriogram and the postmortem specimen. *Circulation* 47:162, 1973.

14. Report of the Ad Hoc Committee on the Indications for Coronary Arteriography. *Circulation* 55:969A, 1977.

15. Conti, C.R. Coronary arteriography. *Circulation* 55:227, 1977.

16. Chaitman, B.R., Fisher, L.D., Bourassa, M.G., Davis, K., Rogers, W.J., Maynard, C., Tyras, D.H., Berger, R.L., Judkins, M.P., Ringqvist, I., Mock, M.B., and Killip, T. Report of the Collaborative Study in Coronary Artery Surgery (CASS). Effect of coronary bypass surgery on survival patterns in subsets of patients with left main coronary artery disease. *Am. J. Cardiol.* 48:765, 1981.

17. Young, S.G. and Froelicher, V.F. Exercise testing: An update. *Mod. Concepts Cardiovasc. Dis.* 52:25, 1983.

18. Isner, J.M., Salem, D.N., Banas, J.S., Jr., and Levine, H.J. Long-term clinical course of patients with normal coronary arteriography: Follow-up study of 121 patients with normal or nearly normal arteriograms. *Am. Heart J.* 102:645, 1981.

19. Heupler, F.A., Jr., Proudfit, W.L., Razavi, M., Shirey, E.K., Greenstreet, R., and Sheldon, W.C. Ergonovine maleate provocative test for coronary arterial spasm. *Am. J. Cardiol.* 41:631, 1978.

20. Cipriano, P.R., Koch, F.H., Rosenthal, S.J., and Schroeder, J.S. Clinical course of patients following the demonstration of coronary artery spasm by angiography. *Am. Heart J.* 101:127, 1981.

21. Cohn, P.F. When is concern about silent myocardial ischemia justified? *Ann. Int. Med.* 100:597, 1984.

22. Graboys, T.B. and Cohn, P.F. The prevalence of angina pectoris and abnormal coronary arteriograms in aortic valvular disease. *Am. Heart J.* 93:382, 1977.

23. Hancock, E.W. Aortic stenosis, angina pectoris, and coronary artery disease. *Am. Heart J.* 93:382, 1977.

24. Friesinger, G.C., Adams, D.F., Bourassa, M.G., Carlsson, E., Elliott, L.P., Gessner, I.H., Greenspan, R.H., Grossman, W., Judkins, M.P., Kennedy, J.W., and Sheldon, W.C. Examination of the Chest and Cardiovascular System Study Group. Optimal resources for examination of the heart and lungs: Cardiac catheterization and radiographic facilities. *Circulation* 68:893A, 1983.

25. Freeman, W.R., Pichard, A.D., and Smith, H. Effect of informed consent and educational background on patient knowledge, anxiety, and subjective responses to cardiac catheterization. *Cath. Cardiovasc. Dis.* 7:119, 1981.

26. Sos, T.A. and Baltaxe, H.A. Cranial and caudal angulation for coronary angiography revisited. *Circulation* 56:119, 1977.

27. Grover, M., Slutsky, R., Higgins, C., and Atwood, J.E. Terminology and anatomy of angulated coronary arteriography. *Clin. Cardiol.* 7:37, 1984.

28. Crocker, R.H., Ockene, I.S., Alpert, J.S., Pape, L.A., and Dalen, J.E. Determinants of total body oxygen consumption in adults undergoing cardiac catheterization. *Cath. Cardiovasc. Diag.* 8:363, 1982.

29. Karliner, J.S., Peterson, K.L., and Ross, J., Jr. Left Ventricular Myocardial Mechanics: Systolic and Diastolic Function. In W. Grossman (ed.), *Cardiac Catheterization and Angiography* (2nd ed.). Philadelphia: Lea & Febiger, 1980, pp. 245–267.

30. Rackley, C.E. Quantitative evaluation of left ventricular function by radiographic techniques. *Circulation* 54:862, 1976.

31. Wynne, J., Green, L.H., Mann, T., Levin, D., and Grossman, W. Estimation of left ventricular volumes in man from biplane cineangiograms filmed in oblique projections. *Am. J. Cardiol.* 41:726, 1978.

32. Bove, A.A., Kreulen, T.H., and Spann, J.F. Computer analysis of left ventricular dynamic geometry in man. *Am. J. Cardiol.* 41:1239, 1978.

33. Cohn, P.F., Gorlin, R., Adams, D.F., Chahine, R.A., Vokonas, P.S., and Herman, M.V. Comparison of biplane and single-plane left ventriculography in patients with coronary artery disease. *Am. J. Cardiol.* 33:1, 1974.

34. Rogers, W.J., Smith, L.R., Hood, W.P., Mantle, J.A., Rackley, C.E., and Russell, R.O. Effect of filming projection and interobserver variability

on angiographic biplane left ventricular volume determination. *Circulation* 59:96, 1979.

35. Elliott, J.P., Green, C.E., Rogers, W.J., Hood, W.P., Mantle, J.A., and Papapietro, S.E. Advantages of the caudocranial left anterior oblique left ventriculogram in adult heart disease. *Am. J. Cardiol.* 49:369, 1982.

36. Horn, H.R., Teichholz, L.E., Cohn, P.F., Herman, M.V., and Gorlin, R. Augmentation of left ventricular contraction pattern in coronary artery disease by an inotropic catecholamine: The epinephrine ventriculogram. *Circulation* 49:1063, 1974.

37. Dyke, S.H., Cohn, P.F., Gorlin, R., and Sonnenblick, E.H. Detection of residual myocardial function in coronary artery disease using postextrasystolic potentiation. *Circulation* 50:694, 1974.

38. Helfant, R., Pine, R., Meister, S., Feldman, M.S., Trout, R.G., and Banka, V.S. Nitroglycerin to unmask reversible asynergy: Correlation with postcoronary bypass ventriculography. *Circulation* 50:108, 1974.

39. Vas, R., Diamond, G.A., Forrester, J.S., Whiting, J.S., Pfaff, M.J., Levisman, J.A., Nakano, F.S., and Swan, H.J.C. Computer-enhanced digital angiography: Correlation of clinical assessment of left ventricular ejection fraction and regional wall motion. *Am. Heart J.* 104:732, 1982.

40. Nichols, A.B., Martin, E.C., Fles, T.P., Stugensky, K.M., Balancio, L.A., Casarella, W.J., and Weiss, M.B. Validation of the angiographic accuracy of digital left ventriculography. *Am. J. Cardiol.* 51:224, 1983.

41. Mancini, G.B.J., Norris, S.L., Peterson, K.L., Gregoratos, G., Widmann, T.F., Ashburn, W.L., and Higgins, C.B. Quantitative assessment of segmental wall motion abnormalities at rest and after atrial pacing using digital intravenous ventriculography. *J. Am. Coll. Cardiol.* 2:70, 1983.

42. Feldman, R.L., Pepine, C.J., Curry, R.C., and Conti, C.R. Case against routine use of glyceryl trinitrate before coronary angiography. *Br. Heart J.* 40:992, 1978.

43. Zir, L.M., Dinsmore, R.E., Goss, C., and Harthorne, J.W. Experience with preformed catheters for coronary angiography by the brachial approach. *Cath. Cardiovasc. Diag.* 1:303, 1975.

44. Price, J.E., Jr., and Rosch, J. Selective coronary arteriography by percutaneous left transaxillary approach using preshaped torque control catheters. *Circulation* 48:1321, 1973.

45. Buxton, A., Goldberg, S., Hirshfeld, J.W., Wilson, J., Mann, T., Williams, D.O., Overlie, P., and Oliva, Philip. Refractory ergonovine-induced coronary vasospasm: Importance of intracoronary nitroglycerin. *Am. J. Cardiol.* 46:329, 1980.

46. Curry, R.C., Pepine, C.J., Sabom, B.S., and

Conti, R.C. Similarities of ergonovine-induced and spontaneous attacks of variant angina. *Circulation* 59:307, 1979.

47. White, C.W., Wright, C.B., Doty, D.B., Hiratza, L.F., Eastham, C.L., Harrison, D.G., and Marcus, M.L. Does visual interpretation of the coronary arteriogram predict the physiologic importance of a coronary stenosis? *N. Engl. J. Med.* 310:819, 1984.

48. American Heart Association Committee Report. A reporting system on patients evaluated for coronary artery disease. *Circulation* 51:5, 1975.

49. Alderman, E.L., Hamilton, K.K., Silverman, J., Harrison, D.C., and Sanders, W.J. Anatomically flexible, computer-assisted reporting system for coronary angiography. *Am. J. Cardiol.* 49:1208, 1982.

50. Faruqui, A.M.A., Maloy, W.C., Felner, J.M., Schlant, R.C., Logan, W.D., and Symbas, P. Symptomatic myocardial bridging of coronary artery. *Am. J. Cardiol.* 41:1305, 1978.

51. Pepine, C.J., Feldman, R.L., Nichols, W.W., and Conti, C.R. Coronary angiography: Potentially serious sources of error in interpretation. *Cardiovasc. Med.* 3:757, 1977.

52. DeRouen, T.A., Murray, J.A., and Owen, W. Variability in the analysis of coronary arteriograms. *Circulation* 55:324, 1977.

53. Fisher, L.D., Judkins, M.P., Lesperance, J., Cameron, A., Swaye, P., Ryan, T., Maynard, C., Bourassa, M., Kennedy, J.W., Gosselin, A., Kemp, H., Faxon, D., Wexler, L., and Davis, K.B. Reproducibility of coronary arteriographic reading in the coronary artery surgery study (CASS). *Cath. Cardiovasc. Diag.* 8:565, 1982.

54. Diamond, G.A., Vas, R., Forrester, J.S., Xiang, H.Z., Whiting, J., Pfaff, M., and Swan, H.J.C. The influence of bias on the subjective interpretation of cardiac angiograms. *Am. Heart J.* 103:68, 1984.

55. Nichols, A.B., Gabrieli, C.F.O., Fenoglio, J.J., Jr., and Esser, P.D. Quantification of relative coronary arterial stenosis by cinevideodensitometric analysis of coronary arteriograms. *Circulation* 69:512, 1984.

56. Spears, J.R., Sandor, T., Als, A.V., Malagold, M., Markis, J.E., Grossman, W., Serur, J.R., and Paulin, S. Computerized image analysis for quantitative measurement of vessel diameter from cineangiograms. *Circulation* 68:453, 1983.

57. Gallagher, K.P., Folts, J.D., and Rowe, G.G. Comparison of coronary arteriography with direct measurement of stenosed coronary arteries in dogs. *Am. Heart J.* 95:338, 1978.

58. Spears, J.R., Marais, H.J., Serur, J., Pomerantzeff, O., Geyer, R.P., Sipzener, R.S., Weintraub, R., Thurer, R., Paulin, S., Gerstin, R., and Grossman, W. In vivo coronary angioscopy. *J. Am. Coll. Cardiol.* 1:1311, 1983.

59. Adams, D.F., Fraser, D.B., and Abrams, H.L. The complications of coronary arteriography. *Circulation* 48:609, 1973.

60. Adams, D.F. and Abrams, H.L. The complications of coronary arteriography. *Circulation* 52 (Suppl. IV):27, 1975.

61. Davis, K., Kennedy, J.W., Kemp, H.G., Jr., Judkins, M.P., Gosselin, A.J., and Killip, T. Complications of coronary arteriography from the Collaborative Study of Coronary Artery Surgery (CASS). *Circulation* 59:1105, 1979.

62. Kennedy, J.W., Baxley, W.A., Bunnel, I.L., Gensini, G.G., Messer, J.V., Mudd, J.G., Noto, T.J., Paulin, S., Pichard, A.D., Sheldon, W.C., and Cohen, M. Mortality related to cardiac catheterization and angiography. *Cath. Cardiovasc. Diag.* 8:323, 1982.

63. Bourassa, M.G., Cantin, M., Sandborn, E.B., and Pederson, E. Scanning electron microscopy of surface irregularities and thrombogenesis of polyurethane and polyethylene coronary catheters. *Circulation* 53:992, 1976.

64. Luepker, R.V., Bouchard, R.J., Burns, R., and Warbasse, J.R. Systemic heparinization during percutaneous coronary angiography: Evaluation of effectiveness in decreasing thrombolic and embolic catheter complications. *Cath. Cardiovasc. Diag.* 1:35, 1975.

65. Roberts, R., Ludbrook, P.A., Weiss, E.S., and Sobel, B.E. Serum CPK isoenzymes after cardiac catheterization. *Br. Heart J.* 37:1144, 1975.

66. Cribier, A., Berland, J., Brunhes, G., Richard, C., and Letac, B. Acute coronary occlusion during coronary angiography in two cases: Treatment by transluminal disobliteration. *Br. Heart J.* 47:244, 1982.

67. Fierens, E. Outpatient coronary arteriography. *Cath. Cardiovasc. Diag.* 10:27, 1984.

68. Gruentzig, A.R., Senning, A., and Siegenthaler, W.E. Nonoperative dilatation of coronary artery stenosis percutaneous transluminal coronary angioplasty. *N. Engl. J. Med.* 301:61, 1979.

69. Goldberg, S., Urban, P., and Greenspon, A. Combination therapy for evolving myocardial infarction: Intracoronary thrombolysis and percutaneous transluminal angioplasty. *Am. J. Med.* 72:994, 1982.

70. Meyer, J., Merx, W., and Schmitz, H. Percutaneous transluminal coronary angioplasty immediately after intracoronary streptolysis of transmural myocardial infarction. *Circulation* 66:905, 1982.

71. Hartzler, G.O., Rutherford, B.D., and McConahay, D.R. Percutaneous transluminal coronary angioplasty with and without thrombolytic therapy for treatment of acute myocardial infarction. *Am. Heart J.* 106:965, 1983.

72. Cowley, M.J., Vetrovec, G.W., Lewis, S.A., Hirsh, P.D., and Wolfgang, T.C. Coronary angioplasty of multiple vessels: acute and long term results. Circulation 70 (suppl II):322, 1984 (abst.).

73. Holmes, D.R., Jr., Vlietstra, R.E., Reeder, G.S., Bresnahan, J.F., Smith, H.C., Bove, A.A., and Schaff, H.V. Angioplasty in total coronary artery occlusion. *J. Am. Coll. Cardiol.* 3:845, 1984.

74. Dorros, G., Cowley, M.J., Simpson, J., Bentivoglio, L.G., Block, P.C., Bourassa, M., Detre, K., Gosselin, A.J., Gruntzig, A.R., Kelsey, S.F., Kent, K.M., Mock, M.B., Mullin, S.M., Myler, R.K., Passamani, E.R., Stertzer, S.H., and Williams, D.O. Percutaneous transluminal coronary angioplasty: Report of complications from the National Heart, Lung, and Blood Institute PTCA Registry. *Circulation* 67:723, 1983.

75. DeWood, M.A., Spores, J., Notske, R., Mouser, L.T., Burroughs, R., and Mohiuddin, S. Prevalence of total coronary occlusion during the early hours of transmural myocardial infarction. *N. Engl. J. Med.* 303:897, 1980.

76. Rentrop, P., Blanke, H., Karsch, K.R., Kaiser, H., Kosterin, G.H., and Leitz, K. Selective intracoronary thrombolysis in acute myocardial infarction and unstable angina pectoris. *Circulation* 63:307, 1981.

77. Ganz, W., Buchbinder, N., Marcus, H., Mondkar, A., Maddahi, J., Charuzi, Y., O'Connor, L., Shell, W., Fishbein, W.C., Kass, R., Miyamoto, A., and Swan, H.J.C. Intracoronary thrombolysis in evolving myocardial infarction. *Am. Heart J.* 101:4, 1981.

78. Mathey, D.G., Kuck, K.H., Tilsner, V., Krebber, H.J., and Bleifeld, W. Nonsurgical coronary artery recanalization in acute transmural myocardial infarction. *Circulation* 63:489, 1981.

79. Spann, J.F., Sherry, S., Carabello, B.A., Denenberg, B.S., Mann, R.H., McCann, W.D., Gault, J.H., Gentzler, R.D., Belber, A.D., Maurer, A.H., and Cooper, E.M. Coronary thrombolysis by intravenous streptokinase in acute myocardial infarction: Acute and follow-up studies. *Am. J. Cardiol.* 53:655, 1984.

80. Anderson, J.L., Marshall, H.W., Bray, B.E., Lutz, J.R., Frederick, P.R., Yanowitz, F.G., Datz, F.L., Klausner, S.C., and Hagan, A.D. A randomized trial of intracoronary streptokinase in the treatment of acute myocardial infarction. *N. Engl. J. Med.* 308:1312, 1983.

81. Khaja, F., Walton, J.A., Brymer, J.F., Lo, E., Osterberger, L., O'Neill, W.W., Coffer, H.T., Weiss, R., Lee, T., Kurian, T., Goldberg, A.D., Pitt, B., and Goldstein, S. Intracoronary fibrinolytic therapy in acute myocardial infarction: Report of a prospective randomized trial. *N. Engl. J. Med.* 308:1305, 1983.

82. Kennedy, J.W., Ritchie, J.L., and Davies, K.B. Western Washington randomized trial of in-

tracoronary streptokinase in acute myocardial infarction. *N. Engl. J. Med.* 309:477, 1983.

83. Goldberg, S., Greenspon, A., and Urban, P. Reperfusion arrhythmia: A marker of restoration of antegrade flow during intracoronary thrombolysis in acute myocardial infarction. *Am. Heart J.* 105:26, 1983.

84. Goldberg, S., Urban, P., and Greenspon, A. Limitation of infarct size with thrombolytic agents: Electrocardiographic indices. *Circulation* 68 (suppl. I):71, 1983.

85. Urban, P., Cowley, M., and Goldberg, S. Clinical course after myocardial reperfusion during myocardial infarction. *Circulation* 68 (suppl. III):210, 1983 (Abstr.).

86. Goldberg, S., Urban, P., and Greenspon, A. Combination therapy for evolving myocardial infarction: Intracoronary thrombolysis and percutaneous transluminal angioplasty. *Am. J. Med.* 72:994, 1982.

87. Meyer, J., Merx, W., and Schmitz, H. Percutaneous transluminal coronary angioplasty immediatley after intracoronary streptolysis of transmural myocardial infarction. *Circulation* 66:905, 1982.

88. Harzler, G.O., Rutherford, B.D., McConahay, D.R., Johnson, W.L., Jr., McCallister, B.R., Gura, G.M., Jr., Lonn, R.C., and Crockett, J.E. Percutaneous transluminal coronary angioplasty with and without thrombolytic therapy for treatment of acute myocardial infarction. *Am. Heart J.* 106:965, 1983.

89. VandeWerf, F., Ludbrook, P.A., Bergmann, S.R., Tiefenbrunn, A.J., Fox, K.A.A., DeGeest, H., Verstraete, M., Collen, D., and Sobel, B.E. Coronary thrombolysis with tissue-type plasminogen activator in patients with evolving myocardial infarction. *N. Engl. J. Med.* 310:609, 1984.

90. Greenspon, A., Weitz, H., and Goldberg, S. Variant angina with coronary thrombus-beneficial effects of early intervention. *Circulation* 68(suppl III):142, 1983.

# 10. DIAGNOSIS OF ACUTE MYOCARDIAL INFARCTION

## Joseph S. Alpert

The first clinical description of a nonfatal myocardial infarction was made in 1910 by two Russian physicians, V.P. Obraztsov and N.S. Strazhesko [1]. Two years later, in the United States, James B. Herrick made similar observations [2]. Herrick was careful to cite the earlier work of the two Russian physicians, which he had read in German translation. The importance of the work of these three authors was that it demonstrated for the first time that coronary arterial occlusion could result in myocardial infarction without necessarily causing the immediate demise of the patient. Coronary thrombi were well known to pathologists at that time, but they were felt to produce either sudden death or no symptoms whatsoever [1].

Until recently, the diagnosis of acute myocardial infarction (AMI) was made on the basis of history and physical examination alone. Such clinical information, later supplemented by certain specific electrocardiographic (ECG) patterns, provided the only means by which this entity was recognized. A modest fever was also known to occur in patients who had sustained an AMI.

The first laboratory tests that were employed to confirm the diagnosis of AMI were determinations of the elevations of the sedimentation rate and the white blood cell count. Recently, a number of other blood tests have been devised that are more specific for myocardial necrosis than these tests. Characteristic elevations of the serum levels of a number of myocardial enzymes have been shown to occur in patients with AMI.

Indeed, highly sensitive assays for some of these substances enable the physician to detect minute quantities of infarcted myocardium. The development of such biochemical tests has resulted in increased reliability in the diagnosis of AMI. Thus, AMI is recognized today in patients who formerly might have been thought to have suffered only an episode of angina pectoris.

The changing sensitivity in the diagnosis of AMI is depicted in figure 10–1. This figure presents a hypothetical graph of the clinical spectrum of all patients with coronary artery disease. At the far left of the bell-shaped population curve are those patients who are asymptomatic despite some degree of coronary arterial stenosis. As one moves along the abscissa horizontally and to the right along the curve, patients manifest increasingly severe clinical syndromes of coronary artery disease: angina pectoris, myocardial infarction, and, eventually, cardiogenic shock secondary to AMI. In a considerable number of patients with myocardial infarction, the diagnosis can be made on the basis of history, physical examination, and ECG changes alone (area A of figure 10–1). In many patients with smaller quantities of infarcted myocardium, the infarction may not be recognized because the diagnostic tools employed (i.e., history, physical examination, and ECG) are only moderately sensitive. Individuals who fall on the curve within area B had the diagnosis of AMI made on the basis of serum enzyme abormalities despite a nondiagnostic history, physical examination, and ECG. All patients who lie on the curve to the left of area B are usually said to have had an anginal episode. Some of these individuals, however, have been falsely diagnosed, since small

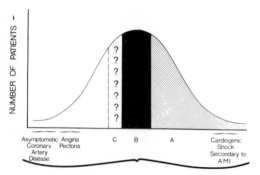

FIGURE 10–1. Hypothetical representation of the population of individuals with coronary artery disease. Along the abscissa are increasingly severe clinical manifestations of coronary heart disease, beginning with asymptomatic coronary atherosclerosis and ending with cardiogenic shock secondary to myocardial infarction. Area A represents individuals with myocardial infarction in whom the clinical presentation is so obvious that the diagnosis can be made with minimal ancillary laboratory information. Area B represents patients with myocardial infarction in whom the clinical findings are more subtle; in this group, ancillary laboratory tests are often required to establish the diagnosis. Area C consists of individuals who, according to our present technology, are felt not to have sustained a myocardial infarction. The question marks imply that individuals in group C have indeed sustained a minor episode of myocardial necrosis.

quantities of their myocardium did, in fact, undergo necrosis.

If a more sophisticated diagnostic technique is employed in evaluating our hypothetical population of patients with suspected AMI, a number of individuals are identified in whom myocardial necrosis has occurred but in whom the diagnosis was not made before the more sophisticated diagnostic modality was employed. The latter patients—that is, those for whom the diagnosis of AMI depends on sophisticated diagnostic technology such as serum enzyme determination—are represented by area B in figure 10–1.

Finally, there are probably still some patients who, according to current diagnostic techniques, are said not to have sustained a myocardial infarction, but in whom a small region of myocardial necrosis did in fact occur (area C of figure 10–1). This last group of patients may be demonstrated to have minor myocardial necrosis

with diagnostic techniques that might be developed in the future.

The hypothetical presentation in figure 10–1 carries an important message: the number of patients in whom myocardial necrosis can be documented is directly proportional to the sensitivity of the diagnostic procedure used to confirm the diagnosis. Much of the recent controversy surrounding diagnosis and treatment of patients with AMI centers on the abilities of particular laboratory tests to confirm the diagnosis of AMI. In some individuals, myocardial infarction may occur without any physical findings or ECG abnormalities whatsoever. The recognition of myocardial necrosis in such individuals depends entirely on various diagnostic laboratory techniques. From this discussion, it can be seen that the sensitivity of the clinician in diagnosing myocardial infarction depends, at least in part, on the sensitivity of various laboratory measurements. Controversies involving the diagnosis of AMI have centered in recent years on these different techniques and their relative merits for increasing diagnostic sensitivity in patients suspected of having AMI. Specifically, clinicians have discussed the role of various precipitating historical factors in initiating AMI, the value of the physical examination in patients with AMI, the relative merits of different blood tests in the diagnosis of AMI, the relative roles of the scalar and vector ECG in the diagnosis of AMI, discrepancies between chest roentgenographic findings and the clinical status of patients with infarction, and the role of cardiac nuclear techniques in the diagnosis of AMI.

With this background in mind, the review of the specific clinical and diagnostic information that leads to the diagnosis of AMI is appropriate. Emphasis will be placed on areas of controversy in which active research is ongoing and conclusions are therefore still tentative.

## Clinical History

### CONTROVERSY SURROUNDING PRECIPITATING FACTORS

In many individuals with AMI, no precipitating factor can be identified. Phipps [3] reported the following patient activities occurring at the onset of acute myocardial infarction: physical exercise in 13 percent, modest or usual exertion in 18 percent, surgical procedure in 6 percent, rest in 51 percent, and sleep in 8 percent. Conversely, other investigators have reported that a significant number of myocardial infarctions occur within a few hours of severe physical exertion [4–7]. Indeed, Fitzhugh and Hamilton [5] pointed out that patients with AMI often performed severe exertion shortly before their infarction and that this exertion occurred at times when the patient was unduly fatigued or emotionally stressed. Thus, heavy exercise would seem to play a role in precipitating myocardial infarction in some patients. Presumably, such infarctions are the result of marked increases in myocardial oxygen consumption in the face of severe coronary arterial narrowing. Supporting this hypothesis is the finding that fatal myocardial infarction during exertion is often associated with extensive coronary arterial narrowing but no occlusion [7].

Some authorities feel that emotional strain may be a precipitating factor in the initiation of acute myocardial infarction [8, 9]; it has even been suggested that severe emotional strain precedes almost all episodes of infarction [8]. A number of reports have documented that upsetting life events are not uncommon in the lives of patients who subsequently suffer a myocardial infarction [10–13]. It must be borne in mind when evaluating such studies that many of these investigations are retrospective in design and frequently lacking in proper controls. In addition, the effect of emotional strain varies from individual to individual. Thus, the exact role that emotional stress plays in precipitating myocardial infarction is still unclear.

Operations and acute blood loss from gastrointestinal or other hemorrhages are frequent precursors to myocardial infarction [14]. Reduced myocardial perfusion secondary to hypovolemia and increased myocardial oxygen demand secondary to fever, tachycardia, and agitation probably lead to such infarctions. Other factors that predispose to myocardial infarction include infections of the respiratory tract, insulin-induced hypoglycemia, high altitude, the administration of various ergot preparations, serum sickness, allergy, and even wasp stings

[15–18]. Negative correlations between cirrhosis of the liver and myocardial infarction have been reported [19, 20]. Although widely held to be true, no correlation between weather conditions and the occurrence of myocardial infarction has been demonstrated.

Recent controversy has surrounded the possibility that coronary spasm plays an important role in the genesis of coronary thrombosis, which, in turn, is known to be a major factor in the pathogenesis of acute myocardial infarction [21]. Many of the above-mentioned factors, i.e., stress, allergic reactions, drugs, etc., might precipitate coronary thrombosis and hence myocardial infarction by causing coronary arterial spasm. In fact, an episode of coronary spasm may be the precipitating factor for coronary thrombosis and subsequent AMI in most patients who develop a myocardial infarct [21].

## PAIN PATTERNS IN ACUTE MYOCARDIAL INFARCTION

The pain of acute myocardial infarction is variable in intensity. Indeed, 20 to 25 percent of infarcts are unrecognized, either because the patient is able to ignore the discomfort or because it is absent altogether. In most patients, however, the pain of AMI is severe and unrelenting. Between 10 and 50 percent of patients with myocardial infarction give a history of prodromal symptoms [22]. This prodrome is usually a mild chest discomfort resembling angina pectoris. In some individuals, however, the prodrome is an unusual sense of severe fatigue. In patients with preexisting stable angina, a period of unstable or accelerating angina may precede the AMI.

The pain of myocardial infarction is usually prolonged, lasting for more than 30 minutes and frequently for a number of hours. The pain is most severe in the region of the sternum, the precordium, or the epigastrium, and it is characterized as constricting, crushing, oppressing, or compressing. Often, patients complain of something sitting on or squeezing the chest. The pain frequently becomes intolerable because of its unrelenting nature. Although the pain is usually described in textbooks as squeezing, choking, viselike, or heavy, it may also be stabbing, knifelike, boring, or burning in nature.

The discomfort of AMI is usually retrosternal

in location, spreading frequently to both sides of the anterior chest, with a predilection for the left side. The discomfort may begin in the epigastrium and simulate abdominal disorders, a symptom that often caused AMI to be diagnosed as acute indigestion in the recent past. The discomfort frequently radiates to the shoulders, upper extremities, neck, jaw, and interscapular region, again favoring the left side. Occasional patients describe the pain as radiating down the inner aspect of the left arm and producing a tingling sensation in the left wrist, hand, and even fingers. In many patients, the site of AMI is a "carbon copy" of the anginal discomfort, only the sensation is more intense [23].

Pericarditis may produce pain as early as the first day after myocardial infarction. Usually, the discomfort of pericarditis is worse during a deep inspiration. It may be relieved in the upright position, particularly if the patient leans forward. Of course, pericarditis occurs only in patients with transmural infarction. The pain of pericarditis is frequently mistaken for the discomfort of postinfarction angina, a syndrome that is disconcerting to patient and physician alike. In a few patients, postinfarction angina may be refractory to therapeutic attempts. Minimal activity, meals, or emotional upset can precipitate this form of unstable angina.

It has been routine clinical teaching that pulmonary hypertension can cause pain resembling that of angina pectoris or myocardial infarction. A recent examination of a large number of patients with pulmonary hypertension of varying severity has demonstrated no difference in the frequency of chest pain between groups of patients with pulmonary hypertension and individuals with normal pulmonary pressure [24]. Thus, it would appear that chest pain in patients with pulmonary hypertension is unrelated to their cardiac disease [24].

## Physical Examination

Patients with acute myocardial infarction appear to be in significant distress. Anguished facial expressions are common, particularly if the pain is persistent. These patients are frequently restless, in sharp distinction to individuals with angina pectoris, who lie quite still, aware that all forms

of activity increase their discomfort. Patients frequently massage or clutch their chests, and the discomfort may be described with a clenched fist held against the sternum, a sign popularized by Dr. Samuel A. Levine. Cold perspiration and skin pallor may be evident.

Blood pressure usually falls acutely after AMI. Some individuals, however, demonstrate a hypertensive response secondary either to pain and agitation or to a neural reflex. As healing occurs, the blood pressure tends to increase and returns to preinfarction levels. Following AMI, previously hypertensive patients often become normotensive without treatment. Patients in shock have systolic blood pressures below 90 mmHg. Individuals with inferior or posterior infarctions, however, may also have systolic blood pressures in the range of 80 to 90 mmHg, a result of the bradycardia-hypotension reflex [25–29]. Such patients demonstrate none of the peripheral manifestations of shock (cold, clammy skin, oliguria, or confusion), and their prognosis is good. Eventually, hypotension resolves in such individuals.

## CONTROVERSIES SURROUNDING PHYSICAL FINDINGS IN ACUTE MYOCARDIAL INFARCTION

It is often stated that the physical examination is not particularly remarkable in patients with AMI. This is occasionally true, but individuals with AMI usually demonstrate a number of physical findings of considerable therapeutic and prognostic significance [30, 31].

Pulsus paradoxus is probably present in patients with AMI more frequently than had been supposed in the past. It is probably the result of right ventricular infarction or marked myocardial stiffness secondary to ischemia and infarction, with resultant imbalance in blood volume distribution during inspiration [32, 33].

Palpation of the carotid pulse gives the examiner an idea of the left ventricular stroke volume: a full pulse implies a larger stroke volume than does a small pulse. Jugular venous pressure is normal in many individuals with AMI, even in the face of left ventricular failure. Jugular venous distention is usually a sign of right ventricular infarction, which occurs on occasion in patients with inferior or posterior left ventricular infarcts

[33]. There may be marked "c–v" waves in the jugular venous pulse of such individuals, and a murmur of tricuspid insufficiency that increases during inspiration may be heard [33].

Chest findings in patients with acute myocardial infarction reflect the presence or absence of left ventricular failure. Moist rales are audible in individuals who develop left ventricular failure after infarction. The prognosis in myocardial infarction is related in part to the percentage of the lung fields over which rales are heard [34]. Wheezing, diffuse bronchial ronchi and poor movement of air may also be present in patients with severe left ventricular failure. This picture mimics that of bronchial asthma and can be quite confusing. Cough with hemoptysis, resembling pulmonary embolism with infarction, can also occur in patients with left ventricular failure following myocardial infarction.

The findings on palpation of the precordium may be normal, but an abnormal pulsation in the region of ECG leads $V_2$ and $V_3$ is often present in patients with anterior infarction. This abnormal precordial impulse is paradoxical and is often clearly separable from the point of maximum impulse (PMI) [30, 31]. In some individuals the abnormal impulse may consist of a diffuse, rippling precordial movement that is approximately 5 to 10 cm in diameter and without discrete PMI.

Heart sounds are frequently quiet in acute myocardial infarction; occasionally they are almost inaudible. The quality of resonance of $S_1$ is abnormal in patients with AMI, with a lowering of the frequency content [35, 36]. As healing occurs, the intensity of the heart sounds increases. Paradoxical splitting of the second heart sound ($S_2$) may occur in acute myocardial infarction, but this finding is not as common as once reported [35].

Systolic murmurs, transient or persistent, are often heard in patients with AMI. Most of these represent mitral regurgitation secondary to papillary muscle dysfunction. Aortic stenosis can also cause ischemic chest pain, however. Aortic stenosis occurs in the same population in which coronary artery disease is common. Therefore, the diagnosis of aortic stenosis should be borne in mind when one notes a systolic murmur in a patient suspected of having had a myocardial infarction. Rarely, diastolic murmurs are produced by blood flowing through a severe coronary arterial stenosis.

Fourth heart sounds are almost universally present in patients with AMI. They reflect modest changes in left ventricular compliance. These same changes in left ventricular stiffness can result in elevation of left ventricular end-diastolic pressure in individuals with ischemic heart disease, even in the absence of heart failure. Unfortunately, fourth heart sounds occur frequently in apparently normal, older individuals [37]. Considerable controversy has surrounded the question of the significance of fourth heart sounds (see chapter 4). Since they are almost always audible in patients with AMI, the absence of a fourth heart sound in an alleged infarction patient in sinus rhythm should lead to a careful review of the diagnosis. On the other hand, the fact that fourth heart sounds are common in healthy, older persons should make one wary of diagnosing significant cardiac disease on the basis of this finding alone.

Third heart sounds reflect left ventricular compliance changes of greater magnitude than those occurring with fourth sounds. Thus, third heart sounds occur in individuals who have sustained extensive myocardial necrosis. Third heart sounds occur more commonly after anterior infarction than after inferior or nontransmural infarction [38]. The mortality of individuals who manifest an $S_3$ during the acute phase of myocardial infarction is 40 percent, compared with 15 percent for patients without a third heart sound [38].

Pericardial rubs occur in as many as 20 percent of patients with acute myocardial infarction [39]. Rubs are notorious for their evanescence, and hence they may occur more commonly. Frequent auscultation in patients with transmural infarction often results in the discovery of a rub that would have gone unnoticed with less persistence. Rubs may be heard soon after the onset of infarction. More commonly, however, they are noted during the second or third day after the infarction. After an extensive infarction, a loud, persistent rub may be heard for many days. Delayed onset of the rub (and of the associated discomfort or pericarditis) is characteristic of the so-called postinfarction (Dressler's) syndrome or postinfarction pericarditis [40–42]. Acute pericarditis, however, may occur late, and the postmyocardial infarction syndrome may occur early. The clinical presentation of these two entities often blends, making it impossible on occasion to discriminate between them.

Pericardial rubs are best heard along the left sternal border or just inside the PMI. Loud rubs may be audible over the entire precordium and even over the back. Occasionally, only the systolic portion of the rub is heard. This may cause confusion, and the diagnosis of ventricular septal rupture or mitral regurgitation may be entertained. Pericarditis and its accompanying rub may be heard after either anterior or inferoposterior infarction. Significant pericardial effusion can occur, particularly in patients receiving anticoagulants. Pericardial rubs may still be heard in individuals with significant pericardial effusion.

## Laboratory Examinations

An increase in the white blood cell count usually occurs after AMI. This elevation may develop within 2 hours of the onset of chest pain. Leukocytosis recedes after a few days and returns to normal within a week after the infarction. The white count varies between 12,000 and 15,000/mm$^3$, occasionally rising as high as 20,000/mm$^3$. There is often an increase in the percentage of polymorphonuclear leukocytes.

The sedimentation rate is also increased following AMI. The sedimentation rate is usually normal for the first few days after infarction, even though fever and leukocytosis are present. The sedimentation rate then rises, peaks on day 4 or 5, and remains elevated for several weeks or more. The increase in the sedimentation rate is secondary to elevated plasma $\alpha_2$-globulin and fibrinogen levels. The extent of elevation of the sedimentation rate does not seem to correlate with the size of the infarction or its prognosis.

### ENZYMATIC DETERMINATIONS

Dying myocardial cells release a number of enzymes into the circulation, and the blood levels of these enzymes can be measured by specific chemical reactions. Determinations of serum activity of creatine phosphokinase (CK), serum glutamic-oxaloacetic transaminase (SGOT), and lactic dehydrogenase (LDH) have become standard criteria in the laboratory diagnosis of myocardial infarction. Although only one of these enzymes need be measured to establish the diagnosis of infarction, most hospitals measure two or three.

Serum glutamic-oxaloacetic transaminase activity exceeds the normal range within 8 to 12 hours following the onset of chest discomfort. Peak SGOT levels occur 18 to 36 hours after infarction, falling to normal within 3 to 4 days. Elevated SGOT activity has been found in 97 percent of 119 autopsy-proved cases of myocardial infarction [43]. False-positive elevations in SGOT occur in patients with primary liver disease, hepatic congestion, skeletal muscle disease, shock, perimyocarditis, pulmonary embolism, and intramuscular injections [44].

Serum lactic dehydrogenase activity exceeds the normal range within 24 to 48 hours after the onset of myocardial infarction. Peak LDH values occur 3 to 6 days after myocardial infarction, falling to normal at 8 to 14 days after infarction. True-positive elevations in serum LDH activity were noted in 86 percent of 282 patients with the clinical diagnosis of myocardial infarction and in 100 percent of 39 patients with autopsy-proved infarction [43]. False-positive elevations of LDH activity occur in patients with hemolysis, megaloblastic anemia, leukemia, liver disease, hepatic congestion, renal disease, neoplasms, pulmonary embolism, myocarditis, skeletal muscle disease, and shock [44].

LDH has five isoenzymes. Fractionation of serum LDH into its five isoenzymes has been said to increase the diagnostic accuracy in AMI. The five LDH isoenzymes are named in order of the rapidity of their migration toward the anode on electrophoresis; thus, $LDH_1$ moves the fastest and $LDH_5$ the slowest. The heart contains mainly $LDH_1$, whereas liver and skeletal muscle contain mostly $LDH_4$ and $LDH_5$. Increased serum $LDH_1$ activity precedes the elevation in serum total LDH and is usually present in the first blood sample taken from a patient with AMI. The true-positive elevations in $LDH_1$ occur in more than 95 percent of patients with myocardial infarction [44]. $LDH_5$ is commonly elevated in patients with congestive heart failure. Unfortunately, hemolysis can also result in elevated serum $LDH_1$ activity. Most conditions that cause elevated serum total LDH activity (e.g., liver and skeletal muscle disease or injury) can be distinguished from AMI by LDH isoenzyme analysis. Serum activity of $\alpha$-hydroxybutyric dehydrogenase (HBD) is often reported in patients with acute myocardial infarction. HBD should not be called a specific enzyme, however, because its measurement is actually a reflection of $LDH_1$ activity.

Creatine phosphokinase (CK) is an enzyme that is said to be particularly specific for the heart. Typically, serum CK activity exceeds the normal range within 6 to 8 hours following the onset of infarction, peaks at about 24 hours, and declines to normal within 3 to 4 days after the onset of chest pain [44]. Females have lower normal CK values than males by about one-third. Before 1972, the elevation of serum CK seemed to be the most sensitive enzymatic criterion of AMI [43–48]. Unfortunately, 15 percent false-positive results occurred in patients with muscle disease, alcohol intoxication, diabetes mellitus, convulsion, and intramuscular injection [44]. Serum CK activity is normal in patients with congestive heart failure, but it may be elevated following pulmonary embolism [44]. Perimyocarditis and skeletal muscle or heart trauma can also result in elevated serum CK. Vigorous exercise may also produce increased serum CK levels.

Three isoenzymes of CK—MM, BB, and MB —have been identified by electrophoresis. Extracts of brain and kidney contain predominantly the BB isoenzyme, whereas skeletal muscle contains mostly MM. Heart muscle contains both MM and MB isoenzymes. MB-CK isoenzyme is also present in modest quantities in the small intestine, tongue, and diaphragm [48, 49]. Despite these small amounts of MB-CK isoenzyme in tissues other than heart, elevated serum activity of MB-CK is almost invariably secondary to AMI. Thus, the measurement of serum MB-CK isoenzyme is said to be the most sensitive and specific serum test for acute myocardial infarction (table 10–1). However, other forms of injury to the myocardium (e.g., myocarditis, trauma, and cardiac surgery) can result in elevated serum MB-CK activity [49–57] and so can

vigorous exercise in professional athletes [58]. Cardiac catheterization does not result in increased activity *unless* an infarction has occurred during the procedure [59]. Techniques for measurement of serum MB-CK levels by radioimmunoassay have been developed [60], which should increase the accuracy and availability of this highly sensitive and specific test.

The isoenzyme MB-CK is considerably more sensitive and specific for the diagnosis of AMI than total CK. Heller and co-workers have demonstrated that patients with elevated serum MB-CK and normal serum total CK represent part of the spectrum of nontransmural myocardial infarction with definite myocardial necrosis [61].

Considerable effort has been expended in order to find a simple, convenient method for measuring the size of a particular myocardial infarct. Besides its relation to prognosis, a convenient measure of infarct size would enable the clinician to test various therapeutic regimens aimed at salvaging acutely ischemic myocardium. One method that has been suggested for quantitating infarct size is to determine the accumulated release of MB-CPK [62]. In this technique, frequent serum determinations of MB-CK are made during the initial days following acute myocardial infarction. The area under the appearance-disappearance curve for serum MB-CK appears to correlate with infarct size. This technique, not without its problems, is discussed further in chapter 13.

OTHER SEROLOGIC TESTS
Release of myoglobin into the circulation from dying myocardial cells can be demonstrated within a few hours after the onset of infarction. Peak levels of serum myoglobin occur earlier than peak values of serum CK [63]. The time of the earliest myoglobin appearance in the serum, its peak level, and the duration of detectable myoglobin release all correlate poorly with these same parameters for serum CK and with clinical estimates of the severity of AMI [63, 64]. Myoglobin seems to appear in the serum in multiple, short bursts that last for an hour or two. This pattern of myoglobin release suggests that myocardial infarction may be occurring in a series of short episodes, rather than as a unified,

TABLE 10–1. Creatine phosphokinase MB isoenzyme versus levels of other serum enzymes in the diagnosis of AMI

| Patient history and ECG findings | Percent with elevated SGOT | Percent with elevated LDH | Percent with elevated total CK | Percent with elevated MB-CK isoenzyme |
|---|---|---|---|---|
| Acute transmural MI | 94 | 100 | 94 | 100 |
| History suggestive of MI and persistent ST-T ECG changes lasting more than 25 hours | 63 | 71 | 70 | 84 |
| History suggestive of MI and elevated SGOT or LDH, but ECG changes nondiagnostic | 80 | 100 | 72 | 100 |

Source: Rapaport, E. *Mod. Concepts Cardiovasc. Dis.* 46:43, 1977, by permission of the American Heart Association, Inc.

single episode of infarction. Myoglobin can also be detected in the serum following damage to skeletal muscle [64].

Alterations in serum concentrations of various trace metals have been reported in patients with AMI. Vallee [65] reported elevations in serum copper concentration in infarction patients that seemed to parallel elevations in the sedimentation rate. Wacker and co-workers [66] observed significant decreases in serum zinc concentration following AMI. The fall in serum zinc levels occurs within 1 day after infarction and is maintained for as long as 2 weeks before returning to the normal range.

WHICH TEST IS MOST SENSITIVE IN THE DIAGNOSIS OF AMI?
Although experience is limited in the measurement of serum myoglobin, nickel, zinc, and copper concentrations in patients with AMI, it appears unlikely that such tests will supplant the measurement of serum MB-CK as the most sensitive diagnostic test for infarcted myocardium. Serum MB-CK levels become elevated following the infarction of as little as 1 gram of myocardium. Since this test is reasonably specific for myocardial injury and readily available to most hospitals, it appears to be the best laboratory determination at present. A promising new test measures serum levels of cardiac myosin light chains [67].

*Electrocardiography*

In the majority of patients with AMI, changes can be documented in serial ECG tracings ob-

tained at least every 12 to 24 hours for 48 to 72 hours after the onset of chest discomfort. Early tracings taken soon after the onset of ischemic discomfort may be within normal limits. Of course, such normal tracings do not rule out the diagnosis of AMI, which may still be confirmed by later ECGs. The earliest abnormalities seen on the ECG of infarction patients are confined to the ST and T segments and are often seen in ECGs obtained during the first few hours after the infarction. Thereafter, significant Q-waves (.04 second or longer in duration and 25 percent or more of the height of the subsequent R-wave), loss of R-wave voltage, or both occur (see figure 13–3). Over hours to days, the T-waves in the affected leads become inverted, and the ST segment returns to (or near to) the baseline.

CONTROVERSIES SURROUNDING THE ECG IN THE DIAGNOSIS OF THE AMI
Many factors limit the ability to use the ECG to diagnose and localize myocardial infarction: the extent of myocardial injury, age of the infarct, site of the infarct, presence of conduction defects, presence of the Wolff-Parkinson-White syndrome, occurrence of previous infarction, and administration of drugs. It is therefore surprising that ECG changes develop with most infarctions found at autopsy.

*Silent Infarctions.* More than 25 percent of electrocardiographically recognized infarctions are discovered first on a routine ECG [68]. In such patients with previously unrecognized infarction, approximately 50 percent give a history of symptoms occurring in the past that are compatible with acute infarction. The other 50 percent of patients, however, have truly silent, asymptomatic infarction. Unrecognized infarction is uncommon in patients with prior angina pectoris; it is more common in individuals with prior diabetes or hypertension. The mechanism of silent infarction is unknown.

*Transmural Versus Nontransmural Myocardial Infarction.* Earlier, widely accepted criteria for the diagnosis of so-called transmural infarction [69] are given in table 10–2. Figure 2–14 depicts so-called anterior and inferolateral infarction and figure 10–2 depicts a posterior infarct. The term *nontransmural infarction* is used to identify individuals with myocardial infarction by history and serum enzyme analysis whose

ECG demonstrates only ST and T-wave changes. Some infarctions produce no ECG change whatsoever.

Electrocardiographic diagnosis of small myocardial infarctions is frequently difficult because ECG evidence of such infarction is often limited to ST segment depression, T-wave inversion, or both. Similar ST segment and T-wave changes can occur in stable or unstable angina pectoris, hyperthyroidism, hyperinsulinism, electrolyte imbalance, shock, and metabolic disorders, as well as following administration of digitalis glycosides [69]. Serial ECGs can be of help in determining whether infarction has occurred: transient changes favor angina whereas persistent changes argue for infarction, provided other causes of ST-T changes have been eliminated. In the final analysis, the diagnosis

TABLE 10–2. Electrocardiographic criteria for localization of Q-wave (transmural) myocardial infarction

ANTERIOR INFARCTION.
1. Anteroseptal infarction:
    A. QS pattern in leads $V_1$, $V_2$, and $V_{3R}$ if taken
    B. Absence of initial Q-waves in $V_5$ and $V_6$
    C. ST elevation and T-wave changes may occur in other leads

2. Anterior or anteroapical infarction:
    A. Initial R-wave maintained in $V_1$, $V_2$, or $V_{3R}$
    B. Appearance of abnormal Q-wave in one or more of leads $V_2$, $V_3$, or $V_4$; alternatively, a decrease in the R-waves without their disappearance in precordial leads $V_5$ through $V_6$.
    C. No abnormal Q-waves in $V_5$, $V_6$, aVL, I, II, III

3. Anterolateral infarction: Abnormal Q-waves in $V_5$ and $V_6$ or in $V_4$, $V_5$, and $V_6$ as well as in leads aVL and I

4. Extensive anterior infarction:
    A. A combination of the findings of 1, 2, and 3
    B. Q-waves are usually present in all precordial leads (except occasionally $V_1$) in lead aVL, and in lead I

5. High anterolateral or high lateral infarction:
    A. Abnormal Q-waves in leads I and aVL
    B. No changes in precordial leads; occasionally, $V_5$ and $V_6$ show minor changes
    C. Leads over the upper left anterior chest, extending into the upper axilla and one or two interspaces above standard leads $V_4$, $V_5$, and $V_6$ may show abnormal Q-waves along with characteristic ST and T changes

INFEROPOSTERIOR INFARCTION.
6. Inferior or diaphragmatic infarction: Appearance of abnormal Q-waves along with characteristic ST and T-wave changes in leads II, III, and aVF or in leads III and aVF

7. Inferolateral infarction: Same criteria as in $V_1$ plus abnormal Q-waves in leads $V_6$, $V_7$, or both and sometimes in leads I, aVL, and $V_5$.

8. Posterior infarction: Appearance of an RSR pattern or a tall, slurred, wide R-wave with an R/S ratio equal to or greater than 1.0 in leads $V_1$, $V_{3R}$, or both

9. Posterolateral infarction: Same criteria as in 8 plus abnormal Q-waves in leads $V_6$, $V_7$, or both and sometimes in leads, I, aVL, and $V_5$.

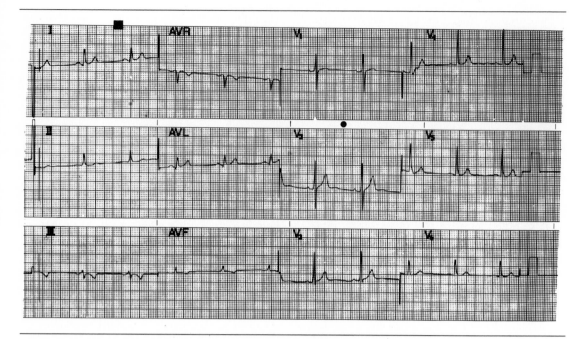

FIGURE 10–2. Electrocardiogram in posterior myocardial infarction. Note the upright T-wave in lead $V_1$, the prominent R-waves in leads $V_1$ and $V_2$, and the flipped T-waves in inferior leads III and AVF.

of such small infarcts must rest on clinical data and laboratory tests rather than on the ECG criteria.

The localization of infarction by ECG has traditionally been employed as though it were quite accurate. In fact, recent work has demonstrated that ECG localization of infarction is accurate only to the extent that infarction can be localized to either the anterior or posterior wall of the left ventricle. Thus, in table 10–2, anteroseptal, anterior, anteroapical, anterolateral, and lateral infarcts occur in the anterior left ventricular wall but are *not* necessarily localized to that region of the anterior wall identified electrocardiographically. This is especially true of the apical infarct [70]. Similarly, inferior, diaphragmatic, posterior, posterolateral, and inferolateral infarcts are noted at postmortem examination to be located in the posterior wall of the left ventricle but *not* necessarily in that subdivision of the posterior wall identified by the ECG. Thus, it is anatomically accurate to identify ECG patterns of infarction only as either anterior or posterior in location. Whether QRS "scoring systems" can aid in this localization is under study [71].

The designations *transmural* (Q-waves or loss of R-waves) and *nontransmural* are also inaccu-

rate in that extensive evidence has been marshaled that demonstrates pathological transmural infarction in the face of only ST and T changes in the ECG and vice-versa [72]. The electrocardiographic findings are so nonspecific with respect to pathological findings that the terms transmural and nontransmural are misnomers. Spodick [72] suggests that the preferable ECG terminology should be Q-wave and non-Q-wave or S-T infarction, since there are a number of clinical, pathological, and prognostic differences between patients with Q-wave infarcts and those with S-T infarctions.

It was once thought that patients with myocardial infarction who manifested only ST and T-wave changes (S-T infarction) demonstrated a more benign clinical course than individuals with Q-waves or loss of R-wave (Q-wave infarction) on the ECG. Recent work has shown that individuals with S-T infarctions have the same extent of coronary atherosclerosis as do patients with Q-wave infarctions [73–75]. Moreover, the long-term prognosis is the same for these two groups of patients [73–75]. An unusual ECG pattern consisting of precordial ST-segment elevation, marked increase in precordial R-wave amplitude with loss of S-waves, and merging of QRS complexes with elevated ST segments has been noted in selected patients, all of whom previously or subsequently developed ventricular fibrillation [76].

*The ECG After the Acute Event. Infarct extension* is often mentioned in the differential diagnosis of chest pain that develops after myocardial infarction. Electrocardiographic mapping of the precordium and serial serum CK determinations have demonstrated that silent extension of infarction may occur in as many as 57 percent of patients with AMI [77]. Symptomatic extension, however, is commonly associated with new ST segment depression or elevation on the routine 12-lead ECG tracing.

*Persistent ST elevation* may also indicate pericarditis or aneurysm formation. Mills and co-workers [78] studied patients with persistent ST segment elevation following AMI. They observed that individuals in whom ST segment elevation persisted for 3 weeks or more invariably had left ventricular aneurysms or extensive scars when subsequently studied by ventriculography [78]. Such persistent ST elevation is *not* the result of continuing ischemia in the peri-infarction zone [79].

Most patients continue to demonstrate the ECG changes from an infarction for the rest of their lives. Occasionally, the ECG changes of acute myocardial infarction disappear, and the tracings appear normal [80]. Resolution of ECG changes can occur in rare instances within the first week after infarction [81].

Precordial ST-segment depression in patients with inferior or posterior Q-wave infarction has been said to reflect associated anterior wall ischemia resulting from a high-grade stenotic lesion of the left anterior descending coronary artery. Multiple investigations have demonstrated that in most instances this is *not* the case. Precordial ST segment depression in patients with inferior/posterior infarction is usually the result of either reciprocal ECG changes, or left ventricular dysfunction secondary to extensive inferior/posterior wall infarction, rather than concomitant anterior wall ischemia [82–85].

*Right Ventricular and Atrial Infarctions.* Right ventricular infarction may be difficult to identify on the ECG because the right ventricular myocardial mass is small in comparison to that of the left ventricle. Recently, however, right ventricular infarction has been identified electrocardiographically. Elevation of ST segments in right precordial leads ($V_1$, $V_{4R}$, $V_{3R}$) has been shown to be sensitive and specific for identification of right ventricular infarction [86]. Atrial infarction can occasionally be inferred from the ECG [87, 88]. Electrocardiographic patterns seen with atrial infarction include depression or elevation of the PQ segment, variation in P-wave contour from baseline morphology, and the occurrence of abnormal atrial rhythms, including atrial flutter, atrial fibrillation, wandering atrial pacemaker, and atrioventricular nodal rhythm.

*Precordial Mapping.* It has been suggested that ECG mapping of precordial Q-wave development and R-wave loss with a 35-lead precordial map reflects the extent of a particular episode of myocardial necrosis. Although still experimental, the results obtained using this atraumatic, noninvasive technique seem to correlate with other assessments of the degree of myocardial injury [89, 90]. Attempts to relate precordial ST segment maps to infarct size have been slightly less successful than using QRS precordial maps because of the development of pericarditis, electrolyte abnormalities, or both in some patients. The subject is discussed further in chapter 13.

*Role of Vectorcardiography.* Some cardiologists feel that vectorcardiography is more sensitive than conventional scalar electrocardiography in recognizing myocardial infarction [91–94]. Vectorcardiographic diagnosis of infarction is not, however, more specific than scalar electrocardiographic diagnosis, in that significant numbers of false-positive diagnoses can and do occur when one is dealing with patients with ventricular hypertrophy, chronic obstructive pulmonary disease, and cardiomyopathy. In addition, many cardiologists are unfamiliar with vectorcardiography, and this tends to limit its usefulness in the diagnosis of AMI. Vectorcardiography, however, is often useful in distinguishing posterior infarction from complete or incomplete right bundle branch block or right ventricular hypertrophy. Moreover, the vectorcardiogram is often helpful in evaluating patients with inferior infarction who satisfy only some of the scalar criteria for inferior infarction. Thus, individuals with diminutive Q-waves in leads II, III, and AVF may have suffered an inferior infarction that can be recognized only by the vectorcardiogram.

## Chest Roentgenography

Chest roentgenograms obtained in patients with AMI are almost always portable films taken in the coronary care unit. Most patients undergo serial chest roentgenography during their stay in the coronary care unit unless their clinical course is completely benign. Two findings are commonly seen in the chest films of infarction patients: signs of left ventricular failure and cardiomegaly.

In general, the chest roentgenogram reflects the hemodynamic status of the left ventricle. Thus, significant elevation in left ventricular filling pressure results in the finding of pulmonary congestion on the chest film [95, 96]. However, the chest film does not always reflect the level of left ventricular filling pressure in patients with AMI. Not infrequently, signs of pulmonary congestion will be present on the chest film, and yet left ventricular filling pressures are normal or nearly so. The converse may also happen. Such discrepancies between left ventricular filling pressure and chest roentgenographic findings are the result of "diagnostic lags" and "posttherapeutic phase lags." Individuals with diagnostic lags have elevated left ventricular filling pressures together with a normal chest roentgenogram. Often, 12 hours pass before roentgenographic findings reflect the hemodynamic status of patients with diagnostic lag. This lag occurs because a period of time is required for interstitial pulmonary edema to accumulate after the left ventricular filling pressure becomes elevated. The posttherapeutic phase lag is the reciprocal of the diagnostic lag: it is the time required for edema fluid to be resorbed after the left ventricular filling pressure has returned to normal. On occasion, it may take up to 4 days for radiographic signs of pulmonary congestion to

clear, despite normalization of the left ventricular filling pressure. Recent experimental work suggests that increased passage of fluid across pulmonary capillary membranes may also be the result of abnormally reduced capillary integrity in the setting of acute myocardial infarction [97].

Cardiomegaly on the chest film is usually a sign of dilatation of one or both ventricular chambers. In patients with AMI, cardiomegaly is usually a sign of prior infarction with resultant compensatory left ventricular dilatation. Patients with cardiomegaly usually have significantly reduced left ventricular function at catheterization. Cardiomegaly on the chest film is also associated with significant increases in left ventricular end-diastolic volume. Patients with increased end-diastolic volumes, however, may still have a normal-sized heart on the chest roentgenogram.

## Hemodynamic Monitoring

Two life-threatening complications of AMI, acute mitral regurgitation and ventricular septal rupture, are distinguished from each other by means of specific hemodynamic criteria. Until recently it was thought that acute mitral regurgitation was characterized by the sudden onset of a loud systolic murmur in association with the development of severe left ventricular failure. Hemodynamic monitoring in such individuals was said to reveal similar values for blood oxygen saturation in all right heart chambers (right atrium, right ventricle, pulmonary artery) and large so-called regurgitant V-waves in the pulmonary capillary wedge pressure tracing. Patients with acute ventricular septal rupture, on the other hand, were said to be characterized by loud systolic murmurs, severe left ventricular failure, absence of V-waves in the pulmonary capillary wedge pressure tracing, and a marked step-up or increase in blood oxygen saturation between the right atrium and the right ventricle [98].

Extensive experience with patients suffering from these two devastating complications of AMI has demonstrated that earlier conceptions of them were partially erroneous. Acute mitral regurgitation may present as severe left ventricular failure with a soft or even absent systolic murmur, although a loud murmur may be present. V-waves are observed in the pulmonary capillary wedge pressure tracing, and there is no blood oxygen saturation step-up in the right heart chambers. Ventricular septal rupture is characterized by a loud and impressive systolic murmur, severe left ventricular failure, a step-up in right heart blood oxygen saturation, and elevated pulmonary capillary wedge pressure *with or without* large V-waves [99]. The association of large V-waves with ventricular septal rupture is not entirely understood, but is probably the result of the larger than normal right ventricular stroke volume pumped into a pulmonary vascular bed with increased blood volume and reduced vascular compliance.

## Echocardiography and Nuclear Cardiology

In recent years two noninvasive techniques, echocardiography and myocardial scintigraphy, have enabled cardiologists to learn a great deal about the pathophysiology of AMI. It has been suggested that these techniques should be employed to aid in the diagnosis of coronary artery disease in both its acute and chronic forms. Since such concepts are discussed at length in chapters 7 and 8, this section will review only pertinent clinical points.

Several studies have demonstrated that routine M-mode echocardiography can detect abnormal wall motion associated with acute myocardial infarction [100–103]. Prognostic information can also be obtained from echocardiographic measurements in patients with AMI. Two-dimensional echocardiography enables one to obtain even more complete visualization of the left ventricle than can be obtained with M-mode echocardiography [104]. M-mode echocardiography visualizes only small regions of the left ventricular septum and posterior wall, while two-dimensional echocardiography reveals large segments of the septal, inferoposterior, and anterolateral walls. Echocardiographic analysis of left ventricular wall motion can be of diagnostic value in patients with ventricular failure of obscure cause in whom the ECG is not diagnostic of infarction [105]. In

such individuals the demonstration of regional left ventricular wall motion abnormalities suggests that the left ventricular failure is secondary to clinically silent myocardial infarction or ischemic cardiomyopathy. Echocardiography can also demonstrate infarct thinning and expansion in selected individuals [106].

Scintigraphy for acute myocardial infarction is based on the selective uptake of a radiopharmaceutical compound by acutely infarcting myocardium ("hot-spot" scintigraphy) [107, 108]. Both animal and clinical studies have demonstrated the utility of hot-spot infarct scintigraphy in detecting and sizing AMI.

Another form of myocardial scintigraphy that can also be used to visualize regions of infarcted myocardium employs radioactive analogs of potassium that are taken up by viable, perfused myocardial cells. Thallium-201 ($^{201}$Tl) is the most popular agent used in this type of scintigraphy [109, 110]. Infarcted zones of myocardium fail to take up thallium and thus produce a "cold spot" for that region of the left ventricle. Unfortunately, transient anginal episodes and old infarcts also produce "cold spots" in the $^{201}$Tl scintigram. Thus, the cold-spot scintigraphic technique is not useful in the early diagnosis of AMI. However, transient $^{201}$Tl defects on exercise scintigrams obtained 7 to 14 days post-AMI identify a subgroup of infarct patients who are at high risk for reinfarction, sudden death, and unstable angina during the subsequent year following infarction [111].

Although a small but significant number of false-positive and false-negative results are obtained, hot-spot scintigraphy can be of clinical utility in the diagnosis of AMI [107, 112]. In certain categories of patients, the usual modalities employed in making the diagnosis of AMI (i.e., history, ECG, and serum enzyme determinations) are rendered unreliable or unobtainable, namely:

1. Patients who have recently undergone cardiac surgery.
2. Patients with left bundle branch block on the ECG.
3. Patients with atypical chest discomfort and equivocal enzymatic and ECG changes.
4. Patients with small infarcts.

5. Patients who seek medical attention 4 to 10 days after a possible or presumptive infarction.
6. Patients with new infarcts or with infarct extensions who have previous or recent myocardial infarctions.

Thus, patients who have recently undergone cardiac surgery may have elevated serum CK (and even MB-CK) levels and an abnormal ECG in the absence of myocardial infarction. Infarct scintigraphy can identify zones of myocardial necrosis in such patients.

It may be difficult to document infarction in individuals with left bundle branch block or equivocal ECG and enzymatic changes. In such patients, as well as in persons with small infarctions in whom the usual diagnostic modalities may be equivocal, infarct scintigraphy may establish or rule out the diagnosis of AMI. In individuals who seek medical attention some days after infarction or in patients with old infarcts or recent extension of infarction, the ECG evidence of infarction, the serum enzyme evidence of infarction, or both may have disappeared or may remain confusing or equivocal. Infarct scintigraphy can help in the diagnosis of AMI in such patients.

The radionuclide technique of gated cardiac blood pool scanning can yield information about left ventricular function heretofore available only at cardiac catheterization. Thus, left ventricular ejection fraction and regional wall motion can be determined with this technique in patients with AMI. Such information is useful for prognosis and can aid in guiding therapy (e.g., digitalization or use of potential myocardial depressants such as beta-blockers) [113]. Localized left ventricular aneurysms can also be identified with gated cardiac blood pool scans. Thus, one can noninvasively identify those individuals with postinfarction left ventricular failure who will be most likely to benefit from a surgical approach to the treatment of their heart failure.

Echocardiography and myocardial scintigraphy are rapidly becoming routine tests in community hospitals throughout the United States; they add an exciting new dimension to the diagnosis and evaluation of patients with AMI. This is especially true when patients are studied with both techniques [114].

## Conclusions

This chapter has reviewed the pertinent clinical aspects concerning the diagnosis of acute myocardial infarction. Like other areas of coronary artery disease, this area is undergoing a transformation that blends traditional clinical techniques with newer and more sophisticated methods. Certain conclusions and tentative summaries of current controversies follow.

In relation to the clinical history, a number of factors such as exertion and psychological stress probably play a role in precipitating AMI in certain individuals. Most attacks, however, occur when the patient is at rest. Coronary spasm may play a role in the pathogenesis of coronary thrombosis and AMI. The physical examination is of definite diagnostic value in patients with AMI, and the presence of a third heart sound represents an important prognostic finding. Similarly, the finding of the systolic murmur of mitral regurgitation or of ventricular septal rupture helps to explain the sudden deterioration of some patients with AMI.

Formerly, the most reliable method of diagnosis of AMI was based on clinical data obtained from the history and physical examination and supported by electrocardiography. In recent years laboratory tests have increased the clinician's sensitivity in making the diagnosis of myocardial infarction. Of particular value in this regard is the measurement of serum levels of the isoenzyme MB-CK, and the most sensitive test for the presence of myocardial necrosis is elevation of the serum level of this isoenzyme. Even slight elevations in serum MB-CK probably represent small amounts of myocardial necrosis.

The scalar ECG, though it has definite limitations, will continue to be favored over the vector ECG in the diagnosis of AMI for the foreseeable future. However, the vectorcardiogram is helpful in diagnosing infarction in individuals with equivocal criteria for inferior or posterior infarction on the scalar ECG. Finally, significant discrepancies can exist between the hemodynamic status of patients with AMI and the finding of left ventricular failure on the chest roentgenogram.

Increases in the sensivity of the diagnosis of AMI will hopefully be forthcoming as experience is gained with a number of echocardiographic and nuclear cardiac techniques, which have been discussed in detail in preceding chapters. The most promising techniques appear to be two-dimensional echocardiography, thallium infarct scintigraphy, and gated cardiac blood pool scanning.

## References

1. Muller, J.E. Diagnosis of myocardial infarction: Historical notes from the Soviet Union and the United States. *Am. J. Cardiol.* 40:269, 1977.
2. Herrick, J.B. Clinical features of sudden obstruction of the coronary arteries. *JAMA* 59:-2015, 1912.
3. Phipps, C. Contributory causes of coronary thrombosis. *JAMA* 106:761, 1936.
4. Master, A.M., Dack, S., and Jaffe, H.L. Factors and events associated with onset of coronary artery thrombosis. *JAMA* 109:546, 1937.
5. Fitzhugh, G. and Hamilton, B.E. Coronary occlusion and fatal angina pectoris: Study of the immediate causes and their prevention. *JAMA* 100:475, 1933.
6. Boas, E.P. Angina pectoris and cardiac infarction from trauma or unusual effort; with consideration of certain medicolegal aspects. *JAMA* 112:1187, 1939.
7. Smith, C., Sauls, H.C., and Ballew, J. Coronary occlusion; a clinical study of 100 patients. *Ann. Intern. Med.* 17:681, 1942.
8. French, A.J. and Dock, W. Fatal coronary arteriosclerosis in young soldiers. *JAMA* 124:1233, 1944.
9. Russed, H.I. Role of heredity, diet and emotional stress in coronary heart disease. *JAMA* 171:503, 1959.
10. Jenkins, C.D. Recent evidence supporting psychologic and social risk factors for coronary disease. *N. Engl. J. Med.* 294:987, 1033, 1976.
11. Rahe, R.H., Romo, M., Bennett, L., and Siltaned, P. Recent life changes, myocardial infarction, and abrupt coronary death. *Arch. Intern. Med.* 133:221, 1974.
12. Theorell, T. and Rahe, R.H. Life change events, ballistocardiography, and coronary death. *J. Human Stress,* Sept. 1975, p. 18.
13. Connolly, J. Life events before myocardial infarction. *J. Human Stress,* Dec. 1976, p. 3.
14. Knapp, R.B., Topkins, M.J., and Artusio, J.F., Jr. The cerebrovascular accident and coronary occlusion in anesthesia. *JAMA* 182:332, 1962.
15. Boas, E.P. Some immediate causes of cardiac infarction. *Am. Heart J.* 23:1, 1942.
16. Goldfischer, J.D. Acute myocardial infarction secondary to ergot therapy. *N. Engl. J. Med.* 262:860, 1960.
17. Roussak, M.J. Myocardial infarction during serum sickness. *Br. Heart J.* 16:218, 1954.
18. Levine, H.D. Acute myocardial infarction following wasp sting. Report of two cases and critical survey of the literature. *Am. Heart J.* 91:365, 1976.
19. Allison, R.B., Rodreguez, F.L., Higgins, E.A., Jr., Leddy, J.P., Abelmann, W.H., Ellis, L.B., and Robbins, S.L. Clinicopathologic correlation in coronary atherosclerosis. Four hundred and thirty patients studied with postmortem coronary angiography. *Circulation* 27:170, 1963.
20. Howell, W.L. and Manion, W.C. The low incidence of myocardial infarction in patients with portal cirrhosis of the liver. *Am. Heart J.* 60:341, 1960.
21. Dalen, J.E., Ockene, I.S., and Alpert, J.S. Coronary spasm, coronary thrombosis, and myocardial infarction: A hypothesis concerning the pathophysiology of acute myocardial infarction. *Am. Heart J.* 104:1119, 1982.
22. Schroeder, J.S., Lamb, I.H., and Hu, M. The prehospital course of patients with chest pain. *Am. J. Med.* 64:762, 1978.
23. Short, D. and Stowers, M. The carbon copy pain of myocardial infarction. *Am. Heart J.* 96:417, 1978.
24. Zimmerman, D. and Parker, B.M. The pain of pulmonary hypertension—fact or fancy? *JAMA* 246:2345, 1981.
25. Thoren, P.N. Activation of left ventricular receptors with nonmedullated vagal afferent fibers during occlusion of a coronary artery in the cat. *Am. J. Cardiol.* 37:1046, 1976.
26. Feola, M., Arbel, E.R., and Glick, G. Attenuation of cardiac sympathetic drive in experimental myocardial ischemia in dogs. *Am. Heart J.* 93:82, 1977.
27. Chadda K.D., Lichstein, E., Gupta, P.K., and Choy, R. Bradycardia-hypotension syndrome in acute myocardial infarction. Reappraisal of the overdrive effects of atropine. *Am. J. Med.* 59:-158, 1975.
28. Maximov, M.J. and Brody, M.J. Changes in regional vascular resistance after myocardial infarction in the dog. *Am. J. Cardiol.* 37:26, 1976.
29. Cohen, L.S. and Costin, J.C. Activation of ventricular mechanoreceptors: Reflex peripheral vasodilatation during myocardial infarction. *Am. J. Cardiol.* 37:128, 1976.
30. Silverman, M.E. and Hurst, J.W. Abnormal physical findings associated with myocardial infarction. *Mod. Concepts Cardiovasc. Dis.* 38:69, 1969.

31. Nellen, M., Maurer, B., and Goodwin, J.F. Value of physical examination in acute myocardial infarction. *Br. Heart J.* 35:777, 1973.

32. Estebar, A., Gomez-Acebo, E., and de la Cal, M.A. Pulsus paradoxus in acute myocardial infarction. *Chest* 81:47, 1982.

33. Cohn, J.N., Guiha, N.H., Broder, M.I., and Limas, C.J. Right ventricular infarction. *Am. J. Cardiol.* 33:209, 1974.

34. Weinblatt, E., Shapiro, S., Frank, C.W., and Sager, R.V. Prognosis of men after first myocardial infarction, mortality and first recurrence in relation to selected parameters. *Am. J. Public Health* 58:1329, 1968.

35. Shaver, J.A. and O'Toole, J.D. The second heart sound: Newer concepts. Part II: Paradoxical splitting and narrow physiological splitting. *Mod. Concepts Cardiovasc. Dis.* 46:13, 1977.

36. Renner, W.F. and Renner, A.B. The quality of resonance of the first heart sound after myocardial infarction: Clinical significance. *Circulation* 59:1144, 1979.

37. Spodick, D.H. and Quarry, V.M. Prevalence of the fourth heart sound by phonocardiography in the absence of cardiac disease. *Am. Heart J.* 87:11, 1974.

38. Riley, C.P., Russell, R.O., Jr., and Rackley, C.E. Left ventricular gallop sound and acute myocardial infarction. *Am. Heart J.* 86:598, 1973.

39. Lichstein, E., Liu, H.M., and Gupta, P. Pericarditis complicating acute myocardial infarction: Incidence of complications and significance of electrocardiogram on admission. *Am. Heart J.* 87:246, 1974.

40. Soloff, L.A. Pericardial cellular response during the post-myocardial infarction syndrome. *Am. Heart J.* 82:812, 1971.

41. Blau, N., Shen, B.A., Pittmann, D.E., and Joyner, C.E. Massive hemopericardium in a patient with post-myocardial infarction syndrome. *Chest* 71:549, 1977.

42. McCabe, J.C., Ebert, P.A., Engle, M.A., and Zabriskie, J.B. Circulating heart-reactive antibodies in the postpericardiotomy syndrome. *J. Surg. Res.* 14:158, 1973.

43. Agress, C.M. and Kim, J.H.C. Evaluation of enzyme tests in the diagnosis of heart disease. *Am. J. Cardiol.* 6:641, 1960.

44. Sobel, B.E. and Shell, W.E. Serum enzyme determinations in the diagnosis and assessment of myocardial infarction. *Circulation* 45:471, 1972.

45. Shell, W.E., Kjekshus, J.K., and Sobel, B.E. Quantitative assessment of the extent of myocardial infarction in the conscious dog by means of analysis of serial changes in serum creatine phosphokinase activity. *J. Clin. Invest.* 50:3614, 1971.

46. Karliner, J.S., Gander, M.P., and Sobel, B.E. Elevated serum glyceraldehyde phosphate dehydrogenase activity following acute myocardial infarction. *Chest* 60:318, 1971.

47. Smith, A.F. Diagnostic value of serum creatine-kinase in a coronary-care unit. *Lancet* 2:178, 1967.

48. Goldbert, D.M. and Windfield, D.A. Diagnostic accuracy of serum enzyme assays for myocardial infarction in a general hospital population. *Br. Heart J.* 34:597, 1972.

49. Roberts, R. and Sobel, B.E. Isoenzymes of creatine phosphokinase and diagnosis of myocardial infarction. *Ann. Intern. Med.* 79:741, 1973.

50. Roberts, R. and Sobel, B.E. Creatine kinase isoenzymes in the assessment of heart disease. *Am. Heart J.* 95:521, 1978.

51. Roberts, R., Gowda, K.S., Ludbrook, P.A., and Sobel, B.E. Specificity of elevated serum MB creatine phosphokinase activity in the diagnosis of acute myocardial infarction. *Am. J. Cardiol.* 36:433, 1975.

52. Rapaport, E. Serum enzymes and isoenzymes in the diagnosis of acute myocardial infarction. *Mod. Concepts Cardiovasc. Dis.* 46:43, 1977.

53. Varat, M.A. and Mercer, D.W. Cardiac specific creatine phosphokinase isoenzyme in the diagnosis of acute myocardial infarction. *Circulation* 51:855, 1975.

54. Alderman, E.L., Matlof, H.J., Shumway, N.E., and Harrison, D.E. Evaluation of enzyme testing for the detection of myocardial infarction following direct coronary surgery. *Circulation* 48:135, 1973.

55. Tonkin, A.M., Lester, R.M., Guthrow, C.E., Roe, C.R., Hackel, D.B., and Wagner, G.S. Persistence of MB isoenzyme of creatine phosphokinase in the serum after minor iatrogenic cardiac trauma. Absence of postmortem evidence of myocardial infarction. *Circulation* 51:627, 1975.

56. Klein, M.S., Coleman, R.E., Weldon, C.S., Sobel, B.E., and Roberts, R. Concordance of electrocardiographic and scintigraphic criteria of myocardial injury after cardiac surgery. *J. Thorac. Cardiovasc. Surg.* 71:934, 1976.

57. Raabe, D.S., Morise, A., Sbarbaro, J.A., and Gundel, W.D. Diagnostic criteria for acute myocardial infarction in patients undergoing coronary artery bypass surgery. *Circulation* 62:869, 1980.

58. Jaffe, A.S., Garfinkel, B.T., Ritter, C.S., and Sobel, B.E. Plasma MB creatine kinase after vigorous exercise in professional athletes. *Am. J. Cardiol.* 53:856, 1984.

59. Roberts, R., Sobel, B.E., and Ludbrook, P.A. Determination of the origin of elevated plasma CPK after cardiac catheterization. *Cath. Cardiovasc. Diag.* 2:329, 1976.

60. Al-Sheikh, W, Heal, A.V., Pefkaros, K.C. et al.:

Evaluation of an immunoradiometric assay specific for the CK–MB isoenzyme. *Am. J. Cardiol.* 54:269, 1984.

61. Heller, G.V., Blaustein, A.S., Wei, J.Y. Implications of increased myocardial isoenzyme level in the presence of normal serum creatine kinase activity. *Am. J. Cardiol.* 51:24, 1983.

62. Hackel, D.B., Reimer, M.D., Ideker, R.E. et al.: Comparison of enzymatic and anatomic estimates of myocardial infarct size in man. *Circulation* 70:824, 1984.

63. Kagen, L., Scheidt, S., and Butt, A. Serum myoglobin in myocardial infarction: The "Staccato Phenomenon." Is acute myocardial infarction in man an intermittent event? *Am. J. Med.* 62:86, 1977.

64. Varki, A.P., Roby, D.S., Watts, H., and Zatuchni, J. Serum myoglobin in acute myocardial infarction: A clinical study and review of the literature. *Am. Heart J.* 96:680, 1978.

65. Vallee, B.L. The time course of serum copper concentrations of patients with myocardial infarctions. *Metabolism* 1:420, 1952.

66. Wacker, W.E.C., Ulmer, D.D., and Vallee, B.L. Metalloenzymes and myocardial infarction. II. Malic and lactic dehydrogenase activities and zinc concentrations in serum. *New Engl. J. Med.* 255:449, 1969.

67. Trahern, C.A., Gere, J.B., Krauth, G.H., and Bigham, D.A. Clinical assessment of serum myosin light chains in the diagnosis of acute myocardial infarction. *Am. J. Cardiol.* 41:641, 1978.

68. Kannel, W.B. and Abbott, R.D.: Incidence and prognosis of unrecognized myocardial infarction. An update on the Framingham Study. *New Engl. J. Med.* 311:1144, 1984.

69. Lipman, B.S., Massie, E., and Kleiger, R.E. *Clinical Scalar Electrocardiography.* Chicago: Year Book, 1972, pp. 219–222.

70. Rothfeld, B., Fleg, J.L., and Gottlieb, S.H. Insensitivity of the electrocardiogram in apical myocardial infarction. *Am. J. Cardiol.* 53:715, 1984.

71. Hinohara, T., Hindman, N.B., White, R.D., Ideker, R.E., and Wagner, G.S. Quantitative QRS criteria for diagnosing and sizing myocardial infarcts. *Am. J. Cardiol.* 53:875, 1984.

72. Spodick, D.H. Q wave infarction versus S-T infarction. Nonspecificity of electrocardiographic criteria for differentiating transmural and nontransmural lesions. *Am. J. Cardiol.* 51:913, 1983.

73. Madigan, N.P., Rutherford, B.D., and Frye, R.L. The clinical course, early prognosis and coronary anatomy of subendocardial infarction. *Am. J. Med.* 60:634, 1976.

74. Rigo, P., Murray, M., Taylor, D.R., Weisfeldt, M.L., Strauss, H.W., and Pitt, B. Hemodynamic and prognostic findings in patients with non-transmural and transmural infarction. *Circulation* 51:1064, 1975.

75. Schulze, R.A., Jr., Pitt, B., Griffith, L.S.C., Ducci, H.H., Achuff, S.C., Baird, M.G., and Humphries, J.O. Coronary angiography and left ventriculography in survivors of transmural and non-transmural myocardial infarction. *Am. J. Med.* 64:108, 1978.

76. Madias, J.E. and Krikelis, E.N. Transient giant R waves in the early phase of acute myocardial infarction: Association with ventricular fibrillation. *Clin. Cardiol.* 4:339, 1981.

77. Reid, P.R., Taylor, D.R., Kelly, D.T., Weisfeldt, M.L., Humphries, J.O., Ross, R.S., and Pitt, B. Myocardial infarct extension detected by precordial ST segment mapping. *N. Engl. J. Med.* 290:123, 1974.

78. Mills, R.M., Young, E., Gorlin, R., and Lesch, M. Natural history of ST segment elevation after acute myocardial infarction. *Am. J. Cardiol.* 35:609, 1975.

79. Gewirtz, H., Horacek, B.L., Wolf, H.K., Rautaharju, P.N., and Smith, E.R. Mechanism of persistent S-T segment elevation after anterior myocardial infarction. *Am. J. Cardiol.* 44:1269, 1979.

80. Kalbfleisch, J.M., Shadaksharappa, K.S., Conrad, L.L., and Sarkar, N.K. Disappearance of the Q-deflection following myocardial infarction. *Am. Heart J.* 76:193, 1968.

81. Haiat, R., Worthington, F.X., Castellanos, A., and Lemberg, L. Unusual normalization of the electrocardiogram on the 6th day of myocardial infarction. *J. Electrocardiol.* 4:363, 1971.

82. Gibson, R.S., Crampton, R.S., Watson, D.D., Taylor, G.J., Carabello, B.A., Holt, N.D., and Beller, G.A. Precordial ST-segment depression during acute inferior myocardial infarction: Clinical, scintigraphic and angiographic correlations. *Circulation* 66:732, 1982.

83. Croft, C.H., Woodward, W., Nicod, P., Corbett, J.R., Lewis, S.E., Willerson, J.T., and Rude, R.E. Clinical implications of anterior S-T segment depression in patients with acute inferior myocardial infarction. *Am. J. Cardiol.* 50:428, 1982.

84. Little, W.C., Rogers, E.W., and Sodums, M.T. Mechanism of anterior ST segment depression during acute inferior myocardial infarction: Observations during coronary thrombolysis. *Ann. Intern. Med.* 100:226, 1984.

85. Ferguson, D.W., Pandian, N., Kioschos, J.M., Marcus, M.L., and White, C.W. Angiographic evidence that reciprocal ST-segment depression during acute myocardial infarction does not indicate remote ischemia: Analysis of 23 patients. *Am. J. Cardiol.* 53:55, 1984.

86. Klein, H.O., Tordjman, T., Ninio, R., et al.

The early recognition of right ventricular infarction: Diagnostic accuracy of the electrocardiographic $V_{4R}$ lead. *Circulation* 67:588, 1983.

87. Lowe, T.E. and Wartman, W.B. Myocardial infarction. *Br. Heart J.* 6:115, 183, 1944.

88. Cushing, E.H., Feil, H.S., Stanton, E.J., and Wartman, W.B. Infarction of the cardiac auricles (atria); clinical, pathological, and experimental studies. *Br. Heart J.* 4:17, 1942.

89. Muller, J.E., Maroko, P.R., and Braunwald, E. Precordial electrocardiographic mapping. Technique to assess efficacy of interventions designed to limit infarct size. *Circulation* 57:1, 1978.

90. Madias, J.E. Precordial ST-segment mapping: 6. Evaluation of serial changes in ST-segment elevations and QRS complexes of precordial maps and standard ECGs in patients with acute myocardial infarction. *Clin. Cardiol.* 7:91, 1984.

91. Chou, T., Helm, R.H., and Kaplan, S. *Clinical Vectorcardiography* (2nd ed.). New York: Grune & Stratton, 1974, pp. 229–233.

92. Benchimol, A. and Desser, K.B. Advances in clinical electrocardiography. *Am. J. Cardiol.* 36:-76, 1975.

93. Stein, P.D. and Simon, A.P. Vectorcardiographic diagnosis of diaphragmatic myocardial infarction. *Am. J. Cardiol.* 38:568, 1976.

94. Howard, P.F., Benchimol, A., Desser, K.B., Reich, F.D., and Graves, C. Correlation of electrocardiogram and vectorcardiogram with coronary occlusion and myocardial contraction abnormality. *Am. J. Cardiol.* 38:582, 1976.

95. Kostuk, W., Barr, J.W., Simon, A.L., and Ross, J., Jr. Correlations between the chest film and hemodynamics in acute myocardial infarction. *Circulation* 48:624, 1973.

96. McHugh, T.J., Forrester, J.S., Adler, L., Zion, D., and Swan, H.J.C. Pulmonary vascular congestion in acute myocardial infarction: Hemodynamic and radiologic correlations. *Ann. Intern. Med.* 79:29, 1972.

97. Slutsky, R.A., Peck, W.W., and Higgins, C.B. Pulmonary edema formation with myocardial infarction and left atrial hypertension: Intravascular and extravascular pulmonary fluid volumes. *Circulation* 68:164, 1983.

98. Meister, S.G. and Helfant, R.H. Rapid bedside differentiation of ruptured interventricular septum from acute mitral insufficiency. *N. Engl. J. Med.* 287:1024, 1972.

99. Pichard, A.D., Kay, R., Smith, H., et al. Large V waves in the pulmonary wedge pressure tracing in the absence of mitral regurgitation. *Am. J. Cardiol.* 50:1044, 1982.

100. Teichholz, L.E., Kreulen, T., Herman, M.V., and Gorlin, R. Problems in echocardiographic volume determinations: Echocardiographic-angiographic correlations in the presence or absence of asynergy. *Am. J. Cardiol.* 37:7, 1976.

101. Corya, B.C., Rasmussen, S., Knoebel, S.B., and Feigenbaum, H. Echocardiography in acute myocardial infarction. *Am. J. Cardiol.* 36:1, 1975.

102. Dortimer, A.C., DeJosepy, R.L., Shiroff, R.A., Litdtke, A.J., and Zelis, R. Distribution of coronary artery disease: Prediction by echocardiography. *Circulation* 54:724, 1976.

103. Nieman, M. and Heikkila, J. Echoventriculography in acute myocardial infarction. II: Monitoring of left ventricular performance. *Br. Heart J.* 38:271, 1976.

104. Pandian, N.G., Skorton, D.J., and Kerber, R.E. Role of echocardiography in myocardial ischemia and infarction. *Mod. Concept. Cardiovasc. Dis.* 53:19, 1984.

105. Horowitz, R.S., Morganroth, J., Parrotto, C., Chen, C.C., Soffer, J., and Pauletto, F.J. Immediate diagnosis of acute myocardial infarction by two-dimensional echocardiography. *Circulation* 65:323, 1982.

106. Eaton, L.W., Weiss, J.L., Bulkley, B.H., et al. Regional cardiac dilatation after acute myocardial infarction. Recognition by two-dimensional echocardiography. *N. Engl. J. Med.* 300:57, 1979.

107. Wynne, J., Holman, B.L., and Lesch, M. Myocardial scintigraphy by infarctavid radiotracers. *Prog. Cardiovasc. Dis.* 20:243, 1978.

108. Croft, C.H., Rude, R.E., Lewis, S.E., Parkey, R.W., Poole, W.K., Parker, C., Fox, N., Roberts, R., Strauss, H.W., Thomas, L.J., Raabe, D.S., Jr., Sobel, B.E., Gold, H.K., Stone, P.H., Braunwald, E., Willerson, J.T., and the MILIS Study Group. Comparison of left ventricular function and infarct size in patients with and without persistently positive technetium-99m pyrophosphate myocardial scintigrams after myocardial infarction: Analysis of 357 patients. *Am. J. Cardiol.* 53:421, 1984.

109. Beller, G.A. and Smith, W. Radionuclide techniques in the assessment of myocardial ischemia and infarction. *Circulation* 53 (Suppl. 1):123, 1976.

110. Okada, R.D., Lim, Y.L., Chesler, D.A., Kaul, S., and Pohost, G.M. Quantitation of myocardial infarction size from thallium-201 images: Validation of a new approach in an experimental model. *J. Am. Coll. Cardiol.* 4:948, 1984.

111. Gibson, R.S., Watson, D.D., Craddock, G.B., et al. Prediction of cardiac events after uncomplicated myocardial infarction: A prospective study comparing predischarge exercise thallium-201 scintigraphy and coronary angiography. *Circulation* 68:321, 1983.

112. Marcus, M.L. and Kerber, R.E. Present status of the [99m]technetium pryophosphate infarct scintigram. *Circulation* 56:335, 1977.

113. Nicod, P., Corbett, J.R., Firth, B.G., et al. Prognostic value of resting and submaximal exercise radionuclide ventriculography after acute myocardial infarction in high-risk patients with single and multivessel disease. *Am. J. Cardiol.* 52:-30, 1983.

114. Wynne, J., Birnholz, J.C., Holman, B.L., Finberg, H., and Alpert, J.S. Radionuclide ventriculography and two-dimensional echocardiography in coronary artery disease. *Am. J. Cardiol.* 41:406, 1978.

# III. PREVENTION AND THERAPY OF CORONARY ARTERY DISEASE

# 11. PREVENTION OF
# CORONARY ATHEROSCLEROSIS

R. Curtis Ellison

Peter F. Cohn

In 1970 the Intersociety Commission on Heart Diseases predicted that "coronary heart disease has reached enormous proportions ... [and] will result in coming years in the greatest epidemic mankind has faced unless we are able to reverse the trend by concentrated research into its cause and prevention" [1]. The scientific community has indeed responded to this call, and although the main thrust of research into heart disease in the United States has been directed toward management of patients who already have coronary artery disease, an increasing amount of money is being allocated to preventive endeavors.

The *primary* prevention of atherosclerosis, the underlying disease process of most coronary artery disease, refers to preventive measures taken prior to the development of any symptoms or other indications that the individual already has the disease. *Secondary* prevention refers to prevention of *further* manifestations of coronary artery disease once the patient has already experienced initial signs, symptoms, or both. The fact that many Americans have findings of early coronary atherosclerosis by the third decade of life (as demonstrated in the International Atherosclerosis Project [2] and in studies of American soldiers killed in recent wars [3]) points to the need for initiating preventive endeavors early in life. In fact, some now refer to atherosclerosis as a *pediatric* disease [4].

As discussed in chapter 3, the well-documented "risk factors" for coronary disease have

evolved from longitudinal studies involving adults. While large groups of young people have recently been assessed for similar factors [5, 6], long-term follow-up—that is, until the onset of clinical coronary disease—has not yet been completed. Many of these factors, however, tend to "track"—that is, peer relationships tend to be similar on subsequent examinations. Therefore, a consideration of "adult" risk factors among children would appear to be a reasonable first approach in considering primary prevention of atherosclerosis.

Points of controversy are probably greater in regard to the prevention of atherosclerosis than to almost any other aspect of coronary artery disease. The nutritional-metabolic theory of atherogenesis, or the "lipid" or "diet-heart" hypothesis, was established early in the twentieth century and has gained support from a very large number of studies in animals and in man since then. As noted in chapter 3, resistance to the theory that diet is of critical importance persists [7].

As Stamler [8] commented, however, the overwhelming body of data in this field, especially from animal experiments and epidemiologic studies, indicates that dietary intake of saturated fats and cholesterol do indeed play a part in the development of coronary artery disease. The decrease in the mortality rates from heart disease in the United States over the past 15 years [9], which have been occurring at a time when the dietary intake of saturated fats and the average blood levels of cholesterol in the population have been decreasing, adds further support to this theory [10]. Nevertheless, questions and controversy remain regarding the magnitude of the effects that can be expected from changes in the American diet, as well do questions as to the age at which certain modifications should be instituted.

The principal controversy regarding the prevention of hypertension deals with the potential role of dietary salt in the causation or development of essential hypertension [11, 12]. As in the case of dietary cholesterol and heart disease, epidemiologic cross-cultural studies are very clear: where dietary sodium is high (and, usually, dietary potassium low), hypertension and its complications are common; in cultures where salt is used sparingly or not at all, hypertension and heart disease are extremely rare. Several problems arise when one attempts to assess the sodium–blood pressure relation critically. First, within a culture, the dietary sodium intake usually varies less than it does within populations. In the United States, for instance, because of the large amounts of added sodium in practically all prepared foods, there is essentially an "obligatory" minimum intake of salt of several grams per day, a level that may already be "excessive" as far as hypertension is concerned. A comparison between blood pressure and salt intake within such a culture may well be unrevealing. Second, methods for assessing dietary intake of sodium among free-living people are cumbersome or inaccurate, due partly to an individual's day-to-day variation in intake [13]. An additional problem may be that the primary effect of sodium on blood pressure is in the very young, when renal, hormonal, and other mechanisms related to the control of blood pressure are being established, whereas almost all studies have been performed in adults. Recent studies in infants do support the hypothesis that early sodium intake may play a role in the genesis of human hypertension [14, 15].

The *value of strenuous physical activity* as a means of preventing heart disease has also led to considerable controversy. Froelicher and Obermann [16], in a 1972 review of over 30 studies relating physical activity and coronary heart disease, concluded that the results are "contradictory and inconclusive." As will be discussed further, however, recent studies by Paffenbarger and associates [17] report beneficial effects of strenuous physical exercise on the incidence of both coronary heart disease and hypertension.

By its very nature, the prevention of coronary artery disease presumes that environment influences its development. The discussion that follows will make quite apparent that a strong genetic component—a predisposition—is also involved for many of the risk factors. The recognition of differential genetic susceptibility serves to clarify certain environmental causal mechanisms; in the clinical situation, it helps to identify individuals who are at higher than average risk for the development of such diseases. In this chapter, current recommendations are outlined. More detailed information on the implementation of preventive strategies is included in articles from a recent Bethesda conference on the prevention of coronary heart disease [18]. Pediatric aspects of prevention are summarized in a book on the subject edited by Lauer and Shekelle [19].

## Experimental Atherosclerosis and Hypertension

### ATHEROSCLEROSIS

Experimental studies in animals have made important contributions to our knowledge of both genetic and environmental factors in the development of atherosclerosis. The first breakthrough came during 1908 to 1912, when Ignatowski, Anitschkow, and their collaborators succeeded in inducing hyperlipidemia and atherosclerosis in rabbits by increasing cholesterol and fat in their diets [20]. Since then, experiments involving dietary alterations have led to the production of atherosclerosis in practically every species of experimental animal known, most recently in nonhuman primates [21]. These studies have pointed out that atherosclerosis results not just from diet alone, but from the complex interplay of diet with other characteristics of the organism, especially certain genetic factors. Despite a large amount of animal research, however, no single hypothesis for the etiology of atherosclerosis has been universally accepted; most investigators believe that a number of mechanisms play a role in its pathogenesis [17].

*Genetic Factors.* Recent studies have indicated that genetic predisposition to atherosclerosis in animals may involve a number of different mechanisms. First, a marked variability exists in the response of individual animals to cholesterol in the diet. In squirrel monkeys, for instance, up to 65 percent of the variability of blood cholesterol can be accounted for by genetic influence [22]. Certain hyperresponders demonstrate up to 3.5 mg/dl increase in blood cholesterol for every 1 mg of cholesterol absorbed, while hyporesponders exhibit very little influence on blood levels due to variations in the dietary cholesterol. Among baboons, the progeny of animals with higher levels of cholesterol while on an atherogenic diet develop higher serum cholesterol during infancy than do the progeny of animals with lower cholesterol levels. The differences in serum cholesterol among the progeny become even more marked in the juvenile period when a moderately atherogenic diet is introduced [17]. Heredity also influences the susceptibility to atherosclerosis at the level of the arterial wall itself. Given certain levels of cholesterol and blood pressure, experimental animals [23] and, presumably, man show marked variability in the degree of coronary atherosclerosis that develops. A third genetic factor related to the development of atherosclerosis may be differences in the size of the low-density lipoprotein (LDL) molecule itself. In macaque monkeys, for example, striking sex differences in the weight of the LDL molecule have been demonstrated. In such animals, there is a close correlation between the LDL size and the severity of coronary artery disease that develops upon stimulation with a high cholesterol diet [24].

Nicolosi and co-workers [25] found that genetic control of the *lipoprotein* response to diet may have important biologic implications. These workers compared the degree and type of hypercholesterolemia that was produced by a high saturated fat diet in two different, but closely related, species of New World monkeys: the squirrel monkey and the cebus monkey. Both squirrel and cebus monkeys responded to coconut oil feeding with an increase in blood cholesterol (to 278 and 280 mg/dl, respectively). The major expansion of the cholesterol pool, however, was my means of an increase in LDL in the squirrel monkeys, but by an increase in high-density lipoprotein (HDL) in the cebus monkeys. The latter ultimately had HDL levels approximately twice those of the former. Much more extensive aortic atherosclerosis was found in the squirrel monkeys than in the cebus monkeys, a finding consistent with recent epidemiologic evidence that suggests that an inverse relation exists between HDL levels and the risk of coronary artery disease in humans [26–28].

*Environmental Influences in Early Life.* Pediatricians and parents have long wanted to know what associations there are, if any, between diet in early life and later atherosclerosis. Early weaning has been shown to lead to higher blood cholesterol in later life in rates [29] and in pigs [30], and it has been suggested that breastfeeding tends to have some protective effect regarding the development of atherosclerosis and coronary disease in humans [17]. This subject, however, has not been studied adequately. Liebman and associates [31] have studied the white Carneau pigeon, an animal that develops severe atherosclerosis similar to that in humans. Young pigeons that are kept lean by underfeeding in the first few weeks of life tend to have much less atherosclerosis in adult life, even after they have resumed an atherogenic diet.

HYPERTENSION

One area of animal research on essential hypertension merits special mention: Dahl and co-workers [32] produced, by selective inbreeding, a salt-sensitive strain of Sprague-Dawley rats that develop severe and lethal hypertension under the influence of increased dietary sodium. Such animals have been extensively studied as a model for some types of genetically influenced essential hypertension in man. While practically all rats, as well as many other experimental animals, will develop essential hypertension with very large amounts of added salt in the diet, the salt-sensitive rats tend to develop severe hypertension on much lower levels of salt intake, levels similar to those of man in many cultures. This was demonstrated dramatically by the development of lethal hypertension in salt-sensitive rats from the ingestion of commercially prepared human baby foods. Furthermore, it was demonstrated that the salt-sensitive rats that were exposed to high sodium in the diet at a very early age (just after weaning) had more rapid progression of their hypertensive disease and much higher mortality than similar rats in whom the sodium "insult" was not begun until 3 to 6 months of age [33,34] (figure 11–1).

## Primary Prevention of Coronary Artery Disease in Humans: Pediatric Aspects

As stated previously, there has been no longitudinal study to demonstrate the relation between

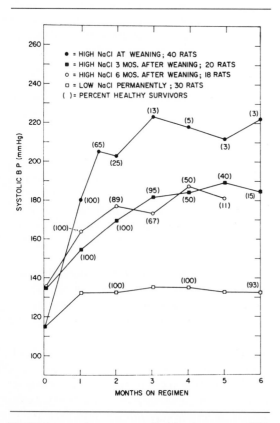

FIGURE 11–1. Average systolic blood pressure (BP) among healthy survivors of groups of rats started on high sodium chloride (NaCl) diets at different ages. For those begun on high NaCl at weaning (solid dots), blood pressure was much higher and the percentage of healthy survivors much lower than for those begun on high NaCl later. (From Dahl, L.K. et al. Effects of chronic excess salt ingestion. *Circ. Res.* 22:11, 1968. Reproduced by permission of the American Heart Association, Inc.)

risk factors present during childhood and subsequent coronary artery disease. The reasons for this are quite simple: large numbers of young people have been screened for risk factors only in recent years; to follow such subjects until clinical coronary disease develops would require a very long follow-up, probably 40 or 50 years. A number of studies, however, would indicate that children with high levels of cholesterol or high blood pressure are at higher than average risk for developing premature cardiovascular disease. Children with above-average levels of cholesterol have a much higher probability of having a family history of early cardiovascular disease than do children with low levels of blood cholesterol [35]. Above-average levels of serum triglyceride do not seem to convey this risk (36), but similar relations have been demonstrated in the families of children with above-average levels of blood pressure. Furthermore, there is a tendency for blood cholesterol, blood pressure, and, especially, body weight to "track" [37–40]. Thus, we may be able to identify "high-risk" individuals at an early age.

The detection of high-risk young people has meaning only insofar as we are able to offer effective means of interrupting the development of atherosclerosis in such individuals. Some general aspects of early intervention should be considered. During the first few decades, atherosclerosis is usually in a very early stage. Certain environmental influences that affect the development of atherosclerotic plaques may be more important at this time than in the situation where significant arterial disease is already present. Similarly, blood pressure is more labile during early life, but it tends to become more fixed during adult life [41]. Many habits, as well as life-style in general, would also appear to be less well established during childhood. Thus, interventions may be more effective during formative years than later in life.

From the point of view of pathology, there may even be critical time periods in early life during which certain environmental influences have their largest effect on disease processes. Even if such is not the case, however, the earlier an intervention is introduced, the longer is the time period over which it can work (given that it is continued). Interventions that are only slightly effective in adult life may be more effective if established early, both because they may be acting at a critical time period in the formation of disease and because they will be working over a much longer period of time.

Neufeld and Goldbourt [42] have concluded that the genetic aspects of coronary artery disease are significant in determining the degree, time course, and severity of the atherosclerotic process. How the genetic and environmental influences interact to produce symptomatic disease is discussed in the following sections.

HYPERCHOLESTEROLEMIA

As noted in chapter 3, a positive relation holds between total cholesterol in the blood and the risk of coronary artery disease in adults. While the increase in risk is most marked at higher levels of cholesterol, there is a progressive increase in risk for values over 200 mg/dl [43–44]. Thus, American adults with levels in the 200 to 240 mg/dl range, which is often considered "within normal limits," are actually at levels that indicate "increased" risk.

Studies of blood lipoproteins have shown that it is primarily the cholesterol carried by the LDL fraction that is related to coronary artery disease risk [45–47]. As noted in chapter 3, the level of HDL has been found to have a strong *inverse* relation to the risk of heart disease [26–28]. In most individuals, however, the largest percentage (usually 60 to 75 percent) of the total cholesterol is carried by the LDL fraction, and there is a close correlation between the two, especially at the higher end of the spectrum [47]. Therefore, assumptions based on population studies in which only total cholesterol was measured are still valid, but where specific measurements of LDL- and HDL-cholesterol are done, the predictive relations between cholesterol levels and the risk of coronary disease are usually improved [47, 48].

*Serum Cholesterol Levels in Children.* School-age children in the United States have levels of blood cholesterol that are considerably higher than those of children in many other parts of the world. In the large studies in Muscatine, Iowa, Lauer and co-workers [5] found the average total cholesterol level to be in the range of 180

mg/dl for children between 6 and 18 years of age; 9 percent were at least 220 mg/dl, and 3 percent were 240 mg/dl or greater (figure 11–2). Similar levels have been found in Louisiana, California, Vermont, and elsewhere in the United States [49–52]. Much lower average levels have been found among children in Africa and in South and Central America [53–55] as well as among certain American Indians [56].

Socioeconomic status has a strong effect on blood cholesterol in young people. For instance, while rural children in Mexico and Guatemala have usually been found to have very low levels of cholesterol (in the range of 100 to 140 mg/dl), more wealthy urban children in the same countries tend to have values closer to those of American school children [54, 55]. In South Africa, white children have 10 times the rate of "hypercholesterolemia" (defined as cholesterol levels greater than 238 mg/dl) than do black children, a difference felt to be due less to racial factors than to socioeconomic and especially *dietary* ones [53]. The "Seven Country Study" [57] demonstrated a close relation between the dietary intake of saturated fat and the average blood level of cholesterol for cohorts of adult subjects in the different countries studied. There is strong evidence that the high levels of cholesterol in the blood of American children are related at least in part to dietary and other aspects of the "American way of life." This is not to deny the large role played by genetics in determining cholesterol levels in children [17]. Both in humans and in experimental animals the response of an individual to a diet is modified by inherited characteristics.

*Effects of Dietary Modification.* The effects on blood levels of cholesterol produced by dietary modification have been demonstrated in young people by Ford et al. [58]. In nonmotivated adolescent males in a boarding school, these workers were able to effect a decrease in blood cholesterol levels of approximately 15 percent by manipulation of saturated and polyunsaturated fats in the school menu pattern. Polyunsaturated fats were utilized as partial replacement for saturated fats in milk, ice cream, cheese, meat products, and bakery items as well as being utilized as cooking oils; a decrease was estimated in die-

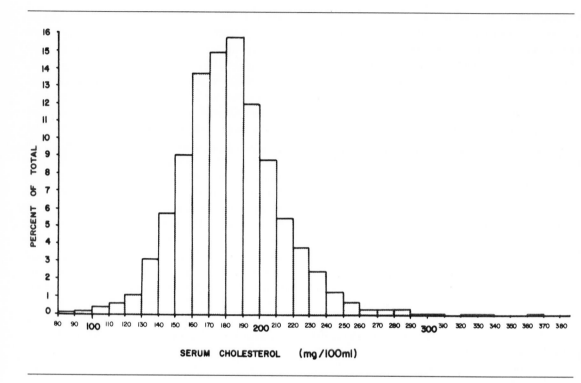

SERUM   CHOLESTEROL   (mg/100ml)

FIGURE 11-2. Histogram of serum cholesterol levels of children in Muscatine, Iowa, study. Ages were 6 through 18 years. Average cholesterol level was 180 mg/dl. (From Lauer, R.M. et al. coronary heart disease risk factors in school: *The Muscatine study. J. Pediatr.* 86:697, 1975.)

tary fat from 39 to 33 percent of total calories and in saturated fatty acids from 15 to 10 percent. Polyunsaturated fatty acids increased from 3 to 10 percent of total calories. With few exceptions, the modified food products were very well accepted by the students.

Commercial food products with higher ratios of polyunsaturated to saturated fatty acids are becoming more widely distributed. "Low-fat" milks, vegetable oil margarines, ice milks, and even some "modified" bakery products are now available and are beginning to make up an increasingly larger percentage of the market. Government regulations, public and health agency pressures, and, especially, economic advantages to the food producers will probably continue to produce changes in the typical American diet so that it becomes more nearly in line with the "prudent" diet advised by the Inter-Society Commission [59].

If such occurs, what will be the effect on coronary artery disease in the country? The National Diet-Heart Study Research Group in 1968 [60] estimated that the coronary artery disease incidence would decrease 24.4 percent, for a 10

percent reduction in mean serum cholesterol in the United States population. Interestingly, recent studies have shown that during the past 15 to 20 years, the mean cholesterol level in the population has indeed decreased by about 10 percent [61–62]. Concurrent with this change in blood cholesterol levels has been an overall decrease in coronary heart disease mortality since 1968 of more than 20 percent for persons 35 to 74 years of age [10].

*Recommendations for the General Population.* One can speculate as to the factors that may have contributed to the recent decline in cardiac mortality. While the concurrent fall in mean cholesterol levels and mortality cannot be cited as definitive proof of the diet-heart theory, there certainly does not appear to be any reason why the advice to the general public regarding a prudent diet should be changed. Increasing the availability and use of low saturated fat food products and decreasing the consumption of dairy products and meat seem to be appropriate measures for the general public to consider for the primary prevention of atherosclerosis. This is being done.

The age at which such dietary measures should begin is not known. Since cholesterol is required for the rapid development of the nervous system during the first year of life, the consensus is that saturated fats should *not* be restricted during early infancy [63–65]. After the first year, however, growth and development appear to be normal on such a restricted diet. Furthermore, Clueck and coworkers [66] have suggested that long-term effects on blood levels of cholesterol may be produced by dietary manipulation in the early years of life. Since areas of significant fibrous plaque formation are often found in Americans by the third decade [2–4], childhood would seem to be the appropriate time to begin such preventive efforts. Thus, the American Heart Association favors "a diet reduced in fat content as a safe and effective element of preventive measures" in healthy children [67].

*Familial Hyperlipidemia.* The measures discussed to this point are those that should be considered for the general pediatric population. However, as many as two million people in the United States are estimated to have some type of familial hyperlipidemia, making such conditions the most common inherited metabolic disease in man. Such individuals require early detection and more extensive therapeutic measures if premature coronary artery disease is to be avoided. The three types of disorders—familial hypercholesterolemia, familial combined hyperlipidemia, and familial hypertriglyceridemia—are all inherited as autosomal dominants. Thus, 50 percent of first-degree relatives receive the affected gene. For familial hypercholesterolemia, penetrance is 100 percent by early infancy, while there is low penetrance until about 25 years of age for the other diseases [68].

The inherited defect in subjects with familial hypercholesterolemia leads to abnormalities in the metabolism of the low-density lipoproteins. As noted in chapter 2, these patients have defi-

cient or absent LDL receptors, making them unable to internalize the LDL, and high levels of circulating lipoproteins in the blood result [68]. As with other types of familial hyperlipidemia, the condition increases the individual's risk for early coronary artery disease [70] (figure 11–3).

Diagnosis of familial hypercholesterolemia is made from a family history of hyperlipidemia, premature coronary artery disease, or sudden death plus the finding of high lipid levels in the subject. Children or young adults with such a family history should have blood studies done; if the subject is less than 12 years of age, only a cholesterol determination (which can be nonfasting) is necessary. For older children or adults, fasting blood levels should be determined for cholesterol and triglycerides. Cholesterol values persistently above 250 mg/dl should be considered indicative of the disease. At the present time, it is recommended that therapy for identified cases begin after the first year of life [71].

The cornerstone of treatment of hypercholesterolemia is a diet that is low in saturated fats, high in polyunsaturated fats, and low in choles-

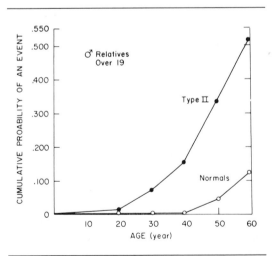

FIGURE 11–3. The cumulative probability of a coronary artery disease (CAD) event, according to age, for males over 19 years of age with familial type II hyperlipoproteinemia, compared to normal relatives. (From Stone, N.J. et al. Coronary artery disease in 116 kindred with familial type II hyperlipoproteinemia. *Circulation* 49:476, 1974. Reproduced by permission of the American Heart Association, Inc.)

terol. Six to 12 months of such dietary therapy should be given before other treatment is considered. If the cholesterol level is not down to less than 250 mg/dl, bile acid-binding resins may be added to the regimen. Other therapies that are sometimes effective include nicotinic acid and D-thyroxine. Such types of treatment are accepted and completely effective, however, in only a small percentage of individuals with hyperlipidemia. In cases where extremely high levels of cholesterol exist, partial ileal bypass [72] is now being considered in many institutions. While few children have had this procedure performed, it has been very successful in adults, leading to a 35 to 40 percent decrease in serum cholesterol over that produced by diet alone [73].

HYPERTENSION

As discussed in chapter 3, for high blood pressure as for blood cholesterol, it appears that "the lower, the better" (see figure 3–7). Heart disease risk is more than twice as high for adults with systolic pressures of 120 to 139 mmHg as it is for those with systolic pressures below 120 mmHg [74].

There are some special circumstances in regard to hypertension as a risk factor when one considers children and young people. First, there is the matter of attempting to *prevent the development of hypertension itself;* this involves the early identification of the "at risk" individual and the institution of appropriate intervention *before* hypertension appears. Second, for young people who have high blood pressure, there is a reluctance to use drug therapy, especially in preadolescent children. This is because of the possible effects on growth and development and the potential for late side effects, which may be of particular importance considering the very long period of time (perhaps 50 years or more) that such patients may require treatment. Thus, nonpharmacologic methods of therapy would be especially desirable for young people with hypertension.

*Prevention of Essential Hypertension.* When considering the prevention of hypertension, a first step should be an evaluation of the factors that have been implicated in its cause. Here, one

must start with heredity. A strong genetic factor is suggested by studies of twins [75, 76] and of adopted versus natural children [77] as well as by the familial aggregation of blood pressure that is apparent by early infancy [78]. The mechanism by which a tendency to hypertension is inherited is not known. Grim and co-workers [79] have recently identified important differences between members of families with essential hypertension and of families without hypertension in the kidneys' ability to handle a sodium load. These workers believe that heritable influences on the renin-angiotensin-aldosterone system may be responsible for the genetic variance observed in blood pressure. Differences between hypertensive families and normotensive families have also been found in sodium transport across cell membranes. Blood pressure, however, is not necessarily fixed on a narrow track by such early factors: correlations between repeated measurements during childhood are usually much lower than during adulthood. Systolic values taken 2 to 4 years apart during childhood, for example, give correlation coefficients of .2 to .3, whereas coefficients of .6 or greater are usually found in adults [41]. This increased lability of blood pressure during the early years of life would suggest that environmental factors may also be acting at this time.

Thus, in addition to an appropriate genetic substrate (a "permissive" factor), certain environmental factors also appear necessary for the development of hypertension. Probably the most important of these is a high dietary intake of sodium. The cross-cultural epidemiologic studies are quite striking: where there is no salt in the diet, there is no hypertension [80, 81]. In fact, the prevalence of elevated blood pressure in a population can be estimated by determining its intake of sodium (figure 11–4). It is not known what level of sodium intake is required for the genetic predisposition for hypertension to be manifest, but it may be as little as 1 or 2 grams of sodium chloride a day for some individuals [11]. This is considerably lower than the 5 to 15 grams per day that is the average level for Americans. It should be realized, however, that the level of sodium in most diets today is not the "natural" level for man; early man probably had an intake of only a few milliequiva-

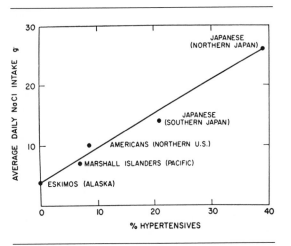

FIGURE 11–4. Average dietary sodium chloride (NaCl) intake and the prevalence of hypertension in different populations. (From Meneely, G.R. and Battarbee, H.D. *Am. J. Cardiol.* 38:768, 1976.)

lents of sodium a day [82]. The human body is remarkably well equipped to function on very low amounts of sodium in the diet; the inability of some individuals to handle the very much larger amounts present in the usual diet of today may well be a major factor in the high prevalence of hypertension in most societies today.

Human infants who are exclusively breast-fed receive about 4 to 6 milliequivalents of sodium per day [83]. Until recently, most proprietary formulas, especially those based on cow's milk, had much higher levels; however, even greater amounts of salt were being given our infants in the strained baby food they received. Salt was being added to the baby food, not because the infant needed it or ate better when it was added [84], but strictly because of the acquired high salt taste preference of the average mother buying the baby food. After Dahl et al.'s startling report in 1970 [85] of the lethal effects of human baby foods on salt-sensitive rats, the amount of salt added was reduced, but only in 1977 did "natural" strained baby foods, with *no* added salt, become readily available from the major food companies.

In a study of infants, Schacter et al. [14] found a positive correlation between sodium intake and blood pressure increase from birth to 6 months of age. Hofman et al. [15] recently re-

ported an experimental study in 476 Dutch infants for whom all supplemental formula and other food were furnished for the first 6 months of life. Infants were randomly assigned to low-sodium or regular-sodium groups; families and physicians were blinded to the assignment. By 6 months of age, the low-sodium group had significantly lower systolic blood pressure and a slower rate of increase than the regular-sodium group. Thus, based on animal data and on preliminary information that breast-fed children and others on low-salt diets from birth may have lower blood pressure in childhood [14, 15, 86], we are now advising that infants from families with a strong history of hypertension be placed on restricted sodium intake from birth. Years of follow-up will be required to test the efficacy of such an endeavor as a means of preventing essential hypertension.

When attempting to prevent hypertension, *weight control* must also be considered. Body weight and ponderousness have long been known to be closely related to blood pressure [87]. In a study evaluating a number of physiologic, psychologic, and social factors as determinants of childhood blood pressure, concurrent ponderousness, independent of *previous* ponderousness, was found to be the major determinant of both systolic and diastolic high blood pressures [12]. The mechanism by which weight (or adiposity) leads to hypertension is not known. Dahl et al. [32] postulated an increased sodium intake associated with greater food intake by obese individuals. However, obese adolescents do not consume more calories than their lean peers [88]. In this study, however, obese subjects consumed no more calories but were found to be excreting more sodium, suggesting that they may be selecting saltier foods to eat. Physicians are well aware of the familial aggregation of obesity; "it runs in the family" is a frequent excuse given for the overweight child. This aggregation, however, has been found to relate not only to heredity [12], but also to shared familial attitudes regarding food and exercise [89]. The latter aspect is particularly well demonstrated by the studies from the veterinary literature that have documented that fat people have fat pets [90].

The prevention of obesity must start early in

life. Knittle [91] has shown that replication of adipose cells occurs primarily in the first year of life and during the growth spurt of adolescence. The prevention of obesity would be expected to be most effective if it is concentrated at such times, since childhood obesity usually leads to lifelong problems with weight control [92].

*Management of Childhood Hypertension.* For the child or adolescent who already has an elevated blood pressure, there is considerable uncertainty as to whether, when, and how it should be managed. In adults with hypertension, a decrease in the blood pressure leads to a decrease in the risk of cardiovascular complications. While similar studies have not been done in young people, it has been demonstrated in the spontaneously hypertensive rat that antihypertensive medications started just after weaning greatly reduce the risk of cardiac hypertrophy; the benefits are less when treatment is started later in life [93]. Potential benefits from early treatment of hypertension could result from the prevention of the arterial or cardiac damage resulting from continuous exposure to such high pressures over a prolonged period of time. On the other hand, hypertension appears to be self-perpetuating, with higher pressures tending to progress even more rapidly over time. Thus, early treatment could be important if it would break the vicious cycle of hypertension and, in effect, "untrack" a young person otherwise destined to have even higher pressures with possible cardiovascular complications later in life. This is especially important since cardiac hypertrophy can be shown by noninvasive means to have already developed in some children with borderline hypertension, i.e., before the elevated pressures becomes fixed [94].

If it is desirable, at least theoretically, to lower the blood pressure of asymptomatic young people with hypertension, questions arise as to when to begin treatment and what type of treatment to use. There is legitimate concern about the administration of antihypertensive drugs to young people, both because such patients are still in their developmental years and because of the potential hazard of administering such agents over a great number of years. Therefore, if adequate compliance could be achieved, it would

seem especially appropriate to try nonpharmacologic methods for controlling blood pressure in such patients. The use of weight reduction (for obese subjects) and the limitation of dietary sodium intake are approaches now being explored. The use of relaxation and meditation and similar techniques, which have been shown to be effective in several small studies in adults with hypertension [95–97], are also currently being tested for their effectiveness in young people. In situations where drugs are considered necessary, propranolol is often selected, since it tends to suppress the hyperdynamic state often found in the young hypertensive subject. This may not always be efficacious, however, since more recent work has case doubt on the importance of the hyperkinetic state as a cause of hypertension in childhood [99].

## EXERCISE, PHYSICAL FITNESS, AND LIFE-STYLE

The preventive programs discussed thus far have dealt largely with the usual physician-patient relationship, and for the most part, they have included a certain negativism: "don't eat salt," "don't eat cholesterol or fat," "don't be obese," and the like. Another quite different approach places the emphasis on good health habits and fitness. Hence, there is more of a positive approach: be fit, be healthy! Compliance is less of a problem, since the activities tend to be self-reinforcing.

The concept of physical fitness as a means of preventing premature coronary artery disease has received considerable emphasis in certain Scandinavian countries but, as of yet, little emphasis in the United States. Several programs in this country have been directed at *young people,* however. Cooper and associates [100] offered a physical fitness program to high school students in Texas, which was to be taken in lieu of their regular gym activity. At the end of 15 weeks of this program, the percentage of students who could complete a 1.5 mile distance in 12 minutes or less increased from 25 to 47 percent, while no significant increase was observed among students undergoing their usual gym activity [100]. A formal program of fitness promotion in Newton, Massachusetts, was begun in 1968. This program, stimulated primarily by physicians in the community, is aimed at an increased awareness of physical fitness on the part of school children as well as in the community as a whole. The town recreational department supported the construction of a "life course" in one of the public parks; success of this endeavor is evidenced by the recent construction of a second such course. A "learning for life" program was instituted in the public schools. This involved (1) the development of new curricula in nutrition and fitness; (2) measurements of fitness, blood pressure, and blood lipids as a teaching exercise; (3) development of systemic fitness training, with testing and retesting; and (4) community outreach through the school system to promote fitness. Long-term follow-up will be required to determine if such endeavors lead to a decrease in coronary artery disease. The subject of physical fitness in children and its implication for the prevention of coronary disease is well summarized by Rowland [39].

## Prevention of Coronary Artery Disease in Adults

Mechanisms of prevention rely on the control of the recognized coronary risk factors cited in chapter 3 and earlier in this chapter, as well as the regulation of other minor or less well-accepted factors ("Type A" behavior, for example). Whether or not such preventive approaches are beneficial in adults, in either the primary or secondary forms, is very controversial [102, 103], but unlike the pediatric experience, there is already a body of literature on the subject. Some of the pertinent questions concerning such studies have been formulated by Borhani [104] in an excellent review. Is risk-factor modification safe and effective? If so, can the disease process be reversed or altered by such modification? Is there yet enough evidence to warrant intensive risk-factor modification in the daily practice of medicine, with its resultant socioeconomic changes in life-style? To help answer these questions, one must first consider the pertinent trials either completed or underway.

PRIMARY PREVENTION TRIALS
Many primary prevention trials are based on the lipid or "diet-heart" hypothesis, which relates dietary fat consumption to the level of serum cholesterol and the incidence of coronary artery disease. The experimental evidence for this hypothesis has been discussed earlier in the chapter, and its epidemiologic significance [105] has been discussed in chapter 3.

Although the National Diet-Heart Study Research Group reported in 1968 [60] that modification of diet in a risk prevention trial was indeed feasible, there are few published studies of such trials, and all are subject to criticism of one type or another. The Anticoronary Club Study in New York City [106], for example, demonstrated that serum cholesterol could be lowered on a diet containing 40 percent fat from 253 to 228 mg/dl and that after 1 year of observation the incidence of new coronary episodes was reduced to 4.3 per thousand as opposed to 10.2 in a control group. This study has been criticized because the participants were volunteers attracted by media advertising and were not randomly assigned to the experimental and control groups. In addition, data analysis was often "after the fact."

The Helsinki study took place in two mental hospitals from 1959 to 1971 and was most recently reviewed by Turpeinen [107]. Patients in one hospital were fed a low-cholesterol diet, whereas patients in the other hospital received a regular diet. Then the diets were reversed midway through the 12-year study. Age-adjusted mortality rates for coronary artery disease were higher when the patients were on the control diet. Interestingly enough, general mortality was also higher. Unfortunately, observed differences in mortality may have been due to different lengths of stay at the various hospitals, change in the rate of intake of high-risk patients, or other factors. The use of mortality as an endpoint was also criticized.

In the Los Angeles study [108], a Veterans Administration hospital was utilized and, again, the same advantages of the low-cholesterol diet were demonstrated. However, cigarette smoking was significantly higher in the control group. The Chicago study [109] also used volunteers, and mortality in the treated group was compared to dropouts from the study and the general population statistics. The study has been criticized on that score as well as on others.

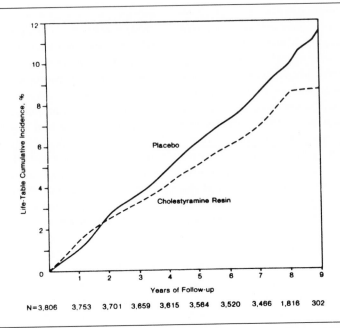

FIGURE 11–5. Life-table cumulative incidence of primary end-point (definite coronary heart disease death and/or definite nonfatal myocardial infarction) in treatment groups, computed by Kaplan-Meier method. N equals total number of Lipid Research Clinics Coronary Primary Prevention Trial participants at risk for their first primary end-point, followed at each time point. (From the Lipid Research Clinics Program. *JAMA* 251:356, 1984.)

In summarizing these reports, Borhani [104] has concluded that primary intervention trials aimed at testing the lipid hypothesis suffer from methodologic shortcomings, including (1) inadequate study design and analysis, (2) small number of patients, (3) failure to use randomization, and (4) lack of double-binding. Some of the statistical procedures are also of doubtful applicability. Despite the suggestive nature of the results of these studies, there was no clear-cut, generally accepted answer to the question of whether primary prevention via cholesterol-lowering measures could alter the incidence of coronary artery disease until the recently released report of the Lipid Research Clinics [110]. This study, using diet, cholestyramine, and placebos in 3,806 asymptomatic type II patients, showed a significant reduction in coronary events (figure 11–5) in the cholestryamine-treated group.

High blood cholesterol level is not the only risk factor being tested. *Mild hypertension* is being studied in the Hypertension Detection and Follow-up Program. The bases for these studies are the epidemiologic studies relating hypertension to coronary artery disease cited in chapter 3 as well as the results of various carefully controlled clinical trials showing a beneficial effect of antihypertensive agents on the inci-

dence of cardiovascular disease [111]. The research protocol involves a 5-year follow-up at 14 centers and four coordinating centers. After participants are identified by population screening, they are randomly assigned to an intensive treatment group (the "stepped-care group," with antihypertensive therapy increased in "steps" until adequate blood pressure lowering occurs) and to a comparison group (called "referred care," since the participants return to their usual source of medical care). Both groups are then followed, and the primary end-point is mortality from all causes. The total group admitted to the study consisted of nearly 11,000 hypertensive subjects aged 30 to 69 drawn from a pool of about 160,000 screened across the country. Those individuals with diastolic blood pressures greater than 95 mmHg at that time were entered into the study and underwent baseline evaluation (including electrocardiogram), were stratified for diastolic blood pressure level (90 to 104 mmHg and more than 115 mmHg), and were then randomly allocated to either "stepped care" or "referred care." The most recent progress report [112] on Stratum One (90 to 104 mmHg) demonstrated that 5-year mortality in the intensively treated patients was 20.3 percent lower than in those given usual care ($P < .01$). Despite these findings, the administration of life-long drug therapy to patients with mild hypertension is still controversial because of its side effects [113].

In addition to hypertension, one of the other nonlipid risk factors that has received attention in primary prevention therapy is *cigarette smoking*. In a study of mortality among British physicians [114], the death rate was highest in smokers, while that of ex-smokers was almost identical to that of the nonsmoking population. Two other large-scale studies have yielded similar results [115, 116], and a variety of groups concerned with preventive medicine and community health have strongly advised against cigarette smoking.

The importance of hypertension and cigarette smoking, as well as the lipid hypothesis, has stimulated interest in evaluating *more than one risk factor simultaneously.* Obvious economic benefits are also to be gained from one comprehensive type of study. Several programs in Europe are now engaged in such trials. The Oslo study group [117] has reported, for example, that changing eating habits and stopping smoking reduced the incidence of myocardial infarction by 47 percent ($p < .05$) compared to a control population (figure 11–6).

In the United States, the program is known as the Multiple Risk Factor Intervention Trial (MRFIT) [118]. Twelve thousand males between 35 and 57 years of age were included in the study, which was performed at 20 centers throughout the United States. Of 360,000 men screened, the 10 to 15 percent felt to be at highest risk (based on the Framingham data described in chapter 3) were randomized into intensive-care and special-care groups, similar to those in the hypertension program described earlier. The study was organized in 1972, and all centers were fully participating by 1974. Goals of the intensive-care group were for individual

patients to lower their cholesterol level by 10 percent and their diastolic blood pressure by 10 percent, with complete (or at least partial) reduction in the level of cigarette smoking. The primary end-point was cardiovascular mortality. Nutrition intervention, a stepped-care blood pressure control protocol, and a variety of anticigarette smoking schemes were employed. Other possible risk factors were also being considered by at least some of the centers. These included behavioral and psychological factors, level of physical activity, and the exercise ECG.

Because of changing life-styles in the general population, however, it was expected that the control group would also show some modification of risk factors. First, life-styles are being affected by the increased emphasis placed on diet and hypertension control by the media, health-care institutions, and so on. Second, since all the patients were volunteers, they would even be more motivated to correct such factors.

As a result of both factors, sizable risk factor reductions were observed in the regular-care group. This in turn was associated with a lower than expected number of deaths, and in fact, mortality was lower than that seen in the special-care group. In that sense the trial was unsuccessful. This is misleading, however, because MRFIT *did* show that a reduction in coronary risk factors could have a beneficial effect on mortality. What was unexpected was the reduction in risk factors seen in the regular-care group. Care in the community was, therefore, better than anticipated. Thus, the "failure" of this trial was paradoxically due to the successful nationwide effort to educate physicians and the public about the desirability of reducing coronary risk bouts. One troublesome feature of the trial was the apparently *increased* mortality in the special-care group. If not merely a statistical fluke, this finding gives credence to those [113] who argue for a nonpharmacological approach to mild hypertension and avoidance of drugs with possibly harmful side effects, such as diuretics.

One of the other major areas for possible primary prevention is concerned with *physical activity.* The beneficial effects of physical training on cardiovascular performance (see chapter 12) have led to increasing interest in using physical activity to ward off, or alter, coronary artery

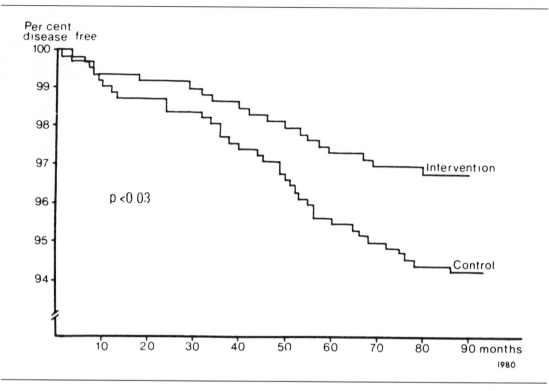

FIGURE 11–6. Life-table analysis of coronary heart disease (fatal and nonfatal myocardial infarction and sudden death) in intervention and control groups in the Oslo study. (From Hjermann, I. et al. *Lancet* 2:1303, 1981.)

disease. Studies suggesting that coronary artery disease can be prevented with increased physical activity have been both retrospective and prospective.

Retrospective studies analyze mortality statistics (usually by death certificates) for coronary artery disease and relate them to the physical activity of the population, usually by considering occupation. Probably the most famous of these is the study by Morris and associates (119) of British bus drivers and conductors, but there is a host of others (excellently reviewed in the study by Froelicher and Oberman [16]) suggesting that increased physical activity on the job decreases the mortality from coronary artery disease. The studies have been criticized [16] because they do not exclude selection bias (e.g., increased cholesterol in one group versus the other) or off-job activities; job transfers and different retirement policies could also explain the difference in observed mortality. In addition to the unreliability of many death certificates, there is always the problem of selection; for example, do people with low-risk factors gravitate to certain jobs? This criticism can also be applied to the studies of Paffenbarger and co-workers [17] relating the physical activity of college alumni to the development of coronary disease: do people with low-risk factors choose a more physically active life-style?

Because of these and other problems associated with such studies, prospective studies were organized. Again, occupation was used as an index of physical activity, and studies were performed in blue-collar versus white-collar workers, active versus less active longshoremen, and so on. Froelicher and Oberman [16] have also reviewed these studies; again, increasing physical activity was found to be inversely related to cardiovascular mortality. However, the detailed methods necessary to characterize the physically active individual either historically or physiologically remain a problem. Some investigations use questionnaires and limited physiologic data, but at the present time, there is only one report of a satisfactorily designed study comparing the incidence of new coronary events in physically active versus inactive men. This is the Puerto Rico Heart Health Program [120], and it appears to confirm the beneficial effects of increased physical activity. With the current mass interest in physical training (e.g., in jogging), it would appear that other such studies will soon be forthcoming.

The last factors to be considered are changes in behavior and psychological makeup, such as modification of the so-called Type A personality discussed in chapter 3. In terms of prevention, there are no data at present in this area.

SECONDARY PREVENTION TRIALS

In secondary prevention trials, the population under study has already experienced a prior myocardial infarction and is randomly assigned to a control group or one of several treatment protocols (e.g., to lower the serum cholesterol or modify other risk factors).

Several studies to decrease serum cholesterol were performed in Great Britain and involved vegetable oils [121, 122] or clofibrate [123, 124] as the cholesterol-lowering agent. Although the serum cholesterol level was usually significantly reduced by dietary management, no differences in mortality between the control and treated groups were observed. Clofibrate also reduced the cholesterol level in one of the studies [124] that did show a reduction in mortality, although whether this was due to the drug's cholesterol-lowering effect is not clear.

In Norway a similar dietary study [125] showed no difference in cardiovascular mortality between patients treated with experimental cholesterol-lowering diets and patients on regular diets. Again, however, the former group had a significant reduction in serum cholesterol levels.

The most extensive, and perhaps the best designed and executed study, took place in the United States, where the Coronary Drug Project [126–129] studied over 8,000 patients. Agents studied included conjugated estrogens, clofibrate, D-thyroxine sodium, and niacin. There was also a placebo group. The estrogen and thyroxine regimens had to be discontinued because of lack of benefit and possible harm [127–128].

Clofibrate and niacin lowered serum cholesterol (and triglyceride) levels, but there was no significant difference in cardiovascular or total mortality over the duration of the study between patients treated with either drug and the placebo group [129]. The results of these trials were interpreted as either negative or inconclusive, with one exception: the NHLBI Type II Coronary Intervention Study [130]. Lack of progression of coronary artery lesions (as demonstrated by angiography) occurred when the serum cholesterol level was lowered by cholestyramine, as opposed to diet alone.

No large-scale secondary prevention trials of hypertension have been conducted, but the results of clinical studies cited earlier suggests that control of hypertension would favorably affect prognosis. When patients who stop smoking after their infarctions are compared to control groups, a reduction in mortality has been reported [131].

Secondary trials in regard to physical activity are best exemplified by rehabilitation programs for patients who have sustained myocardial infarctions. These are discussed in chapter 17, but it should be noted that such studies are largely uncontrolled and rely on volunteers. The volunteers are not only highly motivated, but they are also "selected" because they have enough cardiac reserve to participate in the program. May et al. [132] have summarized the results of six studies (including the National Exercise and Heart Disease Project) involving 2,752 patients: none of the trials showed a statistically significant difference in total mortality between exercise and control groups nor was there any beneficial effect on reinfarction rates. The feasibility of modifying Type A behavior patterns has been demonstrated in a preliminary study by Friedman et al. [133].

## Conclusions

As far as the *pediatric population* is concerned, there is increasing evidence that early life should be the time when primary prevention of coronary artery disease is begun. Fatty streaks and other early signs of atherosclerosis are frequently found in children, and irreversible fibrous lesions in the coronary arteries may be present by the third decade. The risk factors for coronary disease that have been derived from studies in adults appear to be a reasonable starting point for primary preventive endeavors in children. The fact that such characteristics tend to "track" from early life into adulthood, that changes are already being produced in the cardiovascular system by such factors, and the possibility that there may be a critical period in early life when such factors may be particularly harmful emphasize the need for concern about this "adult" disease on the part of pediatricians and family practitioners.

Admittedly, our current recommendations are based in part on human studies considered by many to be inconclusive; however, they are based on sound theory with extensive support from animal experiments. Very long follow-up periods will be required to demonstrate directly the efficacy of preventive endeavors that are being initiated in young people of today.

The widespread screening of children for risk factors is not now recommended; however, the family history of each child should be reviewed carefully to determine which subjects are candidates for familial hypercholesterolemia, and appropriate blood studies should be obtained in them. For children in general, the use of low-fat milk and vegetable margarines, as well as other measures leading to a reduction in saturated fat intake, are advised. Breast-feeding and the use of unsalted baby foods are measures during infancy that may have long-term beneficial effects in preventing hypertension. Attention to possible obesity should also begin shortly after birth; the first year of life and adolescence would appear to be especially important times for the prevention of obesity later in life. The institution of good health habits of exercise and fitness during the early years could also be important in the prevention of vascular diseases. A more community-directed approach by the physician, rather than the usual doctor-patient relationship, may be most efficacious along these lines. The *education* of children and their parents in regard to diet, exercise, smoking, and other aspects of life-style has the greatest promise for preventing coronary artery disease in future generations.

In the *adult population*, there is no clear consensus regarding how primary prevention should be carried out. Few would argue with Werko [134] that in terms of priorities, cigarette smoking should be discouraged and that hypertension should be treated (though at what level to begin treatment is still controversial). It is the lipid hypothesis that is the basis for the most disagreement in terms of preventive approach. As we have noted, based on experimental data in animals and epidemiologic data in various human societies, a reasonable case can be made for associating dietary fat intake, high serum cholesterol levels, and coronary atherosclerosis [8]. Unfortunately, the results of the primary prevention trials in adults have not supplied strong support for this concept, except for the Lipid Research Clinic's study [110]. The others have been criticized on a variety of grounds, including methodological as well as statistical ones. The well-designed MRFIT program was inconclusive because the control group was as health conscious as the study group. This in itself is an indication of how far risk factor reduction has been accepted by the general population.

For the present, recommendations as to diet in asymptomatic adults lack clear consensus. It is hard to believe, however, that reduction of serum cholesterol levels, especially those of 250 mg/dl or greater, by dietary changes (i.e., without drugs) can be of any *harm,* and conceivably they might do good. Similarly, regularly planned physical activity may also be beneficial to cardiovascular performance, even though there is only limited evidence suggesting it can reduce the incidence of coronary disease. Unlike changing one's diet, however, physical activity can be potentially dangerous, especially in individuals with silent ischemia. Pretraining exercise tests are therefore recommended. The much more common problem of orthopedic difficulties secondary to physical exercise is also to be considered.

Secondary prevention poses even more problems. Hypertension and cigarette smoking are recognized as "treatable," but it may be "too late" to start thinking about lipid levels in most adults with clinical coronary disease, especially in those with extensive disease. If a marked reduction in lipid levels is achieved, however, there is now reason to believe that there will be regression of atheromas—or at least less progression—in already diseased vessels [130]. Although physical training in this type of patient is potentially more dangerous than in a person without disease, properly designed exercise programs do appear to improve the patient's clinical picture, even though there is no conclusive evidence that they improve longevity.

## References

1. Executive Board, World Health Organization 1969. Report of Inter-Society Commission for Heart Disease Resources. *Circulation* 42:1, 1970.
2. McGill, H.C., Jr. (ed.). *Geographic Pathology of Atherosclerosis.* Baltimore: Williams & Wilkins, 1968.
3. McNamara, J.J., Molot, M.A., Stremple, J.F., and Cuttin, R.T. Coronary artery disease in combat casualties in Vietnam. *JAMA* 216:-1185, 1971.
4. Voller, R.D., Jr. and Strong, W.B. Pediatric aspects of atherosclerosis. *Am. Heart J.* 101:-815, 1981.
5. Lauer, R.M., Connor, W.E., Leaverton, P.E., Reiter, M.A., and Clarke, W.R. Coronary heart disease risk factors in school: The Muscatine study. *J. Pediatr.* 86:697, 1975.
6. Voors, A.W., Foster, T.A., Frerichs, R.R., Webber, L.S., and Berenson, G.S. Studies of blood pressures in children, ages 5–14 years, in a total biracial community—the Bogalusa heart study. *Circulation* 54:319, 1976.
7. Mann, G.V. Diet Heart: End of an era. *N. Engl. J. Med.* 297:644, 1977; and resulting correspondence, 298:106, 1978.
8. Stamler, J. Lifestyles, major risk factors, proof and public policy. *Circulation* 58:3, 1978.
9. Kannel, W.B. and Thom, T.J. Declining cardiovascular mortality. *Circulation* 70:331, 1984.
10. Walker, W.J. Changing United States life-style and declining vascular mortality: A retrospective. *N. Engl. J. Med.* 308:649, 1983.
11. Freis, E.D. Salt, volume and the prevention of hypertension. *Circulation* 53:589, 1976.
12. Ellison, R.C., Newburger, J.W., and Gross, D.M. Pediatric aspects of essential hypertension. *J. Am. Dietetic Assoc.* 80:21, 1982.
13. Cooper, R., Soltero, I., Liu, K., Berkson, D., Levinson, S., and Stamler, J. The association between urinary sodium exretion and blood pressure in children. *Circulation* 62:97, 1980.
14. Schacter, J., Kuller, L.H., Perkins, J.M., and Radin, M.E. Infant blood pressure and heart rate: Relation to ethnic group (black or white),

nutrition and electrolyte intake. *Am. J. Epidemiol.* 110:205, 1979.
15. Hofman, A., Hazebroek, A., and Valkenburg, H.A. A randomized trial of sodium intake and blood pressure in newborn infants. *JAMA* 250:370, 1983.
16. Froelicher, V.F. and Oberman, A. Analysis of epidemiological studies of physical inactivity as risk factor for coronary artery disease. *Prog. Cardiovasc. Dis.* 15:41, 1972.
17. Paffenbarger, R.S., Jr., Wing, A.L., and Hyde, R.T. Physical activity as an index of heart attack risk in college alumni. *Am. J. Epidemiol.* 108:-161, 1978.
18. Bethesda Conference Report: Prevention of Coronary Heart Disease. *Am. J. Cardiol.* 47:-713, 1981.
19. Lauer, R.M. and Shekelle, R.B. (eds.). *Childhood Prevention of Atherosclerosis and Hypertension.* New York: Raven Press, 1980.
20. Katz, L.N. and Stamler, J. *Experimental Atherosclerosis.* Springfield, Ill.: Thomas, 1953.
21. Cox, G.E., Taylor, C.B., Cox, L.G., and Caunts, M.D. Atherosclerosis in rhesus monkeys. I. Hypercholesteremia induced by dietary fat and cholesterol. *Arch. Pathol.* 66:32, 1958.
22. Clarkson, T.B., Bullock, B.C., Lofland, H.B., and Goodman, H.O. Genetic control of plasma cholesterol. *Arch. Pathol.* 92:37, 1971.
23. Clarkson, T.B. *Genetic Studies of Atherosclerosis in Animals.* Task force on genetic factors in atherosclerotic disease. DHEW Publ. No. (NIH) 76-922, 1975.
24. Rudel, L.L., Pitts, L.L., and Nelson, C.A. Characterization of plasma low density lipoproteins of nonhuman primates fed dietary cholesterol. *J. Lipid Res.* 18:211, 1977.
25. Nicolosi, R.J., Hojnacki, J.L., Llansa, N., and Hayes, K.C. Diet and lipoprotein influence on primary atherosclerosis. *Proc. Soc. Exp. Biol. Med.* 156:1, 1977.
26. Miller, G.J. and Miller, N.E. Plasma high-density-lipoprotein concentration and development of ischaemic heart-disease. *Lancet* 1:16, 1975.
27. Rhoads, G.G., Gulbrandsen, C.L., and Kagan, A. Serum lipoproteins and coronary heart disease in a population study of Hawaii Japanese men. *N. Engl. J. Med.* 294:293, 1976.
28. Gordon, T., Castelli, S.P., Hjortland, M.C., Kannel, W.B., and Dawber, T.R. High density lipoprotein as a protective factor against coronary heart disease: The Framingham study. *Am. J. Med.* 62:707, 1977.
29. Reiser, R. Control of adult serum cholesterol by the nutrition of the suckling: A progress report. *Circulation* 44 (Suppl.2):7, 1971.
30. Reiser, R. and Sidelman, Z. Control of serum cholesterol homeostasis by cholesterol in the

milk of the suckling rat. *J. Nutr.* 103:1009, 1972.

31. Liebman, J., Leash, A., Bonyo, R., and Wallace, W.M. The effect of early underfeeding on the weight on the white Carneau pigeon. *Atherosclerosis* 11:439, 1970.

32. Dahl, L.K., Heine, M., and Tassinari, L. Effects of chronic excess salt ingestion. Evidence that genetic factors play an import role in susceptibility to experimental hypertension. *J. Exp. Med.* 15:1173, 1966.

33. Dahl, L.K. Salt and hypertension. *Am. J. Clin. Nutr.* 25:231, 1972.

34. Dahl, L.K., Knudsen, K.D., Heine, M.A., and Leitl, G.J. Effects of chronic excess salt ingestion. *Circ. Res.* 22:11, 1968.

35. Moll, P.P., Sing, C.F., Weidman, W.H., Gordon, H., Ellefson, R.D., Hodgson, P.A., and Kottke, B.A. Total cholesterol and lipoproteins in school children: Prediction of coronary heart disease in adult relatives. *Circulation* 67:127, 1983.

36. Schrott, H.G., Clarke, W.R., Abrahams, P., Wiebe, D.A., and Lauer, R.M. Coronary artery disease mortality in relatives of hypertriglyceridemic school children: The Muscatine study. *Circulation* 65:300, 1982.

37. Clarke, W.R., Schrott, H., Leaverton, P.E., Connor, W.E., and Lauer, R.M. Tracking of blood lipids and blood pressures in school age children: The Muscatine study. *Circulation* 58:626, 1978.

38. Lauer, R.M., Clarke, W.R., and Beaglehole, R. Level, trends, and variability of blood pressure during childhood: The Muscatine study. *Circulation* 69:242, 1984.

39. Clarke, W.R., Schrott, H.G., Connor, W.E., and Lauer, R.M. Obesity and its effects on childhood blood pressures: The Muscatine study. *Circulation* 56 (Suppl. 3):21, 1977.

40. Zinner, S.H., Rosner, B.R., and Kass, E.D. Eight-year follow-up of blood pressures in childhood. *CVD Epidemiology Newsletter,* Abst. No. 7, p. 18, Jan. 1976.

41. Rosner, B., Hennekens, C.H., Kass, E.D., and Miall, W.E. Age-specific correlation analysis of longitudinal blood pressure data. *Am. J. Epidemiol.* 106:306, 1977.

42. Neufeld, H.N. and Goldbourt, U. Coronary heart disease: Genetic aspects. *Circulation* 67:943, 1983.

43. Keys, A., Taylor, H.L., Blackburn, H., Brozek, J., Anderson, J.T., and Simonson, E. Coronary heart disease among Minnesota business and professional men followed fifteen years. *Circulation* 28:381, 1963.

44. Chapman, J.M. and Massey, F.J. The interrelationship of serum cholesterol, hypertension, body weight, and risk of coronary disease. Results of the first ten years' follow-up in the Los Angeles heart study. *J. Chronic Dis.* 17:933, 1964.

45. Gofman, J.W., Hanig, M., Hones, H.B., Lauffer, M.A., Lawry, E.Y., Lewis, L.A., Mann, G.V., Moore, F.E., Olmstead, F., Yeager, J.F., Andrus, E.C., Barach, J.H., Beams, J.W., Fertig, J.W., Gofman, J.W., Lauffer, M.A., Page, I.H., Shannon, J.A., Stare, F.J., and White, P.D. Evaluation of serum lipoprotein and cholesterol measurements as predictors of clinical complications of atherosclerosis. Report of a cooperative study of lipoproteins and atherosclerosis. *Circulation* 14:691, 1956.

46. Fredrickson, D.S., Levy, R.I., and Lees, R.S. Fat transport in lipoproteins: An integrated approach to mechanisms and disorders. *N. Engl. J. Med.* 276:34, 1967.

47. Kannel, W.B. and Schatzkin, A. Risk factor analysis. *Prog. Cardiovasc. Dis.* 26:309, 1983.

48. Castelli, W.P., Doyle, J.T., Gordon, T., Hames, C.G., Hjortland, M.C., Hulley, S.B., Kagan, A., and Zukel, W.J. HDL cholesterol and other lipids in coronary heart disease: The cooperative lipoprotein phenotyping study. *Circulation* 55:767, 1977.

49. Berenson, G.S., Foster, T.A., Frank, G.C., Frerichs, R.R., Srinivasah, S.R., Voors, A.W., and Webber, L.S. Cardiovascular disease risk factor variables at the pre-school age—the Bogalusa heart study. *Circulation* 57:603, 1978.

50. McGandy, R.B. Adolescence and the onset of atherosclerosis. *Bull. N.Y. Acad. Med.* 47:590, 1971.

51. Starr, P. Hypercholesterolemia in school children. *Am. J. Clin. Pathol.* 56:515, 1971.

52. Clarke, R.P., Merrow, S.B., Morse, E.H., and Keyser, D.E. Interrelationships between plasma lipids, physical measurements, and body fatness of adolescents in Burlington, Vermont. *Am. J. Clin. Nutr.* 23:754, 1970.

53. Duplessis, J.P., Viver, F.R., and DeLange, D.J. The biochemical evaluation of nutrition status of urban school children aged 7–15 years; serum cholesterol and phospholipid levels and serum and urinary amylase activities. *S. Afr. Med. J.* 41:1212, 1967.

54. Golubjatnikov, R.T., Paskey, T., and Inhorn, S.L. Serum cholesterol levels of Mexican and Wisconsin schools. *Am. J. Epidemiol.* 96:36, 1972.

55. Scrimshaw, H.S., Balsan, A., and Arroyava, G. Serum cholesterol levels in school children from three socio-economic groups. *Am. J. Clin. Nutr.* 5:629, 1957.

56. Savage, P.J., Turner, J.N., and Bennett, P.H. Cholesterol and triglyceride levels in Pima Indians over a spectrum of glucose tolerance. *CVD Epidemiology Newsletter,* Abst. No. 94, p. 54.

57. Keys, A. Coronary heart disease in seven countries. *Circulation* 41 (Suppl. 1):1, 1970.

58. Ford, C.H., McGandy, R.B., and Stare, F.J. An institutional approach to the dietary regulation of blood cholesterol in adolescent males. *Prev. Med.* 1:426, 1972.

59. Inter-Society Commission for Heart Disease Resources. Primary prevention of the atherosclerotic diseases. *Circulation* 42:1, 1970.

60. National Diet-Heart Study Research Group. The national diet-heart study final report. *Circulation* 37 (Suppl. 1):1, 1968.

61. Chandler, C.A. and Marston, R.M. Fat in the U.S. diet. *Nutrition Program News.* Washington, D.C.: U.S. Department of Agriculture, May–August, 1976.

62. Statistical Abstract of the United States: 1975 (96th ed.). Washington, D.C.: U.S. Department of Commerce, Bureau of the Census, 1975, p. 2.

63. Fumagalli, R., Smith, M.F., Urna, G., and Padetti, R. The effect of hypocholesteremic agents on myelinogenesis. *J. Neurochem.* 16:1329, 1968.

64. Fomon, S.J. A pediatrician looks at early nutrition. *Bull. N.Y. Acad. Med.* 47:569, 1971.

65. Segall, M.D., Fosbrooke, A.S., Lloyd, J.D., and Wolff, O.H. Treatment of familial hypercholesterolemia in children. *Lancet* 1:641, 1970.

66. Clueck, C.J., Tsang, R., Fallat, R., and Mellies, J.J. Diet in children heterogeneous for familial hypercholesterolemia. *Am. J. M. Dis. Child.* 1313:162, 1977.

67. American Heart Association Committee Report. Diet in the healthy child. *Circulation* 67:1411a, 1983.

68. Frederickson, D.S. and Breslow, J.L. *Primary Hyperlipoproteinemia in Infants.* National Heart and Lung Institute, *DHEW Publication* No. (NIH) 7082, 1973, 315.

69. Goldstein, J.L. and Brown, M.S. Lipoprotein receptors, cholesterol metabolism and atherosclerosis. *Arch. Pathol.* 99:181, 1975.

70. Stone, N.J., Levy, R.I., Fredrickson, D.S., and Verter, J. Coronary artery disease in 116 kindred with familial type II hyperlipoproteinemia. *Circulation* 49:476, 1974.

71. Fomon, S.J. *Infant Nutrition* (2nd ed.). Philadelphia: Saunders, 1974, p. 80–81.

72. Buchwald, H., Moore, R.B., Frantz, I.D., and Varco, R.L. Cholesterol reduction by partial ileal bypass in a pediatric population. *Surgery* 68:1101, 1970.

73. Buchwald, H., Moore, R.B., and Varco, R.L. Surgical treatment of hyperlipidemia. *Circulation* 49 (Suppl. 1):1, 1974.

74. Kannel, W.B. Role of blood pressure in cardiovascular morbidity and mortality. *Prog. Cardiovasc. Dis.* 17:5, 1974.

75. Havlik, R.J., Garrison, R.J., Katz, S.H., Ellison, R.C., Feinleib, M., and Myrianthopoulos, N.C. Detection of genetic variance in blood pressure of seven-year old twins. *Am. J. Epidemiol.* 109:512, 1979.

76. Levine, R.S., Hennekens, C.H., Duncan, R.C., Robertson, E.G., Gourley, J.E., Cassady, J.C., and Gelband, H. Blood pressure in infant twins: Birth to 6 months of age. *Hypertension* 2:1, 1980.

77. Biron, P., Mongeau, J., and Bertrand, D. Familial Aggregation of Blood Pressure in Adopted and Natural Children. In O. Paul (ed.), *Epidemiology and Control of Hypertension.* Miami: Symposia Specialists, 1975.

78. Zinner, S.H., Lee, Y.H., Rosner, B., Oh, W., and Kass, E.H. Factors affecting blood pressures in newborn infants. *Hypertension* 2:99, 1980.

79. Grim, C.E., Luft, F.C., Miller, J.Z., Rose, R.J., Christian, J.C., and Weinberger, M.H. An approach to the evaluation of genetic influences on factors that regulate arterial blood pressure in man. *Hypertension* 2:34, 1980.

80. Prior, A.M., Evans, J.G., Harvey, H.P.B., Davidson, F., and Lindsey, M. Sodium intake and blood pressure in two Polynesian populations. *N. Engl. J. Med.* 279:515, 1968.

81. Page, L.B., Danion, A., and Moellering, R.C., Jr. Antecedents of cardiovascular disease in six Solomon Island societies. *Circulation* 49:1132, 1974.

82. Denton, D. Instinct, appetites and medicine. *Aust. N.Z. J. Med.* 2:203, 1972.

83. American Academy of Pediatrics, Committee on Nutrition. Salt intake and eating patterns of infants and children in relation to blood pressure. *Pediatrics* 53:115, 1974.

84. Fomon, S.J., Thomas, L.N., and Filer, L.J., Jr. Acceptance of unsalted strained foods by normal infants. *J. Pediatr.* 76:242, 1970.

85. Dahl, L.K., Heine, M., Leitl, G., and Tassinari, L. Hypertension and death from consumption of processed baby foods by rats. *Proc. Soc. Exp. Biol. Med.* 133:14, 1970.

86. Ellison, R.C., Gordon, M.J., Sosenko, J.M., and Trudy, J. Breast feeding and later blood pressure in the child. Presented at the *18th Conference on Cardiovascular Disease Epidemiology,* Orlando, Fla., March 1978.

87. Siervogel, R.M., Frey, M.B., Kezdi, P., Roche, A.F., and Stanley, E.L. Blood pressure, electrolytes, and body size: Their relationships in young relatives of men with essential hypertension. *Hypertension* 2:83, 1980.

88. Ellison, R.C., Sosenko, J.M., Harper, G.P., Gibbons, L., Pratter, F.E., and Miettinen, O.S. Obesity, sodium intake and blood pressure in adolescents. *Hypertension* 2 (Suppl 1):1, 1980.

89. Stuart, R.B. and Davis, B. *Slim Chance in a Fat*

*World: Behavior Control of Obesity.* Champaign, Ill.: Research Press Company, 1972. chap. 1.

90. Mason, E. Obesity in pet dogs. *Vet. Rec.* 86:612, 1970.

91. Knittle, J.L. Obesity in childhood: A problem in adipose tissue cellular development. *J. Pediatr.* 81:1048, 1972.

92. Lloyd, J.K., Wolff, O.H., and Whelan, W.S. Childhood obesity. *Br. Med. J.* 2:660, 1967.

93. Pfeffer, M.A. and Pfeffer, J.M. Personal communication.

94. Miall, W.E. and Lovell, H.G. Relation between change of blood pressure and age. *Br. Med. J.* 2:660, 1967.

95. Culpepper, W.S. III, Sodt, P.C., Messerli, F.H., Ruschhaupt, D.G., and Arcilla, R.A. Cardiac status in juvenile borderline hypertension. *Ann. Intern. Med.* 98:1, 1983.

96. Benson, H., Marzetta, B.R., and Rosner, B.A. Decreased Blood Pressure Associated With the Regular Elicitation of the Relaxation Response: A Study of Hypertensive Subjects. In R.S. Eliot (ed.), *Contemporary Problems in Cardiology. Vol. 1. Stress and the Heart.* Mt. Kisco, N.Y.: Futura, 1974, 293.

97. Patel, C. 12-month follow-up of yoga and biofeedback in the management of hypertension. *Lancet* 1:62, 1975.

98. Shapiro, A.P., Schwartz, G.E., Ferguson, D.C.E., Redmond, D.P., and Weiss, S.M. Review of behavioral methods in the treatment of hypertension: A review of their clinical status. *Ann. Intern. Med.* 86:626, 1977.

99. Hofman, A., Ellison, R.C., Newburger, J., and Miettinsen, O.S. Blood pressure and hemodynamics in teenagers. *Br. Heart J.* 48:377, 1982.

100. Cooper, K.H., Purdy, J.D., Friedman, A., Bohannon, R.L., Harris, R.A., and Arends, J.A. An aerobic conditioning program for the Fort Worth, Texas, school district. *Res. Q.* 46:345, 1975.

101. Rowland, T.W. Physical fitness in children: Implications for the prevention of coronary artery disease. *Current Problems in Pediatrics* XI, No. 9, 1981.

102. Corday, E. and Corday, S.R. Prevention of heart disease by control of risk factors: The time has come to face the facts. *Am. J. Cardiol.* 35:330, 1975.

103. Ahrens, E.H. The management of hyperlipidemia: Whether, rather than how. *Am. J. Cardiol.* 40:251, 1977.

104. Borhani, N.O. Primary prevention of coronary heart disease: A critique. *Am. J. Cardiol.* 40:251, 1977.

105. Kannel, W.B. Some lessons in cardiovascular epidemiology from Framingham. *Am. J. Cardiol.* 37:269, 1976.

106. Rinzler, S. Primary prevention of coronary heart disease by diet. *Bull. N.Y. Acad. Med.* 44:937, 1968.

107. Turpeinen, O. Effect of cholesterol-lowering diet on mortality from coronary heart disease and other causes. *Circulation* 59:1, 1979.

108. Dayton, S., Pearce, M., Hashimoto, S., Dixon, W.J., and Tomiyasy, U. A controlled trial of a diet high in saturated fat in preventing complications of atherosclerosis. *Circulation* 40(Suppl. 11):63, 1969.

109. Stamler, J. Acute myocardial infarction, progress in primary prevention. *Br. Heart J.* 33:145, 1971.

110. Lipid Research Clinics Program. The Lipid Research Clinics Coronary Primary Prevention Trial Results. I. Reduction in incidence of coronary heart disease. *JAMA* 251:351, 1984.

111. Veterans Administration Cooperative Study Group on Antihypertensive Agents. Results in patients with diastolic blood pressures averaging 90–114 mmHg. *JAMA* 213:1143, 1970.

112. Hypertension Detection and Follow-up Program Cooperative Group. The effect of treatment on mortality in "mild" hypertension: Results of the hypertension detection and follow-up program. *N. Engl. J. Med.* 307:976, 1982.

113. Geyer, R.P. Sounding board: Should mild hypertension be treated? *N. Engl. J. Med.* 307:306, 1983.

114. Doll, R. and Hill, A.B. Mortality in relation to smoking. Ten years' observation of British doctors. *Br. Med. J.* 1:1399, 1964.

115. Kahn, H.A. The Dorn study of smoking and mortality among U.S. veterans. *Natl. Cancer Inst. Monogr.* 19:1, 1966.

116. Hammond, E.C. Smoking in relation to the death rates of one million men and women. *Natl. Cancer Inst. Monogr.* 19:127, 1977.

117. Hjermann, I., Holme, I., Velve Byre, K., and Leren, P. Effect of diet and smoking intervention on the incidence of coronary heart disease: Report from the Oslo study group of a randomized trial in healthy men. *Lancet* 2:1303, 1981.

118. The Multiple Risk Factor Intervention Trial (MRFIT): Risk factor changes and mortality results. *JAMA* 248:1465, 1982.

119. Morris, J.N., Heady, J.A., Raffle, P.A., Roberts, C.G., and Parks, J.W. Coronary heart disease and physical activity of work. *Lancet* 2:1111, 1953.

120. Garcia-Palmieri, M.R., Costas, R. Jr., Cruz-Vidal, M., Sorlie, P.D., and Havlik, R.J. Increased physical activity: A protective factor against heart attacks in Puerto Rico. *Am. J. Cardiol.* 50:749, 1982.

121. Rosa, G.A., Thomson, W.B., and Williams,

R.T. Corn oil in treatment of ischemic heart disease. *Br. Med. J.* 1:1531, 1965.

122. Controlled trial of soya-bean oil in myocardial infarction. Report of a research committee of the Scottish Society of Physicians. *Br. Med. J.* 4:775, 1971.

123. Trial of clofibrate in the treatment of ischemic heart disease. Five-year study by a group of physicians of the Newcastle-upon-Tyne region. *Br. Med. J.* 4:767, 1971.

124. A co-operative trial in the primary prevention of ischemic heart disease using clofibrate. Report from the Committee of Principal Investigators. *Br. Heart J.* 40:1069, 1978.

125. Leren, P. The effect of plasma cholesterol lowering diet in male survivors of myocardial infarction. A controlled clinical trial. *Acta. Med. Scand.* (Suppl.) 466:13, 1966.

126. Coronary Drug Project Research Group. The Coronary Drug Project—design, methods and baseline results. *Circulation* 47(Suppl. 1):1, 1973.

127. Coronary Drug Project Research Group. The CDP initial findings leading to modifications of its research protocol. *JAMA* 214:1303, 1970.

128. Coronary Drug Project Research Group. The CDP findings leading to further modifications of its protocol with respect to dextrothyroxine. *JAMA* 220:996, 1972.

129. Coronary Drug Project Research Group. Clofi-brate and niacin in coronary heart disease. *JAMA* 231:360, 1975.

130. Brensike, J.F., Levy, R.I., Kelsey, S.F., Passamani, E.R., Richardson, J.M., Loh, I.K., Stone, N.J., Aldrich, R.F., Battaglini, J.W., Moriarty, D.J., Fisher, M.R., Friedman, L., Friedewald, W., Detre, K.M., and Epstein, S.E. Effects of therapy with cholestyramine on progression of coronary arteriosclerosis: Results of the NHLBI Type II Coronary Intervention Study. *Circulation* 69:313, 1984.

131. Mulcahy, R. Influence of cigarette smoking on morbidity and mortality after myocardial infarction. *Br. Heart J.* 49:410, 1983.

132. May, G.S., Eberlein, K.A., Furberg, C.D., Passamani, E.R., and DeMets, D.L. Secondary prevention after myocardial infarction: A review of long-term trials. *Prog. Cardiovasc. Dis.* 24:331, 1982.

133. Friedman, M., Thoresen, C.E., Gill, J.J., Ulmer, D., Thompson, L., Powell, L., Price, V., Elek, S.R., Rabind, D.D., Breall, W.S., Piaget, G., Dixon, T., Bourg, E., Levy, R.A., and Tasto, D.L. Feasibility of altering type A behavior pattern after myocardial infarction. Recurrent coronary prevention project study: Methods, baseline results and preliminary findings. *Circulation* 66:83, 1982.

134. Werko, L. Risk factors and coronary heart disease: Facts or fancy? *Am. Heart J.* 91:87, 1976.

# 12. THERAPY OF ANGINA PECTORIS

Peter F. Cohn

Chapter 2 has described the pathoanatomy of coronary artery disease in humans and has discussed the pathophysiologic mechanisms that form the basis for many of the clinical manifestations of this disease. In the present chapter, the therapy of angina pectoris will be reviewed, including the chronic (stable), unstable, and variant types. Among the points of controversy that will be commented on in this chapter are the modification of risk factors and the role of exercise, clinical value of the calcium-antagonists compared to $\beta$-adrenergic blocking agents, role of coronary angioplasty, prognosis of medically treated patients in the present era, selection of less disabled patients for coronary artery bypass surgery, reappearance of symptoms after surgical therapy, management of coronary artery disease associated with other disease states (both cardiac and noncardiac), and the role of medical and "prophylactic" coronary artery bypass surgery in patients with coronary artery disease who need to undergo *noncardiac* surgery.

## General Approach to the Patient

Depending on the philosophy of the physician caring for the patient with angina pectoris, general therapeutic measures are directed toward either (1) adjusting the patient's life-style to his or her disease or (2) preserving the patient's life-style as much as possible. In either case, factors that precipitate anginal attacks are eliminated or minimized as much as possible.

PHYSICIAN-PATIENT COMMUNICATION
Psychological reassurance concerning the patient's prognosis (perhaps the term *general out-*

look* should be used instead when talking to the patient) combined with a reasonable summary of the pertinent clinical aspects of the disease are important factors to be communicated directly to the patient. Not enough emphasis can be placed on the dictum that good communication with the patient (and his or her family, whenever possible) is essential to good medical care. The physician should use a mixture of common sense, tact, and compassion in explaining the prognosis and the various problems the patient might experience, as well as the therapeutic modalities available for his or her use. The importance of thinking of the anginal attack as part of a "warning system" to prevent the patient from causing undue strain to the heart should be stressed.

Another important aspect of the physician's role is to discuss such things as the kind of work that the patient does; the patient's leisure time, eating habits, and vacation plans; and, with discretion, the amount and intensity of sexual activity. Any major change in life-style should be recommended only after careful and thorough analysis of these factors in relation to symptoms and medication. Whether or not the type of personality (Type A versus Type B) is a risk factor for coronary artery disease is still considered controversial (see chapter 3) despite the reports of the Western Collaborative Group [1]. How Type A personalities can be modified (if, indeed, they do represent added risk) is also unclear, though attempts are being made to devise appropriate protocols [2]. Certain changes in life-style, however, may be necessary, such as modifying certain strenuous activities if they constantly and repeatedly produce angina. These may be minor in many instances; for example, the golfer's activities could be modified to include a golf cart instead of walking. Activities in which the arms are raised above the level of the head (e.g., painting or carpentry) often bring on angina more readily than other activities (presumably because of the added work needed to overcome the effect of gravity), and these may have to be reduced or eliminated. The diurinal variation of angina must also be taken into account: activities that do not precipitate angina in the morning may do so in the afternoon in patients with chronic stable angina [3]. On the other hand, variant angina may be worse in the morning. Rigorous "straining" exercises of the isometric type in which there are sustained muscle contractions (rather than rhythmic, alternating contractions, as in walking) should be cautioned against. Such activities raise blood pressure and may also induce arrhythmias. They include weight-lifting, pushing stalled cars, lifting heavy objects, water-skiing, and certain aspects of snow-shoveling.

Decisions regarding change of work and retirement should only be made as a last resort. These are instances in which full family participation in the decision is advisable.

ANGINA-PROVOKING SITUATIONS
Eliminating or reducing the factors that precipitate anginal episodes is of extreme importance, but each patient must learn what the activity level is in his or her own case by trial and error. Since, as discussed in chapter 2, most anginal episodes are precipitated by increases in the mechanical work of the heart due to increases in heart rate and blood pressure, the patient should avoid sudden bursts of activity, particularly after long periods of rest. Thus, morning activities such as showering, shaving, and dressing should be paced: the more slowly the activity is performed, the better. At certain times, the prophylactic use of nitroglycerin is advocated, as will be discussed subsequently. The rise in blood pressure caused by cold weather can be minimized by using a face mask or scarf to cover the mouth or nose. Uncomfortably hot or humid environments may also precipitate episodes of angina, and air-conditioning may be a necessity rather than a luxury for patients with coronary artery disease. Large meals can have a similar effect, especially if followed by exertion, and the pa-

tient should be so informed. Emotional outbursts should be curtailed in particularly angina-prone individuals (though this is easier said than done). Caffeine ingestion, as in coffee and tea, may have to be stopped or minimized, and for that matter, any drug used for noncardiac disease that increases myocardial oxygen needs (e.g., amphetamines, isoproterenol mists, thyroid hormones) will have to be regulated carefully. Fever, anemia, and thyrotoxicosis may all have a deleterious effect in coronary artery disease. Such conditions must be specifically tested for and, if present, attended to promptly to prevent further myocardial ischemia.

Sexual intercourse is also a stressful activity and one that represents an important problem because it is not often adequately discussed with the patient (see chapter 17). With proper precautions (e.g., prophylactic nitroglycerin, empty stomach, perhaps less strenuous positioning, and the like), most patients with coronary disease should be able to continue with a reasonable degree of sexual activity.

THE ROLE OF EXERCISE
If effort brings on angina, is there still a place in patients with coronary artery disease for physical conditioning through a regular exercise protocol? Although some experimental evidence shows that coronary collateral blood flow can improve with physical training [4], more recent studies do not show an effect [5]; most investigators attribute the beneficial effects of physical training to an improvement in cardiovascular performance rather than to collateral formation [6, 7]. Specifically, in patients with coronary artery disease and angina pectoris, Redwood and associates [8] noted that a 6-week training program seemed to improve exercise performance by reducing the responses of heart rate and arterial pressure to bicycle exercise (figure 12–1) and by prolonging the time at which angina occurred (figure 12–2). Their study also suggested that myocardial oxygen delivery may actually be enhanced in some manner by the extensive exercise program, since trained patients were able to attain a *higher* double-product before angina occurred. Others [9] have found that the anginal threshold (i.e., the double-product at which pain

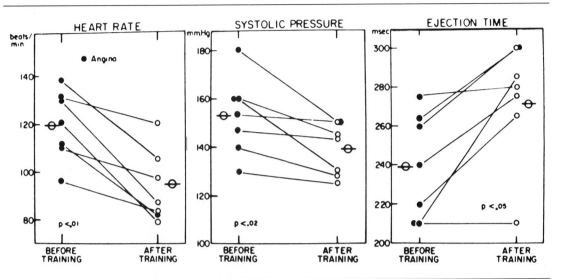

FIGURE 12–1. Effect of 6 weeks of physical training on the response of heart rate, systolic blood pressure, and ejection time to exercise. In each panel, the points to the left represent pretraining values obtained during exercise at the onset of angina; points to the right represent posttraining values measured at the same intensity and duration of exercise as in the pretraining studies. Mean values are presented by the circles with bars. The decreases in heart rate and blood pressure more than compensate for the increase in ejection time and account for the more efficient circulatory response to exercise. (From Redwood, D.R. et al. Reproduced by permission of the *New England Journal of Medicine*, 286:959, 1972.)

occurs) is the same after training. All agree that training prolongs the *time* before angina is experienced. For these reasons, patients are urged to participate in regular exercise programs in conjunction with their drug therapy.

An individual exercise prescription is necessary to minimize harmful effects of too strenuous a conditioning program. The individual protocol is best devised *after* the patient has had a maximal exercise tolerance test. In addition to evaluating total body oxygen consumption, the exercise test can also be useful in noting whether contraindications to an exercise program are present, such as easily provoked angina (particularly in the face of concurrent drug therapy) or arrhythmias. The actual exercise protocol [10] involves a warm-up phase, workout, and cool-

down. The warm-up and cool-down phases are usually about 5 minutes. The purpose of the former (e.g., walking and limbering up exercises) is to stretch and loosen the noncardiac musculoskeletal tissues as well as to allow for a gradual circulatory readjustment so that widespread vasodilation does not cause hypotension, arrhythmias, or syncope when the intense physical activity is suddenly stopped. For the same reason, a hot shower is not recommended *immediately* after exercise. The actual workout phase usually consists of about 20 to 30 minutes of activity at 75 percent of the *patient's* maximal exercise tolerance. Three to five exercise periods a week are usually sufficient to achieve a good conditioning effect. The types of exercise vary from walking and jogging to swimming, bicycling, and rowing.

Perhaps the best way to begin physical training with anginal patients is with a graduated walking program. Level ground surfaces should be utilized, and when outdoors, moderate temperatures are preferred. Reasonable goals can be set up for each week of training [10]. In addition to a conditioning effect of skeletal and cardiac muscle, a regular exercise program can help the individual to "feel better" in general, especially since patients who are involved in exercise programs (either as individuals or as members of groups) are apt to be conscious of proper weight

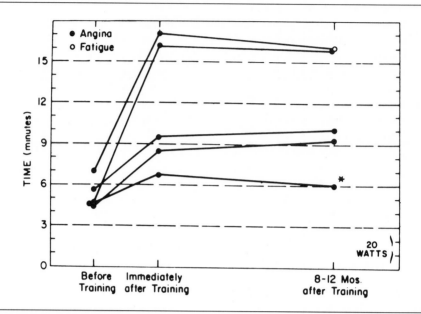

FIGURE 12–2. Duration of exercise required for onset of angina (or fatigue) to occur in each of five patients before training, immediately after training, and 8 to 12 months later. Increased exercise capacity was usually maintained for 8 to 12 months (these patients continued to do daily exercises at home). The asterisk marks the patient who had a myocardial infarction between the immediate posttraining and later posttraining studies. (From Redwood, D.R. et al. New Engl. J. Med. Reproduced by permission of the *New England Journal of Medicine*, 286:959, 1972.)

and health habits and often reduce cigarette smoking or give it up entirely. They also derive psychological benefits because they are participating in their own management. The subject of physical training (especially after a myocardial infarction) is discussed more fully in chapter 16 as well as in specific monographs [11].

MODIFICATION OF RISK FACTORS
As discussed in detail in chapter 3, four major risk factors are generally associated with development of coronary atherosclerosis: cigarette smoking, hypertension, diabetes mellitus, and hyperlipidemia. Modification of these factors is advisable, although once coronary artery disease is present, how much clinical benefit can be achieved is not clear. (The reader is referred to chapter 11 for a discussion of the various secondary prevention trials.) Modification of such factors may be relatively simple or exceedingly difficult.

*Cigarette Smoking.* Patients who smoke should be counseled by their physicians about the dangers of cigarette smoking. Harmful effects are due not only to nicotine ingestion (which causes stimulation of catecholamine release with resultant increase in myocardial irritability, heart rate, and blood pressure as well as possible coronary

vasoconstriction and intravascular platelet aggregation) but also to inhalation of carbon monoxide (which increases the level of carboxyhemoglobin, thereby reducing the amount of oxygen available to the myocardium) [12–14]. Exercise tolerance has been shown to be significantly reduced in coronary patients with elevated blood levels of carboxyhemoglobin from smoking [15]. Whether the threshold for ventricular arrhythmias is lowered in dogs exposed to increased concentrations of this substance is unclear [16, 17]. Also not clear is whether nicotine or carbon monoxide is the more harmful agent, but even with the lesser amount of these substances present in newer cigarettes, the risk of myocardial infarction is unchanged from that found in smokers of the "older" cigarettes [18]. The immediate and long-range harmful effects on both the heart and the lungs should be stressed, and helpful techniques for stopping smoking, including the use of various commercially available "group-therapy" sessions and other psychological support devices, should be provided. As discussed in chapters 3 and 11, epidemiologic studies show that ex-smokers reduce their risk of developing coronary artery disease to approximately that of nonsmokers; the data are less clear regarding smokers with already-present coronary artery disease, although stopping smoking will obviously eliminate the harmful effects of nicotine. Patients with coronary disease can still suffer the ill effects of carbon monoxide because it is also produced by automobile exhausts and by *other* people's cigarettes. [19]. The physician must be able to draw a line between aggressive counseling of patients who continue to smoke and harassment, since the latter may serve only to antagonize the patient and endanger physician-patient rapport.

*Hypertension.* Elevated blood pressure can readily be detected on routine office examianations. In most cases, it can be treated with a variety of medications that are, in large part, not harmful, depending on the drugs and dosages employed. Although a detailed discussion of current concepts in the treatment of hypertension is beyond the scope of this chapter, several excellent reviews [21] and the Report of the Joint National Committee on Detection, Evaluation and Treatment of High Blood Pressure [22] provide pertinent guidelines. These studies recommend that virtually all patients with diastolic pressures of 105 mmHg or greater should be treated, whereas treatment should be individualized for patients with diastolic pressures between 90 and 104 mmHg. Detection and confirmation of the blood pressure measurement are described in the Report of the Joint National Committee, as are recommendations for minimum baseline laboratory tests [22]. Basic laboratory tests include hematocrit, urinalysis, and serum blood urea nitrogen (BUN) and potassium measurement.

The first line of therapy is to achieve proper weight, since many hypertensive patients manifest varying degrees of obesity. As discussed in chapter 11, most investigators agree that patients with diastolic pressures over 95 mmHg

should be treated, initially with thiazide diuretics, with propranolol added if necessary (figure 12–3). (However, Kaplan [23], among others, has questioned the initial use of diuretics.) Patients with higher diastolic blood pressures will usually require the addition of methyldopa, reserpine, or the newer agent clonidine to the above regimen; those with initial pressures of 130 mmHg or more may require urgent treatment and hospitalization. Hydralazine is the next drug to be added, but because it increases cardiac work (and hence myocardial oxygen requirements), it should not be used in patients with coronary artery disease unless a $\beta$-adrenergic blocking agent (e.g., propranolol) is also employed. Without the "protective" cardiac effect of propranolol, tachycardia and arrhythmias may result and pose clinical problems. Newer vasodilators, such as prazosin and minoxidil, are also available. Finally, guanethidine, or the newest agent captopril [24], may be used if the level of blood pressure is still unsatisfactory. Since some of these drugs have troublesome side effects, the reader is referred to the reviews for further information as well as for recommended dosages.

To summarize, because of the serious cardiovascular consequences of hypertension, control of even mild hypertension (as defined above) is recommended.

*Diabetes Mellitus.* Still controversial is the question of whether strict adherence in controlling hyperglycemia will prevent or even reduce vascular complications [25]. The use of constant-infusing insulin pumps may help to solve this question, since the level of control is better than with prior methods. The current recommendation is that patients with ischemic heart disease be screened for diabetes and treated at least with diet therapy if abnormalities of glucose tolerance are revealed. Those with overt diabetes require close follow-up to prevent the more immediate life-threatening complications of the disease (e.g., ketoacidosis and coma), but control should never be at the price of hypoglycemic attacks. Consultation either with internists specializing in diabetic problems or with endocrinologists is recommended for difficult-to-control patients.

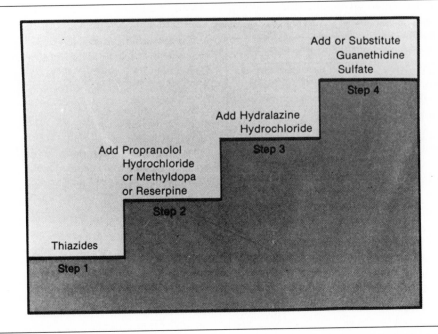

Add or Substitute
Guanethidine
Sulfate

Step 4

Add Hydralazine
Hydrochloride

Step 3

Add Propranolol
Hydrochloride
or Methyldopa
or Reserpine

Step 2

Thiazides

Step 1

FIGURE 12–3. Antihypertensive regimen recommended by the Joint National Committee. In this stepped-care approach, the newer agents, clonidine and prazosin, may be added or substituted for the drugs shown in Step 2 or 3 and captopril for drugs in Step 4. (From Report of the Joint National Committee on Detection, Evaluation, and Treatment of High Blood Pressure. *JAMA* 237:255, 1977. Copyright 1977, American Medical Association.)

*Hyperlipidemia.* Hyperlipidemia is perhaps the most difficult risk factor to "control." Although considerable evidence demonstrates that hyperlipidemia, especially hypercholesterolemia, is associated with coronary atherosclerosis (see chapters 3 and 11 for more detailed discussion), there is no unanimity of opinion that it is the primary inciting agent. Whether, as well as how, to treat "elevated" lipid levels is still not clear [26]. In fact, the definition of an "elevated" lipid level itself is controversial because the risk rises with increasing levels, rather than emerging at any arbitrary level. Radical changes in dietary habits are often difficult in middle-aged people, and whether regression of coronary atherosclerosis can occur with diet therapy alone is questionable. As determined by coronary arteriography, it appears to be a relentless process once the initial lesions have formed in any of the coronary vessels. Regression of coronary atherosclerosis has been demonstrated in nonhuman primates [27], but even with ileal bypass procedures (which produce the greatest reduction in serum cholesterol levels), regression of coronary artery disease in humans has not been clearly shown. On the other hand, lowering lipid levels medically has been associated with regression of *femoral* atherosclerosis in humans [28]. Dietary modification of hyperlipidemia is probably best utilized to *prevent* the development of coronary atherosclerosis; it should be most aggressively followed in the younger age groups, excluding infancy, as described in chapter 11.

Should patients over the age of 50 with *clinically apparent* ischemic heart disease (but not necessarily severe hyperlipidemia) have special diets? As discussed in chapter 11 (see Secondary Prevention Trials), improvement in *clinical status* and *survival* with dietary management of hyperlipidemia was reported in some patients following myocardial infarction, but not confirmed in other similar studies. Simply stated, there are no convincing data in this area. There are, however, certain positive reasons for advising low saturated fat diets and reduction of dietary cholesterol in patients with clinical coronary artery disease. These reasons include the obvious ones: the diets themselves are not harmful, they may lead to weight loss that will improve the feeling of general well-being in the patient, and perhaps most importantly from the physician's point of view, they are evidence to the patient that the doctor is concerned about doing something positive for his condition. A psychological "uplift" may be achieved when the patient can be told that his cholesterol level is falling or his weight reduction is proceeding nicely. Reduction in saturated fats can be achieved by following the kind of diets recommended by the American Heart Association [29] in which animal and hydrogenated vegetable fats are replaced with special margarines, shortenings, and vegetable oils, as well as by consultation with a dietitian-nutritionist.

The use of lipid-lowering drug regimens is perhaps best suited to patients under the age of 50 with markedly elevated lipid levels (i.e., the top 5 to 10 percent of the population), because troublesome side effects are often associated with many of these agents. Two recent reviews [30, 31] have summarized the treatment of hyperlipidemia and provide recommendations for treatment. For patients with increased levels of very low density lipoproteins (VLDL), clofibrate or nicotine acid administration is suggested, whereas for patients with increased levels of low-density lipoproteins (LDL), bile-acid binding resins are preferred. These appear useful in retarding the progression of the disease, as determined by angiography [32]. For a more detailed discussion of dosage, recommendations, and side effects, the reader is referred to the reviews cited earlier [30, 31]. At the present time, few data are available concerning pharmacologic agents that can *raise* the level of high-density lipoproteins (HDL), which may protect against coronary atherosclerosis (see chapter 3).

In addition to the modification of risk factors, there is growing interest in the use of *physical training* as a means of either preventing development of coronary artery disease or reducing its morbid complications once clinical manifestations occur. As discussed in chapters 3 and 11, the relation of exercise (or physical activity in general) to the development of coronary artery

disease is unclear, despite the observations that coronary artery disease appears to be more common in individuals with a sedentary life-style, that physical training can cause a lowering of blood pressure in hypertensive individuals, that it can raise the level of "protective" HDL-cholesterol [33], and that physical training, as previously noted, has a beneficial effect on cardiac performance [6, 7]. Whether the widespread adoption of regular exercise of the dynamic type (e.g., swimming, running, walking, or bicycling) will influence the incidence of coronary artery disease in the future remains to be determined (see chapter 11), but a regular exercise program does have a place in the management of symptomatic patients, as discussed earlier.

Another possible risk factor that could be modified is *obesity,* which is associated with glucose intolerance, hypertension, and reduced levels of HDL-cholesterol [34]. Obesity indirectly increases the work of the heart because of the greater total body effort needed to perform routine activities.

## Medical Management of Chronic (Stable) Angina Pectoris

### NITRATES

Nitrates are the medications most commonly employed by physicians to treat patients with angina pectoris. Their clinical effectiveness was first described in 1867 by Brunton [35]. The basic pharmacologic action of the drugs is to relax smooth muscle [36]. In both normal subjects and those with coronary artery disease, the vasodilatory effects of nitrates are evident in both systemic arteries and veins, but they appear to be predominant in the venous circulation [37]. The decrease in venous tone reduces the return of blood to the heart, and there is a concomitant reduction in external [38] and internal ventricular dimensions [39, 40]. The absolute reduction in end-diastolic size is particularly marked [38, 40] (figure 12–4).

In addition to their action on systemic arteries and veins, the vasodilating effects of the nitrates can also be readily demonstrated on the larger (i.e., conductance) vessels of the heart itself

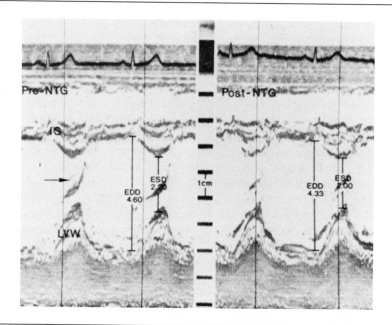

FIGURE 12-4. Echocardiograms before and after administration of nitroglycerin (NTG). The attenuated echoes from the anterior mitral leaflet (arrow) observed in the left ventricular cavity in both panels confirm that the echocardiographic beam traverses the same sector before and after NTG. Both the end-diastolic cavity dimension (EDD) and the end-systolic cavity dimension (ESD) declined, whereas heart rate was nearly constant. LVW = left ventricular wall. (From DeMaria, A.N. et al. *Am. J. Med.* 57:754, 1974.)

[41], although beneficial effects on myocardial blood flow have been more difficult to establish. How, then, do the nitrates relieve angina? Most investigators believe that the nitrates are effective in relieving myocardial ischemia (and angina pectoris) mainly because they decrease the mechanical activity (work) of the heart, and thus its oxygen requirements, through their systemic effects, that is, by "unloading" of the heart via reduction in left ventricular systolic and diastolic pressure and volume (table 12-1) [40–44]. The heart rate may increase when blood pressure falls reflexly, but the nitrates are not thought to have any direct effect on the contractile state of the heart, although there has been some evidence to the contrary [45].

Posture is important in evaluating the hemodynamic effects of the nitrates. In the supine position, venous return is normally greater and exercise tolerance lower [46]. Accordingly, the hemodynamic and angina-relieving effects of this class of drugs are most marked when patients are sitting or standing [47]. By reducing the work of the heart, the nitrates can increase exercise capacity in patients with coronary artery disease [47–49]; hence a greater total *body* workload can be achieved before the cardiac threshold is reached at which angina occurs (figure 12-5). In addition, atrial pacing studies indicate that following administration of these drugs, hemodynamic abnormalities are not as readily apparent, and the heart can be paced to higher rates without episodes of angina [46, 50]. The nitrates have also been shown to improve abnor-

TABLE 12-1. Effects of nitrates of cardiac dynamics

CHANGES THAT TEND TO DECREASE
  MYOCARDIAL OXYGEN CONSUMPTION
  Reduction in blood pressure
  Reduction in ejection time
  Reduction in ventricular volumes

CHANGES THAT TEND TO INCREASE MYOCARDIAL
  OXYGEN CONSUMPTION
  Reflex increase in heart rate
  Reflex and direct (?) increase in contractile state

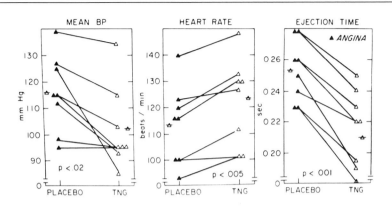

FIGURE 12-5. Comparison of mean blood pressure (BP), heart rate, and ejection time measured after equal amounts of exercise following a placebo (left of each panel) and following nitroglycerin (TNG). A significant fall in BP and ejection time and a rise in heart rate occurred during exercise after nitroglycerin. The net effect of these changes was clinically beneficial, since no patients experienced angina during the TNG exercise protocol, but they did with the placebo (solid triangles). (From Goldstein, R.E. and Epstein, S.E. *Prog. Cardiovas. Dis.* 14:360, 1972. Reproduced by permission.)

malities of ventricular wall motion in patients with coronary artery disease, as demonstrated by contrast ventriculography (see fig. 2–13) [51, 52], echocardiography [40], and radionuclide ventriculography [53] (including cineventriculography) [54].

In addition to the effects of these drugs on cardiac hemodynamics, there is also evidence that they can have a beneficial effect on regional myocardial blood flow. Studies performed in animals demonstrate redistribution of flow to ischemic areas, particularly in the subendocardium [55–58], which is perhaps mediated in part by an increase in collateral flow [59, 60] (figure 12–6). As discussed in chapter 2, most coronary blood flow studies in patients with coronary artery disease that have employed techniques for evaluating myocardial blood flow do not measure *regional* flow, and the results of the studies that measure total or average flow have been conflicting. Some have reported increased flow following administration of sublingual or intravenous preparations [42, 61, 62]. Most report no change or decreased flow [63]. Studies

done in patients at the time of coronary artery bypass surgery, however, have shown a beneficial effect on regional perfusion [64, 65], and such results have also been demonstrated in catheterization laboratory studies employing xenon-133 and a scintillation camera [66, 67].

In the studies from the Peter Bent Brigham Hospital [67], regional myocardial blood flow increased in areas subserved by stenotic coronary arteries when well-developed collateral vessels were available to those regions (figure 12–7). It is doubtful that this effect alone would be sufficient to relieve most effort-related angina, but it is possible (see figure 12–6) that the action of the nitrates on the coronary vessels may complement their systemic effects, perhaps in regions of the heart where the hemodynamic effects not only have reduced myocardial oxygen requirements but have also established a favorable milieu for improved myocardial perfusion by reducing wall tension and extravascular diastolic resistance [45]. The action of the nitrates on the coronary vessels themselves is of more clinical value when there is evidence that coronary *spasm* is occurring, as in Prinzmetal's angina or in those unstable or those chronic angina patients with a strong vasotonic component to their ischemia. Furthermore, recent studies have demonstrated that sublingual and intracoronary nitroglycerin can also dilate the stenosis; this may turn out to be a major component of the drug's beneficial acts [68]. Coronary artery spasm due to nitrate *withdrawal* has been postulated as the cause of a chest pain syndrome in workers engaged in the manufacture of these

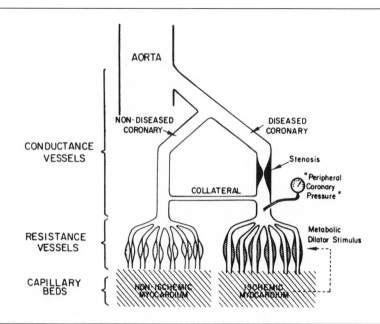

FIGURE 12–6. Relation between ischemic and nonischemic portions of the coronary circulation. Because of the high proximal resistance within a diseased coronary artery, the arterioles beyond the obstruction are obliged to remain dilated to sustain flow. Metabolic byproducts from the ischemic myocardium probably are the major stimulus to the local vasodilation. Further dilation is not likely to be beneficial and may be harmful if there is also dilation of nonischemic beds with diversion of coronary blood flow. Nitrates do not apparently have this adverse effect, but they may instead augment collateral flow to ischemic areas and increase the "peripheral coronary pressure" as indicated by the manometer, as well as having beneficial effects on cardiac dynamics and metabolism (see text). (From Goldstein, R.E. and Epstein, S.E. *Prog. Cardiovas. Dis.* 14:360, 1972. Reproduced by permission.)

drugs [69]. Constant exposure to nitrates apparently results in a reduction in coronary tone in some individuals. When these workers are away from the factory for the weekend and the nitrate effect has dissipated, there is presumably a "rebound" vasoconstriction in normal coronary arteries that can cause an anginalike syndrome that mimics ischemic heart disease.

*Types of Preparations and Routes of Administration.* *Nitroglycerin* given sublingually is the drug of choice for treatment of the acute angina attack or for prophylactic administration prior to an activity known to precipitate angina in a given patient. The usual dose is .3 to .4 mg (or less if headache is troublesome), and most patients will respond within 3 minutes to one or two tablets. Intolerance is rarely a problem with intermittent usage. Except for specially stabilized preparations, nitroglycerin tablets for sublingual use

tend to lose their potency, especially if exposed to light, and they should be kept in dark containers. The effect of *oral,* sustained-release nitroglycerin preparations is still unclear [69], but the value of *intravenous* nitroglycerin is now well established in the treatment of unstable angina [70]. *Intracoronary* nitroglycerin [71] has been used to diagnose and relieve coronary spasm, to prevent spasm during percutaneous transluminal coronary angioplasty, and to exclude or reverse spasm in patients with acute myocardial infarction.

*Cutaneous* nitroglycerin was described in 1955 but did not become popular until several studies in the mid-1970s showed effects lasting for several hours [72, 73]. Initially, the nitroglycerin-lanolin compound was spread over the chest, back, abdomen, or thighs in ½-to 2-inch doses. More recently, slow-release preparations of cutaneous nitroglycerin have become available.

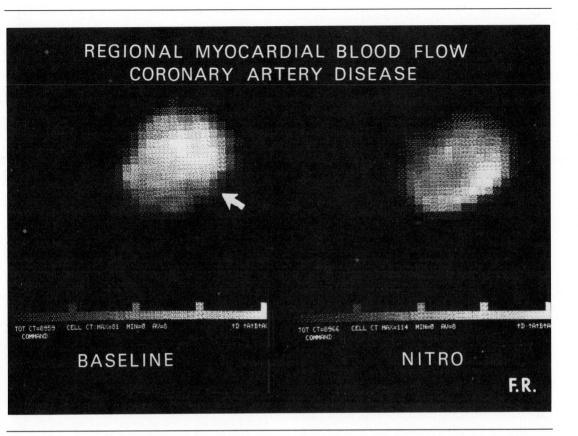

REGIONAL MYOCARDIAL BLOOD FLOW
CORONARY ARTERY DISEASE

BASELINE

NITRO

F.R.

FIGURE 12–7. Radioisotope (xenon-133) images before (A) and after (B) sublingual administration of nitroglycerin. The increasing intensity of the gray-to-white scale reflects increasing flow rates (not concentration of the radioisotope). After nitroglycerin, the underperfused area (arrow) supplied by the distal left circumflex artery is no longer apparent. The reduction in perfusion in the upper regions suggests that there has been redistribution of flow after nitroglycerin administration. On arteriography, this patient demonstrated excellent collateral pathways from a nondiseased left anterior descending artery to a significantly diseased left circumflex artery. (From Cohn, P.F. et al. *Am. J. Cardiol.* 39:672, 1977.)

These systems use nitroglycerin reservoirs that (hopefully) permit an even and gradual absorption over a 24-hour period. They are aesthetically more pleasing than the lanolin components, but as has been pointed out [74] their efficacy has yet to be demonstrated in rigorous protocols. They are also more expensive than the lanolin ointment. Nitroglycerin is also available in a transmucosal (buccal) form [75]. These tablets, inserted under the upperlip, allow gradual and uniform release of the drug. Another ingenious new delivery system for nitroglycerin incorporates the drug into an oral spray [76]. This has the potential to be the most rapidly acting of all of the nitroglycerin preparations.

Adverse reactions to nitroglycerin are not uncommon and include headache, flushing, and hypotension. The latter is only rarely severe, but it can be potentially dangerous if the chest pain is due to a myocardial infarction rather than to angina.

*Other nitrate preparations* are available in chewable, sublingual, and oral form. One of the most popular of such preparations is isosorbide dinitrate, available in 2.5 to 5.0 mg sublingual doses, 5 to 10 mg chewable form, 5 to 40 mg tablets, and controlled-release capsules for oral administration. Initially, the oral nitrates were not felt to be of any benefit because of inadequate gastrointestinal absorption and rapid hepatic breakdown. More recent studies, however, have shown that oral nitrates can increase exercise tolerance and can thus be of potential clinical benefit to patients with coronary artery disease [77, 78]. Improvement in exercise tolerance is a better end-point than merely recording either patients' subjective responses to the drug or how much less nitroglycerin they require (both of which can be shown to be "improved" by placebos), and hence it offers more reliable evidence of potential clinical benefit. Whether oral nitrates cause tolerance to nitroglycerin and other nitrate preparations is not clear. Some studies [79] show no tolerance, while others do [80].

Whether or not oral nitrate preparations actually provide "longer" duration of action than does sublingual nitroglycerin is also a subject of continuing controversy. There is less disagreement about the duration of action of the ointment than about that of the oral agents (figure 12–8), but some groups have found the exercise test data for oral nitrates to be disappointing. At issue seems to be the type of exercise testing protocol employed as well as the dosage of the oral agents. Whereas the literature concerning the usual 5 to 10 mg doses does not show much benefit over placebos, studies using larger doses (10 to 30 mg) have demonstrated increased exercise capacity in patients with coronary artery disease (figure 12–9) [78].

Even though the issue is still not settled, the following summary appears reasonable: First, nitroglycerin ointment and high-dose oral nitrate preparations take about 30 minutes to produce a noticeable effect, maximal effect is present at 1½ to 3 hours, and by 4 hours, little effect remains. Whether "sustained release" preparations give even longer-acting benefits is conjectural. Second, sublingual and transmucosal nitroglycerin and sublingual isosorbide dinitrate have a rapid onset of activity (several minutes); maximal activity lasts for about 10 minutes with nitroglycerin (with lesser effects lasting for an additional hour). Transmucosal (buccal) nitroglycerin may be effective for 3 to 5 hours.

Although the controversy as to the efficacy of "long-acting" nitrates continues, the contemporary physician would be wise to learn how to employ the full armamentarium of the nitrate preparations in treating patients with coronary

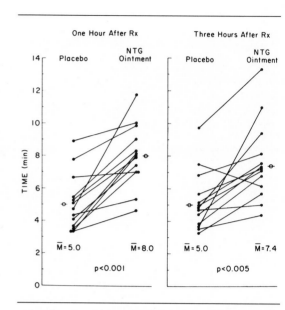

FIGURE 12–8. Duration of exercise at onset of angina (in minutes) is compared after administration of placebo (left of each panel) and after application of nitroglycerin (NTG) ointment. The average dose of the 2 percent NTG ointment was approximately ½ inch applied to the patient's back. Responses in each patient are plotted. Mean values (M) demonstrate that a significant increase in exercise capacity was present 1 hour after the ointment was applied and persisted at least 3 hours afterward. (From Reichek, N. et al. Long-acting nitroglycerin for angina, 1982; old dog, new tricks. *Circulation* 50:348, 1974. Reproduced by permission of the American Heart Association, Inc.)

artery disease. This is especially true since by virtue of their unloading effect on the heart, they are also useful for treating congestive heart failure. Suggested guidelines for drug management of patients with angina will be offered after discussion of the other commonly used pharmacologic agents.

### β-ADRENERGIC BLOCKING AGENTS

At one time, the only FDA-approved drug of this type for angina was propranolol. Now, there are a host of such agents (vide infra). However, propranolol remains the standard by which other agents of this type are compared. In over a decade of use, this drug has proved to be a highly effective and safe agent for treatment of most patients with angina pectoris [81, 82]. The mechanism of action of this drug in treating an-

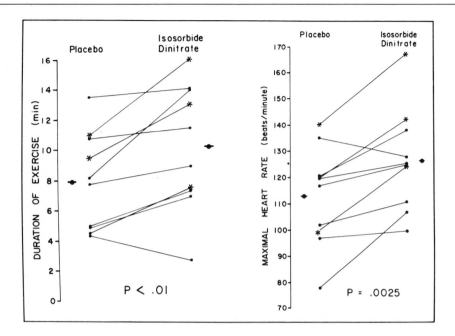

FIGURE 12–9. Duration of exercise and maximal heart rate attained during exercise 2 hours after a placebo was given and 2 hours after oral administration of 7.5 to 20 mg of isosorbide dinitrate in 10 patients. Patients indicated by solid dots experienced angina with both bouts of exercise; patients denoted with asterisks had "silent" ischemia (ischemic ECG changes without pain), and the test was stopped at that point. Compared to the placebo, both the duration of exercise and the maximal heart rate achieved were significantly increased by oral nitrate ingestion. (From Glancy, D.L. et al. *Am. J. Med.* 62:39, 1977.)

TABLE 12–2. Effects of $\beta$-adrenergic blocking agents on cardiac dynamics

CHANGES THAT TEND TO DECREASE
MYOCARDIAL OXYGEN CONSUMPTION
Reduction in heart rate
Reduction in contractility
Slight (if any) reduction in blood pressure

CHANGES THAT TEND TO INCREASE MYOCARDIAL
OXYGEN CONSUMPTION
Increase in ventricular volumes
Increase in ejection time

gina is through reducing myocardial oxygen requirements for any given level of activity. This reduction is accomplished mainly by reducing heart rate, with a lesser effect on arterial blood pressure, and myocardial contractility (table 12–2). Investigations into the effect of propranolol on resting left ventricular function have yielded conflicting results. Some studies have demonstrated that the drug increases ventricular volume [83] and thereby increases myocardial oxygen requirements, though in most patients the effect of these actions is usually minimal. Furthermore, even though propranolol may have a small depressant effect on global and segmental ejection fraction [84] during exercise, it can be beneficial in the presence of ischemia-producing

lesions [85, 86]. In addition to improvement of symptoms, enhanced exercise tolerance with reduction in ST segment depression [87] has been demonstrated, as has a modification in the anginal threshold determined by atrial pacing [88]. It has also been suggested that propranolol may reverse abnormal platelet aggregation by reducing platelet thromboxane $A_2$ generation [89].

Despite differences in mode of action, chronic administration either of propranolol or the nitrates reduces the frequency of anginal episodes when the effects are compared in the same group of patients [90]. Some investigators have reported an additive effect of the two drugs in increasing exercise tolerance under laboratory conditions, but this has not been confirmed by other groups. Certainly, the reflex tachycardia that may accompany nitrate-induced arterial hypotension is blocked by propranolol. Propranolol also can be combined with calcium-antagonists to provide additive antianginal effects [91].

Adverse reactions to propranolol include fatigue, gastrointestinal upset, sexual dysfunction, intensification of insulin-induced hypoglycemia by masking of hypoglycemic symptoms, bronchoconstriction, bradyarrhythmias, heart block, and hypotension [92]. In patients who already have a compromised left ventricle, congestive heart failure may ensue or may be made worse. This effect can be somewhat tempered by the use of digitalis or, in some cases, prevented by the "prophylactic" digitalization of those patients with large hearts who require propranolol for control of angina. Propranolol can also potentiate coronary vasoconstriction, and thus be harmful in some patients with increased coronary vasomotor tone [93]. Peripheral vasoconstriction can precipitate episodes of Raynaud's phenomenon and cause uncomfortable coldness in the arms and legs. Sudden withdrawal of the drug in ambulatory patients has been reported to result in acute ischemic episodes [94]. There are several possible mechanisms for this phenomenon. Since the drug prevents angina, patients who feel better increase their activities to a level that formerly would have resulted in chest pain. When the drug is discontinued, they are usually still operating at this higher level of exertion but without the drug's protective effects. Because the greatest benefit in activity tolerance occurs in patients who were previously most disabled, the withdrawal effect would be most marked in those readily prone to myocardial ischemia. Some groups have reported an increase in platelet aggregation and shortened platelet-survival time following abrupt withdrawal of the drug [95]. Other suggested mechanisms involve an unmasking of increased sympathetic tone, adverse alterations in oxygen affinity for hemoglobin, increased beta-receptor sensitivity, increased number of beta-receptors, and progression of atherosclerosis. The latter is not related to the drug's effects but to the natural history of the disease. The withdrawal phenome-

non is much less marked in hospitalized patients [96], thus suggesting that the higher "set" of activity level is the mechanism. This is also supported by recent evidence showing that there is no physiologic basis for a rebound mechanism due to heightened beta-receptor sensitivity [97]. Either tapering the propranolol dose or using a prolonged small-dose schedule can prevent the syndrome [98].

As a reasonable therapeutic goal, the resting heart rate should be less than 60 beats per minute and less than 100 after maximal exercise. Substantial training effects can still be achieved in coronary patients despite the reduced heart rate [99]. The usual dosage varies from 40 to 480 mg per day; higher dosages may be of even more benefit to cardiac function during exercise, even when medium doses relieve symptoms [100]. Serum levels of at least 30 ng/ml are usually required to achieve a 25 percent or greater reduction in frequency of angina [101]. Dosage need not be q.i.d.; b.i.d. dosage is also effective [102]. A long-acting once-a-day peparation is also available [103].

Five other $\beta$-adrenergic drugs are also approved for use in the United States (table 12–3). Labetalol, a drug with both alpha-adrenergic and beta-adrenergic blocking effects, has recently been added to the list. These beta-blockers differ from propranolol in one way or another. Propranolol is a noncardioselective beta-blocker with some quinidinelike antiarrhythmic activity but no intrinsic sympathometic activity (ISA), i.e., partial beta-antagonist activity. Nadolol and timolol have similar features to propranolol but are longer acting and are recommended in one-daily (40- to 240 mg) and two-daily doses (10–30 mg), respectively. Timolol, like propranolol, is also approved for use in postmyocardial infarction patients (see chapter 13) and, like propranolol, has been shown to reduce ischemia-induced left ventricular dysfunction [104, 105]. Metoprolol and atenolol are beta-cardioselective agents with proven effectiveness in treating angina [104, 106, 107]. The usual dose of metoprolol is 50 to 200 mg twice a day. Atenolol, like nadolol, is hydrophilic, which means less sleep disturbances and longer half-life (i.e., one daily dosage at 50 to 100 mg). Pindolol is not cardioselective but does have the strongest ISA of any currently

TABLE 12–3. Different pharmacodynamic properties of FDA-approved β-adrenergic blocking agents

| Agent | β-blocking potency ratio (propranolol = 1.0) | Relative cardiac selectivity | Intrinsic sympathomimetic activity (ISA) | Membrane stabilizing activity |
|---|---|---|---|---|
| Atenolol | 1.0 | + | 0 | 0 |
| Metoprolol | 1.0 | + | 0 | 0 |
| Nadolol | 1.0 | 0 | 0 | 0 |
| Pindolol | 6.0 | 0 | + | + |
| Propranolol | 1.0 | 0 | 0 | + + |
| Timolol | 6.0 | 0 | 0 | 0 |

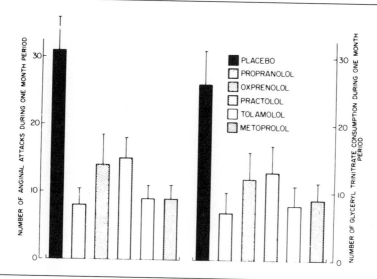

FIGURE 12–10. Comparison of effects of five β-adrenoreceptor antagonists with different actions during sustained treatment (22 patients). Data represent mean ± standard error of the mean. The number of anginal attacks and nitroglycerin consumption were significantly reduced during treatment with all five drugs in comparison to treatment with a placebo (p < 0.01). The differences between the five drugs were not significant. Propranolol and oxprenolol are non-cardioselective; practolol, metoprolol, and tolamolol are cardioelective; oxprenolol and practolol have ISA (see text). (From Thadani, U. et al. *Am. J. Med.* 68:-246, 1980.)

available drug and is an effective antianginal agent [108], even though only the exercise heart rate, not the resting heart rate, is blocked. Usual dosage is 5 to 30 mg twice a day. Are there any inherent advantages to cardioselectivity or partial agonist activity? Cardioselectivity should be of advantage in certain patients (asthmatics, for example) but often when the

dose of the agent is increased, cardioselectivity is lost. ISA would be expected to be most suited to the patient who needs bronchodilation or who has depressed left ventricular function, and exercise studies appear to show that this type of beta-blocker does maintain left ventricular function better than beta-blockers without this property [109]. As far as clinical antianginal effects alone are concerned, however, there does not appear to be any advantage to cardioselectivity or ISA [110] (figure 12–10).

CALCIUM-ANTAGONISTS
(CALCIUM-CHANNEL BLOCKING AGENTS)
These agents inhibit contraction of cardiac and vascular smooth muscle cells by decreasing the cellular uptake of calcium via the "slow channel" [111]. The resulting systemic vasodilation causes unloading of the left ventricle, and the coronary vasodilation leads to increased myocar-

dial perfusion. These actions, plus the negative inotropic effects of these drugs (table 12–4), often alleviate myocardial ischemia, hence their value as antianginal agents [111, 112]. At the present time, nifedipine, verapamil, and diltiazem have been approved by the FDA. Their clinical efficacy in stable, chronic angina has been shown in a variety of studies either alone [113–115] or combined with β-adrenergic blocking agents [91, 116, 117] (figure 12–11). As will be discussed subsequently, they are especially valuable in the treatment of unstable angina and Prinzmetal's angina. Nifedipine is the most potent vasodilator of the three; its side effects include headache, flushing, and leg edema. Usual dosage is 10 to 40 mg orally four times a day. Verapamil slows atrioventricular conduction and must be used cautiously in patients with cardiac conduction problems. Dosage is 80 to 120 mg three times a day. Diltiazem may actually increase oxygen delivery in addition to lowering arterial pressure during exertion. Its action on the coronary vasculature is relatively selective, which may explain the low incidence of adverse effects compared to the other two drugs, but like verapamil, it can slow heart rate and atrioventricular conduction. Dosage is 30 to 90 mg four times a day.

OTHER ANTIANGINAL THERAPIES
*Digitalis* is used in patients with ischemic heart disease to treat congestive heart failure. It can also be used to treat angina pectoris, however, *if* there is cardiomegaly or left ventricular failure. In this situation, the net effect of decreasing heart size and reducing myocardial oxygen requirements offsets the drug's positive inotropic

TABLE 12–4. Effects of calcium-antagonists on cardiac dynamics

| |
|---|
| CHANGES THAT TEND TO DECREASE MYOCARDIAL OXYGEN CONSUMPTION |
| Reduction in blood pressure |
| Reduction in contractility* |
| Reduction in heart rate* |
| |
| CHANGES THAT TEND TO INCREASE MYOCARDIAL OXYGEN CONSUMPTION |
| Reflex increase in heart rate |

*Especially verapamil, and to a lesser extent diltiazem.

actions and the intrinsic increase in myocardial oxygen requirements. Since most patients with angina pectoris do *not* have cardiomegaly or failure, it is not surprising that variable responses in angina relief and in increased exercise tolerance have been observed following digitalization. The beneficial effect in patients without congestive heart failure may be explained by the observation that the end-diastolic volume falls in such patients, even when initially normal [112]. In patients with angina and left ventricular dysfunction but without clinical congestive heart failure, it has also been demonstrated that when digoxin therapy is *combined* with propranolol, exercise tolerance can be improved [119]. Finally, digitalis should be employed if the patient's angina is provoked by tachyarrhythmias that can be prevented by digitalis (see below).

*Anticoagulant therapy* with warfarin derivatives is no longer recommended in patients with chronic angina pectoris. Because of the possibility that increased platelet aggregation may contribute to ischemic episodes, there is continuing interest in studying the clinical effectiveness of agents that prevent or reduce platelet aggregation. Acetylsalicylic acid (aspirin) inhibits several phases of platelet aggregation and has been used to treat a variety of disorders that may involve increased platelet aggregation; these include transient cerebral ischemic attacks, thromboembolus formation after insertion of prosthetic heart valves, and most importantly for purposes of this chapter, coronary artery disease. Multicenter trials to assess the value of this drug in reducing morbidity and mortality in patients who have already experienced prior myocardial infarction have been inconclusive [120]. (Another drug with similar antiplatelet properties, the uricosuric agent sulfinpyrazone, has also demonstrated some "protective" benefits in patients with coronary artery disease, though not all are convinced [121].) Frishman and associates [122] evaluated exercise tolerance in patients with stable angina pectoris before and after aspirin therapy. Although platelet aggregation was reduced, exercise tolerance, the anginal threshold, and ischemic ECG abnormalities were not altered. Therefore, whether treatment with aspirin will be beneficial in either short- or

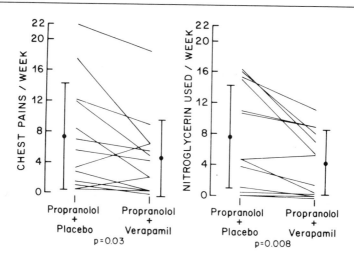

FIGURE 12–11. Number of episodes of chest pain/-week (left) and the number of nitroglycerin tablets used/week (right) during propranolol-placebo and propranolol-verapamil therapy. Each line represents the data from one patient, and the means ± 1 standard deviation is displayed on either side of each set of lines. During propranolol-verapamil therapy, the number of episodes of chest pain and nitroglycerin tablets consumed was lower than during propranolol-placebo therapy. (Reprinted with permission from the American College of Cardiology. From Winniford, M.D. et al. *J. Am. Coll. Cardiol.* 1:482, 1983.)

long-term treatment of coronary artery disease is still unclear. The problem deserves further investigation because of the drug's antiplatelet actions, its low cost, and its relatively few side effects.

*Antithyroid drugs,* radioiodine, or both have also been used in the past, but their role has been replaced by current medical therapy or myocardial revascularization surgery.

*Alcohol* has been traditionally advocated as an antianginal remedy, but no convincing data have been presented as to its efficacy, and one recent study [123] even suggests it may be harmful.

*Antiarrhythmic agents* can be useful in those patients whose angina results from one or more types of arrhythmias. To the previously cited example of digitalis usage for tachyarrhythmias such as paroxysmal atrial tachycardia or fibrillation, one can add quinidine or procainamide for ventricular tachycardia, as well as the newer agents described in chapter 15.

*Diuretics* can be used in conjunction with digitalis when congestive heart failure is thought to be responsible in whole or part for anginal episodes. Such agents may be particularly useful in those patients with nocturnal angina whose pain is precipitated by the increased venous return associated with the supine position.

*Sedatives and tranquilizers* are most helpful in those patients whose angina is precipitated or exacerbated by stress, tension, or emotional problems in general.

The *intra-aortic balloon assist device* is usually reserved for patients with unstable angina or postinfarction shock. External counterpulsation devices are obviously more suitable for patients with chronic angina, but their clinical benefit is yet to be clearly proved [124], and they are under continuing study.

*Percutaneous transluminal coronary angioplasty (PTCA)* was introduced in humans by Gruntzig in 1978 [125]. With this technique, a balloon catheter is introduced into a coronary artery and through the area of stenosis (see chapter 9 and figures 9–13 through 9–20). When successful, this procedure disrupts the intima and splits the atherosclerotic plaque. Coronary occlusion can occur in 5 percent of patients, usually due to dissection of the vessel. Immediate surgery must be performed in these instances. Mortality rates are about 1 percent [126]. PTCA is successful in 60 to 80 percent of patients [127] and symptomatic relief is often combined with improvement in left ventricular function, thallium-stress tests, etc. [128, 130]. About 20 percent of the successfully treated patients will develop restenosis and over half can benefit from repeat angioplasty. At the present time the procedure is recommended mainly for those patients who have a proximal, discrete stenosis in one of the major coronary arteries. Most patients have moderately severe angina. Only 5 to 10 percent of patients who are candidates for coronary bypass surgery are suitable for PTCA. Another catheter-related technique uses laser irradiation to vaporize atherosclerotic plaques and intracoronary thrombi [131]. This technique may prove to be helpful antianginal treatment in selected patients.

GUIDELINES FOR PATIENT MANAGEMENT
As noted earlier, reassurance, modification of risk factors, avoidance of angina-provoking situations whenever possible, and a properly designed exercise program are important adjuncts to drug therapy.

Whether or not patients should "walk through" angina is debatable, with many physicians concerned about unduly increasing the risks of morbid events. Patients should be advised to sit up or even stand during anginal episodes, but not to become supine, in order to minimize the effect of venous return on the heart. Nitroglycerin is the first line of therapy (see below); patients who forget to carry their medication can be advised to do a Valsalva maneuver (or even hold their breath) to slow the heart rate and hopefully obtain relief. Although administration of nitroglycerin was discussed earlier in the chapter, some additional points are worth emphasizing.

Patients should be carefully instructed on the use of nitroglycerin, both as a remedial and as a prophylactic (anticipatory) measure, before starting any activity that they think or know from experience might bring on angina. Some patients feel that taking the medication is a sign of "weakness" and prefer to "tough it out" instead. This attitude may invite danger (e.g., arrhythmias or infarction) and should be discouraged. Furthermore, the drug should be kept on the person *at all times* and refilled every 6 months because of deterioration. Some physi-

cians have the patients take the drug for the first time in their presence to make sure they are taking it properly and to familiarize them with its noncardiac effects. Finally, the drug should be taken with the patients sitting (but not supine) to maximize its venous pooling effects and to prevent syncope that might occur in the standing position due to hypotension.

Drug therapy may be limited to nitroglycerin on only an "as necessary" (P.R.N.) regimen if pain episodes are relatively infrequent (once or twice a week). In a minority of patients with angina of several years' duration, the pain may spontaneously remit and no further therapy may be needed [132]. In others, it will progress and require more intensive drug therapy to relieve or at least stabilize symptoms. Thus, if nitroglycerin is required on a daily basis, "long-acting" oral, cutaneous, or sublingual nitrate preparations; moderate doses of $\beta$-blockers (at least 20); or both should also be employed.

Because of their physiologic effects (see tables 12–1 and 12–2), nitrates and $\beta$-blockers often act synergistically for the benefit of the patient, but the patient should be made aware that $\beta$-blockers and the nitrate preparations are purely "preventive" drugs and are not effective for the acute anginal episodes. Increasing the doses of these drugs will depend on the clinical response or if an exercise testing protocol is followed, on improvement in exercise tolerance, in the degree of ST segment depression, or both. Propranolol may be increased 10 to 20 mg per dose for stable angina. Heart rate may decrease to the 40s during sleep, but this in itself is not cause for concern unless it is accompanied by hypotension, syncope, or heart block. If angina persists at high doses of propranolol (more than 320 to 400 mg/day) and of long-acting oral nitrates (more than 30 to 80 mg/day) plus nitroglycerin ointment, then a calcium-channel blocker should be added. Nifedipine is preferred because it has no negative chronotropic action. In those situations in which there appears to be a vasotonic component to the patient's angina (i.e., it occurs at variable thresholds of exertion) and heart rate reduction is also needed, diltiazem or verapamil may be used instead of beta-blockers.

If the patient is still symptomatic, then PTCA or surgery should be considered. The decision as

to when the patient should undergo cardiac catheterization varies from physician to physician.
Some clinicians take a more aggressive stance
regarding younger patients (under 50 years old)
because of the prognostic data that can be obtained from the coronary arteriograms (see
below), while others prefer to wait for refractoriness to medical therapy to develop. In patients *not* considered technically suitable for
PTCA or surgery, the use of very large doses of
β-blockers combined with calcium-antagonists
may be necessary to control angina. Occasionally, severe symptomatic bradycardia or heart
block may result in elderly patients, and insertion of a permanent demand pacemaker may be
necessary.

A final word is important concerning the assessment of therapy by the clinician. Despite
necessary emphasis on more objective parameters, how the patient *feels* is still the keystone in
this evaluation. Specifically, is the patient now
able to perform work and leisure activities more
comfortably than formerly? Is there an improved sense of well-being? If objective measurements are needed, perhaps the easiest technique is simply to have the patient record how
many anginal attacks requiring nitroglycerin are
experienced on a daily or weekly basis as various
therapeutic regimens are offered. The best objective measurement is probably the graded exercise test. Many cardiologists consider this procedure to be an extremely useful part of the
assessment of therapy because it can be standardized and repeated at regular intervals. Improvement in total exercise time, the depth of ST depression, and other physiologic measurements
(see chapter 6) help to document the beneficial
subjective effects of therapy.

## Prognosis in Medically Treated Patients

Many investigators believe that the natural history of coronary artery disease can be best documented by using a life-table analysis with death
as the end-point. Criteria for patient selection
for such analyses have varied, however.

In the prearteriographic era, the underlying
pathoanatomy could only be estimated, and the
selection of patients for prospective analyses was
based on signs or symptoms of the disease (e.g.,

angina, myocardial infarction, and the like). The
advent of coronary angiography and left ventriculography allowed angiographic parameters
(i.e., the location and extent of vessel disease,
abnormalities of wall motion, and the ejection
fraction) to be used as patient selection criteria.
What role various modalities of medical therapy
have played in the "natural history" of coronary
artery disease can also be assessed by the life-
table technique, although this is difficult at times
because of nonstandardization of drug regimens, combinations of drugs, and so on.

### USING SIGNS AND SYMPTOMS AS
### CRITERIA FOR PATIENT SELECTION
Of the nonarteriographic studies, the Framingham Study discussed in chapter 3 is considered
the most ideal. The sample population in that
geographic area was followed prospectively
over a 10-year period [133]. The annual mortality was 4 percent once angina had developed
and following a nonfatal myocardial infarction,
5 percent. Other contemporary studies reported
similar results [134], but higher mortality rates
were reported in earlier studies [135]. The adverse influence of hypertension on the prognosis
of patients with coronary artery disease was reported by Frank et al. [136]). Effects of other
risk factors, such as smoking and hyperlipidemia, on the mortality of patients with *established* coronary artery disease are not clear,
but a recent study from Finland suggests an adverse effect [137].

An abnormal ECG appears to worsen prognosis according to studies done by several groups
[138]. The most ominous changes include ventricular ectopic activity [139]. The risk of sudden death is two to three times greater in patients who exhibit ventricular premature beats
even during standard ECGs [140], and the frequency, configuration, and timing of the ventricular premature beats all influence this relation [141] (see chapter 5 for further discussion).
Left ventricular hypertrophy, prior infarction,
and conduction defects, particularly those involving the left bundle branch system, also carry
augmented risk [138] in patients with clinical
evidence of coronary artery disease. ECG evidence of myocardial ischemia (i.e., resting ST
segment depression [138]) also carries a risk of

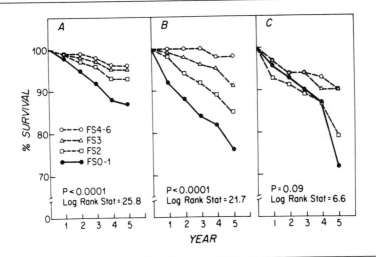

FIGURE 12–12. Cumulative survival rates based on the final exercise stage (FS) achieved for the patients with less than 1 mm (A), 1 to 2 mm (B), and greater than 2 mm (C) ST segment depression during exercise testing. A high-risk subgroup (n=492, annual mortality rate above 5 percent) comprised patients with 1 mm or greater ST depression and a final exercise stage of 1 or less, whereas a low-risk subgroup (n =1,302, annual mortality rate less than 1 percent) consisted of patients with less than 1 mm ST depression and a final exercise stage of 3 or higher. (Reprinted with permission from the American College of Cardiology. From Weiner, et al. *J. Am. Coll. Cardiol.* 3:772, 1984.)

increased mortality in such patients. ST segment depression during or after exercise is clearly of prognostic value in patients *suspected* of having coronary artery disease [142], and its prognostic value in those subjects *already* demonstrating overt coronary artery disease has also been reported [143] (figure 12–12). As noted previously in chapter 6, when marked ST depression is related to coronary arteriographic findings, the basis for the prognostic data present in the markedly abnormal exercise response becomes more apparent.

## USING ANGIOGRAPHIC FINDINGS AS CRITERIA FOR PATIENT SELECTION

With the advent of coronary arteriography and left ventriculography, it became possible to relate the natural history of ischemic heart disease to both the severity of coronary artery disease and left ventricular wall motion abnormalities. A combination of early studies from several major centers indicated that if only one of the three major coronary arterial branches was significantly stenosed, the annual mortality rate was approximately 2 percent [144]. If two of the three major arteries were stenosed, the rate was approximately 7 percent, and if all three were stenosed, the rate was approximately 11 percent. The Cleveland Clinic experience is one of the largest in the world. In 1973, Bruschke and associates [145] published a follow-up study of about 600 patients with symptomatic coronary artery disease seen at the Cleveland Clinic. Five-year mortality in one-vessel disease was 15 percent; two-vessel disease, 38 percent; and three-vessel disease, 54 percent. In general, the results of the 5-year follow-up studies were also found in the 10-year follow-up [146], and in the 15-year followup published in 1983 [147] (figure 12–13A). Interestingly, the series from the multihospital VA trial [148] shows a yearly mortality of only 4 percent, and this probably reflects the effects of newer therapy (with beta-blockers) on prognosis. This effect is also seen in other more recent studies, the largest of which is the Coronary Artery Surgery Study (CASS). This multicenter study enrolled over 20,000 patients from 1975 to 1979. The cumulative 4-year survival of medically managed patients in this study

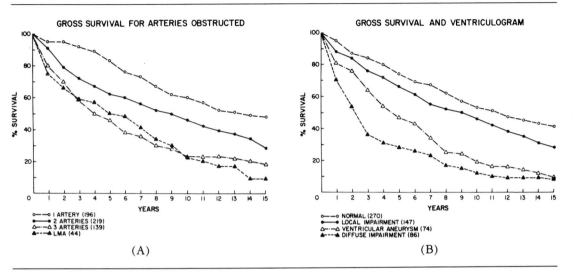

FIGURE 12–13. (**A**) Total survival rate related to the number of arteries significantly narrowed. (**B**) Total survival rate and ventriculographic findings. Diffuse impairment and ventricular aneurysm are not mutually exclusive (22 patients had both). (From Proudfit, W.J., et al. Fifteen year survival study of patients with obstructive coronary artery disease. *Circulation* 68:-986, 1983. Reprinted by permission of the American Heart Association, Inc.)

was analyzed to determine the survival of specific subsets of patients with one-, two-, and three-vessel disease [149]. The results were 92 percent, 84 percent, and 68 percent, respectively (figure 12–14), a considerably better rate from that cited in the Cleveland Clinic studies. These figures are similar to those obtained from the Duke University data bank [150]. The Duke group has also reported survival in patients with various types of single-vessel disease. Patients with right coronary disease had the best 5-year prognosis (96 percent); those with proximal left anterior descending lesions, the worst (90 percent), but the latter figure is still better than would have been expected from the earlier Cleveland Clinic studies.

Stenotic lesions of the main left coronary artery are particularly life-threatening; the Cleveland Clinic study reported a 5-year mortality of 57 percent [152], and more recent results are similar, especially with high-grade lesions [153, 154].

Of major importance in the work from the Cleveland Clinic was the inclusion for prognostic purposes of left ventricular wall motion abnormalities ranging from mild to diffuse [147, 155] (figure 12–13B). Thus, the 5-year mortality was 10 percent in patients with single-vessel disease and normal wall motion, compared to 60 percent for those with diffuse scar, and the 5-year mortality was 35 percent in patients with three-vessel disease and normal wall motion, compared to 90 percent for those with diffuse scar. Similarly, at the Peter Bent Brigham Hospital [156], a significant increase was observed in short-term (2-year) mortality in patients with three-vessel disease and an abnormal ejection fraction (less than .50), compared to those patients with three-vessel disease and values above .50 (36 versus 12 percent; p < .001). Similar findings emphasizing the importance of a reduced ejection fraction were reported by Gross and co-workers [157] in a series of 231 patients rejected for coronary artery surgery, and in 733 medically treated patients in the Seattle Heart Watch Study [158].

These and other studies cumulatively show that the prognosis for a patient with ischemic heart disease depends both on the severity and extent of the coronary artery disease and on the degree of impairment of left ventricular function. Additive effects on mortality due to cigarette smoking, hypertension, diabetes mellitus, or other nonangiographic factors appeared to be minimal in those studies that evaluated such factors. Severity of symptoms influences prognosis,

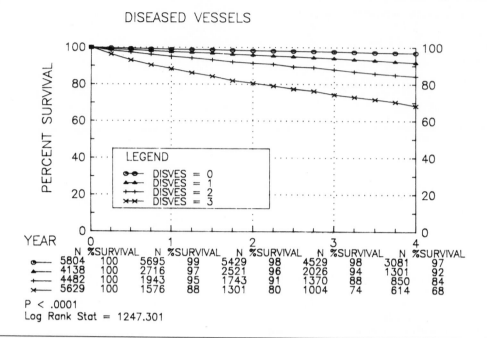

P < .0001
Log Rank Stat = 1247.301

FIGURE 12–14. Cumulative 4-year survival of all of the medically treated CASS registry patients. Four groups are shown on the basis of angiographic extent of coronary obstructive disease. DISVES = diseased vessels. (From Mock, M.B. et al. Survival of medically treated patients in the Coronary Artery Surgery Study (CASS) Registry. *Circulation* 66:562, 1982. Reprinted by permission of the American Heart Association, Inc.)

however, and asymptomatic or mildly symptomatic patients have about half the mortality of more severely symptomatic persons [159, 160] (figure 12–15).

One of the additional benefits of the angiographic approach has been the ability to characterize progression of atherosclerosis in those patients presenting with the clinical manifestations of coronary artery disease. Coronary atherosclerosis is a dynamic, rather than static, disorder, and the development of new lesions or progression of older ones obviously can influence prognosis. The rate of progression differs from patient to patient; lipid abnormalities may or may not be associated with a higher rate of progression—this is still unclear. Clinical indications of progression include myocardial infarction and, in one instance [161], worsening angina pectoris. Interestingly, the chances of a *new* atherosclerotic lesion developing are almost the same as those of a preexisting one becoming more severe. The longer time intervals between studies directly influence chance of detecting

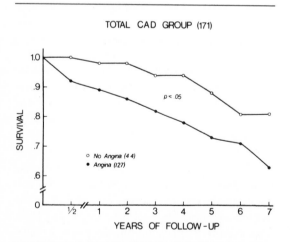

FIGURE 12–15. Survival curves for 44 patients without anginal symptoms and 127 matched patients with anginal symptoms in the Duke-Harvard Coronary Artery Disease (CAD) Data Bank. (From Cohn, P.F. et al. *Am. J. Cardiol.* 47:233, 1981.)

progression. By contrast, adults with *normal* coronary arteries and chest pain syndromes were unlikely to develop coronary atherosclerosis when repeat arteriograms were performed an average of 42 months after the initial study [162].

## EFFECT OF MEDICAL THERAPY ON PROGNOSIS

In the earlier angiographic studies, the widespread use of propranolol had not yet been adopted. Therefore, the 6 to 7 percent annual mortality reported by most of these studies may reflect the *lack* of currently available maximal medical therapy. As we have noted, the multihospital VA study [148] did include larger numbers of patients treated with this drug, and this may account for the improvement in longevity reported. The other recent studies [149–151] also used beta-blockers. More direct evidence that $\beta$-adrenergic blocking agents may improve mortality in coronary artery disease has been reported in several studies. This effect was most marked in relation to sudden death, as well as to overall cardiac mortality [163, 164]. Other new agents such as the calcium-antagonists may also improve survival, but no data are yet available.

As noted previously, another recent pharmacologic approach in reducing cardiac deaths after myocardial infarction employs drugs such as aspirin and sulfinpyrazone that interfere with platelet aggregation and thereby prevent the development of intra-arterial platelet-fibrin thrombi. Goldman and Pichard [165] discuss at length the results of the inconclusive clinical trials with these agents in a recent comprehensive review.

## Medical Therapy of Unstable Angina Pectoris

The syndrome of unstable angina pectoris has been known by a variety of names, including "acute coronary insufficiency," "preinfarction angina," and "intermediate syndrome." The unique clinical presentation of unstable angina pectoris has already been summarized in chapter 4 and the pathophysiological mechanisms for this syndrome have been discussed in chapter 2. Before proceeding to a discussion of medical therapy, however, it would be useful to again note the differences between stable and unstable angina.

The chest discomfort in unstable angina is similar in quality to that of stable angina, but often it is more intense; it is usually described as pain, rather than an oppressive feeling, may persist for as long as 30 minutes, and unlike chronic angina, occasionally awakens the patient from sleep or occurs at rest. In the crescendo type of unstable angina, more severe, prolonged, or frequent angina is superimposed on the patient's preexistent stable angina pattern. Several clues in the history suggest the development of unstable angina; these include an abrupt and persistent reduction in the threshold of physical activity that provokes the patient's angina; radiation of the discomfort to a new site; and onset of new features associated with the pain, such as diaphoresis, nausea, or palpitation. Patients in whom unstable angina is superimposed on long-standing, stable angina almost always have significant multivessel obstructive disease, while patients with new onset of severe angina may have a strong dynamic (vasoconstrictive) component superimposed on fixed obstructive disease, involving only a single coronary artery [166].

It is becoming increasingly apparent that a reduction of myocardial oxygen supply, i.e., coronary vasospasm, may be responsible for many cases of angina at rest and not merely those associated with Prinzmetal's type [167]. Thus, in carefully monitored patients, Chierchia and his colleagues [168] observed that a reduction of coronary sinus oxygen saturation, signifying a reduction of coronary blood flow in the presence of constant oxygen needs, is followed in turn by the characteristic electrocardiographic changes and chest discomfort, and only then does blood pressure and/or heart rate rise. It now appears that in some patients, oxygen demands rise, even at rest, and outstrip the limited oxygen availability. In others, oxygen requirements remain constant, but the oxygen supply is reduced as a consequence of coronary vasoconstriction, platelet aggregates, and/or thrombus formation [168]. Both mechanisms (increased demand and reduced supply) probably operate simultaneously in some patients. Indeed, the elevation of arterial pressure and heart rate and coronary vasoconstriction may result from a generalized increase in sympathetic discharge and might well occur simultaneously.

In considering therapy, it is important to remember that unstable angina pectoris is a serious, potentially dangerous condition and requires immediate attention. Once diagnosed, the patient should be admitted to the hospital and immediately placed at bed rest. Removal from an emotionally taxing situation and institution of a quiet atmosphere with physical and emotional rest, the physician's reassurance, and mild sedation (or antianxiety drugs) are all helpful in diminishing episodes of rest pain in most patients. In some, the pain will completely disappear. Conditions that may be responsible for transient increases in myocardial oxygen demands, such as tachyarrhythmias, infection, fever, thyrotoxicosis, anemia, exacerbation of preexisting heart failure, and concurrent illnesses, should be treated appropriately. Control of these aggravating factors will be helpful in an additional number of patients [169].

The electrocardiogram should be monitored continuously and serial CK-MB enzymes obtained to rule out a myocardial infarction. Patients with transient ST elevations and/or ventricular tachycardia are in a high-risk subgroup [170], as are patients with nondiagnostic CK-MB elevations [171, 172]. Invasive monitoring is usually *not* necessary, unless a serious hemodynamic disturbance is suspected.

SPECIFIC DRUG THERAPY

*Nitrates* continue to be a mainstay of treatment. In addition to frequently relieving and preventing the pain of unstable angina, they improve global and regional left ventricular function. As with chronic angina, nitrates may be given sublingually, orally, or topically, and they may be of the short- or long-acting variety. The route of administration is probably not very important, except that intravenous nitroglycerin offers the advantage of more consistent control of ischemic episodes during the first 24 hours of treatment [69, 70]. The dose of nitrates should be sufficient to lower arterial pressure by 15 mmHg or to 100 to 110 mmHg systolic, whichever represents a smaller reduction.

*Beta-adrenergic blockers* also play a key role in the pharmacological treatment of unstable angina pectoris. In patients who are already on beta-blockers when unstable angina develops, the drug should be continued unless contraindications have developed. The dosage of the beta-blocker should be adjusted so that resting heart rate drops to between 50 and 60 beats/min. This usually requires 240 to 320 mg of propranolol per day (or the equivalent for other beta-blockers). Beta-blockade may improve pulmonary congestion if the elevated pulmonary venous pressure is due to an ischemia-induced reduction of left ventricular compliance or left ventricular systolic failure. These drugs should be discontinued or the dose reduced and treatment with diuretics instituted if heart failure is precipitated by beta-blockade in patients with previous infarction. Similarly, if angina is made worse rather than better because of these drugs due to their potential for increasing vasomotor tone [93], then they should be stopped. This is not a common occurrence, however, since most patients with fixed lesions seem to benefit from the effects of beta-blockers on heart rate regardless of their vasotonic actions.

*Calcium-channel blockers* are an extremely helpful addition to the treatment of unstable angina, either as initial therapy or along with conventional pharmacotherapy (nitrates, and beta-blockers) when the latter has not been totally successful. This was demonstrated in 19 patients by Moses et al. [173] and then in a large, 138-patient double-blind, randomized, placebo-controlled trial by Gerstenblith et al. [174]. They observed that treatment failure (defined as sudden death, myocardial infarction or bypass surgery within 4 months) occurred in 43 of 70 patients (61 percent) given conventional treatment and placebos and in a significantly lower number, 30 of 68 (44 percent), given nifedipine in addition to conventional treatment. The benefits were particularly striking in patients with ST segment elevation during angina. Nifedipine was also compared with conventional therapy (propranolol and nitrates) in a double-blind randomized study of 126 patients with unstable angina [175]. No significant overall differences in the frequency of anginal attacks per day or the number of required sublingual tablets were observed between nifedipine and conventional therapy. However, in those patients who had already received beta-blockade by the time they presented with unstable angina, nifedipine appeared to be superior to conventional therapy; in those patients with unstable angina who had not received beta-blockers at the time they presented with unstable angina, nifedipine appeared to be superior to conventional therapy; in those patients with unstable angina who had not received beta-blockers at the time of presentation, conventional therapy appeared to be superior to nifedipine. Thus, when calcium-channel blockers are added to conventional therapy of unstable angina, they appear to exert an additional beneficial effect. Their role is especially important in patients who have not responded to conventional pharmacotherapy and/or in patients with ST segment elevations.

Even more than chronic angina, unstable angina may be associated with enhanced platelet reactivity, as reflected in increased plasma concentrations of platelet factor 4 and $\beta$-thromboglobulin, as well as release of thromboxane $B_2$ into the coronary sinus [176]. It is possible that platelet aggregation at the site of critical obstruction in the coronary vascular bed may intensify ischemia [177]. Because of these considerations, a large randomized trial, lasting 12 weeks, was organized in which men with unstable angina regularly took aspirin, a potent antiplatelet drug. One aspirin tablet (324 mg) resulted in a 50 percent reduction in mortality and nonfatal myocardial infarction [178].

Patients in whom medical management fails require *intra-aortic balloon counterpulsation,* which results in the prompt relief of chest pain. This relief is due to reduction in afterload and augmentation of regional coronary blood flow [179]. In many instances the pain recurs when intra-aortic balloon pulsation is discontinued; therefore, this technique is useful primarily because it allows the safe performance of coronary arteriography.

Urgent coronary artery bypass grafting should be performed in patients with no contraindication to operation who are medical failures, have a suitable coronary anatomy, and require intra-aortic balloon counterpulsation to control or prevent recurrent ischemic episodes. Patients

with left main coronary artery disease should also be operated on. Other patients are gradually ambulated, and if rest angina or angina on mild effort recurs despite maximal medical therapy, coronary arteriography is carried out. If the coronary anatomy is suitable for bypass grafting, they are operated on during the same hospitalization whenever possible. Patients with unstable angina and one-vessel disease and discrete proximal lesions may undergo *transluminal angioplasty* (see chapter 9) with excellent results [180]. Other patients who improve on medical management may be discharged from the hospital, and the decision regarding surgical treatment can be made on the basis of their symptoms and anatomic findings, just as is done for patients with chronic stable angina.

PROGNOSIS

In the preangiographic era, most studies of unstable angina were retrospective surveys relating prodromal events to subsequent myocardial infarction; therefore, unstable angina pectoris was considered to be "preinfarction angina," a term that has outlived its usefulness. In Fulton's study of 167 patients, only 16 percent developed a myocardial infarction and 2 percent died within 3 months [181]. Krauss et al. [182] reviewed 100 patients with angina at rest; immediate hospital mortality was only 1 percent and the myocardial infarction rate was 7 percent. The study by Gazes et al. [183] is the first reported *long-term* follow-up study and included 140 patients with unstable angina diagnosed prior to 1961 and followed for 10 years. At 3 months, the incidence of myocardial infarction was 21 percent and the mortality was 10 percent; at 1 year the mortality was 18 percent, at 5 years it had risen to 39 percent, and at 10 years, to 52 percent. Although the overall survival rate was 82 percent at 1 year, it was only 57 percent in the subgroup of patients with persistent pain after 48 hours of bed rest, compared with 96 percent in those whose pain was quickly relieved. Patients with unstable angina at highest risk of death and/or infarction appear to be those whose pain does not respond rapidly and in whom the pattern of unstable angina is superimposed on previously stable coronary disease.

Clearly, the prognosis of unstable angina has

improved over the past 20 years. In the most detailed angiographic survey, the National Co-operative Study Group entered a total of 288 patients into a randomized medical surgical pro-tocol between 1972 and 1976 [184–187]. Med-ical in-hospital mortality was 3 percent and the rate of in-hospital infarction, 8 percent. Follow-up results were complicated by the high cross-over rate (37 percent) from medical to surgical therapy. This will be discussed further in the subsequent section on cardiac surgery.

## Medical Therapy of Prinzmetal's (Variant) Angina Pectoris

As noted in chapter 4, Prinzmetal's angina is a form of unstable angina in that it occurs almost exclusively at rest. Unlike other forms of unsta-ble angina, it is always characterized by ST seg-ment elevations on the electrocardiogram and is always due to coronary spasm, either superim-posed on fixed lesions or in completely normal vessels. Attacks of Prinzmetal's angina tend to be clustered between midnight and 9 a.m. [185] and are often part of a generalized vasospastic disorder [189]. The pathoanatomy and physio-logical mechanisms of this syndrome were dis-cussed in more detail in chapter 2. The use of ergonovine to precipitate episodes of spasm in the catheterization laboratory was discussed in chapter 9.

The management of this syndrome depends on its correct diagnosis—either clinically or by demonstration of spasm at angiography. Use of nitrates is paramount, as in other forms of an-gina, but it is the direct coronary vasodilatory action of these drugs that is dominant, rather than their systemic effects. Although all types of preparations are useful, the intracoronary form may have to be used in some refractory patients, especially in those who develop spasm while in the catheterization laboratory [190]. Beta-blockers are contraindicated in cases of frank spasm because of their propensity to potentiate coronary vasoconstriction. The calcium-channel blockers are now the drugs of choice (in addi-tion to nitrates) in treating this disorder. In a multicenter trial with nifedipine, the frequency of anginal episodes and use of nitroglycerin dramatically declined [191] (figure 12–16).

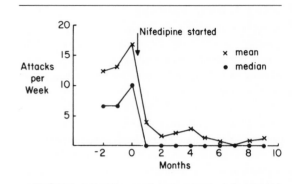

FIGURE 12–16. Mean and median weekly attack rates at various times before and during nifedipine therapy in 127 patients. A prompt, dramatic, and sustained decrease in attack frequency occurred during nifedi-pine treatment. (From Antman, E. et al. Reproduced, by permission of the *New England Journal of Medi-cine,* 302:1269, 1980.)

Long-term results are also impressive, though the dose may have to be altered [192]. Long-term results are also favorable with diltiazem [193] and verapamil [194] with or without ni-trates. Other drug therapy includes α-adrener-gic blockade with prazosin [195]. Coronary ar-tery bypass surgery, and other procedures such as sympathetic denervation, may be helpful in selected patients and are discussed in a subse-quent section.

Prognosis is variable and, in general, patients without fixed lesions do better. In a study by Waters et al. [196] of 132 consecutive patients, 18 patients died or experienced a myocardial infarction within 1 month after initial hospitali-zation. Serious arrhythmias and sudden death occurred in 19 of 114 patients followed by Miller et al. [197]. Therefore, despite the ad-vent of newer drugs, this syndrome is still a dan-gerous one in some individuals. In others, even those who survive an infarct, the disease may stabilize and symptoms may even diminish with time.

## Medical Therapy of Silent Myocardial Ischemia

The clinical features of this interesting syndrome were discussed at length in chapter 4. At pre-sent, the explanation for the lack of symptoms during ischemic episodes remains unresolved (see chapter 2). Prognosis appears to be better than in symptomatic patients [198] (see figure 12–15); treatment is controversial. Beneficial effects of "prophylactic" therapy with beta-blockers and calcium-antagonists are still in the experimental stage. Recommendations for surgical management appear restricted to those patients with either left main or three-vessel disease. In patients with silent myocardial ischemia following myocardial infarction, prognosis is probably similar to that of patients who have either stable or unstable angina in the postinfarction state. Therefore, more aggressive treatment in these persons may be warranted.

## Surgical Management of Ischemic Heart Disease

This discussion represents a "medical" viewpoint on this subject, though not the only one. A "surgical" viewpoint and discussion of technical aspects is given in chapter 14. To introduce the subject, a brief historical perspective is necessary.

Since 1937, numerous surgical procedures have been proposed for revascularization of the myocardium. McIntosh and Garcia [199] describe these procedures in their extensive review. These procedures include suturing the omentum directly to the epicardium, manipulating coronary venous pathways, applying irritants (e.g., phenol, talc, or asbestos) to the epicardium with the anticipation that new blood vessels will form, and ligating the distal internal mammary artery in order to increase blood flow through the vessel's pericardial branches.

A more physiologic approach based on the myocardial sinusoidal circulation was demonstrated by Vineberg in a canine preparation with an experimentally occluded coronary artery. Implantation of a systemic artery deep into the myocardium beyond the area of obstruction resulted in the formation of new blood vessels that communicated with the distal branches of the obstructed coronary artery. In 1964, Vineberg and Walker [200] reported on the geneally good clinical course of 140 patients who had received the implanted vessel over the preceding 13 years. Sustained relief of angina and sub-

sequent reduction in mortality or in the rate of recurrent myocardial infarction (compared to nonrandomized "control" patients) were not clearly demonstrated to result from the operation [199].

The Cleveland Clinic group has introduced or popularized several surgical procedures that have directly involved the coronary arteries, including roofing over an atheromatous plaque with a pericardial patch graft, resecting the obstructed portion of the coronary artery and interposing a venous graft, and performing mechanical endarterectomy [201, 202]. The last procedure was supplanted by gas endarterectomy [203], but none of these operations has been shown to be of sustained benefit, and they are often associated with a high operative mortality. By the late 1960s, the use of portions of saphenous vein as aortocoronary bypass grafts was reported by Favaloro [204] and Johnson and his associates [205], and soon after Green [206] introduced the use of the internal mammary artery for the same purpose. For discussion of the technical aspects and comparative advantages of the saphenous vein and internal mammary artery procedures, the reader is again referred to chapter 14.

### PATIENT SELECTION CRITERIA

To undergo this procedure, patients with chronic angina must usually satisfy certain clinical, angiographic, and hemodynamic criteria [207]. Unfortunately, the criteria may differ from one institution to another, making comparisons of clinical benefit difficult.

*Clinical Factors.* There is still general agreement with the 1972 report [208] of the American Heart Association's committee on coronary artery surgery that the most widely accepted indication for coronary artery bypass surgery in chronic angina is "significant disability from moderate to severe angina pectoris, unresponsive to optimal medical care." The terms *significant disability, moderate to severe angina,* and *optimal medical care* are, of course, subject to varying interpretations. Using the framework of the New York Heart Association's functional classification for purposes of this review, we can define "significant disability from moderate to severe angina" as functional class III or IV, that is, symptomatic status at one's ordinary activity or at rest. Similarly, "mild symptomatic angina" can be defined as functional class II, that is, symptomatic status at more than one's ordinary type of activity. Even within this framework, however, classification of the same patient may differ from physician to physician, which reemphasizes one of the major problems in the selection of patients for surgery: the lack of objective criteria as to the severity of angina. "Optimal medical care" would hopefully involve control of blood pressure, arrhythmias, and metabolic abnormalities (such as carbohydrate intolerance and hyperlipidemias), abstinence from smoking, and, most importantly, medication with beta-blocking agents and calcium-antagonists (in addition to nitrates) for control of anginal symptoms.

In published reports in the early 1970s, most patients selected for operation did have moderate to severe angina [209, 210]. With the reduction in perioperative mortality, less symptomatic patients are now operated on more frequently.

The fact that different groups of patients may be operated on for different reasons makes interpretation of the results in regard to selectivity of clinical factors very difficult. Thus, one might envision successful coronary artery bypass to result in relief of angina symptoms, reversion to normal of an abnormal exercise test, prevention of future myocardial infarctions, increased life expectancy, or some combination of these factors. Not only is this problem compounded by a paucity of data concerning optimum medical care and the degree of preoperative ECG exercise abnormalities, but most often the reasons for referral (when other than the relief of angina) are not elucidated in the reports.

*Angiographic Factors.* There is "general agreement that the best candidates for bypass surgery are those with severe (greater than 75 percent) stenosis of the luminal diameter in the proximal segments of major branches of the coronary arteries" [208], as demonstrated by superior quality angiograms taken in multiple views. Examples of such lesions are provided in figures 9–8 to 9–10. Although there is some evidence that performing coronary artery bypass surgery on

lesions of less than this degree will lead to lower patency rates, many centers do consider operable lesions to include 50 to 75 percent luminal stenosis.

The state of the distal vasculature is equally important. This can be evaluated directly by angiographic assessment and indirectly by flow measurements. An early report from the Montreal Heart Institute [211] involving 154 venous grafts studied 2 months and 1 year after operation concluded that late patency of the grafts was related to coronary arterial runoff as determined by the diameter of the coronary vessel, the size of the distal vascular bed, and, to a lesser degree, distal coronary atherosclerosis. This report indicated that the best results (75 to 80 percent graft patency) were found in vessels greater than 1.5 mm diameter that perfused a large peripheral vascular bed and were free of distal atheromas occluding more than 25 percent of the vessel lumen. Diameters measured at angiography correlated satisfactorily with those obtained at operation in many of these patients. In addition to such direct assessments, flow rates measured at the time of operation have indicated that rates less than 40 ml/min—the average is nearly 70 ml/min in the saphenous veins—are often associated with graft closure, but at higher rates this is less common [212]. The possible causes for reduced flow include a small coronary artery pressure gradient, technically poor anastomosis, and a small myocardial mass perfused by the graft, which, in turn, may be due to diseased distal vasculature.

*Hemodynamic Factors (Including Ventricular Wall Motion).* The relation between clinical congestive heart failure, abnormal hemodynamic parameters, extensive wall motion abnormalities on the ventriculogram, and poor results from bypass procedures is now well appreciated after early reports addressed this issue [213–215].

When ventricular volumes were determined and the systolic ejection fraction calculated, the results were similar to what was observed in medically treated patients: there was a decided increase in morbidity and mortality at ejection fraction values less than .50 (and especially at values less than .30), although anginal symptoms were usually relieved. At the Peter Bent Brigham Hospital in the early 1970s [214], 35 percent of patients with ejection fractions less than .50 had a poor surgical result (defined as perioperative mortality or development or persistence of heart failure), compared to 3 percent of patients with ejection fractions greater than .50. (A number of patients in this series also had aneurysmectomies.) Similarly, a report from Duke [215] mentioned an operative mortality of 55 percent in patients with ejection fractions less than .25. Mortality is currently less mainly because of the use of the intra-aortic balloon device. The CASS registry cites an operative mortality of 6.7 percent for ejection fractions less than 20 percent, 4.4 percent for ejection fractions 20 to 30 percent, and 1.9 percent for ejection fractions greater than 50 percent [216].

In evaluating patients with asynergy, it is important to utilize biplane ventriculographic techniques whenever possible. As discussed in chapter 9, the biplane study allows evaluation of more areas of ventricular wall than does a single-plane projection. Furthermore, techniques that allow ventricular wall motion to be analyzed in a *second state* (after inotropic stimulation or unloading of the ventricle) should also be utilized whenever possible, since they can demonstrate enhancement of otherwise depressed wall motion (see chapter 2). *Contractile reserve* is the term used to describe the ability of ventricular wall segments that contract abnormally at rest to demonstrate augmented contractility, often with an increase in overall ejection fraction [215]. There is evidence that localized zones that respond to an inotropic stimulation or to a decrease in preload and afterload may also show more normal wall motion on postoperative catheterization studies, presumably as a result of the myocardial revascularization procedure [217]. Demonstration of augmentation of contractility and similar improvement after revascularization is, in turn, related to the finding that many hypokinetic (and even akinetic) areas of the ventricular wall are composed of either muscle or a mixture of muscle and fibrous scar but are not totally scarred [217].

Although surgical risk is higher in patients with depressed left ventricular function, many such patients will experience relief of anginal pain, relief of failure symptoms, or both. Employing inotropic stimulation, further discrimination can be made among the patients in this higher risk group to achieve optimal selection of surgical candidates [218]. Long-term (5-year) results also can be predicted with this technique [219] (table 12–5).

## BENEFICIAL AND ADVERSE EFFECTS OF CORONARY ARTERY BYPASS SURGERY

*Perioperative Morbidity and Mortality.* Perioperative mortality (usually up to 30 days after surgery) following myocardial revascularization for the treatment of stable and unstable angina pectoris has been steadily declining. Many centers report operative mortalities of 1 to 3 percent in patients with good myocardial contractility. In the CASS registry [216], the overall perioperative mortality in 6,630 patients was 2.3 percent. It was higher in the aged, in women, in patients with left main lesions, and in those requiring emergency surgery. Kouchoukos et al. [220] contrasted mortality in the early 1970s (2.7 percent) with that in the late 1970s (1.2 percent). Improved perioperative management, rather than patient selection, was held responsible for the 55 percent decline in mortality.

The average rate of perioperative *myocardial infarctions* that could be expected with elective coronary artery bypass surgery was formerly 10 to 15 percent and is now closer to 5 percent in the CASS experience [221]. The most accurate method for diagnosing such events relies on ECG evidence of new and persistent Q-waves, especially when they are combined with marked elevation of cardiac enzymes and abnormal myocardial scintigrams [222]. In some cases, the Q-waves are apparently due to the venting procedure that may be employed during cardiac surgery and thus are not always representative of "true" infarctions [223]. The degree of preoperative left ventricular dysfunction, duration of bypass time, and number of grafts influenced the prevalence of perioperative infarctions in one series [215]. Whether *nonfatal* postoperative infarction is associated with a worse long-term prognosis or is relatively benign is not clear, though the latter is suggested by two large studies [221, 224].

TABLE 12-5. Survival data in surgically treated patients based on change in ejection fraction with inotropic stimulation ($\Delta EF$)

|  | Group A ($\Delta EF \geq 0.10$) | Group B ($\Delta EF < 0.10$) | p value |
|---|---|---|---|
| Total patients (n) | 20 | 15 | |
| CONDITION (n, %)[a] | | | |
| Improved | 10, 50% | 2, 13% | < 0.02 |
| Stable | 2, 10% | 2, 13% | |
| Worse | 4, 20% | 1, 7% | |
| DEATH (n, %)[b] | | | |
| Late | 2, 10% | 4, 27% | |
| Early | 2, 10% | 6, 40% | < 0.05 |
| 5-year survival (n, %) | 16, 80% | 5, 33% | < 0.01 |

[a]Improved, stable, worse refers to change in New York Heart Association functional class for failure symptoms.
[b]Early death = death in 60 days or less; late death = death between 60 days and 5 years.
p = probability value comparing Groups A and B.
Source: Nesto, R. et al. *Am. J. Cardiol.* 50:39, 1982.

Overall *vein graft patency rates* reported at 6 to 12 months following surgery range from 70 to 86 percent, and 84 to 95 percent [199, 225] of patients have at least one graft patent. Graft occlusion is not uncommon after 1 year, based on 10–12-year follow-up studies [226]. Distal arterial runoff is perhaps the most important single factor in influencing graft patency. Angiographic criteria described earlier in this section are useful in estimating the amount of runoff, as are blood flow measurements made at time of surgery [212]. Why some vein grafts develop fibrous intimal proliferation is still unclear, as is the relationship between such lesions and atherosclerosis in the grafts. Elevated blood lipids may be a factor [227]. While prevention of late graft closure remains unresolved, one large study suggests that early graft closure can be prevented by antiplatelet agents [228].

*Progression of disease in the native coronary circulation* may also contribute to poor clinical results. The tendency for *proximal* lesions to progress to complete stenosis may be of little importance if the graft is patent, but progression of disease *distal* to the graft may have more serious effects (figure 12–17). At an average follow-up of 1 year, the frequency of distal progression is about 25 to 30 percent [220], a rate not significantly different from that in nongrafted arteries [230]. It is important to stress that progression of disease in *unoperated vessels* may be a major reason for return of angina, in addition to graft closure [226].

*Other Adverse Effects.* Arterial hypertension developing early after coronary artery surgery is not uncommon and may require intensive therapy with both intravenous nitroglycerin and nitroprusside [231]. Constrictive pericarditis is a rare complication (.2 percent incidence rate), but should be considered in those postoperative patients who present with deteriorating cardiac function [232]. Recurrent cellulitis in the leg with the vein graft site has recently been reported in five "toxic" patients with high fevers; penicillin therapy is usually required [233].

*Symptomatic Results.* The consensus of various centers is that approximately 70 to 95 percent of patients operated on will report either complete or significant relief of anginal symptoms compared to the preoperative state [199, 225]. In most cases, however, this is a subjective impression and subject to criticism by those who are skeptical of the need for surgery and aware of the placebo effect of a thoracotomy.

When exercise testing is done pre- and postoperatively in such patients, the results often *do* substantiate the belief that both clinical and physiologic improvements have occurred. Miller and Bruce [234], for example, described a patient with subjective relief of anginal symptoms who also clearly demonstrated objective

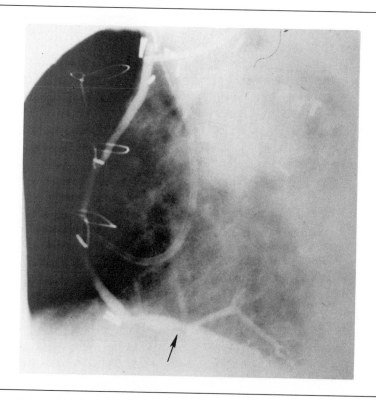

FIGURE 12–17. Angiogram demonstrating progression of disease distal to the insertion of a patent saphenous vein bypass graft. The lesion in the right coronary artery (arrow) was not present preoperatively.

improvement in cardiac function when evaluated by maximal treadmill testing and other hemodynamic studies.

The ST segment response to exercise can also be used as an indicator of improved myocardial perfusion following surgery. An example is depicted in figure 12–18, in which a "positive" test (i.e., one with ischemic ST segment depression) became "negative" (i.e., the ST segment remained isoelectric).

In addition to the ST segment response, other exercise studies [235, 236] have also shown improvement in exercise duration and workload postoperatively, but not to the degree that the patients reported relief of anginal symptoms. Techniques that combine pre- and post-operative exercise testing with pre- and postoperative myocardial imaging with thallium-201 can often indicate noninvasively whether the improved symptomatic state is due to improved regional myocardial perfusion via patent grafts [237]. This is a potentially important approach, since, as noted earlier, there is a varying incidence of nonfatal operative and perioperative infarctions that may paradoxically "improve" patients by eliminating or reducing the ischemic focus. The occurrence of such infarctions not only may alleviate the angina, but also the exercise tests may convert from positive to negative [238]. Therefore, factors other than the myocardial revascularization procedure per se (i.e., infarction, cardiac denervation, or placebo effect) *may* be responsible for either diminution in symptoms or a negative exercise test. Increased exercise capacity can more reasonably be attributed to physiologic improvement because of successful revascularization, however, and it is therefore a more reliable measurement in this regard than is reduction in symptoms.

These qualifications notwithstanding, reports of significant *short-term* improvement in anginal symptoms following bypass procedures are widespread. For a variety of reasons, however, the procedure has *not* contributed to a large

# PREOPERATIVE

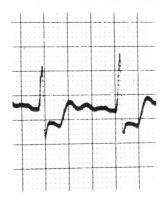

# POSTOPERATIVE

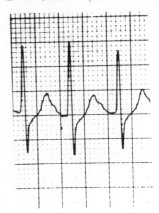

FIGURE 12–18. Preoperative and postoperative exercise ECG in a patient with multivessel coronary artery disease. Preoperatively, marked ischemic ST depression in lead $V_4$ was present (in panel on left) after 7 minutes of exercise at a rate of 108 beats/min. Postoperatively, there is no ST segment depression in the same lead after 10 minutes of exercise at a heart rate of 165 beats/min. The test was stopped because of fatigue.

number of patients returning to work or remaining gainfully employed [239]. There is also a tendency for gradual deterioration to occur in results as a function of time (some of which is probably related to disease in nongrafted vessels) [226]; however, the rate of late deaths appears unchanged.

Whether or not coronary artery bypass surgery improves left ventricular function (as demonstrated by postoperative catheterization studies) is difficult to evaluate because of the incidence of operative or perioperative myocardial infarctions, the progression of disease in native coronary arteries, and closure of bypass grafts. Thus, improvement in function, no change, and worsening have been reported in varying degrees from several centers. When more quantitative data are obtained with radionuclide studies [240–242] or echocardiography [243], the results are generally favorable.

Improvement in cardiac failure symptoms is also variable. The best clinical results appear to be obtained in patients undergoing complete revascularization who have *associated* angina, only intermittent episodes of failure, and limited areas of severe asynergy.

*Longevity.* Lack of controlled studies in most reports (see the next section for the exceptions) makes evaluation of surgical results difficult, even those of long duration and with hundreds of consecutive cases [244]. Hammermeister

[245] recently reviewed the effect of coronary bypass surgery on survival and noted the importance of left ventricular function as a predictor of late, as well as perioperative, mortality. Interestingly, although female sex has been cited as a risk factor for perioperative mortality [216], 10-year survival was similar in the Cleveland Clinic experience [246].

High-grade lesions of the main left coronary artery are considered particularly life-threatening, and they are associated with a very poor prognosis when treated medically. The Cleveland Clinic reported a 5-year survival of 43 percent [145]. Prognosis is especially poor with more than 70 percent stenosis, compared to 50 to 70 percent stenosis [153]. The surgical experience with direct myocardial revascularization procedures in this group of patients has been encouraging, however. Two-year survival was 86 percent in a series of 149 patients [247] and 3-year survival was 91 percent in 1,492 patients in the CASS registry [248] (figure 12–19). Perioperative mortality is usually somewhat higher than with other lesions (3 to 5 percent).

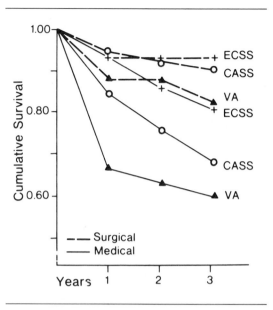

FIGURE 12–19. Cumulative 3-year survival rates of medically and surgically treated patients with left main coronary artery disease in three studies: the most recent study (CASS), the European study (ECSS), and the Veterans Administration (VA) study. In the European study, only patients less than 65 years old with an ejection fraction of .5 or greater were entered. In CASS, a larger spectrum of disease severity is represented. (From Chaitman, B.R. et al. *Am. J. Cardiol.* 48:765, 1981.)

## Results of Studies Comparing Medical Versus Surgical Therapy for Chronic Angina

Cardiologists have displayed and continue to display skepticism toward surgical procedures for treating coronary artery disease. In the light of the generally disappointing results of the earlier procedures, a certain degree of skepticism is clearly warranted. However, for the contemporary cardiologist evaluating the patient with coronary artery disease as a possible candidate for coronary bypass grafting, certain conclusions appear reasonable in light of the available data from randomized studies.

The data regarding *clinical* factors clearly demonstrate that compared to medical treatment, myocardial revascularization significantly alleviated anginal symptoms in the great majority of patients with chronic angina. Besides the randomized, multihospital VA cooperative study [249], the finding of more *symptomatic* relief with surgery has also been reported from several small randomized series [250–252]. Available exercise data from these studies show similar results. In two randomized trials [253, 254], for example, exercise performance was evaluated pre- and 5 years posttherapy; following coronary bypass surgery, maximal exercise performance was superior to that of comparable, medically treated contols. But what of longevity? In the large multihospital VA study [148], mortality at the end of 3 years was 12 percent in the surgical group, compared to 13 percent in the medically treated group. In the initial analyses there were no significant differences in any subgroup, but none of the patients in this series had left main artery disease. Earlier results from the study had indicated that in this one subgroup, surgery did significantly prolong life compared to medical therapy [235] (see figure 12–19), and patients with left main artery disease were no longer randomized. In more recent analyses [256, 257], a multivariate risk function was designed to separate patients into low- and high-risk subgroups based on simple clinical variables. High-risk patients without left main disease did better after surgery in terms of longevity. Also, when only the 10 hospitals (of 13 total) with low perioperative mortality (3.3 percent) were compared, surgically treated three-vessel disease also showed a significant increase in survival. Another large-scale, randomized trial took place in Europe. In both its initial and latest analyses [258], a significant increase in survival was found in the three-vessel disease subgroup (figure 12–20). In two other large computer-matched (but non-randomized) studies from Duke University [259] and the Seattle Heart Watch Registry [245], similar results in the three-vessel disease subgroup were also reported. By contrast, in the latest multicenter study (CASS) no significant differences were found in mortality or recurrent myocardial infarction in the total group or the three-vessel subgroup [260] (figure 12–21). However, these patients had mild angina, unlike the VA and European studies. Based on these studies, I feel it is valid to recommend that most symptomatic patients with three-vessel disease—plus, of course, those who have left main lesions—be

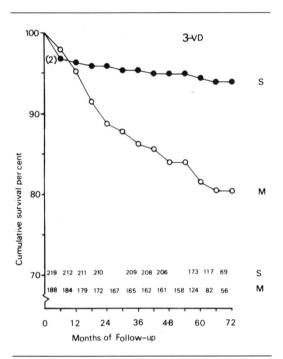

FIGURE 12-20. Cumulative survival curves for the patients with three-vessel disease (3-VD). M=medical group; S=surgical group (including two (2) perioperative deaths) in the European Coronary Surgery Study. (From the European Coronary Surgery Study Group. Prospective randomized study of coronary artery bypass surgery in stable angina pectous: A progress report on survival. *Circulation* 65: (Suppl 11):67, 1982. Reprinted by permission of the American Heart Association, Inc.)

operated on to increase longevity, rather than merely to ease refractory symptoms. For a more detailed discussion of many of the various medical-surgical trials noted above, the reader is again referred to the excellent recent review on the subject by Hammermeister [245].

### SURGERY FOR UNSTABLE ANGINA PERCTORIS AND PRINZMETAL'S ANGINA

Earlier in this chapter we outlined our procedure for selecting unstable angina patients for surgery. This policy, one of medical "cooling down" whenever possible and then elective surgery within several weeks, is generally followed at most centers. Though some physicians prefer to discharge their patients and wait for a return of severe symptoms, the experience of the National Cooperative Study [184–187] and other

studies [261] that many patients will have such episodes within 6 months of discharge argue for a more aggressive policy. Patients who are refractory to medical therapy or who have left main lesions are operated on as emergencies.

As Rahimtoola notes in his recent review [262], patients undergoing surgery without medical cooling down have higher perioperative morbidity and mortality rates than patients operated on later. Surgically treated patients have better relief of symptoms than do medically treated patients. The high numbers of early "crossovers" to surgery (37 percent in the National Cooperative Study) make it difficult to compare survival rates using the two modes of therapy. There is no question, however, that with suitable preoperative medical treatment and improved methods of myocardial protection, 10-year survival rates greater than 80 percent can be expected [264].

Coronary artery bypass surgery in Prinzmetal's angina is usually of no value in patients without obstructive coronary lesions, though occasional exceptions have been reported [265]. In patients with spasm superimposed on obstructive lesions, benefit can be more substantial, especially when cardiac sympathetic denervation (plexectomy) is also performed [266]. In considering patients for surgical therapy, it must be reemphasized that the natural history of this syndrome is such that spontaneous remissions are frequent and cardiac mortality is low in successfully treated patients [267, 268].

## Management of Coronary Artery Disease Associated with Valvular Heart Disease and Certain Noncardiac Disorders

### VALVULAR HEART DISEASE AND IDIOPATHIC HYPERTROPHIC SUBAORTIC STENOSIS

*Mitral Valve Disease.* Coronary artery disease was once considered an uncommon occurrence in patients with *rheumatic mitral valve disease.* For example, in 1942, Levine and Kauvar [269] diagnosed coronary artery disease clinically in only 10 of 314 adults with mitral stenosis (3.1 percent).

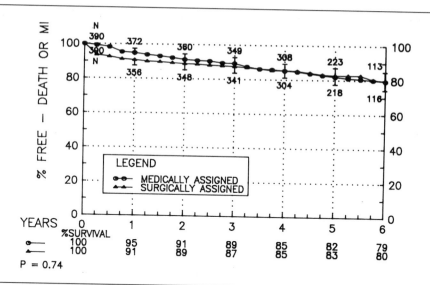

FIGURE 12–21. Survival and absence of myocardial infarction (MI) according to number of diseased vessels in patients with coronary artery disease who were randomly assigned to medical or surgical therapy (life-table method). The probability of remaining alive and free of myocardial infarction was similar in the medical and surgical groups who had one-vessel disease, two-vessel disease, and three-vessel disease. (From the CASS Principal Associates. Reprinted, by permission of the *New England Journal of Medicine*, 310:750, 1984.)

More recent angiographic [270] and autopsy [271] studies continue to show that atherosclerotic coronary artery disease occurs with reduced frequency in patients with rheumatic mitral valve disease, but the concomitant appearance of these two disease processes is *not* as rare as was once believed. For example, Befeler and associates performed coronary arteriography on 26 male patients with mitral stenosis and found five who had significant coronary artery disease. This is not surprising, since with modern medical and surgical therapy the life expectancy of patients with rheumatic mitral valve disease has improved, and more patients with mitral valve involvement are now reaching the age range in which atherosclerotic coronary artery disease becomes manifest. In addition, coronary artery obstruction due to *embolization* occurs with some regularity in patients with mitral valve disease, especially those with atrial fibrillation.

In managing patients with *both* rheumatic mitral valve disease and angina due to coronary artery disease, care must be taken when digitalis is used to control rapid ventricular responses to atrial fibrillation. Digitalis can increase myocardial oxygen requirements and theoretically worsen angina, although by slowing the heart rate, this deleterious effect is usually effectively "balanced" and angina abates. Beta-blockers may be preferable because they have the opposite effect on oxygen requirements while still being useful for control of the arrhythmias. In some patients, both digitalis and beta-blockers may be necessary.

Any patient scheduled to undergo cardiac catheterization and possible mitral valve surgery in whom coronary artery disease is even suspected should probably have coronary arteriography performed as a part of the catheterization procedure. Furthermore, if significant coronary artery obstruction is found, a reasonable argument could be made for performing coronary artery bypass surgery at the time of mitral valve replacement or commisurotomy to ensure a maximal operative result and smooth postoperative course.

The major type of *nonrheumatic mitral valve disease* is the mitral valve prolapse (Barlow's) syndrome. Since the patients may have ventricular arrhythmias and, less commonly, a chest pain syndrome, there is always the question of whether concomitant coronary artery disease is present. The association of the two diseases varies from series to series. Coronary artery disease is very uncommon, for example, when the patient population consists of premenopausal females. Propranolol has been effective in relieving the clinical symptoms in Barlow's syndrome, as it has in coronary artery disease. Coronary arteriography is usually not recommended unless severe angina persists despite adequate medical therapy or the mitral regurgitation is severe enough to warrant evaluation for mitral valve surgery and the patient also has an anginal syndrome.

*Aortic Valve Disease.* The frequency of angina pectoris in patients with significant aortic valve disease due to various causes has been reported to be 40 to 80 percent in those with predominant *aortic stenosis* [272, 273], and only 3 to 30 percent in those with predominant *aortic regurgitation* [272]. More recent studies have shown that angina pectoris can occur with approximately equal frequency in patients with aortic stenosis (48 to 63 percent), aortic regurgitation (35 to 62 percent), and mixed aortic stenosis and regurgitation (30 to 67 percent) [274, 275] (figure 12–22). It should be emphasized that angina may occur as a result of the aortic valve disease *with or without* the concomitant presence of coronary artery disease.

The frequency of associated coronary artery disease in patients with aortic valve disease has varied widely in the numerous published reports. Graboys and Cohn [274] found coronary artery disease in 31 percent of 67 patients (see figure 12–22), which is similar to the 39 percent frequency reported by Hakki et al. [275]. Bonchek and associates [276], however, found only a 10 percent frequency of severe coronary artery disease in patients with aortic valve, and Basta and co-workers [272] found a 13 percent frequency. There is also controversy as to whether severe coronary artery disease can exist in conjunction with aortic valve disease *without* causing angina; some studies report this to be rare [274, 275], while others report it to be more common [273] but still relatively infrequent.

In the medical management of angina due to aortic stenosis *alone,* the use of beta-blockers would be contraindicated because of the drugs' depressant effects on myocardial contractility in a situation in which the heart needs greater, rather than reduced, force to eject blood through the narrowed orifice. However, the drugs might be of value when *both* diseases are present, the angina is due *mainly* to the coronary artery disease, and the aortic stenosis is not severe. Because of their potential for hypotension, vasodilators (such as nitrates and calcium-antagonists) are better tolerated in patients with predominant aortic regurgitation, in contrast to those with predominant aortic stenosis.

It is recommended that all patients with aortic valve disease who have symptoms or signs of ischemic heart disease and who are being evaluated for aortic valve surgery should undergo coronary arteriography at the time of cardiac catheterization. If significant coronary artery disease is found, coronary artery bypass surgery should be performed at the time of aortic valve surgery (see chapter 14). It is still unclear whether all patients with aortic valve disease, including those without angina, should have coronary arteriography performed prior to aortic valve surgery. Some have argued that accurate definition of the coronary ostia is sufficient reason to perform coronary arteriography in those centers where the ostia are cannulated during aortic valve surgery; others see no need for it [277].

Patients with *idiopathic hypertrophic subaortic stenosis* often have chest pain. As with Barlow's syndrome, the frequency of coexistence of coronary artery disease varies with the age and sex of the population under study. The frequency of coronary artery disease can be as high as 25 percent in patients over 40 years of age; it is unusual to find females under 40 years of age with both conditions [278]. If the patients represent difficult therapeutic problems because of chest pain, coronary arteriography is strongly recommended. If severe coronary artery disease is present, therapy with $\beta$-adrenergic blockade and calcium antagonists may not be sufficient, and revascularization surgery (possibly combined with septal incision or partial resection) may be indicated.

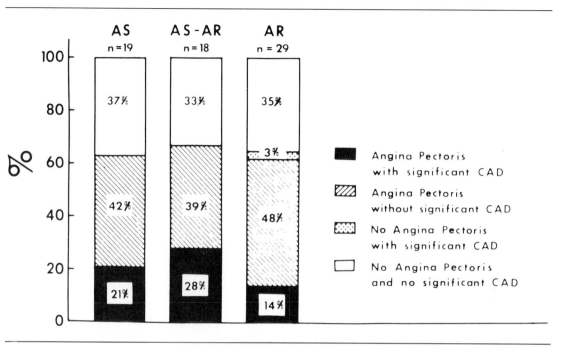

FIGURE 12–22. Prevalence of both angina pectoris and coronary artery disease (CAD) in patients with aortic stenosis (AS) and regurgitation (AR). There is no significant variation in any of the three subgroups. (From Graboys, T.B. and Cohn, P.F. The prevalence of angina pectoris and abnormal coronary arteriograms in severe aortic valvular disease. *Am. Heart J.* 93:683, 1977.)

## ATHEROSCLEROTIC CORONARY ARTERY DISEASE IN ASSOCIATION WITH CHRONIC RENAL FAILURE, HEMODIALYSIS, AND RENAL TRANSPLANTATION

Patients undergoing chronic hemodialysis for renal failure as well as those who have received kidney transplants may have an acceleration of atherogenesis involving all arteries [279]. Furthermore, the frequency of cardiovascular morbidity and mortality is drastically increased in chronic hemodialysis and renal transplant patients [279]. The influence of coronary artery disease on such patients is especially strong if the patients are diabetic. One study [280], which employed coronary arteriography in diabetic patients (without clinically apparent coronary artery disease) before renal transplantation, demonstrated that the 2-year survival was 88 percent in 12 patients with angiographically determined coronary artery disease, compared to 22 percent in nine patients with coronary artery disease (p < .025).

The underlying mechanism of the accelerated atherogenesis has not been elucidated completely. Very low density lipoproteins (VLDL) are consistently elevated in dialysis patients. In addition, hemodialysis and renal transplant patients have reduced high-density lipoprotein (HDL) cholesterol levels as well as high ratios of low-density lipoprotein (LDL) to HDL-cholesterol. Since experimental evidence suggests that HDL retards the development of atherosclerosis and LDL has the opposite effect, these higher ratios of LDL- and HDL-cholesterol may be causally related to the high cardiovascular morbidity and mortality among dialysis and transplant patients.

Medical management of patients with chronic renal disease and angina poses special problems (a low hematocrit may exacerbate angina, as can fluid shifts during dialysis), and because of the previously noted cardiac morbidity in such patients, nephrologists may prefer a more aggressive approach to the cardiac disease (i.e., myocardial revascularization). A growing number of hemodialysis and renal transplant patients have successfully undergone coronary arteriography and subsequent saphenous vein bypass surgery because of severe angina pectoris. The increase in surgical risk is not significant, and the cardiac surgery may improve their long-term outlook.

## NONCARDIAC SURGERY IN PATIENTS WITH ATHEROSCLEROTIC CORONARY ARTERY DISEASE

During the first postoperative week, the metabolic requirements of the issues directly affected by a noncardiac surgical procedure increase markedly. In response, cardiac output increases concomitantly. In the patient with coronary artery disease, the requirements for an augmented cardiac output may lead to an imbalance between myocardial oxygen supply and demand, resulting in the development of myocardial ischemia. Several complications may develop perioperatively that are stressful to the cardiovascular systems of all patients but that are especially dangerous to patients with angina due to coronary artery disease [281]. First, hemorrhage with resultant hypotension may compromise myocardial blood flow. Second, impaired ventilation, which is most likely to occur in patients undergoing noncardiac intrathoracic and high intra-abdominal surgery, may cause hypoxemia, which, if severe, can lead to myocardial injury. Third, infection in the immediate postoperative period places an added burden on the cardiovascular system and is especially deleterious to the patient with underlying coronary artery disease.

Since the 1930s, numerous studies have attempted to define the risk of surgery in patients with coronary artery disease and to compare that risk to that of patients of similar ages without clinical evidence of coronary disease. Despite the limitations of this type of study, a consistent trend appears in almost all of them: for any noncardiac surgical procedure, the morbidity and mortality in patients with coronary disease is severalfold higher than in patients of similar age without coronary disease [281].

What are the factors that contribute to this two- to threefold increase in perioperative mortality among patients with coronary artery disease? Perioperative mortality in patients with coronary disease apparently is *not* affected by the clinical manner in which the patient manifests the disease. Thus, surgical mortality is similar in patients with a previous myocardial infarction and in those with angina pectoris. Some studies have demonstrated that perioperative mortality in patients with coronary artery disease is related directly to the *duration* and *magnitude* of the surgical procedure [282].

If the patient with coronary artery disease is to undergo a major noncardiac operation, there is no difference in morbidity or mortality between spinal and general anesthesia. The latter is sometimes associated with depression of myocardial performance, but the former can also be complicated by hypotension. Therefore, there is no rationale for recommending spinal rather than general anesthesia, but because of the variability in individual cases, coordinated management between cardiologist and anesthesiologist is essential [282].

In general, surgical morbidity and mortality are especially high in those patients who undergo surgery during the first 3 months after a myocardial infarction; therefore, elective procedures should be postponed for that period of time, since risk declines from that point on.

*Is There a Role for "Prophylactic" Coronary Artery Bypass Surgery in Patients with Coronary Artery Disease Who Require a Major Noncardiac Operation?* Preliminary studies indicate that coronary artery bypass surgery lowers the risk of subsequent noncardiac operations in patients with coronary artery disease. McCollum and associates [283] reviewed the records of 60 patients who underwent coronary artery bypass surgery and who subsequently required from one to three major noncardiac operations. None died during the operative procedure or during the early postoperative period. Edwards and coworkers [284] found similar results in 53 patients requiring major vascular reconstructive procedures. At the Peter Bent Brigham Hospital, this approach has been employed several times in patients with recent episodes of unstable angina pectoris or in patients with chronic and severe (but not necessarily intractable) angina [281]. These latter patients have either left main coronary artery stenosis or significant stenosis of two (and usually all three) major coronary arteries. They have successfully undergone coronary arteriography and "prophylactic" coronary artery bypass surgery prior to femoral-popliteal bypass surgery, abdominal aortic aneurysm resection, cholescystectomy with common duct exploration, and renal transplantation. Whether this approach will become more widespread in the future depends on many factors, including the results of various studies investigating the longevity of surgically treated versus medically treated patients with coronary artery disease. At the present time, it should be considered only in those centers with a very low perioperative mortality rate for myocardial revascularization procedures. Since both *carotid* and coronary artery disease are manifestations of the same underlying disease process, it is not surprising that there is a relatively high incidence of critical carotid arterial disease in patients who are candidates for coronary bypass surgery and vice versa; in one series 12 percent of such patients had serious carotid artery obstruction [285]. Although there is no agreement about the ideal manner in which these patients should be managed, many surgeons now prefer to perform combined carotid end-arterectomy and coronary artery bypass surgery at the same sitting in patients who require both procedures.

*When Should Digitalis be Administered?* Digitalis administration prevents supraventricular arrhythmias after *cardiac* surgery [286]. However, the administration of the drug to patients with coronary artery disease (as well as other forms of cardiac disease) who are scheduled for noncardiac surgery is a subject of considerable controversy. There is no argument that digitalis should be administered to patients who need to undergo noncardiac surgery *if* either overt congestive heart failure or atrial tachyarrythmias are present, but should it be given "prophylactically" to *all* patients with clear-cut coronary artery disease? Over the past 10 years, it has become clear that digitalis intoxication is far more common than was previously believed. Thus, the *prophylactic* administration of digitalis to patients with coronary artery disease who are about to undergo *noncardiac* surgery probably does not produce enough advantages to outweigh its disadvantages. If digitalis is administered in such small increments that toxicity is

truly negligible, its inotropic and antiarrhythmic properties are probably negligible as well. On the other hand, if doses are given sufficient to produce a clear pharmacologic effect, the chance of toxicity may be considerable, especially in the immediate postoperative period. In this period, electrolyte shifts of major proportion are occurring, and these can, for example, provoke digitoxic arrhythmias by reducing serum potassium levels.

*Should β-Blockers be Discontinued?* In the operative and immediate postoperative period, these drugs can depress myocardial contractility and, in conjunction with the depressant properties of all general anesthetics, lead to profound hemodynamic instability. As a result, it may be *theoretically* desirable to discontinue them 12 to 24 hours preoperatively so that intraoperative myocardial depression due to β-blockers is not a problem. However, we agree with those [287] who advocate continuing use in angina patients undergoing either cardiac or noncardiac surgery. Continuing use up to the time of surgery and restarting afterward (by intravenous therapy, if necessary) provides protection against perioperative ischemia and arrhythmias. If the attending physician, the surgeon, and the anesthesiologist *do* prefer they be discontinued, then it is probably best that the β-blocker dosage be tapered gradually over the 2 to 4 days immediately preoperatively and that this tapering be done in the hospital with the patient's activities limited. In contrast, patients with unstable angina who require noncardiac surgery should *never* have their β-blocker discontinued at all and should be seriously considered for myocardial revascularization procedures prior to general surgery.

## Conclusions

In treating patients with angina, two approaches are now feasible: (1) to reduce the mechanical work of the heart and (2) to augment myocardial blood flow in ischemic regions. All of the major antianginal drugs (the β-adrenergic blocking agents, the calcium-antagonists, and the nitrates) appear to decrease cardiac mechanical activity, and the calcium-antagonists and the nitrates may also augment flow to underperfused areas. The primary action of the nitrates is still not resolved, but the present prevailing opinion is that the drugs' systemic effects are of major importance. The emergence of PTCA is an exciting advance; how widespread its application remains unclear. The role of digitalis therapy seems limited to certain situations in which cardiomegaly, tachyarrhythmia, or left ventricular dysfunction is present. The advantages of physical conditioning programs seem real, although the mechanism of their benefit is uncertain and their long-term effects on longevity are still unresolved. Treatment of risk factors in the patient already presenting with angina is generally advised for a variety of reasons, but whether regression of atheromas—or even prevention of development of new lesions—can occur has also not been substantiated in humans.

The role of the coronary bypass procedure in regard to *longevity* has become better defined in patients with three-vessel disease. There is no question that it reduces symptoms over the short term in patients who appear difficult to control on a medical regimen, but the indications for or against myocardial revascularization in patients *without* intractable angina and left main or three-vessel disease will continue to vary from physician to physician.

Management of suspected coronary artery disease when it occurs in association with other cardiac diseases—particularly aortic valvular disease—may be difficult, and coronary arteriography may be necessary to confirm the diagnosis. For certain noncardiac diseases, the use of "prophylactic" coronary artery bypass surgery for severe coronary artery disease may become more prevalent as the operative mortality for myocardial revascularization becomes lower.

## References

1. Rosenman, R.H., Brand, R.J., Scholtz, R.I., and Friedman, M. Multivariate prediction of coronary heart disease during 8.5 year follow-up in the Western Collaborative Group Study. *Am. J. Cardiol.* 37:903, 1976.
2. Friedman, M., Thoresen, C.E., Gill, J.J., Ulmer, D., Thompson, L., Powell, L., Price, V., Elek, S.R., Rabind, D.D., Breall, W.S., Piaget, G., Dixon, T., Bourg, E., Levy, R.A., and Tasto,

D.L. Feasibility of altering type A behavior pattern after myocardial infarction. Recurrent coronary prevention project study: Methods, baseline results and preliminary findings. *Circulation* 66:83, 1982.
3. Joy, M., Pollard, C.M., and Numan, T.O. Diurnal variation in exercise responses in angina pectoris. *Br. Heart J.* 48:156, 1982.
4. Heaton, W.H., Marr, K.C., Capurro, N.L., Goldstein, R.E., and Epstein, S.E. Beneficial effect of physical training on blood flow to myocardium perfused by chronic collaterals in the exercising dog. *Circulation* 57:575, 1978.
5. Schaper, W. Influence of physical exercise on coronary collateral blood flow in chronic experimental two-vessel occlusion. *Circulation* 65:905, 1982.
6. Clausen, J.P. Circulatory adjustments to dynamic exercise and effect of physical training in normal subjects and in patients with coronary artery disease. *Prog. Cardiovasc. Dis.* 18:459, 1976.
7. Hagberg, J.M., Ehsani, A.A., and Holloszy, J.O. Effect of 12 months of intense exercise training on stroke volume in patients with coronary artery disease. *Circulation* 67:1194, 1983.
8. Redwood, D.R., Rosing, D.R., and Epstein, S.E. Circulatory and symptomatic effects of physical training in patients with coronary artery disease and angina pectoris. *N. Engl. J. Med.* 286:959, 1972.
9. Clausen, J.P. and Trap-Jensen, J. Heart rate and arterial blood pressure during exercise in patients with angina pectoris: Effect of training and of nitroglycerin. *Circulation* 53:436, 1976.
10. Fox, S.M., Naughton, J.P., and Gorman, P.A. Physical activity and cardiovascular health: The exercise prescription. *Mod. Concepts Cardiovasc. Dis.* 41:21, 1972.
11. Amsterdam, E.A., Wilmore, J.H., and DeMaria, A.N. *Exercise in Cardiovascular Health and Disease.* New York: Yorke Medical Books, 1977, p. 313.
12. Kannel, W.B. Update on the role of cigarette smoking in coronary artery disease. *Am. Heart J.* 101:319, 1981.
13. Folts, J.D. and Bonebrake, F.C. The effects of cigarette smoke and nicotine on platelet thrombus formation in stenosed dog coronary arteries: Inhibition with phentolamine. *Circulation* 65:465, 1982.
14. Klein, L.W., Pichard A.D., Holt, J., Smith, H., Gorlin, R., and Teichholz, L.E. Effects of chronic tobacco smoking on the coronary circulation. *J. Am. Coll. Cardiol.* 1:421, 1983.
15. Aronow, W.S. Smoking, carbon monoxide, and coronary heart disease. *Circulation* 48:1169, 1973.
16. Aronow, W.S., Stemmer, E.A., Wood, B.,

Zweig, S., Tsao, K., and Raggio, L. Carbon monoxide and ventricular fibrillation threshold in dogs with acute myocardial injury. *Am. Heart J.* 95:754, 1978.

17. Foster, J.R. Arrhythmogenic effects of carbon monoxide in experimental acute myocardial ischemia: Lack of slowed conduction and ventricular tachycardia. *Am. Heart J.* 102:876, 1981.

18. Kaufman, D.W., Helmrich, S.P., Rosenberg, L., Miettinen, O.S., and Shapiro, S. Nicotine and carbon monoxide content of cigarette smoke and the risk of myocardial infarction in young men. *N. Engl. J. Med.* 308:409, 1983.

19. Aronow, W.S. Effect of passive smoking on angina pectoris. *N. Engl. J. Med.* 299:21, 1978.

20. Frolich, E.D. Newer concepts in antihypertensive drugs. *Prog. Cardiovasc. Dis.* 20:385, 1978.

21. Stokes, G.S., Oates, H.F., and MacCarthy, E.P. Antihypertensive therapy: New pharmacological approaches. *Am. Heart J.* 100:741, 1980.

22. Report of the Joint National Committee on Detection, Evaluation and Treatment of High Blood Pressure: A cooperative study. *JAMA* 237:255, 1977.

23. Kaplan, N.M. New choices for the initial drug therapy of hypertension. *Am. J. Cardiol.* 51:-1786, 1983.

24. Case, D.B., Atlas, S.A., Sullivan, and Laragh, J.H. Acute and chronic treatment of severe and malignant hypertension with the oral angiotensin-converting enzyme inhibitor captopril. *Circulation* 64:765, 1981.

25. Kaplan, S.A., Lippe, B.M., Brinkman, C.R. III, Davidson, M.B., and Geffner, M.E. Diabetes mellitus. *Am. Intern. Med.* 96:635, 1982.

26. Havel, R.J. Treatment of hyperlipidemias: Where do we start? *Am. J. Med.* 73:301, 1982.

27. St. Clair, R.W. Atherosclerosis regression in animal models: Current concepts of cellular and biochemical mechanisms. *Prog. Cardiovasc. Dis.* 26:109, 1983.

28. Blankenhorn, D.H., Brooks, S.H., Selzer, R.H., and Barndt, T., Jr. The rate of atherosclerotic change during treatment of hyperlipoproteinemia. *Circulation* 57:355, 1978.

29. Grundy, S.M., Bilheimer, D., Blackburn, H., Brown, W.V., Kwiterovich, P.O., Jr., Mattson, F., Schoenfeld, G., and Weidman, W.H. Rationale of the diet-heart statement of the American Heart Association: Report of Nutrition Committee. *Circulation* 65:839A, 1982.

30. Brown, W.V., Goldberg, I.J. and Ginsberg H.N. Treatment of common lipoprotein disorders *Prog. Cardiovasc. Dis.* 27:1, 1984.

31. Jones, P. and Gotto, A.M. Jr. Drug treatment of hyperlipidemia. *Mod. Concepts Cardiovasc. Dis.* 53:53, 1984.

32. Brensike, J.F., Levy, R.I., Kelsey, S.F., Pass-

amani, E.R., Richardson, J.M., Loh, I.K., Stone, N.J., Aldrich, R.F., Battaglini, J.W., Moriarty, D.J., Fisher, M.R., Friedman, L., Friedewald, W., Detre, K.M., and Epstein, S.E. Effects of therapy with cholestyramine on progression of coronary atherosclerosis: Results of NHLBI Type II Coronary Intervention Study. *Circulation* 69:313, 1984.

33. Hartung, G.H., Squires, W.G., and Gotto, A.M., Jr. Effect of exercise training on plasma high-density lipoprotein cholesterol in coronary disease patients. *Am. Heart J.* 101:181, 1981.

34. Gordon, T., Castelli, W.P., Hjortland, M.C., Kannel, W.B., and Dawber, T.R. Diabetes, blood lipids, and the role of obesity in coronary heart disease risk for women. *Ann. Intern. Med.* 87:393, 1977.

35. Brunton, T.L. On the use of nitrate of amyl in angina pectoris. *Lancet* 2:97, 1867.

36. Cohn, P.F. and Gorlin, R. Physiologic and clinical actions of nitroglycerin. *Med. Clin. North Am.* 58:407, 1974.

37. Mason, D.T. and Braunwald, E. The effects of nitroglycerin and amyl nitrate on arteriolar and venous tone in the human forearm. *Circulation* 32:755, 1965.

38. Williams, J.F., Jr., Glick, G., and Braunwald, E. Studies on cardiac dimensions in intact unanesthetized man. V. Effects of nitroglycerin. *Circulation* 49:146, 1974.

39. Burggraf, G.W. and Parker, J.O. Left ventricular volume changes after amyl nitrite and nitroglycerin in man as measured by ultrasound. *Circulation* 49:146, 1974.

40. DeMaria, A.N., Vismara, L.A., Audtiore, K., Amsterdam, E.A., Zelis, R., and Mason, D.T. Effects of nitroglycerin on left ventricular cavity size and cardiac performance determined by ultrasound in man. *Am. J. Med.* 57:754, 1974.

41. Feldman, R.L., Pepine, C.J., and Conti, C.R. Magnitude of dilatation of large and small coronary arteries by nitroglycerin. *Circulation* 64:-324, 1981.

42. Fuchs, R.M., Brinker, J.A., Guzman, P.A., Kross, D.E., and Yin, F.C.P. Regional coronary blood flow during relief of pacing-induced angina by nitroglycerin: Implications for mechanism of action. *Am. J. Cardiol.* 50:19, 1982.

43. Slutsky, R., Battler, A., Gerber, K., Gordon, D., Froelicher, V., Karliner, J., and Ashburn, W. Effect of nitrates on left ventricular size and function during exercise: Comparison of sublingual nitroglycerin and nitroglycerin paste. *Am. J. Cardiol.* 45:831, 1980.

44. Flessas, A.P. and Ryan, T.J. Effects of nitroglycerin on isometric exercise. *Am. Heart J.* 105:-239, 1983.

45. Greenberg, H., Dwyer, E.M., Jr., Jameson, A.G., and Pinkernell, B.H. Effects of nitroglyc-

erin on the major determinants of myocardial oxygen consumption. An angiographic and hemodynamic assessment. *Am. J. Cardiol.* 36:-426, 1975.

46. Lecerof, H. Influences of body position on exercise tolerance, heart rate, blood pressure and respiration rate in coronary insufficiency. *Br. Heart J.* 33:78, 1971.

47. Christensson, B., Karlefors, T., and Westling, H. Hemodynamic effects of nitroglycerin in patients with coronary heart disease. *Br. Heart J.* 27:511, 1965.

48. Thadani, U., Fung, H.L., Darke, A.C., and Parker, J.O. Oral isosorbide dinitrate in the treatment of angina pectoris: Dose-response relationship and duration of action during acute therapy. *Circulation* 62:491, 1980.

49. Degre, S.G., Strappart, G.M., Sobolski, J.C., Berkenboom, G.M., Stoupel, E.E., and Vandermoten, P.P. Effect of oral sustained-released nitroglycerin on exercise capacity in angina pectoris: Dose-response relation and duration of action during double-blind crossover randomized acute therapy. *Am. J. Cardiol.* 51:1595, 1983.

50. Chiong, M.A., West, R.O., and Parker, J.O. Influence of nitroglycerin on myocardial metabolism and hemodynamics during angina induced by atrial pacing. *Circulation* 45:1044, 1972.

51. McAnulty, J.H., Hattenhauer, M.T., Rosch, J., Kloster, F.E., and Rahimtoola, S.H. Improvement in left ventricular wall motion following nitroglycerin. *Circulation* 51:140, 1975.

52. McEwan, M.P., Berman, N.D., Morch, J.E., Feiglin, D.H., and McLaughlin, P.R. Effect of intravenous and intracoronary nitroglycerin on left ventricular wall motion and perfusion in patients with coronary artery disease. *Am. J. Cardiol.* 47:102, 1981.

53. Salel, A.F., Berman, D.S., DeNardo, G.L., and Mason, D.T. Radionuclide assessment of nitroglycerin influence on abnormal left ventricular segmental contraction in patients with coronary artery disease. *Circulation* 53:975, 1976.

54. Borer, J.S., Bacharach, S.L., Green, M.B., Kent, K.M., Johnston, G.S., and Epstein, S.E. Effect of nitroglycerin on exercise-induced abnormalities of left ventricular regional function and ejection in coronary artery disease. Assessment of radionuclide cineangiography in symptomatic and asymptomatic patients. *Circulation* 57:314, 1978.

55. Bache, R.J., Ball, R.M., Cobb, F.R., Rembert, J.C., and Greenfield, J.C., Jr. Effects of nitroglycerin on transmural myocardial blood flow in the unanesthetized dog. *J. Clin. Invest.* 55:1219, 1975.

56. Fam, W.M. and McGregor, M. Effect of coronary vasodilator drugs on retrograde flow in areas of chronic myocardial ischemia. *Circ. Res.* 15:355, 1964.

57. Macho, P. and Vatner, S.F. Effects of nitroglycerin and nitroprusside on large and small coronary vessels in conscious dogs. *Circulation* 64:-1101, 1981.

58. Weintraub, W.S., Akizuki, S., Agarwal, J.B., Bodenheimer, M.M., Banka, V.S., and Helfant, R.H. Comparative effects of nitroglycerin and nifedipine on myocardial blood flow and contraction during flow-limiting coronary stenosis in the dog. *Am. J. Cardiol.* 50:281, 1982.

59. Cohen, M.V., Downey, J.M., Sonnenblick, E.H., and Kirk, E.S. The effects of nitroglycerin on coronary collaterals and myocardial contractility. *J. Clin. Invest.* 52:2836, 1973.

60. McGregor, M. The nitrates and myocardial ischemia. *Circulation* 66:689, 1982.

61. Cowan, C., Duran, P.V.M., Corsini, G., Goldschlager, N., and Bing, R.J. The effects of nitroglycerin on myocardial blood flow in man. Measured by coincidence counting and bolus injections of rubidium. *Am. J. Cardiol.* 24:154, 1969.

62. Knoebel, S.B., McHenry, P.L., Bonner, A.J., and Phillips, J.F. Myocardial blood flow in coronary artery disease. Effect of right atrial pacing and nitroglycerin. *Circulation* 47:690, 1973.

63. Ganz, W. and Marcus, H.S. Failure of intracoronary nitroglycerin to alleviate pacing-induced angina. *Circulation* 46:880, 1972.

64. Goldstein, R.E., Stinson, E.B., Schere, J.L., Seningen, R.P., Grehl, T.M., and Epstein, S.E. Intraoperative coronary collateral function in patients with coronary occlusive disease. Nitroglycerin responsiveness and angiographic correlations. *Circulation* 49:298, 1974.

65. Horwitz, L.D., Gorlin, R., Taylor, W.J., and Kemp, H.G. Effects of nitroglycerin on regional myocardial blood flow in coronary artery disease. *J. Clin. Invest.* 50:1578, 1971.

66. Maseri, A. Regional Myocardial Blood Flow in Man—Evaluation of Drugs. In Strauss, H.W., Pitt, B., and James, A.E. (eds.), *Cardiovascular Nuclear Medicine.* St. Louis: Mosby, 1974, p. 171.

67. Cohn, P.F., Maddox, D.E., Holman, B.L., Markis, J.E., Adams, D.F., and See, J.R. Effect of sublingually administered nitroglycerin on regional myocardial blood flow in patients with coronary artery disease. *Am. J. Cardiol.* 39:672, 1977.

68. Brown, B.G., Bolson, E., Petersen, R.B., Pierce, C.D., and Dodge, H.T. The mechanisms of nitroglycerin action: Stenosis vasodilatation as a major component of the drug response. *Circulation* 64:1089, 1981.

69. Berkenboom, G.M., Sobolski, J.C., and Degre,

S.G. Oral sustained-release nitroglycerin in chronic stable angina: A multicenter, double-blind, randomized crossover trial. *Am. J. Cardiol.* 53:15, 1984.

70. Kaplan, K. Davison, R., Parker, M., Przybylek, J., Teagarden, J.R., and Lesch, M. Intravenous nitroglycerin for the treatment of angina at rest unresponsive to standard nitrate therapy. *Am. J. Cardiol.* 51:694, 1983.

71. Feldman, R.L., Marx, J.D., Pepine, C.J., and Conti, C.R. Analysis of coronary responses to various doses of intracoronary nitroglycerin. *Circulation* 66:321, 1982.

72. Reichek, N., Goldstein, R.E., Redwood, D.R., and Epstein, S.E. Sustained effects of nitroglycerin ointment in patients with angina pectoris. *Circulation* 50:348, 1974.

73. Parker, J.O., Augustine, R.J., Burton, J.R., West, R.O., and Armstrong, P.W. Effect of nitroglycerin in ointment on the clinical and hemodynamic response to exercise. *Am. J. Cardiol.* 38:162, 1976.

74. Parker, J.O. and Fung, H.-L. Transdermal nitroglycerin in angina pectoris. *Am. J. Cardiol.* 54:471, 1984.

75. Abrams, J. New nitrate delivery systems: Buccal nitroglycerin. *Am. Heart J.* 105:848, 1983.

76. Kimchi, A., Lee, G., Amsterdam, E., Fujii, K., Krieg, P., and Mason, D.T. Increased exercise tolerance after nitroglycerin oral spray: A new and effective therapeutic modality in angina pectoris. *Circulation* 67:122, 1983.

77. Udhoji, V.N. and Heng, M.K. Hemodynamic effects of high-dose sustained-action oral isosorbide dinitrate in stable angina. *Am. J. Med.* 76:234, 1984.

78. Markis, J.E., Gorlin, R., Mills, R.M., Williams, R.A., Schweitzer, P., and Ransil, B.J. Sustained effect of orally administered isosorbide dinitrate on exercise performance of patients with angina pectoris. *Am. J. Cardiol.* 43:265, 1979.

79. Lee, G., Mason, D.T., and DeMaria, A.N. Effects of long-term oral administration of isosorbide dinitrate on the antianginal response to nitroglycerin. Absence of nitrate cross-tolerance and self-tolerance shown by exercise testing. *Am. J. Cardiol.* 41:82, 1978.

80. Dalal, J.J., Yao, L., and Parker, J.O. Nitrate tolerance: Influence of isosorbide dinitrate on the hemodynamic and antianginal effects of nitroglycerin. *J. Am. Coll. Cardiol.* 2:115, 1983.

81. Warren, S.G., Bremer, D.L., and Orgain, E.S. Long-term propranolol therapy for angina pectoris. *Am. J. Cardiol.* 37:420, 1976.

82. Michaelson, S.P. and Wolfson, S. Role of propranolol in treatment of angina pectoris. *Cardiovasc. Med.* 3:331, 1978.

83. Parker, J.O., West, R.O., and DiGiorgi, S. Hemodynamic effects of propranolol in coronary heart disease. *Am. J. Cardiol.* 21:11, 1968.

84. Friedman, M.J., Temkin, L.P., Goldman, S., and Ovitt, T.W. Effects of propranolol on resting and postextrasystolic potentiated left ventricular function in patients with coronary artery disease. *Am. Heart J.* 105:81, 1983.

85. Marshall, R.C., Wisenberg, G., Schelbert, H.R., and Henze, E. Effect of oral propranolol on rest, exercise and postexercise left ventricular performance in normal subjects and patients with coronary artery disease. *Circulation* 63:572, 1981.

86. Rainwater, J., Steele, P., Kirch, D., LeFree, M., Jensen, D., and Vogel, R. Effect of propranolol on myocardial perfusion images and exercise ejection fraction in men with coronary artery disease. *Circulation* 65:77, 1982.

87. Hossack, R.F., Bruce, R.A., and Kusumi, F. Comprehensive analysis of exertional ECG changes before and after oral propranolol. *Clin. Cardiol.* 2:270, 1979.

88. Armstrong, P.W., Chiong, M.A., and Parker, J.O. Effects of propranolol on the hemodynamic coronary sinus blood flow and myocardial metabolic response to atrial pacing. *Am. J. Cardiol.* 40:83, 1977.

89. Mehta, J. and Mehta, P. Effects of propranolol therapy on platelet release and prostaglandin generation in patients with coronary heart disease. *Circulation* 6:1294, 1982.

90. Battock, D.J., Alvarez, H., and Chidsey, C.A. Effects of propranolol and isosorbide dinitrate on exercise performance and adrenergic activity in patients with angina pectoris. *Circulation* 39:157, 1969.

91. Winniford, M.D., Huxley, R.L., and Hillis, L.D. Randomized, double-blind comparison of propranolol alone and a propranolol-verapamil combination in patients with severe angina of effort. *J. Am. Coll. Cardiol.* 1:492, 1983.

92. Shand, D.G. Propranolol. *N. Engl. J. Med.* 293:280, 1975.

93. Kern, M.J., Ganz, P., Horowitz, J.D., Gaspar, J., Barry, W.H., Lorell, B.H., Grossman, W., and Mudge, G.H., Jr. Potentiation of coronary vasoconstriction by beta-adrenergic blockade in patients with coronary artery disease. *Circulation* 67:1178, 1983.

94. Miller, R.R., Olson, H.G., Amsterdam, E.A., and Mason, D.T. Propranolol withdrawal rebound phenomenon. Exacerbation of coronary events after abrupt cessation of antianginal therapy. *N. Engl. J. Med.* 293:416, 1975.

95. Goldstein, R.E., Corash, L.C., Tallman, J.F., Jr., Lake, C.R., Hyde, J., Smith, C.C., Capurro, N.L., and Anderson, J.C. Shortened platelet survival time and enhanced heart rate responses after abrupt withdrawal of propranolol from normal subjects. *Am. J. Cardiol.* 47:115, 1981.

96. Shiroff, R.A., Mathis, J., Zelis, R., Schneck, D.W., Babb, J.D., Leaman, D.M., and Hayes, A.H., Jr. Propranolol rebound—a retrospective study. *Am. J. Cardiol.* 41:778, 1978.

97. Lindenfeld, J., Crawford, M.H., O'Rourke, R.A., Levine, S.P., Montiel, M.M., and Horwitz, L.D. Adrenergic responsiveness after abrupt propranolol withdrawal in normal subjects and in patients with angina pectoris. *Circulation* 62:704, 1980.

98. Rangno, R.E., Nattel, S., and Lutterodt, A. Prevention of propranolol withdrawal mechanism by prolonged small dose propranolol schedule. *Am. J. Cardiol.* 49:828, 1982.

99. Pratt, C.M., Welton, D.E., Squires, W.G., Jr., Kirby, T.E., Hartung, G.H., and Miller, R.R. Demonstration of training effect during chronic β-adrenergic blockade in patients with coronary artery disease. *Circulation* 64:1125, 1981.

100. Morris, K.G., Higginbotham, M.B., Coleman, R.E., Shand, D.G., and Cobb, F.R. Comparison of high-dose and medium-dose propranolol in the relief of exercise-induced myocardial ischemia. *Am. J. Cardiol.* 52:7, 1983.

101. Alderman, E.L., Davies, R.O., Crowley, J.J., Lopes, M.G., Brooker, J.Z., Friedman, J.P., Graham, A.F., Matlof, H.J., and Harrison, D.C. Dose response effectiveness of propranolol for the treatment of angina pectoris. *Circulation* 51:964, 1975.

102. Thadani, U. and Parker, J.O. Propranolol in angina pectoris: Comparison of therapy given two and four times daily. *Am. J. Cardiol.* 46:117, 1980.

103. Parker, J.O., Porter, A., and Parker, J.D. Propranolol in angina pectoris: Comparison of long-acting and standard-formulation propranolol. *Circulation* 65:1351, 1982.

104. Frishman, W.H. Atenolol and timolol, two new systemic β-adrenoceptor antagonists. *N. Engl. J. Med.* 36:1456, 1982.

105. Brown, E.J., Jr., Holman, B.L., Wynne, J., Swinford, R., and Cohn, P.F. Effect of timolol on exercise-induced reduction in regional ejection fraction in patients with coronary artery disease. *Chest* 84:258, 1983.

106. McLeod, A.A. and Shand, D.G. Atenolol: A long-acting beta-adrenoceptor antagonist. *Ann. Intern. Med.* 96:244, 1982.

107. DiBianco, R., Singh, S.N., Shah, P.M., Newton, G.C., Miller, R.R., Nahormek, P., Costello, R.B., Laddu, A.R., Gottdiener, J.S., and Fletcher, R.D. Comparison of the antianginal efficacy of acebutolol and propranolol: A multicenter, randomized, double-blind placebo-controlled study. *Circulation* 65:1119, 1982.

108. Parker, J.O. Comparison of slow-release pindolol, standard pindolol, and propranolol in angina pectoris. *Am. J. Cardiol.* 51:1062, 1983.

109. Taylor, S.H., Silke, B., and Lee, P.S. Intravenous beta-blockade in coronary heart disease: Is cardioselectivity or intrinsic sympathomimetic activity hemodynamically useful? *N. Engl. J. Med.* 306:631, 1982.

110. Thadani, U., Davidson, C., Singleton, W., and Taylor, S.H. Comparison of five beta-adrenoreceptor antagonists with different ancillary properties during sustained twice daily therapy in angina pectoris. *Am. J. Med.* 68:243, 1980.

111. Braunwald, E. Mechanism of action of calcium-channel-blocking agents. *N. Engl. J. Med.* 307:1618, 1982.

112. Maseri, A., Parodi, O., and Fox, K.M. Rational approach to the medical therapy of angina pectoris: The role of calcium antagonists. *Prog. Cardiov. Dis.* 25:269, 1983.

113. Weiner, D.A. and Klein, M.D. Verapamil therapy for stable exertional angina pectoris. *Am. J. Cardiol.* 50:1153, 1982.

114. Go, M., Jr. and Hollenberg, M. Improved efficacy of high-dose versus medium- and low-dose diltiazem therapy for chronic stable angina pectoris. *Am. J. Cardiol.* 53:669, 1984.

115. Sherman, L.G. and Liang, C.S. Nifedipine in chronic stable angina: A double-blind placebo-controlled crossover trial. *Am. J. Cardiol.* 51:706, 1983.

116. Bassan, M., Weiler-Ravell, D., and Shalev, O. The additive antianginal action of oral nifedipine in patients receiving propranolol. *Circulation* 66:710, 1982.

117. Arnman, K. and Ryden, L. Comparison of metoprolol and verapamil in the treatment of angina pectoris. *Am. J. Cardiol.* 49:821, 1982.

118. DeMots, H., Rahimtoola, S.H., Kremkau, E.L., Bennett, W., and Mahler, D. Effects of ouabain on myocardial oxygen supply and demand in patients with chronic coronary artery disease. A hemodynamic, volumetric and metabolic study in patients without heart failure. *J. Clin. Invest.* 58:312, 1976.

119. Crawford, M.H., LeWinter, M., O'Rourke, R.A., Karliner, J.S., and Ross, J.E., Jr. Combined propranolol and digoxin therapy in angina pectoris. *Ann. Intern. Med.* 83:449, 1975.

120. Aspirin Myocardial Infarction Study Research Group. A randomized, controlled trial of aspirin in persons recovered from myocardial infarction. *JAMA* 243:661, 1980.

121. Hood, W.B., Jr. More on sulfinpyrazone after myocardial infarction (editorial). *N. Engl. J. Med.* 306:988, 1982.

122. Frishman, W.H., Christodoulou, J., Webster, B., Smithen, C., Killip, T., and Scheidt, S. Aspirin therapy in angina pectoris: Effect on platelet aggregation exercise tolerance, and electrocar-

diographic manifestations of ischemia. *Am. Heart J.* 92:3, 1978.

123. Orlando, J., Aronow, W.S., Cassidy, J., and Prakash, R. Effect of ethanol on angina pectoris. *Ann. Intern. Med.* 84:652, 1976.

124. Solignac, A., Ferguson, R.J., and Bourassa, M.G. External counterpulsation: Coronary hemodynamics and use in treatment of patients with stable angina pectoris. *Cath. Cardiolvasc. Diag.* 3:37, 1977.

125. Gruntzig, A. Transluminal dilatation of coronary artery stenoses. *Lancet* 1:263, 1978.

126. Dorros, G., Cowley, M.J., Simpson, J., Bentivoglio, L.G., Block, P.C., Bourassa, M., Detre, K., Gosselin, A.J., Gruntzig, A.R., Kelsey, S.F., Kent, K.M., Mock, M.B., Mullin, S.M., Myler, R.K., Passamani, E.R., Stertzer, S.H., and Williams, D.O. Percutaneous transluminal coronary angioplasty: Report of complications from the National Heart, Lung, and Blood Institute PTCA Registry. *Circulation* 67:723, 1983.

127. Kent, K.M., Bentivoglio, L.G., Block, P.C., Cowley, M.J., Dorros, G., Gosselin, A.J., Gruntzig, A., Myler, R.K., Simpson, J., Stertzer, S.H., Williams, D.O., Fisher, L., Gillespie, M.J., Detre, K., Kelsey, S., Mullin, S.M., and Mock, M.B. Percutaneous transluminal coronary angioplasty: Report from the Registry of the National Heart, Lung, and Blood Institute. *Am. J. Cardiol.* 49:2011, 1982.

128. Kent, K.M., Bonow, R.O., Rosing, D.R., Ewels, C.J., Lipson, L.C., McIntosh, C.L., Bacharach, S., Green, M., and Epstein, S.E. Improved myocardial function during exercise after successful percutaneous transluminal coronary angioplasty. *N. Engl. J. Med.* 306:441, 1982.

129. Scholl, J.M., Chaitman, B.R., David, P.R., Duprias, G., Brevers, G., Val, P.G., Lesperance, J., and Bourassa, M.G. Exercise electrocardiography and myocardial scintigraphy in the serial evaluation of the results of percutaneous transluminal coronary angioplasty. *Circulation* 66:380, 1982.

130. Williams, D.O., Riley, R.S., Singh, A.K., and Most, A.S. Coronary circulatory dynamics before and after successful coronary angioplasty. *J. Am. Coll. Cardiol.* 1:1268, 1983.

131. Lee, G., Ikeda, R., Herman, I., Dwyer, R.M., Bass, M., Hussein, H., Kozina, J., and Mason, D.T. The qualitative effects of laser irradiation on human arteriosclerotic disease. *Am. Heart J.* 105:885, 1983.

132. Kannel, W.B. and Sorlie, P. Remission of clinical angina pectoris. The Framingham Study. *Am. J. Cardiol.* 42:119, 1978.

133. Kannel, W.B. and Feinleib, M. Natural history of angina pectoris in the Framingham Study: Progress and survival. *Am. J. Cardiol.* 29:154, 1972.

134. Frank, C.W., Weinblatt, E., and Shapiro, S. Angina pectoris in men: Prognostic significance or related medical factors. *Circulation* 47:509, 1973.

135. White, P.D., Bland, E.F., and Miskall, E.W. Prognosis of angina pectoris: Long-term follow-up of 497 cases including note on 75 additional cases of angina pectoris decubitus. *JAMA* 123:801, 1943.

136. Frank, C.W., Weinblatt, E., Shapiro, S., and Sager, R.V. Prognosis of men with coronary heart disease as related to blood pressure. *Circulation* 38:432, 1968.

137. Heliovaara, M., Karvonen, M.J., Punsar, S., and Haapakoski, J. Importance of coronary risk factors in the presence or absence of myocardial ischemia. *Am. J. Cardiol.* 50:1248, 1982.

138. Blackburn, H. The prognostic importance of the electrocardiogram after myocardial infarction: Experience in the coronary drug project. *Ann. Intern. Med.* 77:677, 1972.

139. Kotler, M.N., Tabatznik, B., Mower, M.M., and Tominaga, S. Prognostic significance of ventricular ectopic beats with respect to sudden death in the late postinfarction period. *Circulation* 47:959, 1973.

140. Kannel, W.B., Boyle, J.T., McNamara, P., Quickenton, P., and Gordon, T. Precursors of sudden coronary death. *Circulation* 51:606, 1975.

141. Lown, B. and Wolf, M. Approach to sudden death from coronary heart disease. *Circulation* 44:130, 1971.

142. Robb, G.P. and Seltzer, F. Appraisal of the double two-step exercise test. A long-term follow-up study of 3325 men. *JAMA* 234:727, 1975.

143. Weiner, D.A., Ryan, T.J., McCabe, C.H., Chaitman, B.R., Sheffield, L.T., Ferguson, J.C., Fisher, L.D., and Tristani, F. Prognostic importance of a clinical profile and exercise test in medically treated patients with coronary artery disease. *J. Am. Coll. Cardiol.* 3:772, 1984.

144. Reeves, T.J., Oberman, A., Jones, W.B., and Sheffield, L.T. Natural history of angina pectoris. *Am. J. Cardiol.* 33:423, 1974.

145. Bruschke, A.V., Proudfit, W.L., and Sones, F.M. Progress study of 490 consecutive nonsurgical cases of coronary diseases followed 5–9 years. I. Arteriographic correlations. *Circulation* 47:1147, 1973.

146. Proudfit, W.L., Bruschke, A.V.G., and Sones, F.M., Jr. Natural history of obstructive coronary artery disease: Ten-year study of 601 nonsurgical cases. *Prog. Cardiovasc. Dis.* 22:53, 1978.

147. Proudfit, W.J., Bruschke, A.V.G., MacMillan, J.P., Williams, G.W., and Sones, F.M., Jr. Fifteen year survival study of patients with obstruc-

tive coronary artery disease. *Circulation* 68:986, 1983.

148. Murphy, M.L., Hultgren, N.H., Detre, K., Thomsen, J., and Takaro, T. Treatment of chronic stable angina. *N. Engl. J. Med.* 297:621, 1977.

149. Mock, M.B., Ringqvist, I., Fisher, L.D., Davis, K.B., Chaitman, B.R., Kouchoukos, N.T., Kaiser, G.C., Alderman, E., Ryan, T.J., Russell, R.O., Jr., Mullin, S., Fray, D., Killip, T., III, and Participants in the Coronary Artery Surgery Study. Survival of medically treated patients in the Coronary Artery Surgery Study (CASS) Registry. *Circulation* 66:562, 1982.

150. Harris, P.J., Lee, K.L., Harrell, F.E., Jr., Behar, V.S., and Rosati, R.A. Outcome in medically treated coronary artery disease: Ischemic events. Nonfatal infarction and death. *Circulation* 62:718, 1980.

151. Califf, R.M., Tomabechi, Y., Lee, K.L., Phillips, H., Pryor, D.B., Harrell, F.E., Jr., Harris, P.J., Peter, R.H., Behar, V.S., Kong, Y., and Rosati, R.A. Outcome in one-vessel coronary artery disease. *Circulation* 67:283, 1983.

152. Lim, J.S., Proudfit, W.L., and Sones, F.M., Jr. Left main coronary arterial obstruction: Long-term follow-up of 141 nonsurgical cases. *Am. J. Cardiol.* 36:131, 1975.

153. Conley, M.J., Ely, R.L., Kisslo, J., Lee, K.L., McNeer, J.F., and Rosati, R.A. The prognostic spectrum of left main stenosis. *Circulation* 57:-947, 1978.

154. Takaro, T., Peduzzi, P., Detre, K.M., Hultgren, H.N., Murphy, M.L., van der Bel-Kahn, J., Thomsen, J., and Meadows, W.R. Survival in subgroups of patients with left main coronary artery disease: Veterans Administration Cooperative Study of Surgery for Coronary Arterial Occlusive Disease. *Circulation* 66:14, 1982.

155. Bruschke, A.V., Proudfit, E.L., and Sones, F.M. Progress study of 490 consecutive nonsurgical cases of coronary disease followed 5–9 tears. II. Ventriculographic and other correlations. *Circulation* 47:1154, 1973.

156. Nelson, G.R., Cohn, P.F., and Gorlin, R. Prognosis in medically treated coronary artery disease. The value of the ejection fraction compared with other measurements. *Circulation* 52:408, 1975.

157. Gross, H., Vaid, A.K., and Cohen, M.V. Prognosis in patients rejected for coronary revascularization surgery. *Am. J. Med.* 64:9, 1978.

158. Hammermesiter, K.E., DeRouen, T.A., and Dodge, H.T. Variables predictive of survival in patients with coronary disease: Selection by univariate and multivariate analyses from the clinical, electrocardiographic, exercise, arteriographic, and quantitative angiographic evaluations. *Circulation* 59:421, 1979.

159. Cohn, P.F., Harris, P., Barry, W.H., Rosati, R.A., Rosenbaum, P., and Waternaux, C. Prognostic importance of anginal symptoms in angiographically defined coronary artery disease. *Am. J. Cardiol.* 47:233, 1981.

160. Kent, K.M., Rosing, D.R., Ewels, C.J., Lipson, L., Bonow, R., and Epstein, S.E. Prognosis of asymptomatic or mildly symptomatic patients with coronary artery disease. *Am. J. Cardiol.* 49:1823, 1982.

161. Moise, Al., Theroux, P., Taeymans, Y., Waters, D.D., Lesperance, J., Fines, P., Descoings, B., and Robert, P. Clinical and angiographic factors associated with progression of coronary artery disease. *J. Am. Coll. Cardiol.* 3:659, 1984.

162. Marchandise, B., Bourassa, M.G., Chaitman, B.R., and Lesperance, J. Angiographic evaluation of the natural history of normal coronary arteries and mild coronary atherosclerosis. *Am. J. Cardiol.* 41:216, 1978.

163. β-Blocker Heart Attack Trial Research Group. A randomized trial of propranolol in patients with acute myocardial infarction. I. Mortality results. *JAMA* 247:1707, 1982.

164. The Norwegian Multicenter Study Group. Timolol-induced reduction in mortality and reinfarction in patients surviving acute myocardial infarction. *N. Engl. J. Med.* 304:801, 1981.

165. Goldman, G.J. and Pichard, A.D. The natural history of coronary artery disease: Does medical therapy improve the prognosis? *Prog. Cardiovasc. Dis.* 25:513, 1983.

166. Victor, M.F., Likoff, M.J., Mintz, G.S., and Likoff, W. Unstable angina pectoris of new onset: A prospective clinical and arteriographic study of 75 patients. *Am. J. Cardiol.* 47:228, 1981.

167. Maseri, A. and Chierchia, S. Coronary artery spasm: Demonstration, definition, diagnosis, and consequences. *Prog. Cardiovasc. Dis.* 25:-169, 1982.

168. Chierchia, S., Brunelli, C., Simonetii, I., Lazzari, M., and Maseri, A. Sequence of events in angina at rest: Primary reduction in coronary flow. *Circulation* 61:759, 1980.

169. Oliva, P.B. Unstable rest angina with ST-segment depression: Pathophysiologic considerations and therapeutic implications. *Ann. Int. Med.* 100:424, 1984.

170. Johnson, S.M., Mauritson, D.R., Winniford, M.D., Willerson, J.T., Firth, B.G., Cary, J.R., and Hillis, L.D. Continuous electrocardiographic monitoring in patients with unstable angina pectoris: Identification of high-risk subgroup with severe coronary disease, variant angina, and/or impaired early prognosis. *Am. Heart J.* 103:4, 1982.

171. Armstrong, P.W., Chiong, M.A., and Parker, J.O. The spectrum of unstable angina: Prognos-

tic role of serum creatine kinase determination. *Am. J. Cardiol.* 49:1849, 1982.

172. Boden, W.E., Bough, E.W., Benham, I., and Shulman, R.S. Unstable angina with episodic ST segment elevation and minimal creatine kinase release culminating in extensive, recurrent infarction. *J. Am. Coll. Cardiol.* 2:11, 1983.

173. Moses, J.W., Wertheimer, J.H., Bodenheimer, M.M., Banka, V.S., Feldman, M., and Helfant, R.H. Efficacy of nifedipine in rest angina refractory to propranolol and nitrates in patients with obstructive coronary artery disease. *Ann. Intern. Med.* 94:425, 1981.

174. Gerstenblith, G., Ouyang, P., Achuff, S.C., Bulkley, B.H., Becker, L.C., Mellits, E.D., Baughman, K.L., Weiss, J.L., Flaherty, J.T., Kallman, C.H., Llewellyn, M., and Weisfeldt, M.L. Nifedipine in unstable angina: A double-blind, randomized trial. *N. Engl. J. Med.* 306:885, 1982.

175. Muller, J.E., Turi, Z.G., Pearle, D.L., Schneider, J.F., Serfas, D.H., Morrison, J., Stone, P.H., Rude, R.E., Rosner, B., Sobel, B.E., Tate, C., Scheiner, E., Robers, R., Hennekens, C.H., and Braunwald, E. Nifedipine and conventional therapy for unstable angina pectoris: A randomized, double-blind comparison. *Circulation* 69:728, 1984.

176. Sobel, M., Salzman, E.W., Davies, G.C., Handin, R.I., Sweeney, J., Ploetz, J., and Kurland, G. Circulating platelet products in unstable angina pectoris. *Circulation* 63:300, 1981.

177. Folts, J.D., Gallagher, K., and Rowe, G.G. Blood flow reductions in stenosed canine coronary arteries: Vasospasm or platelet aggregation? *Circulation* 65:248, 1982.

178. Lewis, H.D., Davis, J.W., Archibald, D.G., Steinke, W.E., Smitherman, T.C., Doherty, J.E., III, Schnaper, H.W., LeWinter, M.M., Linares, E., Pouget, J.M., Sabharwal, S.C., Chesler, E., and DeMots, H. Protective effects of aspirin against acute myocardial infarction and death in men with unstable angina: Results of a Veterans Administration Cooperative Study. *N. Engl. J. Med.* 309:396, 1983.

179. Fuchs, R.M., Brin, K.P., Brinker, J.A., Guzman, P.A., Heuser, R.R., and Yin, F.C.P. Augmentation of regional coronary blood flow by intra-aortic balloon counterpulsation in patients with unstable angina. *Circulation* 68:117, 1983.

180. Williams, D.O., Riley, R.S., Singh, A.K., Gewirth, H., and Most, A.S. Evaluation of the role of coronary angioplasty in patients with unstable angina pectoris. *Am. Heart J.* 102:1, 1981.

181. Fulton, M., Lutz, W., Donald, K.W., Kirby, B.J., Duncan, B., Morrison, S.L., Kerr, F., Julian, D.G., and Oliver, M.F. Natural history of unstable angina. *Lancet* 1:860, 1972.

182. Krauss, K.R., Hutter, A.M., and DeSanctis, R.W. Acute coronary insufficiency: Course and follow-up. *Circulation* 45 (Suppl. I):66, 1972.

183. Gazes, P.C., Mobley, E.M., Jr., Faris, H.M., Jr., Duncan, R.C., and Humphries, G.B. Preinfarctional (stable) angina—a prospective study; Ten year follow-up. Prognostic significance of electrocardiographic changes. *Circulation* 48:331, 1973.

184. Unstable Angina Pectoris: National Cooperative Study Group to Compare Medical and Surgical Therapy. I. Report of protocol and patient population. *Am. J. Cardiol.* 37:896, 1976.

185. Unstable Angina Pectoris: National Cooperative Study Group to Compare Surgical and Medical Therapy. II. In-hospital experience and initial follow-up results in patients with one, two and three vessel disease. *Am. J. Cardiol.* 42:839, 1978.

186. Unstable Angina Pectoris: National Cooperative Study Group to Compare Surgical and Medical Therapy. III. Results in patients with S-T segment elevation during pain. *Am. J. Cardiol.* 45:819, 1980.

187. Unstable Angina Pectoris: National Cooperative Study Group to Compare Medical and Surgical Therapy. IV. Results in patients with left anterior descending coronary artery disease. *Am. J. Cardiol.* 48:517, 1981.

188. Araki, H., Koiwaya, Y., Nakagaki, O., and Nakamura, M. Diurnal distribution of ST-segment elevation and related arrhythmias in patients with variant angina: A study by ambulatory ECG monitoring. *Circulation* 67:995, 1983.

189. Miller, D., Waters, D.D., Warnica, W., Szlachcic, J., Kreeft, J., and Theroux, P. Is variant angina the coronary manifestation of a generalized vasospastic disorder? *N. Engl. J. Med.* 304:763, 1981.

190. Pepine, C.J., Feldman, R.L., and Conti, C.R. Action of intracoronary nitroglycerin in refractory coronary artery spasm. *Circulation* 65:411, 1982.

191. Antman, E., Muller, J., Goldberg, S., MacAlpin, R., Rubenfire, M., Tabatznik, B., Liang, C.S., Heupler, F., Achuff, S., Reichek, N., Geltman, E., Kerin, N.Z., Neff, R.K., and Braunwald, E. Nifedipine therapy for coronary-artery spasm: Experience in 127 patients. *N. Engl. J. Med.* 302:1269, 1980.

192. Hill, J.A., Feldman, R.L., Conti, C.R., Hill, C.K., and Pepine, C.J. Long-term responses to nifedipine in patients with coronary spasm who have an initial favorable response. *Am. J. Cardiol.* 52:24, 1983.

193. Schroeder, J.S., Lamb, I.H., Bristow, M.R., Ginsburg, R., Hung, J., and McAuley, B. Pre-

vention of cardiovascular events in variant angina by long-term diltiazem therapy. *J. Am. Coll. Cardiol.* 1:1507, 1983.

194. Freedman, S.B., Richmond, D.R., and Kelly, D.T. Long-term follow-up of verapamil and nitrate treatment for coronary artery spasm. *Am. J. Cardiol.* 50:711, 1982.

195. Winniford, M.D., Filipchuk, N., and Hillis, L.D. Alpha-adrenergic blockade for variant angina: A long-term, double-blind, randomized trial. *Circulation* 67:1185, 1983.

196. Waters, D.D., Szlachcic, J., Miller, D., and Theroux, P. Clinical characteristics of patients with variant angina complicated by myocardial infarction or death within 1 month. *Am. J. Cardiol.* 49:658, 1982.

197. Miller, D.D., Waters, D.D., Szlachcic, J., and Theroux, P. Clinical charcteristics associated with sudden death in patients with variant angina. *Circulation* 66:588, 1982.

198. Cohn, P.F. Prognosis and treatment of asymptomatic coronary artery disease. *J. Am. Coll. Cardiol.* 1:959, 1983.

199. McIntosh, H.D. and Garcia, J.A. The first decade of aortocoronary bypass grafting, 1967–1977. A review. *Circulation* 57:405, 1978.

200. Vineberg, A. and Walker, J. The surgical treatment of coronary artery heart disease by internal mammary artery implantation: Report of 140 cases followed up to thirteen years. *Dis. Chest* 45:190, 1964.

201. Favaloro, R. Direct and indirect coronary surgery. *Circulation* 41:1197, 1972.

202. Effler, D.B. Myocardial revascularization surgery since 1945. Its evolution and impact. *J. Thorac. Cardiovasc. Surg.* 72:823, 1976.

203. Sawyer, P.N., Kaplitt, M.J., Sobel, S., and DiMaio, D. Application of gas endarterectomy to atherosclerotic peripheral vessels and coronary arteries. Clinical and experimental results. *Circulation* 36(Suppl. I):163, 1967.

204. Favaloro, R.G. Saphenous vein graft in the surgical treatment of coronary artery disease: Operative technique. *J. Thorac. Cardiovasc. Surg.* 58:178, 1969.

205. Johnson, W.D., Flemma, R.J., Lepley, D., Jr., and Ellison, E.H. Extended treatment of severe coronary artery disease: A total surgical approach. *Ann. Surg.* 170:460, 1969.

206. Green, G.E. Internal mammary artery to coronary artery anastomosis: Three year experience with 165 patients. *Ann. Thorac. Surg.* 14:260, 1972.

207. Cohn, P.F. Clinical, angiographic and hemodynamic factors influencing selection of patients for coronary artery bypass surgery. *Prog. Cardiovas. Dis.* 18:223, 1975.

208. Report of Inter-Society Commission for Heart Disease Resources. Optimal resources for coronary artery surgery. *Circulation* 46:325, 1972.

209. Alderman, E.L., Matlof, H.J., Wexler, L., Shumway, N.E., and Harrison, D.C. Results of direct coronary artery surgery for the treatment of angina pectoris. *N. Engl. J. Med.* 388:535, 1973.

210. Morris, G.C., Jr., Reul, G.J., Howell, J.F., Crawford, E.S., Chapment, D.W., Beazley, H.L., Winters, W.L., Peterson, P.K., and Lewis, J.M. Follow-up results of distal coronary artery bypass for ischemic heart disease. *Am. J. Cardiol.* 29:180, 1972.

211. Lesperance, J., Bourassa, M.G., Biron, P., Campeau, L., and Saltiel, J. Aorta to coronary artery saphenous vein grafts. Preoperative angiographic criteria for successful surgery. *Am. J. Cardiol.* 30:459, 1972.

212. Grondin, C.M., Lapage, G., Castonguay, Y.R., Meere, C., and Grondin, P. Aortocoronary bypass graft. Initial blood flow through the graft, and early postoperative patency. *Circulation* 44:815, 1971.

213. Spencer, F.C., Green, G.E., Tice, D.A., Wallsh, E., Mills, N.L., and Glassman, E. Coronary artery bypass grafts for congestive heart failure. A report of experiences with 40 patients. *J. Thorac. Cardiovasc. Surg.* 62:529, 1971.

214. Oldham, H.N., Jr., Kong, Y., Bartel, A.G., Morris, J.J., Jr., Behar, V.S., Peter, R.H., Rosati, R.A., Young, W.G., Jr., and Sabiston, D.C., Jr. Risk factors in coronary artery bypass surgery. *Arch. Surg.* 105:918, 1972.

215. Cohn, P.F., Gorlin, R., Herman, M.V., Sonnenblick, E.H., Horn, H.R., Cohn, L.H., and Collins, J.J., Jr. Relation between contractile reserve and prognosis in patients with coronary artery disease and a depressed ejection fraction. *Circulation* 51:414, 1975.

216. Kennedy, J.W., Kaiser, G.C., Fisher, L.D., Fritz, J.K., Myers, W., Mudd, J.G., and Ryan, T.J. Clinical and angiographic predictors of operative mortality from the Collaborative Study in Coronary Artery Surgery (CASS). *Circulation* 63:793, 1981.

217. Helfant, R.H. Asynergy in coronary heart disease. Evolving clinical and pathophysiologic concepts. *Ann. Intern. Med.* 87:475, 1977.

218. Cohn, L.H., Collins, J.J., Jr., and Cohn, P.F. Use of the augmented ejection fraction to select patients with severe left ventricular dysfunction for coronary revascularization. *J. Thorac. Cardiovasc. Surg.* 72:835, 1976.

219. Nesto, R.W., Cohn, L.H., Collins, J.J., Jr., Wynne, J., Holman, L., and Cohn, P.F. Inotropic contractile reserve: A useful predictor of increased 5 year survival and improved postoperative left ventricular function in patients with

coronary artery disease and reduced ejection fraction. *Am. J. Cardiol.* 50:39, 1982.

220. Kouchoukos, N.T., Oberman, A., Kirklin, J.W., Russeel, R.O., Jr., Karp, R.B., Pacifico, A.D., and Zorn, G.L. Coronary bypass surgery: Analysis of factors affecting hospital mortality. *Circulation* 62(Suppl I):84, 1980.

221. Chaitman, B.R., Alderman, E.L., Sheffield, L.T., Tong, T., Fisher, L., Mock, M.B., Weins, R.D., Kaiser, G.C., Roitman, D., Berger, R., Gersh, B., Schaff, H., Bourassa, M.G., Killip, T., and participating CASS medical centers. Use of survival analysis to determine the clinical significance of new Q waves after coronary bypass surgery. *Circulation* 67:302, 1982.

222. Raabe, D.S., Jr., Morise, A., Sbarbaro, J.A., and Gundel, W.D. Diagnostic criteria for acute myocardial infarction in patients undergoing coronary artery bypass surgery. *Circulation* 62:869, 1980.

223. Aintablian, A., Hamby, R.I., Hoffman, I., Weisz, D., Voletti, C., and Wisoff, B.G. Significance of new Q waves after bypass grafting: Correlations between graft patency, ventriculogram, and surgical technique. *Am. Heart J.* 95:429, 1978.

224. Gray, R.J., Matloff, J.M., Conklin, C.M., Ganz, W., Charuzi, Y., Wolfstein, R., and Swan, H.J.C. Perioperative myocardial infarction: Late clinical course after coronary artery bypass surgery. *Circulation* 66:1185, 1982.

225. Rahimtoola, S.H. Coronary bypass surgery for chronic angina—1981. A perspective. *Circulation* 65:225, 1982.

226. Campeau, L., Lespérance, J. and Bourassa, M.G. Natural history of saphenous vein aortocoronary bypass grafts. *Mod. Concepts Cardiovasc. Dis.* 53:59, 1984.

227. Palac, R.T., Meadows, W.R., Hwang, M.H., Loeb, H.S., Pifarre, R., and Gunnar, R.M. Risk factors related to progressive narrowing in aortocoronary vein grafts studied 1 and 5 years after surgery. *Circulation* 66 (Suppl I):40, 1982.

228. Chesebro, J.H., Fuster, V., Elveback, L.R., Clements, I.P., Smith, H.C., Homles, D.R., Jr., Bardsley, W.T., Pluth, J.R., Wallace, R.B., Puga, F.J., Orszulak, T.A., Piehler, J.M., Danielson, G.K., Schaff, H.V., and Frye, R.L. Effect of dipyridamole and aspirin on late vein-graft patency after coronary bypass operations. *N. Engl. J. Med.* 310:209, 1984.

229. Levine, J.A., Bechtel, D.J., Gorlin, R., Cohn, P.F., Herman, M.V., Cohn, L.H., and Collins, J.J., Jr. Coronary artery anatomy before and after direct revascularization surgery: Clinical and cinearteriographic studies in 67 selected patients. *Am. Heart J.* 89:561, 1975.

230. Palac, R.T., Hwang, M.H., Meadows, W.R., Croke, R.P., Pifarre, R., Loeb, H.S., and Gunnar, R.M. Progression of coronary artery disease in medically and surgically treated patients 5 years after randomization. *Circulation* 64(Suppl II):17, 1981.

231. Flaherty, J.T., Magee, P.A., Gardner, T.L., Potter, A., and MacAllister, N.P. Comparison of intravenous nitroglycerin and sodium nitroprusside for treatment of acute hypertension developing after coronary artery bypass surgery. *Circulation* 65:1072, 1982.

232. Ribeiro, P., Sapsford, R., Evans, T., Parcharidis, G., and Oakley, C. Constrictive pericarditis as a complication of coronary artery bypass surgery. *Br. Heart J.* 51:205, 1984.

233. Baddour, L.M. and Bisno, A.L. Recurrent cellulitis after saphenous venectomy for coronary bypass surgery. *Ann. Intern. Med.* 97:493, 1982.

234. Miller, D.W., Jr. and Bruce, R.A. Physiologic improvement following coronary artery bypass surgery. *Circulation* 57:831, 1978.

235. Weiner, D.A., McCabe, C.H., Roth, R.L., Cutler, S.S., Berger, R.L., and Ryan, T.J. Serial exercise testing after coronary artery bypass surgery. *Am. Heart J.* 101:149, 1981.

236. Sarma, R.J. and Sanmarco, M.E. Reversal of exercise-induced hemodynamic and electrocardiographic abnormalities after coronary artery bypass surgery. *Circulation* 65:684, 1982.

237. Wainwright, R.J., Brennand-Roper, D.A., Maisey, M.N., and Sowton, E. Exercise thallium-201 myocardial scintigraphy in the follow-up of aortocoronary bypass graft surgery. *Br. Heart J.* 43:56, 1980.

238. Block, T.A., Munag, J.A., and English, M.T. Improvement in exercise performance after unsuccessful myocardial revascularization. *Am. J. Cardiol.* 40:673, 1977.

239. Johnson, W.D., Kayser, K.L., Pedraza, P.M., and Shore, R.T. Employment patterns in males before and after myocardial revascularization surgery: A study of 2229 consecutive male patients followed for as long as 10 years. *Circulation* 65:1086, 1982.

240. Reduto, L.A., Lawrie, G.M., Reid, J.W., Whissenand, H.H., Noon, G.P., Kanon, D., DeBakey, M.E., and Miller, R.R. Sequential postoperative assessment of left ventricular performance with gated cardiac blood pool imaging following aortocoronary bypass surgery. *Am. Heart J.* 101:59, 1981.

241. Lim, Y.L., Kalff, V., Kelly, M.J., Mason, P.J., Currie, P.J., Harper, R.W., Anderson, S.T., Federman, J., Sterling, G.R., and Pitt, A. Radionuclide angiographic assessment of global and segmental left ventricular function at rest and during exercise after coronary artery bypass graft surgery. *Circulation* 66:972, 1982.

242. Brundage, B.H., Massie, B.M., and Botvinick, E.H. Improved regional ventricular function

after successful surgical revascularization. *J. Am. Coll. Cardiol.* 3:902, 1984.

243. Rubenson, D.S., Tucker, C.R., London, E., Miller, D.C., Stinson, E.B., and Popp, R.L. Two-dimensional echocardiographic analysis of segmental left ventricular wall motion before and after coronary artery bypass surgery. *Circulation* 66:1025, 1982.

244. Lawrie, G.M., Morris, G.C., Jr., Calhoon, J.H., Safi, H., Zamora, J.L., Beltengady, M., Baron, A., Silvers, A., and Chapman, D.W. Clinical results of coronary bypass in 500 patients at least 10 years after operation. *Circulation* 66(Suppl I):1, 1982.

245. Hammermeister, K.E. The effect of coronary bypass surgery on survival. *Prog. Cardiovasc. Dis.* 25:297, 1983.

246. Loop, F.D., Golding, L.R., Macmillan, J.P., Cosgrove, D.M., Lyte, B.W., and Sheldon, W.C. Coronary artery surgery in women compared with men: Analysis of risks and long-term results. *J. Am. Coll. Cardiol.* 1:383, 1983.

247. Oberman, A., Kouchoukos, N.T., Harrell, R.R., Holt, J.H., Jr., Russell, R.O., Jr., and Rackley, C.E. Surgical versus medical treatment in disease of the left main coronary artery. *Lancet* 2:591, 1976.

248. Chaitman, B.R., Fisher, L.D., Bourassa, M.G., Davis, K., Rogers, W.J., Maynard, C., Tyras, D.H., Berger, R.L., Judkins, M.P., Ringqvist, I., Mock, M.B., and Killip, T., and participating CASS medical centers. Effect of coronary bypass surgery on survival patterns in subsets of patients with left main coronary artery disease. Report of the Collaborative Study in Coronary Artery Surgery (CASS). *Am. J. Cardiol.* 48:765, 1981.

249. Peduzzi, P. and Hultgren, H.N. Effect of medical vs. surgical treatment on symptoms in stable angina pectoris. The Veterans Administration Cooperative Study of Surgery for coronary arterial occlusive disease. *Circulation* 60:888, 1979.

250. Aranow, W.S. and Stemmer, E.A. Two-year follow-up of angina pectoris: Medical or surgical therapy. *Ann. Intern. Med.* 82:208, 1975.

251. Mathur, V.S. and Guinn, G.A. Prospective randomized study of coronary bypass surgery in stable angina. The first 100 patients. *Circulation* 52(Suppl. I):33, 1975.

252. Kloster, F., Kremkau, L., Rahimtoola, S., Rosch, J., Ritzman, L., and Kanarek, P.H. Prospective randomized study of coronary bypass surgery for chronic stable angina. *N. Engl. J. Med.* 300:149, 1979.

253. Fowles, R.E., Fitzgerald, J.W., Barry, W.H., and Hultgren, H.N. Long-term effects of coronary surgery versus medical therapy on exercise performance. *Am. J. Cardiol.* 41:396, 1978.

254. Pantely, G.A., Kloster, F.E., and Morris, C.D. Late exercise test results from a prospective randomized study of bypass surgery for stable angina. *Circulation* 68:413, 1983.

255. Takaro, T., Hultgren, H.N., Lipton, M.J., and Detre, K.M. The VA cooperative randomized study of surgery for coronary arterial occlusive disease. II. Subgroup with significant left main lesions. *Circulation* 54(Suppl. 3):116, 1976.

256. Detre, K., Peduzzi, P., Murphy, M., Hultgren, H., Thomsen, J., Oberman, A., Takaro, T., and the Veterans Administration Cooperative Study Group for Surgery for Coronary Arterial Occlusive Disease. Effect of bypass surgery on survival in patients in low- and high-risk subgroups delineated by the use of simple clinical variables. *Circulation* 63:1329, 1981.

257. The Veterans Administration Coronary Artery Bypass Surgery Cooperative Study Group. Eleven-year survival in the veterans administration randomized trial of coronary bypass surgery for stable angina. *New Engl. J. Med.* 311:1333, 1984.

258. European Coronary Surgery Study Group: Prospective randomized study of coronary artery bypass surgery in stable angina pectoris: A progress report on survival. *Circulation* 65(Suppl. II):67, 1982.

259. Whalen, R.E., Harrell, F.E., Jr., Lee, K.L., and Rosati, R.A. Survival of coronary artery disease patients with stable pain and normal left ventricular function treated medically or surgically at Duke University. *Circulation* 65(Suppl. II):49, 1982.

260. CASS principal investigators and their associates. Myocardial infarction and mortality in the coronary artery surgery study (CASS) randomized trial. *N. Engl. J. Med.* 310:750, 1984.

261. Brown, C.A., Hutter, A.M., DeSanctis, R.W., Gold, H.K., Leinbach, R.C., Roberts-Niles, A., Austen, W.G., and Buckley, M.J. Prospective study of medical and urgent surgical therapy in randomizable patients with unstable angina pectoris: Results of in-hospital and chronic mortality and morbidity. *Am. Heart J.* 102:959, 1981.

262. Rahimtoola, S.H. Coronary bypass surgery for unstable angina. *Circulation* 69:841, 1984.

263. Hultgren, H.N., Shettigar, U.R., and Miller, D.C. Medical versus surgical treatment of unstable angina. *Am. J. Cardiol.* 50:663, 1982.

264. Rahimtoola, S.H., Ninley, D., Grunkemeier, G., Tepley, J., Lambert, L., and Starr, A. Ten-year survival after coronary bypass surgery for unstable angina. *N. Engl. J. Med.* 308:676, 1983.

265. Sussman, E.J., Goldberg, S., Poll, D.S., Macvaugh, H., III, Simson, M.B., Silber, S.A., and

Kastor, J.A. Surgical therapy of variant angina associated with nonobstructive coronary disease. *Ann. Intern. Med.* 94:771, 1981.

266. Betriu, A., Pomar, J.L., Bourassa, M.G., and Grondin, C.M. Influence of partial sympathetic denervation on the results of myocardial revascularization in variant angina. *Am. J. Cardiol.* 51:661, 1983.

267. Waters, D.D., Bouchard, A., and Theroux, P. Spontaneous remission is a frequent outcome of variant angina. *J. Am. Coll. Cardiol.* 9:195, 1983.

268. Bott-Silverman, C. and Heupler, F.A., Jr. Natural history of pure coronary artery spasm in patients treated medically. *J. Am. Coll. Cardiol.* 2:200, 1983.

269. Levine, S.A. and Kauvar, A.J. Association of angina pectoris or coronary thrombosis with mitral stenosis. *J. Mt. Sinai Hosp.* 8:754, 1942.

270. Befeler, B., Kamen, A.R., and MacLeod, M.B. Coronary artery disease and left ventricular function in mitral stenosis. *Chest* 57:435, 1970.

271. Tadavarthy, S.M., Vlodaver, Z., and Edwards, J.E. Coronary atherosclerosis in subjects with mitral stenosis. *Circulation* 54:519, 1976.

272. Basta, L.L., Raines, D., Najjar, S., and Kioschos, J.M. Clinical hemodynamic and coronary angiographic correlates of angina pectoris in patients with severe aortic valve disease. *Br. Heart J.* 37:150, 1975.

273. Moraski, R.E., Russell, R.O., Jr., Mantle, J.A., and Rackley, C.E. Aortic stenosis, angina pectoris, coronary artery disease. *Cath. Cardiovasc. Dis.* 2:157, 1976.

274. Graboys, T.B. and Cohn, P.F. The prevalence of angina pectoris and abnormal coronary arteriograms in severe aortic valcular disease. *Am. Heart J.* 93:683, 1977.

275. Hakki, A.H., Kimbiris, D., Iskandrian, A.S., Segal, B.L., Mintz, G.S., and Bemis, C.E. Angina pectoris and coronary artery disease in patients with severe aortic valvular disease. *Am. Heart J.* 100:441, 1980.

276. Bonchek, L.I., Anderson, R.P., and Rosch, J. Should coronary arteriography be performed routinely before valve replacement. *Am. J. Cardiol.* 31:462, 1973.

277. Exadactylos, N., Sugrue, D.D., and Oakley, C.M. Prevalence of coronary artery disease in patients with isolated aortic valve stenosis. *Br. Heart J.* 51:121, 1984.

278. Lardani, H., Serrano, J.A., and Villamil, R.J. Hemodynamics and coronary angiography in idiopathic hypertrophic subaortic stenosis. *Am. J. Cardiol.* 41:476, 1978.

279. Scharf, S., Wexler, J., Longnecker, R.E., and Blaufox, M.D. Cardiovascular disease in patients on chronic hemodialytic therapy. *Prog. Cardiovasc. Dis.* 25:343, 1980.

280. Weinrauch, L.A., D'Elia, J.A., Healy, R.W., Gleason, R.E., Takacs, F.J., Libertino, J.A., and Leland, O.S. Asymptomatic coronary artery disease: Angiography in diabetic patients before renal transplantation. Relation of findings to postoperative survival. *Ann. Intern. Med.* 296:1436, 1977.

281. Hillis, L.D. and Cohn, P.F. Noncardiac surgery in patients with coronary artery disease: Risks, precautions, and perioperative management. *Arch. Intern. Med.* 138:972, 1978.

282. Wells, P.H. and Kaplan, J.A. Optimal management of patients with ischemic heart disease for noncardiac surgery by complementary anesthesiologist and cardiologist interaction. *Am. Heart J.* 102:1029, 1981.

283. McCollum, C.H., Garcia-Rinaldi, R., Graham, J.M., and DeBakey, M.E. Myocardial revascularization prior to subsequent major surgery in patients with coronary artery disease. *Surgery* 81:302, 1977.

284. Edwards, W.H., Mulherin, J.L., and Walker, W.E. Vascular reconstructive surgery following myocardial revascularization. *Ann. Surg.* 187:653, 1978.

285. Barnes, R.W., Liebman, P.R., Marszalek, P.B., Kirk, C.L., and Goldman, M.H. The natural history of asymptomatic carotid disease in patients under going cardiovascular surgery. *Surgery* 90:1075, 1981.

286. Chee, T.P., Prakash, N.S., Desser, K.B., and Benchimol, A. Postoperative supraventricular arrhythmias and the role of prophylactic digoxin in cardiac surgery. *Am. Heart J.* 104:974, 1982.

287. Oka, Y., Frishman, W., Becker, R.M., Kadish, A., Strom, J., Matsumoto, M., Orkin, L., and Frater, R. Clinical pharmacology of the new beta-adrenergic blocking drugs. Part 10. Beta-adrenoceptor blockade and coronary artery surgery. *Am. Heart J.* 99:255, 1980.

# 13. THERAPY OF ACUTE MYOCARDIAL INFARCTION

Kanu Chatterjee

William W. Parmley

A fatal outcome in patients with acute myocardial infarction results from arrhythmias and pump failure. Although mortality due to primary arrhythmias seems to have been reduced by electrocardiographic monitoring and more aggressive antiarrhythmic therapy, the mortality associated with the low-output syndrome that complicates acute myocardial infarction is still very high.

Recent experimental and clinical research has provided newer knowledge about the pathophysiology of acute myocardial infarction and its consequences; progress in the therapy of complications of acute myocardial infarction, however, has been relatively slower. Until recently, one of the major difficulties in managing acutely ill cardiac patients has been the inability to define precisely the underlying mechanism and the degree of depression of cardiac function in an individual patient. The development of balloon-tip flotation catheters (Swan-Ganz type), however, has greatly facilitated safe, reliable, and continuous hemodynamic monitoring, even in critically ill cardiac patients.

Over the last few years, there has also been increasing interest in limiting infarct size, as it seems almost certain that the larger the infarct, the worse the immediate and late prognosis. It seems logical, therefore, that therapeutic approaches to reduce the extent of

myocardial ischemic injury should play an important role in the rational management of patients with acute myocardial infarction. The lack of sensitive methods for measuring infarct size imposes a great limitation on the evaluation of any therapy designed to reduce infarct size. Furthermore, some therapies that appear to be sound on a physiologic basis have not been particularly useful in clinical practice. Apparently, therefore, despite a better understanding of the pathophysiology of acute myocardial infarction, considerable controversy remains regarding appropriate therapy for the consequences of acute myocardial infarction.

The present chapter will offer general guidelines for care of the patient with acute myocardial infarction (e.g., regarding diet, ambulation, and the like), discuss the theory and practice of limiting infarct size, discuss indications of hemodynamic monitoring, and present an overview of the practical management of low output state and cardiogenic shock in patients with acute myocardial infarction.

Areas of controversy include techniques and limitations of estimating infarct size, possible harmful effects of some inotropic and vasodilating agents, whether to use anticoagulation therapy, how early to allow patients to ambulate and to discharge them from the hospital, the role of surgery, and the importance of right ventricular infarcts. Because the therapy of arrhythmias in the setting of an acute infarction will be discussed at length in chapter 15, it will not be presented in this chapter.

357

## General Approach to the Management of Patients with Acute Myocardial Infarction

The following guidelines, adapted from those of Alpert and Francis [1], represent a useful therapeutic regimen:

1. *Vital signs:* The frequency of taking vital signs (respiratory rate, blood pressure, and pulse) varies from hospital to hospital, but a reasonable schedule is every 30 minutes times four, then every 60 minutes times two. If the patient is stable, a frequency of every 2 hours for the first 24 hours and every 4 hours thereafter is recommended. Temperature may be taken two to four times a day.

2. *Diet:* A recommended diet consists of 1,500 calories of soft food with increased bulk (to prevent constipation) and no added salt. The convalescent period following an acute myocardial infarction represents a good time to introduce a patient to a diet that is low in cholesterol and saturated fat and high in unsaturated fat. The patient should probably have no oral intake for the first 4 to 6 hours, and the feedings should be small, either four or six times a day for the first several days. Oral fluid intake should be moderate, about 2 liters per day.

3. *Electrocardiograms:* Daily recordings are recommended.

4. *Portable chest roentgenogram:* This should be obtained on admission and as necessary, depending on clinical status.

5. *Oxygen supplementation:* This can be accomplished by nasal prongs (2 liters/min or as required).

6. *Daily weights and intake and output recordings are recommended.*

7. *Intravenous infusion:* A 5 percent saline-in-water solution at "keep-open" rate is advisable. Either a short plastic line inserted in a peripheral vein or a central venous line may be used.

8. *Laboratory tests:* Various combinations of cardiac enzymes (creatine phosphokinase, serum glutamic-oxaloacetic transaminase, and lactic dehydrogenase) are usually obtained for diagnosis (see chapter 8) and for estimating the size of the infarct (discussed subsequently). Daily electrolyte determinations are advisable in those patients who are prone to arrhythmias; periodic determination

of other tests (hematocrit, white blood cell count, prothrombin time, and tests of renal function) are also recommended.

9. *Medications:* A daily *stool softener* is recommended; for patients who are constipated, a gentle laxative such as milk of magnesia (at night) is also useful. Mild *sedatives* such as diazepam (5 mg) or chlordiazepoxide (10 mg) may be ordered four times a day if necessary. Flurazepam (30 mg) is recommended for sleep at night. *Analgesics,* such as morphine or hydromorphone (Dilaudid), are preferred for pain associated with anterior or lateral infarcts. The increased parasympathomimetic actions of these drugs, however, may add to the increased vagal tone seen with inferior infarction, and meperidine (Demerol) is preferred in that setting. Also, nitrous oxide gas has been shown to be a useful analgesic in patients with acute infarction [2].

*Anticoagulation* is a controversial point. "Minidose" heparin every 8 to 12 hours subcutaneously for the first 4 to 5 days has been recommended to reduce the prevalence of thrombophlebitis and pulmonary embolism. This seems reasonable in light of the small risks of adverse side effects, although the protective effects remain to be more definitively documented. The role of longer-duration anticoagulation with warfarin derivatives in uncomplicated myocardial infarctions has once again become a subject of controversy since recent investigations suggested that there still may be a place for this kind of therapy [3].

In regard to *ambulation,* there is little uniformity of opinion as to when a patient should be allowed to ambulate and be discharged from the hospital or advised to return to work. The traditional approach has been to prescribe prolonged bed rest, even for the uncomplicated patients, because of the fear that early ambulation may cause extension of the infarction, precipitate heart failure or arrhythmias, or enhance the risk of the development of ventricular aneurysm and rupture. Recent studies have indicated, however, that patients with uncomplicated myocardial infarction not only can start ambulating on the second day after the infarction, but they can also be discharged from the hospital at the end of the first week without suffering any untoward consequences [4]. In the absence of hypotension, congestive heart failure, shock, recurrent dysrhythmias, or postinfarction angina, early discharge from the hospital has not been associated with any higher risk of reinfarction, ventricular rupture, or sudden death. Early discharge, however, cannot be recommended for those patients who develop complications during the acute phase. Patients who are not in the "good risk" group should remain in the hospital for 2 or 3 weeks, depending on the individual problems in each patient. There is growing evidence that in certain patients the risk of late, in-hospital death following discharge from the coronary care unit is higher. Patients with anteroseptal myocardial infarction and bundle branch block have been found to be most vulnerable, and prolonged hospitalization (up to 6 weeks) has been advocated by some [5]. Left ventricular failure is usually present in the majority of these patients. Whether more aggressive therapy for pump failure, prolonged hospitalization, or both can influence the prognosis remains uncertain; nevertheless, it seems likely that a rapid increase in physical activity in the immediate postinfarction period in such patients may aggravate failure.

## Reduction of Infarct Size: Theory and Practice

As noted in the following section, pump failure complicating acute myocardial infarction carries a very poor prognosis, and the management of such patients still remains a therapeutic challenge. The extent of myocardial necrosis is the major determinant of the severity of pump failure; damage to approximately 20 percent of the left ventricular mass precipitates congestive heart failure, and necrosis of 40 percent of the left ventricle is associated with cardiogenic shock [6]. Logically, therefore, attempts to limit infarct size should be one of the major therapeutic goals if a significant improvement in the prognosis of patients with pump failure is to occur.

METHODS TO DETERMINE THE EXTENT OF ISCHEMIA
In experimental models, various methods to determine the extent of myocardial ischemic injury have been tested, and the influence of many

therapeutic modalities to reduce infarct size has been evaluated. Extrapolating the results obtained in experimental animals to humans, however, is difficult. Studies related to myocardial infarction in animals are usually performed after acute coronary artery occlusion in the presence of an otherwise normal coronary circulation. In patients with obstructive coronary artery disease, inhomogeneity in the degrees of myocardial ischemia may exist because of multivessel involvement. Recent studies indicate that complete thrombotic occlusion of the coronary artery resulting in total interruption of blood flow is the mechanism of myocardial infarction in the vast majority of patients [7]. However, in a few patients, a new infarct may not always result from a sudden, discrete occlusion of a coronary artery. Prolonged ischemia from an imbalance of myocardial oxygen supply and demand, without an acute and complete coronary artery occlusion, may cause myocardial infarction. The status of the collateral vessels at the time of the infarct and the presence or absence of coronary artery spasm may influence the extent of myocardial ischemic injury.

The roles of platelets, vasoactive peptides, proteolytic enzymes, and changes in the microvasculature in initiating and defining the extent of myocardial infarction also remain uncertain and may be different in humans than in experimental animals. Besides, the methods for determining infarct size that are suitable in experimental models are not always clinically applicable. Many of these suggested techniques for measuring infarct size lack sensitivity and therefore impose serious limitations in evaluating the influence of any therapeutic intervention designed to reduce myocardial ischemic injury. Two methods—ST segment mapping and creatine phosphokinase curves—are most commonly used to measure the extent of myocardial ischemic injury and infarct size both in experimental animals and in patients.

*ST Segment Mapping.* In 1920, Pardee [8] suggested that ST segment changes on the electrocardiogram (ECG) indicated myocardial injury. Since then, a strong but empirical correlation between the height of ST elevation and the extent of myocardial injury and its clinical consequences has been observed in many patients. In the last decade, the feasibility of utilizing the change in ST segments to measure infarct size more precisely has been explored in experimental models [9].

It has been demonstrated that the sum of ECG ST elevations on an epicardial grid measured 15 minutes after coronary artery occlusion in dogs correlates well with the extent of myocardial damage determined 24 hours to several days later by creatine phosphokinase histochemical techniques and electromicroscopic techniques (figure 13–1). A close correlation between *epicardial* and *precordial* ST segment elevations has been demonstrated in experimental myocardial infarction [10]. Thus, precordial ST seg-

ment mapping with the use of a multiple-lead electrode blanket (figure 13–2) has been proposed for clinical use in patients with acute myocardial infarction to determine the extent of myocardial damage [11].

It must be emphasized, however, that there are serious limitations, both theoretical and practical, in the use of ST segment shifts in the ECG as quantitative indicators of myocardial ischemic injury. In experimental myocardial infarction, a poor correlation between the decrement of myocardial tissue flow and the magnitude of changes in ST segments has been reported [12–15]. ST segments may remain isoelectric in many epicardial sites overlying myocardial tissue, with flows of as little as 10 percent of nor-

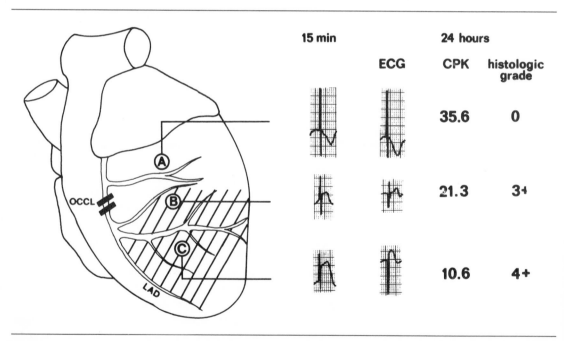

FIGURE 13-1. The heart and its arteries in a canine preparation. The left anterior descending (LAD) artery was occluded at its midportion (OCCL). The shaded area represents the zone of ST segment elevation 15 minutes after occlusion. To the right of the heart are examples of epicardial electrograms, myocardial creatine phosphokinase (CPK) values (IU/mg protein), and histologic grades from another similarly prepared dog. Site A (from nonischemic myocardium) exhibited no ST segment changes 15 minutes after occlusion, and 24 hours later it showed a normal QRS configuration, normal CPK activity, and appeared normal histologically. Site B (border zone) showed moderate ST segment elevation at 15 minutes, while at 24 hours, there was a significant Q-wave and partial loss of R-wave voltage. The CPK activity was moderately depressed, and the histologic section was graded 3 + (51 to 75 percent) necrosis. Site C (center of the ischemic zone) had marked ST segment elevation at 15 minutes, and at 24 hours it demonstrated a total loss of R-wave with a QS complex. The myocardial CPK activity was greatly depressed, and the histologic section was graded 4 + (more than 75 percent) necrosis. (From Muller, J.E. et al. A technique to assess the efficacy of interventions designed to limit infarct size. *Circulation* 57:1, 1978. Reproduced by permission of the American Heart Association, Inc.)

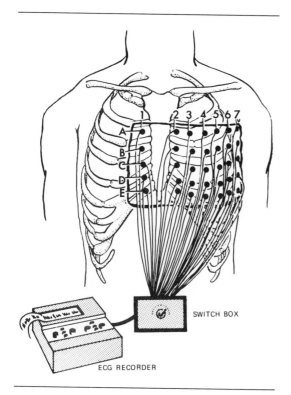

FIGURE 13–2. The 35-electrode map on a patient's chest. A representative ECG obtained from the map is depicted in figure 13–3. (From Muller, J.E. et al. A technique to assess the efficacy of interventions designed to limit infarct size. *Circulation* 57:1, 1978. Reproduced by permission of the American Heart Association, Inc.)

mal [14, 15]. ST segments shifts following experimental coronary artery occlusion also do not correlate well with biochemical and metabolic indexes of ischemia. Significant depression of high-energy phosphate stores may occur in hypoxic hearts prior to any changes in ST segments [16]. Furthermore, no clear relation has been observed between the degree of ST segment elevation and the amount of lactate accumulation or of adenosine triphosphate and creatine phosphate depletion from the injured myocardium [17].

The precise mechanism of ST segment elevation in ischemia has not been delineated. Seemingly, it is a complex electrophysiologic event involving current flow from abnormal to normal tissue during electrical diastole and from normal to abnormal tissue during systole. Any changes in resting membrane potential or action potential duration, irrespective of the cause, may therefore affect ST segments.

Considerable clinical problems are also associated with using ST segment elevation as a measure of the extent of myocardial damage. ST segment elevations associated with pericarditis, a frequent complication of transmural myocardial infarction, may cloud the significance of ST segment elevations as indicators of myocardial ischemic injury. Furthermore, in most patients with acute myocardial infarction a substantial spontaneous decline in the magnitude of ST segment elevation occurs within a few hours after the onset of chest pain, with marked individual variation. Between 6 and 24 hours after the onset of chest pain, a 32 percent average decrease in ST segment elevations has been reported [18]. Even within 6 hours of the onset of chest pain, there may be a significant spontaneous reduction in ST segment elevation (approximately 30 percent) [19]. It is apparent, therefore, that the effect of interventions to reduce infarct size cannot be assessed by ST segment mapping with any precision within the first few hours of the onset of infarction, the time period during which the greatest promise of limiting the extent of myocardial ischemia exists. Therefore, some investigators have suggested that rather than concentrating on the decrease in ST segment elevation, the physician should be aware that a *second* increase in ST segment elevation indicates extension of necrosis [20].

Because of these problems in the clinical use of precordial ST segment mapping to estimate infarct size, QRS changes have been evaluated for determination of the extent of myocardial injury. It has been suggested that the depth of the Q-wave and the loss of the R-wave may be better predictors of ischemic damage (figure 13–3) [21,22]. Further studies, such as those documenting the natural course of the QRS complex [22], will be needed to assess the sensitivity of QRS changes as a measure of infarct size before such techniques can be applied clinically. Furthermore, it has been demonstrated that changes in ventricular volumes and dimensions, in addition to myocardial damage, can markedly influence epicardial QRS amplitude [23, 24].

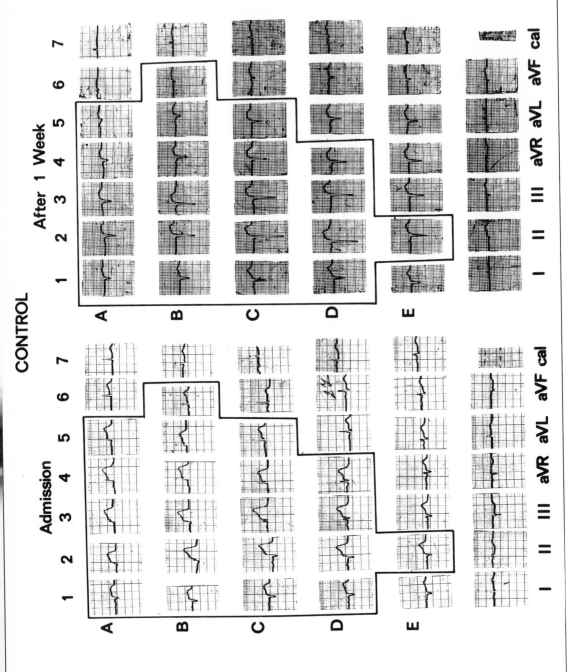

*Creatine Phosphokinase Disappearance Curves.* Determination of the creatine phosphokinase disappearance curve is the other technique that has been used to estimate infarct size, both in experimental animals and in patients with acute myocardial infarction. The enzyme creatine phosphokinase is formed in cardiac muscle and in virtually every other tissue of the body. It is especially abundant in skeletal muscle and the brain. Early experimental studies have demonstrated that the creatine phosphokinase content of infarcted myocardium shows a good inverse correlation with infarct size as determined morphologically. A close direct correlation was also found between the creatine phosphokinase content and the blood flow to ischemic and infarcted myocardium [25]. Further studies in experimental animals have confirmed the basic correlation between creatine phosphokinase depletion from damaged myocardium and infarct size as determined by various techniques [26, 27]. In experimental myocardial infarction, a correlation among serial serum creatine phosphokinase levels, the magnitude of creatine phosphokinase depletion from infarcted myocardium, and the morphologically determined infarct size at postmortem examination has also been demonstrated.

Serial determinations of serum creatine phosphokinase levels over a period of time allow one to predict mathematically the absolute amount of creatine phosphokinase entering the circulation on the basis of the area under the curve of the enzyme levels plotted against time. A good correlation among the estimated total serum creatine phosphokinase, the extent of myocardial infarction, and the myocardial creatine phosphokinase depletion has been reported in

FIGURE 13–3. An example of the use of 35-lead precordial ECG mapping to evaluate the development of myocarcial necrosis in a patient with an anterior myocardial infarction. Figure 13–2 shows the location of sites A through E and 1 through 7. The sites with ST segment elevation of 0.15 mV or more on admission are outlined. Note the unfavorable progression from ischemic injury to necrosis with 100 percent loss of R-wave voltage by 1 week in sites within the outline. (From Muller, J.E. et al. A technique to assess the efficacy of interventions designed to limit infarct size. *Circulation* 57:1, 1978. Reproduced by permission of the American Heart Association, Inc.)

experimental myocardial infarction in dogs [28]. It has also been suggested that the ultimate size of the infarct can be predicted from the initial portion of the creatine phosphokinase curve determined during the first 5 hours in dogs and the first 7 hours in humans [29]. This technique has the potential of providing an early estimation of the expected infarct size, and it can therefore be useful in the evaluation of therapy through the observation of deviations from the predicted infarct size. Indeed, in experimental animals, a good correlation between predicted and observed infarct size has been reported [29]. On the other hand, in patients with acute myocardial infarction, it has been reported that the prediction of infarct size from 7-hour curves may have errors of between 30 and 40 percent of the actual infarct size [30].

There are also several theoretical and practical problems in using the creatine phosphokinase curves for the estimation of infarct size. The serum creatine phosphokinase level at any given time is the result of the amount of the enzyme entering the blood and the amount leaving the blood. The rate of entry of the enzyme into the blood may vary if the infarction is not complete at a discrete point in time. Furthermore, the amount of creatine phosphokinase released from the myocardium not only depends on the extent of myocardial injury, but also on the rate of washout of the enzyme from the underperfused infarcted areas. Destruction of the enzyme in the cardiac lymph and venous blood is also an important variable that may introduce a significant error in estimating accurately the amount of enzyme released from the infarcted myocardium. The rate of removal of creatine phosphokinase from the blood may also vary. The function of the reticuloendothelial system, which plays an important role in the clearance of the enzyme, may be variable in individual patients. The disappearance rate of the enzyme may also be delayed in shock or by certain pharmacologic agents. Recent studies have outlined the many variables that enter into the estimation of infarct size from creatine phosphokinase curves and have indicated that large errors in calculated infarct size could occur if the variables deviated by as little as one standard deviation [31]. These studies have also indicated that the factors that might influence the entry of the enzyme into the blood and its disappearance from the blood may vary, and thus a poor correlation between enzymatic and histologic estimates of the extent of myocardial infarction may be observed [32]. Nevertheless, enzymatic indices have been reported to correlate with prognosis in one study of 560 patients [33].

When the total creatine phosphokinase curves are used for the estimation of infarct size, variable errors may be introduced because of the release of enzyme from skeletal muscle, which might occur in the presence of pump failure and shock or after intramuscular injection. To circumvent this difficulty, the MB isozyme of creatine phosphokinase has been used, which provides a better approach to the evaluation of the extent of myocardial ischemic injury. A batch absorption technique and a radioimmunoassay have been developed that permit the rapid and accurate measurement of MB isozymes. A major clinical problem in using the enzymatic models for predicting infarct size is that frequently the patients are admitted late after the onset of infarction, when the serum creatine phosphokinase level has already risen. Therefore, the early portion of the curve is frequently missed. Another difficulty is that for the prediction of infarct size, 7 to 9 hours must elapse before the curve can be constructed and intervention begun. Whether the enzymatic predictive models are of practical value for intervention therapy to decrease infarct size is still unclear.

*Other Techniques.* Recently, scintigraphic techniques have been used to estimate infarct size in experimental animals and have been extended to clinical practice. Technetium-99m pyrophosphate scintigraphy provides a sensitive and relatively specific indicator of the presence of acute infarction (see chapter 8). Experimental studies have shown a good correlation between acute infarct size, as judged from the area of abnormal myocardial uptake of radionuclide on the technetium-99m pyrophosphate scintigram, and the extent of histologically determined infarct size or gross infarct weight [36]. Thallium-201 myocardial perfusion defects also correlate well with histologic estimates of infarct size in dogs [37].

In clinical studies, however, no consistent correlation has been observed between the infarct size determined by scintigraphic techniques and that determined by enzymatic or ECG techniques. In some investigations, a good correlation between the infarct area determined with technetium-99m pyrophosphate and the infarct size estimated from serial serum creatine phosphokinase values has been observed [38]; in others, however, no such correlation has been found [39]. Clearly, therefore, without further evaluation, the sensitivity of the scintigraphic techniques for the estimation of infarct size remains unproved, and its routine clinical application cannot be recommended at the present time. Presently, positron radioisotope imaging, computerized tomography, and nuclear magnetic resonance are under investigation as potential techniques to determine infarct size. However, their roles in clinical practice are yet to be determined.

It is apparent that for clinical use, no accurate technique is presently available for either measuring or predicting the ultimate infarct size. Although promising techniques are being developed—including ECG mapping, MB isozyme creatine phosphokinase analysis, and radioisotopic myocardial scanning—no reliable and sensitive method is as yet available to apply to the individual patient.

EFFECTS OF THERAPY ON THE EXTENT OF MYOCARDIAL ISCHEMIA
Although the influence of various types of therapeutic interventions on the extent of myocardial ischemic injury has been investigated on experimental animals [40, 41], clinical experience is extremely limited. Attempts to limit infarct size have been based on the physiologic principles of (1) decreasing myocardial oxygen requirements, (2) increasing myocardial oxygen supply, (3) augmenting anaerobic metabolism, and (4) protecting against autolytic and heterolytic processes.

*β-Adrenergic Blocking Agents.* The principle of decreasing myocardial oxygen demand has been utilized to reduce the extent of myocardial injury and to preserve the viability of ischemic myocardium. β-adrenergic blocking agents, such as propranolol and practolol, reduce heart rate and contractility and thereby reduce myocardial energy demands. Furthermore, it has been suggested that propranolol decreases platelet adhesiveness [42] and improves perfusion to ischemic subendocardial tissue [43]. In some studies, an improvement in myocardial ischemia was observed with the use of $\beta$-adrenergic blocking agents: reduction in epicardial ST segment elevation and a decrease in the expected infarct size in propranolol-treated animals were reported [44]. In other studies, however, no beneficial influence of propranolol on myocardial damage was noted on the basis of regional myocardial blood flow or of tissue creatine phosphokinase depletion [45]. In some patients with acute myocardial infarction, the administration of propranolol has been shown to cause an increase in myocardial lactate extraction (which provides biochemical evidence of lessening ischemia) [46], a decrease in precordial ST segment elevations [47], and a reduction in cardiac enzyme levels [48].

A number of prospective, randomized studies have attempted to determine the influence of $\beta$-adrenergic blocking agents, administered within a few hours of onset of myocardial infarction, on the extent of "infarct size" in patients with evolving myocardial infarction. Both cardioselective and nonselective beta-blocking agents have been used, and generally beneficial effects have been reported [49, 50]. In the study reported by Herlitz et al. [49], metoprolol, a relatively cardioselective $\beta_1$-adrenergic receptor blocking agent was initially administered intravenously (15 mg total : 3 bolus of 5 mg at 2-minute intervals) within 12 hours of the onset of chest pain, followed by 50 mg orally four times daily for 2 days, and thereafter 100 mg twice daily for 3 months. A reduction in the enzymatically and electrocardiographically determined myocardial infarction size was noted after early beta-blockade with metoprolol in patients with recent myocardial infarction. The international collaborative study group also reported a reduction of infarct size estimated by enzymatic and electrocardiographic techniques using timolol [50], a nonselective beta-blocker. In this study, two bolus injections of 1 mg of timolol were given within 5 hours of the onset

of symptoms, followed by 0.6 mg/hour infusion for 24 hours. Oral therapy with timolol, 10 mg twice daily, was then continued for the rest of the hospital stay. Approximately a 30 percent reduction of maximal cumulative creatine kinase release and a 20 to 25 percent smaller change in QRS-vector variables were noted in the timolol-treated patients. Early intervention with beta-blockers in these studies was associated with shorter duration of chest pain and decreased need of analgesics. Significant adverse effects, such as congestive heart failure, occurred infrequently with beta-blocker therapy in these patients.

Contrary to these reports, administration of intravenous propranolol followed by oral therapy early after the onset of myocardial infarction was not associated with any beneficial effects [51]. Infarct size in gram-equivalents, estimated from plasma MB creatine kinase (CK) activity, was almost identical in placebo-treated and propranolol-treated groups. Peak plasma levels of MB-CK were similar in the two groups. There was also no difference in the area of myocardial pyrophosphate uptake and in the magnitude of R-wave loss on electrocardiograms. Left ventricular ejection fraction was also similar in propranolol- and placebo-treated groups. Thus, the role of beta-blockade for reduction of the extent of myocardial injury remains unproved, and its routine application cannot be recommended. However, as beta-blockade therapy has been shown to decrease the incidence of reinfarction, sudden death, and overall mortality in patients following first infarction [52–54], beta-blockers, unless contraindicated, should be employed. For secondary prevention and to improve late prognosis, beta-blocker therapy can be started within 2 to 3 weeks after infarction.

*Vasodilator Drugs.* The rationale for the use of vasodilator agents for the preservation of ischemic myocardium is based on the principle that, in general, such drugs reduce myocardial oxygen demand and hence can alter the myocardial oxygen supply-and-demand ratio more favorably. In the presence of pump failure, most vasodilator agents (except phentolamine) do not cause any change in heart rate. Indeed, in some patients the heart rate may decrease during vasodilator therapy. Myocardial wall tension decreases as both the intraventricular pressure and the ventricular end-diastolic volume and radius decrease (Laplace relation). As most vasodilator agents do not possess any direct inotropic effect, overall myocardial oxygen demand tends to decrease, and therefore a favorable effect on the extent of myocardial ischemic injury is expected during vasodilator therapy. As discussed subsequently in this chapter, however, no convincing data are yet available to suggest that there is a significant and consistent reduction in infarct size during vasodilator therapy, irrespective of the vasodilator agent used. Furthermore, a reduction in coronary perfusion due to a reduction in aortic diastolic pressure and maldistribution of myocardial blood flow is a potentially deleterious effect of vasodilator therapy, and this effect must be considered during evaluation of the effects of vasodilator agents on myocardial ischemic injury.

Presently, nitrates are frequently used for "afterload" reduction in patients with acute myocardial infarction, whether in the presence or absence of symptoms of continued myocardial ischemia. In patients without heart failure, however, nitrates induce reflex tachycardia, which in itself increases myocardial oxygen demand. Nitrates may also cause redistribution of blood flow within the myocardium, which in some circumstances might be favorable and in others, unfavorable [55]. To combat such potentially deleterious effects, nitrates have been combined with $\alpha$-adrenergic agonists such as methoxamine, and in studies of experimental myocardial infarction, such combinations have been shown to improve myocardial ischemia [56]. In patients with acute myocardial infarction, however, no consistent results have been observed with this combination. In some prospective, randomized studies, a reduction of infarct size calculated from CK and CK-MB activity curves was observed with intravenous nitroglycerin [57]. However, in other similar studies no significant change in infarct size was noted. Furthermore, nitroglycerin therapy did not influence the immediate or late prognosis [58, 59].

Controversy also exists regarding the possible beneficial and deleterious effects of sodium ni-

troprusside. Like nitrates, nitroprusside causes reflex tachycardia in the absence of heart failure. Moreover, reduction in coronary perfusion, maldistribution of myocardial blood flow, and reduction in collateral flow to the ischemic myocardium are the potential adverse effects of nitroprusside on coronary hemodynamics and myocardial metabolism. Nitroprusside, on the other hand, can also decrease myocardial oxygen requirements and improve subendocardial perfusion presumably by increasing transmyocardial pressure gradient. It is not surprising, therefore, that with nitroprusside variable and conflicting results have been reported regarding reduction of the extent of myocardial injury. In some investigations an increase in ST segment elevation and a higher level of serum creatine kinase occurred, indicating an extension of myocardial injury [60–62]. Other studies that employed similar techniques to measure infarct size, however, observed a beneficial response [63–65]. As reduction of perfusion pressure is a potential hazard of vasodilator therapy, and since no conclusive evidence exists for the reduction in infarct size, routine use of nitroprusside or nitroglycerin cannot be recommended in patients with acute myocardial infarction.

The influence of other vasodilator agents such as phentolamine, trimethaphan, hydralazine, or minoxidil on the extent of myocardial ischemia in patients with acute myocardial infarction has not been thoroughly investigated; however, their overall effects on myocardial metabolism are likely to be similar. It is apparent that the exact role of vasodilator therapy in preserving ischemic myocardium in patients with acute myocardial infarction remains uncertain at this time, and such therapy should be considered only in the presence of heart failure.

*Glucose-Insulin-Potassium Infusion.* Another possible therapeutic approach to decrease myocardial energy demands is the use of glucose-insulin-potassium (GIK) infusion. One of the major metabolic effects of GIK infusion is a reduction of the level of circulating free fatty acids, which is frequently elevated in the early stages of acute myocardial infarction. Elevated free fatty acids have been shown in experimental animals to increase myocardial oxygen demand and to enhance myocardial ischemia [66]. Reduction in free fatty acid levels should therefore be beneficial, and, indeed, in experimental myocardial infarction, GIK infusion has been shown to decrease the extent of myocardial ischemic injury [67, 68]. GIK infusion, however, may produce a beneficial response in myocardial ischemia by other mechanisms. It is presumed that GIK infusion causes an increase in glycolytic adenosine triphosphate levels, and the myocardium may derive significant energy from augmented anaerobic metabolism. It has also been suggested that GIK may cause a decrease in cellular acylcoenzyme A levels, and therefore improved adenine nucleotide translocase activity may result. Despite these potentially beneficial effects of GIK infusion on myocardial ischemia, there is no evidence that it causes significant reduction in infarct size in patients with acute myocardial infarction [69, 70]. Hemodynamic deterioration, as evidenced by an increase in left ventricular filling pressure and cardiac work, has also been observed during GIK infusion [69].

*Other Approaches.* Coronary blood flow and energy supply to the myocardium can be enhanced by several theoretically possible means. Myocardial revascularization, retroperfusion, elevation of arterial oxygen tension, and the use of thrombolytic agents (see chapter 9) have the potential of increasing oxygen supply to the myocardium directly. An increase in oxygen and energy supply to the ischemic myocardium may be caused indirectly by promoting collateral flow (e.g., by increased coronary perfusion pressure, administration of vasodilators, counterpulsation, or use of hyaluronidase), by increasing capillary flow in an area of myocardial swelling (e.g., by mannitol or hypertonic glucose administration), as well as by enhancing the transport of nutrients from the capillaries into the myocardial cells. The benefits of these therapeutic approaches that potentially increase myocardial energy supply, however, have not been established in patients with acute myocardial infarction.

MYOCARDIAL REVASCULARIZATION. Surgery has been performed early in the course of acute infarction in an attempt to salvage ischemic myocardium, but no consistent beneficial response has been observed [71–73]. Furthermore, revascularization in the presence of acute myocardial infarction carries significant risks for extending the infarct by precipitating hemorrhage in the infarcted area, for inducing more arrhythmias, as well as for incurring higher operative mortality (see chapter 14). It is apparent that without further definitive studies, revascularization surgery should be performed only for the treatment of complications of acute infarction, such as papillary muscle infarct, ventricular septal rupture, or postinfarction angina.

MECHANICAL ASSISTANCE. Use of intra-aortic balloon counterpulsation or external counterpulsation combined with vasodilator administration produces beneficial hemodynamic responses: a decrease in left ventricular filling pressure along with an increase in cardiac output and an augmentation of coronary artery perfusion pressure have been reported [74, 75]. The increased collateral flow to the ischemic myocardium resulting from increased perfusion pressure and the concomitant decrease in myocardial oxygen demand (through reduction of preload and afterload) obtained with the use of counterpulsation devices should also improve myocardial metabolism and hence reduce the extent of myocardial ischemic injury. Indeed, in experimental myocardial infarction, a reduction in infarct size, which was determined by ECG and histopathologic techniques, has been reported following the use of counterpulsation [76, 77]. In some patients, severe angina that has been unresponsive to conventional therapy has improved during counterpulsation, thus suggesting that counterpulsation has beneficial effects on myocardial ischemia [74]. Clinical studies, however, are still too limited [78] to advocate its use in patients with uncomplicated myocardial infarction. Furthermore, the potential risks of inducing leg ischemia, aortic dissection, and other complications [79] during the use of intra-aortic balloon counterpulsation must be evaluated before its routine application can be considered.

HYPEROSMOTIC AGENTS. Experimental studies have shown that the endothelial cells of the small vessels begin to swell within 20 to 120 minutes following the onset of myocardial ischemia [80]. This cell swelling may impede the passage of red blood cells and cause a further reduction of oxygen supply to the ischemic myocardium. It has been proposed that the use of hyperosmotic agents such as mannitol and hypertonic glucose can reduce intracellular edema, and hence it has the potential of improving blood flow to ischemic zones.

Earlier animal studies indeed reported improved regional coronary blood flow in ischemic myocardium after treatment with mannitol during acute and chronic myocardial ischemia [81]. In addition, improved cardiac performance and a decrease in the histopathologically estimated infarct size were observed during mannitol-induced hyperosmolarity [82, 83]. More recent studies, however, have not only failed to demonstrate any reduction of the ultimate infarct size, but have also shown that mannitol might hinder the development of collateral vessels [84]. Mannitol causes major shifts of fluid to the intravascular space, and its administration carries certain potential hazards [83]; mannitol therapy, therefore, cannot be recommended at the present time.

HYALURONIDASE. The enzyme hyaluronidase, which depolymerizes mucopolysaccharides, has been shown to decrease myocardial ischemic injury in experimental infarction. Based on epicardial ST segment changes, myocardial creatine phosphokinase depletion, and histologic examination, significant reduction in myocardial necrosis 24 hours after coronary artery occlusion has been reported in hyaluronidase-treated animals [85, 86]. It has also been suggested that hyaluronidase reduces the ultimate extent of necrosis and results in a larger quantity of normally contracting myocardium when the infarction has healed.

The mechanism of the beneficial effects of hyaluronidase in experimental myocardial infarction has not been clarified. It has been shown to penetrate the ischemic zone, probably by depolymerizing the mucopolysaccharides. It has been hypothesized that this action may facilitate the transport of substrates to the ischemic myocardium. It might also help to wash out potentially harmful metabolites from the infarcted myocardium. The effects of hyaluronidase on myocardial ischemic injury have been investigated only in a small number of patients with acute myocardial infarction [87]. Decreased Q-wave development and less loss of R-waves were observed in the hyaluronidase-treated patients. On the other hand, in a double-blind, prospective, randomized study, quantitative analysis of infarct size estimated from the creatine kinase curves did not demonstrate any beneficial effect of hyaluronidase [88]. In this study, only a small number of patients were randomized. Thus, routine clinical usage of this agent must await larger, controlled studies.

OXYGEN. Another relatively innocuous therapeutic approach to increase oxygen supply to ischemic myocardium is to increase arterial oxygen tension ($PO_2$). In experimental myocardial infarction, exposure of the animal to 40 percent oxygen has produced a reduction in the extent of myocardial ischemic injury [89]. In patients with acute myocardial infarction, administration of 100 percent oxygen for 1 hour has been shown to reduce precordial ST segment elevations [90]. The mechanism by which increased arterial $PO_2$ may produce beneficial effects on myocardial ischemia remains unclear. Whether the mechanism is through an enhanced diffusion gradient for oxygen or through increased collateral blood flow brought on by reflex vasoconstriction of normal vessels is not known [91]. It appears, however, that oxygen therapy, which has been long employed and well tolerated by patients, may have some beneficial effect on myocardial ischemia.

ANTIINFLAMMATORY AGENTS. Experimental studies indicate that the inflammatory reactions that follow the initial myocardial damage might produce secondary adverse effects on the extent of myocardial injury. Increase in capillary permeability, interstitial edema, leukotaxis, phagocytosis, and injury to cell membranes all might be contributory. Interventions that decrease such inflammatory reactions therefore have the potential to limit infarct size.

The effects of *cobra venom factor,* which inhibits the action of the complement system, and of *aprotinin,* an inhibitor of the kallikrein system, have been investigated in experimental myocardial infarction, and their beneficial effects in limiting myocardial ischemic injury have been reported. No clinical studies, however, have yet been performed with these two anti-inflammatory agents to evaluate their effectiveness in reducing myocardial injury in patients with acute myocardial infarction.

*Glucocorticoids,* because of their probable anti-inflammatory effects, have received considerable attention both in experimental animals and in patients, and their potentially beneficial effects in reducing the extent of myocardial infarction have been explored. Myocardial ischemia has been shown to disrupt cellular membranes and to release lysosomal hydrolytic enzymes that may cause further cellular damage [92]. It has been suggested that steroids might stabilize lysosomal and other cellular membranes and thereby prevent secondary damage to the myocardium following the onset of infarction [93–97]. No convincing evidence is available, however, to suggest that with such therapy, viability of the ischemic myocardium can be maintained or the extension of infarction can be retarded.

In some investigations of experimental myocardial infarction, the administration of corticosteroids has caused a reduction in the extent of myocardial ischemic injury as determined by histopathologic and ECG techniques [93, 94, 98, 99]; in others, which used the same techniques for measurements of infarct size, no beneficial effects were observed [100, 101]. Similarly, in patients with acute myocardial infarction, the use of corticosteroids has produced conflicting data with respect to preservation of ischemic myocardium. In studies with similar protocols utilizing single or multiple doses of methylprednisolone and using the same enzymatic techniques (creatine phosphokinase levels) to estimate infarct size, a reduction in infarct size has been observed [102], but in others no change in infarct size was noted [103, 104]. Differences in the protocols and in the timing of the intervention following the onset of symptoms may account for some of the discrepancies in these results; nevertheless, it is apparent that a significant and clinically relevant reduction in the extent of myocardial injury is unlikely to occur with the use of corticosteroids.

Furthermore, the possible adverse effects of therapy with steroids should not be overlooked. A deleterious hemodynamic response [105] and impairment of healing of the infarct are potentially hazardous side effects of corticosteroid therapy. Experimental work has shown definite retardation in the healing of myocardial infarcts in dogs, especially with larger doses of steroids [106]. Isolated clinical studies have indicated an increased propensity to develop ventricular aneurysm and ventricular rupture in patients with acute myocardial infarction who are receiving steroid therapy [103, 107]. Experimental studies suggest that a high dose of methylprednisolone, not a low dose, causes marked scar thinning [108].

At the present time, no standard therapy with proved, beneficial effects seems to be available for reducing the extent of myocardial ischemic injury in patients with acute myocardial infarction. This frustration, however, should not make a physician underestimate the very important concept of infarct size reduction. When making clinical decisions, the physician must consider the effects of all conventional and unconventional therapy employed for the management of such patients on the ultimate extent of myocardial damage, even though a clear answer might not be available. Prompt treatment of life-threatening dysrhythmias is indicated not only to prevent immediate catastrophe, but also to prevent infarction extension if at all possible. Similarly, before the institution of inotropic therapy, one must consider that increased contractility may enhance myocardial ischemia and influence the prognosis adversely. Irrespective of the inotropic agents used, an augmented contractile state increases myocardial oxygen demand and therefore may cause the extension of myocardial injury. Digitalis, isoproterenol, dopamine, and other inotropic drugs have been shown to cause deterioration in myocardial metabolism as well as an increase in infarct size. Avoidance of inotropic agents, whenever possible, is therefore clearly warranted.

During vasodilator therapy for pump failure, the physician's awareness regarding the possibility of enhancing existing myocardial ischemia because of an excessive reduction in coronary perfusion pressure is absolutely essential. It must also be emphasized that a given therapy that might be beneficial to one patient may prove harmful to others. A reduction in arterial pressure in hypertensive patients is likely to cause a decrease in myocardial injury; on the other hand, in normotensive or hypotensive patients a reduction in arterial pressure by a similar magnitude may cause enhancement of myocardial ischemia. It is apparent that for proper management, therapy needs to be tailored according to the needs of the individual patient.

## Effects of Inotropic and Vasodilator Drugs in Patients with Acute Myocardial Infarction

### INOTROPIC AGENTS

Inotropic agents are usually employed for treatment of low output state, although they have the potential for increasing myocardial ischemia. Among the variety of inotropic drugs employed are digitalis, isoproterenol, norepinephrine, glucagon, dopamine, and dobutamine. No data in the post-infarction state are available for the newly approved drug, amrinone.

*Digitalis.* Despite considerable investigation, the role of digitalis in the treatment of myocardial infarction remains uncertain. In experimental studies, the inotropic effects of digitalis are easily demonstrated, both in isolated papillary muscle preparations and in the intact normal heart [109]. Also, in patients without heart failure, there is an increase in contractility as suggested by an increase in the maximum rate of rise of left ventricular pressure (dP/dt) and in the maximum velocity of contractile element shortening (vmax). These occurred without changes in heart rate, arterial pressure, or left ventricular filling pressure [110–112]. Changes in contractility, however, may not necessarily be expressed by changes in cardiac output [113].

In patients with chronic congestive heart failure, some improvement in pump function, as evidenced by an increase in stroke work and a fall in left ventricular filling pressure, has been observed [114, 115], although controversy still exists regarding the efficacy of digitalis therapy in chronic heart failure [116]. In patients with acute myocardial infarction with or without heart failure, no consistent beneficial hemodynamic response has been observed. Most clinical studies have revealed little or no increase in cardiac output or stroke volume following the administration of intravenous digitalis preparations [117–120]. Although some patients

showed a modest decrease in left ventricular filling pressure [121], the majority had little or no change. Furthermore, when digitalis-induced improvement in left ventricular function occurred in patients with acute myocardial infarction, it was most often seen in patients without evidence of pump failure; in patients with significant failure or shock, improvement in left ventricular function was only rarely observed [122].

Figure 13–4 illustrates the hemodynamic effects of digitalis in 25 patients with acute myocardial infarction. Based on clinical criteria, patients were classified as having shock, heart failure, or no heart failure. The group with no heart failure responded with 18 percent and 38 percent increases in cardiac and stroke work indexes, respectively, whereas individuals with heart failure and shock showed no physiologically important changes in either cardiac output or left ventricular filling pressure. Digitalis administration in acute myocardial infarction, therefore, appears to produce beneficial hemodynamic effects only in those patients who do not require it. Paradoxically, those who do need the drug showed essentially no hemodynamic improvement.

In some patients with acute myocardial infarction, left ventricular filling pressure may de-

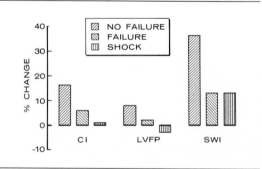

FIGURE 13–4. Changes in left ventricular function following the intravenous administration of digitalis to patients with acute myocardial infarction. Only in patients without heart failure was there a significant increase in cardiac index (CI). No significant changes in left ventricular filling pressure (LVFP) occurred in any group. Changes in stroke work index (SWI) were greatest in those individuals in whom use of the drug was not indicated on clinical grounds. (From Forrester, J.S. and Chatterjee, I. In Vogel, J.H.K. (ed.), *Advances in Cardiology* (Vol. II). Basel: Karger, 1974.)

crease, even though the cardiac output may not change. It might be reasoned, therefore, that digitalis therapy may still be useful because of the reduction in diastolic pressure and volume, which might have a myocardial oxygen-sparing effect [123]. Evaluation of the changes in coronary blood flow and myocardial metabolism, however, indicates that adverse metabolic responses to digitalis may occur in patients with acute myocardial infarction. We investigated changes in coronary blood flow, myocardial oxygen consumption, and transmyocardial lactate extraction in nine patients with acute myocardial infarction [122]. Each patient demonstrated increases in coronary blood flow and in myocardial oxygen consumption following digitalis administration, and one patient developed angina. The increase in coronary blood flow and myocardial oxygen consumption following administration of digitalis in acute infarction can be explained by its positive inotropic effect.

Increases in left ventricular dP/dt and in maximum velocity of contractile element shortening without a significant change in heart rate and arterial pressure have been observed in patients with acute infarction who were treated with digitalis [121]. The magnitude of the increase in myocardial oxygen demand due to the enhanced contractile state may exceed its expected reduction resulting from a relatively minor decrease in left ventricular filling pressure; this thus accounts for the net increase in coronary blood flow and myocardial oxygen consumption. These data therefore suggest that digitalis produces little or no beneficial hemodynamic response in acute infarction. Furthermore, its administration may increase the degree of myocardial ischemia. A decrease in left ventricular filling pressure, which appears to be the only potentially beneficial hemodynamic effect of digitalis in patients with acute infarction, can be achieved more effectively and safely with the use of a diuretic such as furosemide [124].

Controversy also exists regarding the possibly deleterious effects of digitalis in inducing serious ventricular arrhythmias in the presence of myocardial ischemia. In experimental models, it has been demonstrated that the dose of digitalis needed to induce ventricular tachycardia is significantly lowered by the presence of myocardial

ischemia [125–127]. In clinical studies, some, but not all, patients have shown an increased propensity to develop ventricular arrhythmias [117, 124, 128–130]. From a clinical point of view, it is apparent that a drug such as digitalis —which produces little or no beneficial hemodynamic effects but might increase myocardial ischemia and precipitate ventricular arrhythmias —has limited value in the management of pump failure complicating myocardial infarction.

*Isoproterenol.* Isoproterenol consistently increases cardiac output by increasing both stroke volume and heart rate [131–133]. These beneficial hemodynamic effects, however, are accompanied by a marked deterioration of myocardial metabolism. Myocardial oxygen consumption increases and transmyocardial lactate extraction decreases, thus indicating enhancement of myocardial ischemia [132]. An increase in myocardial ischemia eventually causes deterioration of mechanical function, which explains the overall ineffectiveness of isoproterenol for the treatment of pump failure complicating myocardial infarction [131].

*Norepinephrine.* With norepinephrine, the magnitude of increase in cardiac output is considerably less than that obtained with isoproterenol [132]. With norepinephrine, however, there is less tachycardia and a significant increase in arterial pressure and systemic vascular resistance [132, 134]. Therefore, the use of norepinephrine has been advocated for temporary support of arterial pressure in patients with hypotension complicating myocardial infarction. An increase in coronary blood flow and myocardial oxygen consumption along with an improved transmyocardial lactate extraction have been observed in some hypotensive patients [132].

Despite such reported improvement in coronary hemodynamics and myocardial metabolism, however, the effectiveness of norepinephrine for the treatment of low cardiac output complicating myocardial infarction remains debatable. Norepinephrine generally becomes increasingly ineffective as the severity of left ventricular dysfunction increases. We investigated the hemodynamic effects of graded doses of norepinephrine administered to 25 patients with acute myocardial infarction [135]. The response to norepinephrine was determined in large part by the resting level of cardiac function. In surviving patients with an adequate initial cardiac output and little or no left ventricular failure, cardiac output increased by 24 percent, and there was no change in systemic vascular resistance. By contrast, in patients with severe pump failure or shock who did not survive, systemic vascular resistance increased markedly, and only a minimal increase in cardiac output occurred. Thus, in patients in whom therapy was most indicated, the drug was least effective (table 13–1).

*Dopamine.* Dopamine, a biologic precursor of norepinephrine, produces hemodynamic effects similar to those of norepinephrine. Dopamine acts on adrenergic receptors by direct stimulation, although some of its effects are due to the release of endogenous norepinephrine. Cardiac effects are beta-receptor mediated and consist of an increase in heart rate and the rate and force of contraction. Dopamine, like norepinephrine, stimulates alpha-receptors in peripheral arterioles and veins and has no effect on peripheral vascular beta-receptors. Although dopamine in adequate doses increases cardiac output and decreases left ventricular filling pressure (which indicates improved cardiac performance), the magnitude of improvement, as with norepinephrine, appears to be dependent on the initial level of cardiac function. The more severe the dysfunction, the less is the response. Indeed, in patients with severe pump failure or shock complicating acute myocardial infarction, the increase in cardiac output with dopamine is primarily due to an increase in heart rate and not to an increase in stroke volume [136]. Furthermore, as with other inotropic agents, dopamine may cause deterioration in myocardial metabolism and enhance existing myocardial ischemia [136].

*Dobutamine.* Dobutamine, another inotropic agent, is frequently used for the treatment of acute and chronic heart failure. Dobutamine is predominantly a $\beta_1$-receptor agonist, and with larger doses also stimulates $\beta_2$-receptors of the peripheral vascular beds. Dobutamine increases cardiac output and stroke volume without producing excessive tachycardia or hypertension. Indeed, hypotension can occur, although very infrequently, when there is marked reduction in systemic vascular resistance. Pulmonary capillary wedge and pulmonary artery pressures tend to decrease in most patients. Dobutamine, in most patients, increases coronary blood flow and myocardial oxygen consumption [137]. A disproportionate increase in myocardial oxygen consumption has the potential to produce deleterious effects on myocardial metabolic function.

The hemodynamic effects of dobutamine and digitalis have been compared in the same patients with acute myocardial infarction [139]. Dobutamine increased cardiac output and decreased pulmonary capillary wedge pressure consistently; digoxin, on the other hand, had

TABLE 13–1. Hemodynamic response to graded doses of norepinephrine in survivors and nonsurvivors with acute myocardial infarction

| | Survivors | | | | Nonsurvivors | | | |
|---|---|---|---|---|---|---|---|---|
| | Control | 3–5 μg | 5–8 μg | 8–10 μg | Control | 3–5 μg | 5–8 μg | 8–10 μg |
| BP | 85.0 | 95.6 | 96.6 | 102.7 | 68.0 | 73.9 | 80.1 | 88.8 |
| HR | 78.3 | 77.8 | 75.5 | 86.6 | 90.6 | 90.7 | 89.3 | 93.7 |
| CO | 4.6 | 5.0 | 4.9 | 5.7 | 3.1 | 3.3 | 3.2 | 3.5 |
| SW | 73.9 | 84.3 | 88.3 | 93.8 | 31.6 | 36.5 | 41.5 | 45.0 |
| SVR | 17.1 | 17.7 | 18.8 | 16.8 | 24.0 | 24.1 | 26.3 | 30.0 |

BP = mean blood pressure (mmHg); CO = cardiac output (liters/min); HR = heart rate (beats/min); SVR = systemic vascular resistance (dynes·sec·cm$^{-5}$); SW = stroke work (g-m/beat).

Source: Chatterjee, K. et al. *Ann. Clin. Res.* 9:124, 1977.

inconsistent effects. It seems, therefore, that if inotropic support is desired for the treatment of pump failure complicating myocardial infarction, dobutamine is preferable to digitalis. Some differences in the hemodynamic effects of dobutamine and dopamine have been observed in a number of studies [140, 141]. For a similar increase in cardiac output, dopamine produced a greater increase in arterial pressure and a smaller decrease in systemic vascular resistance. Another difference was that dopamine tended to increase pulmonary capillary wedge and pulmonary artery pressures, while with dobutamine, pulmonary capillary wedge and pulmonary artery pressures tend to decrease or remain unchanged.

The decision to use dobutamine or dopamine should be based on the hemodynamic abnormalities. In the presence of hypotension, and particularly when pulmonary capillary wedge pressure is not markedly elevated, dopamine is preferable to dobutamine. When pulmonary capillary wedge pressure is elevated, and in the absence of hypotension, dobutamine can be used effectively to increase cardiac output.

It needs to be emphasized that the use of inotropic agents can be associated with deleterious effects on myocardial metabolic function in patients with acute myocardial infarction and severe coronary artery disease due to excessive increases in myocardial oxygen requirements. Thus, the potential benefits and the risks should always be considered during inotropic therapy of heart failure complicating acute myocardial infarction.

## VASODILATORS

The vasodilators are frequently referred to as drugs that reduce impedance or afterload. These descriptive terms indicate that one of their primary actions is to reduce the resistance of ejection, which can thereby increase cardiac output. Recently, it has been appreciated that some drugs have predominant vasodilating effects, which also produce important hemodynamic effects such as reducing ventricular filling pressures. Therefore, the term *vasodilator* is an appropriate one, since it encompasses both primary effects of these drugs: arteriolar and venous dilation. The predominant mechanism

through which vasodilators increase cardiac output is by reducing systemic arteriolar tone and systemic vascular resistance. The terms *afterload* and *impedance reduction* have been used to describe this particular action of vasodilator drugs. It must be emphasized, however, that the precise quantification of afterload in the intact heart is difficult.

To extend the concept of afterload from an isolated heart muscle system to the intact heart, one has to determine the instantaneous wall stress faced by the muscle fibers in the ventricular wall. This determination would require instantaneous measurements of intraventricular pressure, wall thickness, fiber direction, and radius of curvature, which would be difficult to calculate for the ejecting heart. Although aortic pressure represents to some extent the afterload faced by the ventricle (since the heart must develop that pressure before it can eject blood into the aorta), the relation between aortic pressure and wall stress is only a general one. Furthermore, in certain circumstances, aortic pressure does not reflect the changes in cardiac performance produced by vasodilator drugs. Vasodilators may decrease systemic vascular resistance and increase cardiac output (blood pressure = cardiac output × systemic vascular resistance) by about the same magnitude. Under such circumstances, the blood pressure may change very little, despite the fact that a marked hemodynamic change has been produced by the vasodilator. This emphasizes the difficulty of using arterial pressure as a measure of the afterload faced by the heart. It is also clear that one should not necessarily judge the therapeutic effects of a vasodilator by how much it reduces arterial pressure. The hemodynamic goal of vasodilator therapy in heart failure is to increase cardiac output and to reduce pulmonary capillary wedge pressure, but not necessarily to reduce blood pressure.

Vasodilator drugs have been referred to as "impedance-reducing agents." *Impedance* is the instantaneous ratio of pulsatile pressure to pulsatile flow. A strict definition requires the calculation of a series of harmonics that describe pressure and flow [142]. Such information cannot be obtained easily in clinical practice, and the influence of vasodilator agents on aortic impedance can only be inferred. The concept, however, has a practical advantage because aortic impedance is somewhat related to systemic vascular resistance, which can be easily quantitated in clinical practice. Whereas impedance is the instantaneous relation between pressure and flow, systemic vascular resistance is the average value of this relation throughout many cardiac cycles.

Although the vasodilator drugs improve cardiac performance primarily by their peripheral vascular effects, other potential mechanisms exist through which vasodilators may favorably affect hemodynamics. First, they may reduce myocardial oxygen demand by decreasing left ventricular diastolic pressure and volume and, to some extent, arterial pressure. Such a decrease in myocardial oxygen demand may alter the myocardial oxygen demand-supply relation more favorably. It has also been suggested that some vasodilators improve collateral blood flow to the ischemic myocardium and hence can improve the mechanical function of the ischemic myocardial segments [143]. Although the concept that improvement of segmental myocardial ischemia during vasodilator therapy can significantly contribute to improvement in overall cardiac function is an important one, the clinical significance of such a concept needs to be explored.

A newly appreciated mechanism that may alter the hemodynamic consequences of vasodilator drugs is the effect such agents have on the compliance of the left ventricle [144]. Evidence suggests that vasodilator drugs may produce an acute increase in left ventricular compliance [145]. Since left ventricular end-diastolic volume is the most important determinant of stroke volume, an increase in stroke volume would occur at a comparatively lower level of filling pressure, with increased compliance.

For the therapy of low output complicating myocardial infarction, several vasodilator agents have been used. Although most vasodilator agents produce similar qualitative hemodynamic effects, the quantitative hemodynamic responses vary. Different pharmacologic properties of these vasodilator agents account to some extent for the differences in their hemodynamic effects. The hemodynamic response may also vary according to the subset of patients treated and the severity of left ventricular dysfunction. The choice of vasodilator agents should depend on the specific hemodynamic deficits present in a given patient and on the hemodynamic effects expected from the use of a particular agent. The major hemodynamic effects of the vasodilator agents used for the treatment of pump failure in patients with acute infarction are summarized below.

*Sodium nitroprusside* has a balanced effect on both the precapillary resistance bed and the postcapillary capacitance bed. Because of its arteriolar dilating effects, there is a decrease in systemic vascular resistance along with an increase in cardiac output. Venodilation causes a reduction in systemic and pulmonary venous pressures. An increase in cardiac output along with a decrease in left ventricular filling pressure indicate improved cardiac performance. Beneficial hemodynamic responses to nitroprusside, however, are not observed in all patients with acute myocardial infarction. The major determinants appear to be the initial level of filling pressure and the magnitude of depression of cardiac function.

The hemodynamic effects of sodium nitroprusside infusion in 27 patients with acute myocardial infarction are summarized in table 13–2 [146]. The patients were divided into three groups according to their initial left ventricular filling pressure and severity of congestive heart failure. Group I included those patients with a normal left ventricular filling pressure (15 mmHg or less); these patients did not have any overt sign of heart failure. Group II patients had moderate left ventricular failure on the basis of clinical and radiologic findings; their initial left ventricular filling pressure was greater than 15 mmHg and their left ventricular stroke work index was 20 g-m/m² or more. Group III patients had an initial left ventricular filling pressure greater than 15 mmHg and a stroke work index less than 20 g-m/m². Clinically, group III patients had the most severe left ventricular failure; all patients had frank pulmonary edema. Furthermore, the majority of patients in group III were relatively hypotensive, and many had clinical features of shock. During nitroprusside infusion, systemic and pulmonary arterial pressures, left ventricular filling pressure, and right atrial pressures decreased in all three groups.

TABLE 13-2. Hemodynamic effects of Nitroprusside infusion in patients with acute myocardial infarction (mean + SEM).

| | Group I (6)[a] | | Group II (9)[a] | | Group III (12)[a] | |
|---|---|---|---|---|---|---|
| | Control | Nitro-prusside | Control | Nitro-prusside | Control | Nitro-prusside |
| Heart rate (beats/min) | $89.0 \pm 7.1$ | $96.7 \pm 8.6$ | $91.3 \pm 4.2$ | $94.7 \pm 3.4$ | $100.2 \pm 4.0$ | $100.5 \pm 4.8$ |
| Mean arterial pressure (mmHg) | $91.0 \pm 2.6$ | $85.8 \pm 3.9$ | $100.6 \pm 4.5$ | $87.7 \pm 4.1$ | $82.4 \pm 2.2$ | $76.2 \pm 2.8^b$ |
| Mean pulmonary arterial pressure (mmHg) | $16.5 \pm 1.7$ | $11.3 \pm 1.0^b$ | $31.8 \pm 1.6$ | $23.9 \pm 2.0^b$ | $37.0 \pm 1.5$ | $24.7 \pm 1.4$ |
| Mean right atrial pressure (mmHg) | $5.2 \pm 1.4$ | $2.8 \pm 1.2$ | $10.4 \pm 1.5$ | $7.2 \pm 1.4^b$ | $12.8 \pm 1.4$ | $8.5 \pm 1.3^b$ |
| Left ventricular filling pressure (mmHg) | $11.2 \pm 4.6$ | $6.3 \pm 1.1^b$ | $23.6 \pm 1.0$ | $15.2 \pm 1.5^b$ | $29.0 \pm 1.6$ | $18.7 \pm 1.8^b$ |
| Cardiac index (liter/min/m²) | $2.9 \pm .2$ | $2.9 \pm .2$ | $2.6 \pm 0.1$ | $3.1 \pm 0.2^b$ | $1.8 \pm 0.1$ | $2.2 \pm 0.1^b$ |
| Stroke work index (g-m/m²) | $38.8 \pm 7.6$ | $34.5 \pm 6.2$ | $33.6 \pm 2.9$ | $34.2 \pm 1.8$ | $13.8 \pm 1.1$ | $17.6 \pm 1.5^b$ |
| Systemic vascular resistance (dynes·sec·cm⁻⁵) | $1,383 \pm 148$ | $1,321 \pm 119$ | $1,577 \pm 141$ | $1,231 \pm 146$ | $1,908 \pm 260$ | $1,431 \pm 137^b$ |
| Pulmonary vascular resistance (dynes·sec·cm⁻⁵) | $64 \pm 12$ | $77 \pm 19$ | $148 \pm 32$ | $84 \pm 21^b$ | $234 \pm 28$ | $114 \pm 14^b$ |

[a]Numbers in parentheses indicate number of patients.
[b]$p < 0.05$; nitroprusside therapy versus control.

Source: Chatterjee, K. et al. *Ann. Clin. Res.* 9:124, 1977.

Significant increases in cardiac output and stroke volume together with a decrease in systemic vascular resistance were observed in group II and III patients. In group I patients, however, stroke volume usually decreased along with the decrease in left ventricular filling pressure, indicating no improvement in left ventricular function (figure 13–5). Furthermore, a reflex tachycardia developed in most patients in this group. A lack of increase in cardiac output was observed not only in the presence of an initially normal left ventricular filling pressure, but also when the left ventricular filling pressure was decreased to a very low level. In patients with a relatively normal cardiac output and systemic vascular resistance, a further improvement in cardiac function might not be observed [147].

The hemodynamic effects of *phentolamine,* an adrenergic-receptor-blocking agent and a direct smooth-muscle relaxant, are very similar to those of nitroprusside [148–152]. Right atrial,

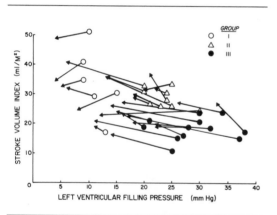

FIGURE 13–5. Influence of nitroprusside infusion on left ventricular performance in a group of patients with acute myocardial infarction. Group I represents patients with an initial left ventricular filling pressure of less than 15 mmHg; these patients did not have clinical left ventricular failure. Groups II and III had left ventricular failure with filling pressures greater than 15 mmHg. Group II had an initial stroke work index greater than 20 m-g/m². In groups II and III, patients demonstrated an increase in stroke volume along with a decrease in left ventricular filling pressure. In group 1, patients showed a low filling pressure; however, there tended to be a reduction in stroke volume together with a reduction in filling pressure. (From Chatterjee, K. and Parmley, W.W. *Prog. Cardiovasc Dis.* 19:301, 1977.)

pulmonary capillary wedge, and mean arterial pressures decrease. In patients with elevated left ventricular filling pressures, cardiac output and stroke volume increase, together with a decrease in systemic vascular resistance. Pulmonary vascular resistance decreases in most patients. In patients with a normal left ventricular filling pressure, stroke volume might not increase, since the left ventricular filling pressure decreases. One difference between the hemodynamic effects of phentolamine and sodium nitroprusside is that with phentolamine, there is a tendency to develop tachycardia (figure 13–6), the mechanism of which is unclear.

*Nitroglycerin,* whether administred sublingually, topically, or intravenously, significantly decreases pulmonary capillary wedge and right atrial pressures [153–158]. In most patients, however, there is little or no decrease in systemic vascular resistance and consequently little or no increase in left ventricular stroke volume and cardiac output. In patients with failure, arterial pressure falls only modestly, and usually there is no tachycardia. In patients with a normal left ventricular filling pressure or in those in whom the left ventricular filling pressure decreases to a very low level, arterial pressure and stroke volume may decrease significantly, and reflex tachycardia develops.

The hemodynamic effects of *isosorbide dinitrate,* whether administered orally or sublingually, are similar to those of nitroglycerin [159]. The essential difference between sublingual nitroglycerin and the nitrates is in their duration of action (sublingual nitroglycerin lasting approximately 20 minutes; sublingual isosorbide dinitrate, an average of 2 hours; and oral isosorbide dinitrate, an average of 4 hours). Hemodynamic effects of *trimethaphan* have been investigated only in a small number of patients with acute infarction [160]. This limited study indicated that trimethaphan produces hemodynamic effects similar to those of nitroglycerin in that systemic and pulmonary venous pressures decrease significantly but cardiac output may not change.

It is apparent that the random choice of vasodilator agents for the treatment of left ventricular dysfunction is inappropriate, and their selection should be made both according to their

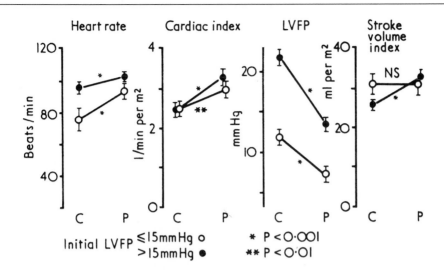

FIGURE 13–6. Hemodynamic effects of phentolamine in patients with acute myocardial infarction summarized from the published literature. Patients were divided on the basis of their initial left ventricular filling pressure into those with left ventricular filling pressures (LVFP) less than 15 mmHg (N=37). Note that the greatest increase in cardiac index and stroke volume index occurred in patients with a high filling pressure. Also, LVFP fell more and heart rate increased less in patients with a high filling pressure. From Chatterjee, K. and Parmley, W.W. *Prog. Cardiovasc. Dis.* 19:301, 1977.)

principal hemodynamic effects and in relation to the specific hemodynamic abnormalities in individual patients. In patients with adequate cardiac output but with an elevated left ventricular filling pressure, nitroglycerin or isosorbide dinitrate are appropriate vasodilator agents. On the other hand, if cardiac output is markedly reduced and left ventricular filling pressure is elevated, nitroprusside or phentolamine are likely to be more effective in correcting the hemodynamic deficits. Tachycardia and the indirect inotropic effects of phentolamine may be disadvantageous, however, because of the possible increase in myocardial oxygen demand.

Although the beneficial hemodynamic effects of various vasodilator agents in patients with low output complicating myocardial infarction are well documented, major controversy exists regarding the possible deleterious effects of vasodilator therapy on coronary hemodynamics

and myocardial ischemia. Some reduction in arterial pressure (i.e., coronary artery perfusion pressure) is common during vasodilatory therapy, irrespective of the vasodilator agent used. Hence, there is the potential risk of reducing coronary blood flow and myocardial perfusion. However, concurrent changes in the determinants of myocardial oxygen demand also occur during vasodilator therapy. In patients with heart failure, the left ventricular end-diastolic pressure and volume consistently decrease, and the heart rate either remains unchanged or decreases (except with phentolamine). In general, the vasodilator agents do not possess any direct inotropic effect. Hence, the net result is likely to be a reduction in myocardial oxygen demand. Therefore, despite some reduction in coronary blood flow due to reduced perfusion pressure, the overall myocardial oxygen supply-demand ratio may still remain favorable during vasodilator therapy.

Myocardial perfusion is also influenced by changes in the resistance of the coronary vascular bed as well as by changes in collateral blood flow. The distribution of blood flow to the endocardium and epicardium is also influenced by changes in the transmyocardial pressure gradient (i.e., the difference between the coronary artery perfusion pressure and left ventricular diastolic pressure).

Both experimental and clinical studies to elucidate the effects of two commonly used vasodilators, nitroprusside and nitroglycerin, on coronary hemodynamics, myocardial metabolism, and the extent of myocardial ischemic injury in the presence of myocardial infarction have yielded conflicting results. Nitroprusside, in the absence of obstructive coronary artery disease, decreases coronary vascular resistance and increases coronary blood flow [161]. In patients with acute myocardial infarction and left ventricular dysfunction, however, coronary blood flow and myocardial oxygen consumption tended to decrease, and this was probably related to a decrease in the determinants of myocardial oxygen demand [144, 146]. Decreased myocardial oxygen consumption was accompanied by an increase in transmyocardial lactate extraction, which indicated improvement in myocardial ischemia [144, 162]. In the presence of heart failure and an elevated left ventricular filling pressure, administration of nitroprusside has been shown to increase subendocardial blood flow, which is presumably related to a significant increase in the transmyocardial pressure gradient [163].

The effects of nitroglycerin on myocardial metabolism and on the extent of myocardial ischemic injury in the presence of acute infarction are also not clearly defined. An increase in subendocardial as well as in collateral blood flow to the ischemic myocardium during nitroglycerin therapy has been reported [143]. Contrary to these results, a reduction in regional myocardial flow to the poststenotic areas following nitroglycerin administration has been observed [164]. A paradoxical effect of nitroglycerin on segmental left ventricular wall motion in patients with obstructive coronary artery disease has also been reported, and a "coronary steal syndrome" has been suggested as the underlying mechanism [165]. It has been reported [61] that this "coronary steal" from the ischemic myocardium may also occur with nitroprusside or phentolamine, resulting in increased myocardial ischemic injury.

The effects of nitroglycerin and nitroprusside on myocardial infarct size, as has been discussed earlier, are variable and remain controversial. It is apparent that irrespective of the vasodilator agent used, the effects on the metabolic and me-

chanical function of ischemic myocardium in patients with coronary artery disease are likely to be variable and will be determined by concurrent changes in the various factors that influence myocardial perfusion and oxygen demand. The possibility of increased hypoxia in some areas of the myocardium because of reduction in perfusion pressure during vasodilator therapy remains a potential hazard. Better knowledge of regional myocardial perfusion and metabolism would be most helpful in determining the degree of reduction of arterial pressure that can be tolerated by individual patients. However, a significant reduction in arterial pressure, particularly in hypotensive or normotensive patients, irrespective of the vasodilator agent used, is likely to cause enhancement of existing myocardial ischemia despite a reduction in myocardial oxygen demand. It should be emphasized that when the objective of treatment is to improve pump function, the beneficial hemodynamic effects of vasodilator therapy can be obtained in many patients without a significant reduction in arterial pressure. The purpose of vasodilator therapy in patients with heart failure is to improve cardiac output by decreasing systemic vascular resistance, not to reduce arterial pressure. Hemodynamic monitoring to detect changes in arterial pressure, cardiac output, and systemic vascular resistance as well as in left ventricular filling pressure is therefore essential during vasodilator therapy.

## Hemodynamic Monitoring

Hemodynamic monitoring allows for the diagnosis of the mechanism and etiology of "low output state," which is necessary for instituting appropriate therapy. Hemodynamic monitoring is also required for the prompt assessment of the results of therapy and for alterations in therapeutic interventions that might be necessary during the management of a low output state. Furthermore, determination of the severity of hemodynamic abnormalities and of the degree of depression of left ventricular function provides useful information regarding immediate and late prognosis of patients with acute myocardial infarction.

Monitoring of arterial pressure, right and left

ventricular filling pressure, and determination of cardiac output are frequently required during the diagnosis and management of low output state. In the presence of peripheral vasoconstriction, monitoring of central arterial pressure (e.g., femoral arterial pressure) is preferable because a significant discrepancy may be observed between peripheral arterial (e.g., radial) and central arterial pressures. Accurate determination of arterial pressure is essential when one institutes vasodilator therapy. Right and left ventricular filling pressures are approximated by determining the right atrial and pulmonary capillary wedge pressures, respectively. In the absence of elevated pulmonary vascular resistance, pulmonary artery end-diastolic pressure corresponds closely to mean pulmonary capillary wedge pressure. Thus, pulmonary capillary wedge pressure can be substituted by pulmonary artery end-diastolic pressure for monitoring left ventricular filling pressure in these patients. However, at the time of initial determination one needs to confirm the lack of significant differences between pulmonary artery diastolic and pulmonary capillary wedge pressures (less than 5 mmHg). Cardiac output is determined most frequently by the thermodilution technique, which allows for frequent and reproducible measurements at the bedside with little or no inconvenience even to critically ill patients. With the advent of triple-lumen balloon flotation catheters equipped with thermistors, right and left ventricular filling pressures and cardiac output can be determined with the use of a single catheter that can be inserted into the pulmonary artery at the bedside without fluoroscopy [166].

Prolonged hemodynamic monitoring with the use of balloon flotation (Swan-Ganz) catheters is well tolerated and the complications are few [167]. The usual complications associated with insertion of central venous lines (arterial injury, pneumothorax, local hematoma, and sepsis), however, do occur during insertion of Swan-Ganz catheters. Transient atrial and ventricular arrhythmias are frequent, but sustained tachyarrhythmias are extremely infrequent. In patients with left bundle branch block, manipulation of the catheter in the right ventricular cavity must be avoided to prevent ventricular asystole, which might result from simultaneous occurrence of

right bundle branch block from the catheter irritating the right ventricular endocardium. Knotting of the catheter and balloon rupture are rare complications during catheter insertion. Pulmonary infarction is another complication that can be prevented if one does not allow the tip of the flotation catheter to migrate to the distal pulmonary artery branches and to the wedge position. Pulmonary artery rupture is the least common but most serious complication of hemodynamic monitoring and can be fatal. It tends to occur most frequently in patients with severe pulmonary hypertension, and sudden overinflation of the balloon by a large volume of air when the catheter is positioned in the smaller pulmonary artery branches is usually the immediate cause. Hence, the catheters should be positioned in the central pulmonary artery branches, and rapid overdistention of the balloon must be avoided. Since the introduction of the heparin-bonded catheters, the incidence of venous thrombosis has markedly declined. The frequency of venous thrombosis with the use of nonheparin-bonded catheters has been reported to be as high as 67 percent [168].

Hemodynamic monitoring can be used for the diagnosis of a number of complications of acute myocardial infarction (table 13–3). Hypovolemic shock is uncommon, and its diagnosis is difficult without determining hemodynamics. Both right atrial and pulmonary capillary wedge pressures are lower than normal in addition to relative hypotension and low cardiac output. Minor differences of opinion exist about the optimal level of filling pressure in patients with acute myocardial infarction [169, 170]. Studies in some patients with acute myocardial infarction have shown that the maximum cardiac index (CI) or stroke index is obtained when the left ventricular end-diastolic pressure ranges between 20 and 24 mmHg [169]. When the mean pulmonary capillary wedge pressure was measured in another group of patients, the maximum stroke volume index was obtained with pulmonary capillary wedge pressures between 14 and 18 mmHg [166]. Since the left ventricular end-diastolic pressure is usually higher than the simultaneously measured mean pulmonary capillary wedge pressure, these two studies are probably not in conflict.

TABLE 13-3. Hemodynamic differentiation of causes of low systemic output commonly encountered in cardiac care units

|  | RAP | PCWP | Equalization of diastolic pressures | PADP vs. PCWP |
|---|---|---|---|---|
| Hypovolemic shock | low | low | absent | PADP = PCWP |
| Cardiogenic shock | normal or high | high | absent | PADP = PCWP |
| Right ventricular infarct | high | normal or high | may be present | PADP = PCWP |
| Precapillary hypertension | high | normal | absent | PADP > PCWP |
| Cardiac tamponade | high | high | present | PADP = PCWP |

RAP = right atrial pressure; PADP = pulmonary arterial diastolic pressure; PCWP = pulmonary capillary wedge pressure.

Figure 13-7 shows changes in stroke work index (SWI) during changes in pulmonary artery occluded pressure, either during volume expansion or following diuretic therapy, in a group of patients with acute myocardial infarction. In patients who initially had a pulmonary artery occluded pressure less than 14 mmHg, there was usually an increase in SWI with a further increase in pulmonary artery occluded pressure. In patients with an initial filling pressure greater than 18 mmHg, there was little or no

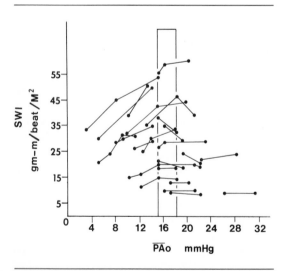

FIGURE 13-7. Relation between stroke work index (SWI) and pulmonary artery occluded pressure ($\overline{PA}$o) in acute infarction. No significant increase in SWI was observed when $\overline{PA}$o exceeded 18 mmHg. In most patients, the maximum level of SWI was attained when the $\overline{PA}$o ranged between 14 and 18 mmHg. (From Crexells, C. et al. Reproduced, by permission of the *New England Journal of Medicine,* 289:1263, 1973.)

increase in the SWI with a further increase in filling pressure. It appears, therefore, that in the majority of patients with acute myocardial infarction, the optimal level of left ventricular filling pressure (pulmonary artery occluded pressure) in terms of maximum cardiac or stroke output ranges between 14 and 18 mmHg. It needs to be emphasized that for accurate diagnosis of hypovolemic shock it is necessary to demonstrate that both right and left ventricular filling pressures are less than optimal. Virtually no information is available regarding the optimal right ventricular filling pressure in patients with acute myocardial infarction; however, normal right ventricular filling pressure usually does not exceed 7 mmHg.

Determination of hemodynamics aids in the diagnosis of predominant right ventricular infarction and primary right ventricular failure. Physical findings, electrocardiogram, echocardiography, and myocardial scintigraphy are all helpful in the diagnosis of predominant right ventricular infarction. However, hemodynamic monitoring is required to determine the severity of right ventricular failure and to assess results of therapy when low cardiac output is present. Disproportionate elevation of right atrial pressure compared to pulmonary capillary wedge pressure is the most frequent hemodynamic abnormality [171–173]. In patients with severe right ventricular infarction and low systemic output, equalization of diastolic pressures (right atrial pressure = pulmonary capillary wedge pressure) simulating effusive constrictive pericarditis is also frequently observed [172]. In these patients, echocardiography to exclude pericardial effusion is recommended. Studies in experimental animal models have demonstrated that the equalization of the diastolic pressures following isolated right ventricular infarction results from increased intrapericardial pressure from acute right ventricular dilation [173]. It is apparent that in the presence of predominant right ventricular infarction with right ventricular dilatation, pulmonary capillary wedge or right atrial pressures do not reflect left or right ventricular filling pressures. Transmural pressures (diastolic pressure–pericardial pressure) is the true ventricular filling pressure; with increased intrapericardial pressure, irrespective of its cause, pulmonary capillary wedge pressure will increase due to increased left ventricular diastolic pressure without any change in transmural pressure. Thus, in patients with right ventricular dilation and primary right ventricular failure, one cannot use pulmonary capillary wedge pressure to assess changes in left ventricular preload. Determinations of left ventricular cavity size by echocardiography or gated blood pool scintigraphy are helpful in these circumstances for evaluation of changes in left ventricular preload.

Two life-threatening complications of myocardial infarction—severe mitral regurgitation due to papillary muscle infarct and large "left-to-right" shunt due to ventricular septal rupture—can also be diagnosed by bedside hemodynamic monitoring. Severe acute mitral regurgitation is recognized by the presence of a giant peaked regurgitant V-wave in the pulmonary capillary wedge pressure tracings or by the reflected V-wave before the dicrotic notch in the pulmonary artery pressure tracings. Left-to-right shunt is diagnosed by the presence of signficantly higher (more than 5 percent vol) oxygen saturation in pulmonary arterial blood compared to that in right atrial blood samples. In the presence of a large left-to-right shunt, the normal V-wave in the wedge pressure tracing may be markedly accentuated and may simulate the regurgitant wave of severe acute mitral regurgitation. The onset of the regurgitant wave, however, is earlier and coincides with the QRS complex of the electrocardiogram, and the peak of the regurgitant wave occurs before the end of the T-wave. The onset of the large V-wave associated with ventricular septal rupture occurs late in systole, usually after the QRS complex. The accentuation of the V-wave in ventricular septal rupture is most likely related to increased venous return to the left atrium due to large left-to-right shunt.

Hemodynamic monitoring is also helpful to assess the severity of left ventricular failure. Despite left ventricular infarction, cardiac output, left ventricular stroke work index, and left ventricular filling pressure may remain normal (compensated subset). In these patients, no specific therapy is indicated unless a further complication is encountered. Some patients develop symptoms of pulmonary congestion without manifestations of hypoperfusion; in these patients, pulmonary capillary wedge pressure is elevated but cardiac output may remain normal (pulmonary congestion with adequate cardiac output). Diuretics, and occasionally nitroglycerin, frequently decrease pulmonary venous pressure and relieve symptoms of pulmonary venous congestion. Higher cardiac output and left ventricular stroke work index associated with tachycardia and normal or low pulmonary capillary wedge pressure may be observed, although infrequently after acute myocardial infarction (hyperdynamic subset). In these patients also, no specific therapy is indicated unless postinfarction angina or other complications ensue. The hemodynamic correlates of clinical manifestations of hypoperfusion and pulmonary congestion following acute myocardial infarction are lower cardiac output and stroke work index and elevated pulmonary capillary wedge pressure. In patients with cardiogenic shock, left ventricular stroke work index is markedly decreased (less than 20 gm-m²) and associated with hypotension and elevated pulmonary capillary wedge pressure. The hemodynamic subsets of patients with acute myocardial infarction based on initial hemodynamic findings are summarized in table 13–4.

It is apparent that hemodynamic monitoring is necessary for the diagnosis and management of the various complications of acute myocardial infarction. However, routine hemodynamic monitoring is not indicated; patients who do not have manifestations of pulmonary venous congestion or hypoperfusion (compensated or hyperdynamic subsets) can be observed clinically. However, when unexplained sinus tachycardia or overt manifestations of hypoperfusion and/or

TABLE 13–4. Hemodynamic subsets in acute myocardial infarction

| LVFP | LVSWI | CI | HR | AP | Subset |
|------|-------|-----|-----|-----|--------|
| normal | normal | normal | normal | normal | compensated |
| decreased | increased | normal | normal or increased | normal or elevated | hyperdynamic |
| decreased | decreased | decreased | increased | decreased | hypovolemia |
| increased | decreased | decreased | increased | normal or decreased | pump failure |

LVFP = left ventricular filling pressure; LVSWI = left ventricular stroke work index; CI = cardiac index; HR = heart rate; AP = atrial pressure.

pulmonary venous hypertension is present, hemodynamic monitoring is often necessary.

## Therapy of Low Output State and Cardiogenic Shock

Low cardiac output following acute myocardial infarction may result from brady- and tachyarrhythmias, by predominant right or left ventricular infarction, or by complications such as pulmonary embolism, cardiac tamponade, and hypovolemia. Cardiogenic shock is the extreme degree of "low output state" associated with hypotension and manifestations of diminished organ perfusion. The development of therapies for low output state depends on its pathogenesis and mechanism.

RIGHT VENTRICULAR INFARCTION
Predominant right ventricular infarction occurs almost exclusively in patients with inferior or inferoposterior myocardial infarction. Clinical evidence of right ventricular failure (e.g., elevated jugular venous pressure, right ventricular gallop, tricuspid regurgitation in the absence of left ventricular failure, and significant pulmonary hypertension) is an important diagnostic clue. Kussmaul's sign is a very sensitive clinical indication for the diagnosis of right ventricular infarction. Precordial ECG leads $V_1$, $V_{3R}$, and $V_{4R}$ frequently show ST elevations and/or loss of R-waves in patients with predominant right ventricular infarction [174]. Echocardiography and blood pool scintigraphy usually reveal a dilated, poorly contracting right ventricle with normal or near normal left ventricular size and systolic function [175]. Technetium-99$^m$ pyrophosphate myocardial scintigraphy, however, provides the definitive diagnosis and demon-

strates pyrophosphate uptake by the right ventricular wall [176, 177].

Although noninvasive investigations are usually adequate for the diagnosis of right ventricular infarction, hemodynamic monitoring is required to assess the severity of low output state and the results of therapy. In patients with low cardiac output in addition to disproportionate elevation of right atrial pressure compared to pulmonary capillary wedge pressure, "equalization of the diastolic pressures" is also seen frequently. In experimental isolated right ventricular infarction in dogs, equalization of the diastolic pressures results from an increased intrapericardial pressure, which imposes a restriction on diastolic filling of the ventricles [173]. That increased intrapericardial pressure contributes to the equalization of the ventricular diastolic pressures is evident from the fact that after pericardiectomy such hemodynamic abnormalities are no longer seen. The pericardium is a stiff structure. Acute right ventricular or right atrial dilation following right ventricular infarction encroaches on intrapericardial volume and causes a disproportionate elevation of intrapericardial pressure and equalization of the diastolic pressures [173, 178].

The important mechanism for the decreased systemic output in the presence of predominant right ventricular infarction appears to be due to decreased left ventricular preload. Decreased left ventricular transmural pressure and left ventricular diastolic volume occur in experimental isolated right ventricular infarction [173]. Decreased left ventricular preload results from decreased right ventricular systolic function as well as from increased intrapericardial pressure, which also compromises ventricular fillings. Intravenous fluid administration, despite elevated right atrial pressures, increases systemic output. The precise mechanism for this improvement is not clear; in experimental right ventricular infarction, volume loading increases left ventricular preload (transmural pressure and diastolic volume). Increased left ventricular preload at least partly results from this improvement in right ventricular systolic function [179]. Passive filling of the left ventricle with volume loading is also a potential mechanism for increasing left ventricular preload. It needs to be emphasized that left ventricular infarction is almost always associated with clinical right ventricular infarction. Therefore, left ventricular failure may coexist with right ventricular failure. Volume loading alone in these circumstances may not be effective in reversing the low output state. Furthermore, excessive fluid administration may cause excessive dilation of the right ventricle and a further increase in intrapericardial pressure, which may compromise left ventricular filling. Thus, although volume loading is usually associated with increased systemic output, excessive fluid administration should be avoided (right atrial pressure should be kept below 25 mmHg).

Vasodilators such as nitroglycerin or nitrates and sodium nitroprusside have the potential to decrease pulmonary vascular resistance (right ventricular afterload) and right ventricular pump function. Consequently, an increase in left ventricular preload may result from the use of these vasodilators. Vasodilators, however, should not be used without concomitant administration of intravenous fluids, because left and right ventricular preload may decline due to decreased venous return.

The role of inotropic therapy in reversing low output states in patients with predominant right ventricular infarction has not been adequately evaluated. Isoproterenol enhances contractile function and decreases pulmonary vascular resistance; however, it also induces life-threatening ventricular arrhythmias. In light of this, its use cannot be recommended despite its theoretical advantages. As dopamine may increase pulmonary artery pressure, its use should be restricted to patients with severe hypotension. Dobutamine, on the other hand, can cause a reduction in pulmonary artery pressure and pul-

monary vascular resistance. Therefore, in the absence of hypotension, dobutamine is preferable if inotropic therapy is needed.

Right ventricular pneumatic pump and pulmonary artery balloon counterpulsation have the potential to improve low output in patients with severe acute right ventricular failure, although such measures are rarely needed for the management of predominant right ventricular infarction.

Severe low output state associated with hypotension can occur when brachyarrhythmias complicate right ventricular infarction. The incidence of complete A-V block in patients with right ventricular infarction is considerably higher than the reported overall incidence in patients with acute myocardial infarction [180]. Loss of timed atrial contraction appears to be particularly detrimental in patients with predominant right ventricular infarction. During ventricular pacing with loss of atrial contribution, stroke volume is significantly lower than during atrioventricular sequential pacing at an identical pacing rate [181]. Due to the synchronous atrial and ventricular diastole during ventricular pacing, ventricular filling is probably further compromised because of the decreased available intrapericardial space. Whatever the mechanism for the deleterious effect of ventricular pacing, atrioventricular sequential pacing should be considered in patients with right ventricular infarction complicated by complete A-V block.

HYPOVOLEMIC SHOCK
Shock syndrome associated with severe hypotension and low cardiac output due to relative or absolute hypovolemia is a relatively rare complication of acute myocardial infarction. Repeated administration of diuretics or nitrates and severe diaphoresis and vomiting may precipitate hypovolemic shock. Patients with hypovolemia need intravenous fluid therapy to increase right and left ventricular preload. The choice of intravenous fluid is not critical. If there is adequate increase in cardiac output, fluid administration should be continued to maintain pulmonary capillary wedge pressure between approximately 15 to 20 mmHg [170]. In most patients with acute myocardial infarction and relatively normal left ventricular size, there usually is no further in-

crease in cardiac output when pulmonary capillary wedge pressure exceeds 18 to 20 mmHg during volume expansion.

In some patients, cardiac output and stroke volume do not increase significantly despite increasing pulmonary capillary wedge pressure to optimal range. Significant left ventricular dysfunction coexists in these patients, and therefore therapy should be similar to that for treatment of "pump failure," maintaining optimal filling pressure.

## LEFT VENTRICULAR FAILURE AND CARDIOGENIC SHOCK

Left ventricular failure is the commonest cause of "low output state" in patients with recent myocardial infarction. The hemodynamic abnormalities of left ventricular failure consist of elevated pulmonary capillary wedge pressure and reduced stroke volume, stroke work, and cardiac output. Cardiogenic shock is the clinical expression of severe left ventricular failure and is associated with hypotension, tachycardia, and manifestations of diminished organ perfusion, such as oliguria, mental obtundation, and cold and clammy skin. Although left ventricular failure can be suspected clinically, hemodynamic monitoring is essential to determine the severity of pump failure and to monitor responses of the therapeutic interventions.

Based upon initial measurements of the left ventricular stroke work index, arterial pressure, systemic vascular resistance and pulmonary capillary wedge pressure, patients with left ventricular failure can be categorized into hemodynamic subsets to guide in the selection of therapy (table 13–5). Patients in subset 1 have mild left ventricular dysfunction; cardiac output is normal or only slightly decreased; and pulmonary capillary wedge pressure is elevated. In these patients, symptoms related to pulmonary venous hypertension rather than to hypoperfusion predominate. Intermittent administration of diuretics will decrease pulmonary venous pressure and relieve symptoms adequately in most patients [183, 184]. Changes in pulmonary capillary wedge pressure should be monitored during diuretic therapy to avoid lowering the filling pressure to hypovolemic levels. If the pulmonary capillary wedge pressure remains elevated despite diuretic therapy, nitroglycerin and other organic nitrates should be considered. Pulmonary and systemic venous pressures tend to decrease with nitrates in almost all patients.

In patients with more severe pump failure, left ventricular stroke work, stroke volume, and cardiac output are markedly decreased, and pulmonary capillary wedge pressure and systemic vascular resistance are elevated. In the absence of hypotension, vasodilator therapy appears to improve left ventricular performance in these patients [18]. Nitroprusside or phentolamine appear to be the preferred vasodilator agents, since these drugs increase cardiac output and decrease pulmonary capillary wedge pressure. Phentolamine, however, can cause tachycardia and, therefore, might increase myocardial oxygen requirements. Moreover, phentolamine therapy is much more expensive than nitroprusside therapy. Hence, nitroprusside is the most frequently used vasodilator agent in these patients.

It needs to be emphasized that hemodynamic monitoring is essential during vasodilator therapy. One of the potential hazards is hypotension. Acute myocardial infarction is frequently observed in patients with multivessel coronary artery disease. To provide adequate myocardial perfusion to the noninfarcted territories through the stenosed but not yet completely occluded coronary arteries, adequate perfusion pressure must be maintained. During myocardial ischemia, autoregulatory reserve of the distal coronary vascular bed is exhausted due to metabolically mediated maximal coronary vasodilation. In such circumstances, maintenance of perfusion pressure becomes more important because coronary blood flow becomes pressure dependent. If marked hypotension occurs, potential exists for enhanced myocardial ischemia, irrespective of the vasodilator agent used. The major objective for vasodilator therapy is to decrease left ventricular resistance to ejection and to increase cardiac output. If the increase in cardiac output is proportional to the decrease in systemic vascular resistance, mean arterial pressure remains unchanged.

The initial infusion rate of the vasodilators (nitroprusside, 10 μg/min; phentolamine, .1 mg/min; nitroglycerin, 10 μg/min) should be small and the dose should be increased gradu-

TABLE 13–5. Suggested therapy according to the severity of left ventricular failure and initial hemodynamic abnormalities

| Subset | Clinical signs | CI (L/min/m²) | PCWP mmHg | SAP mmHg | Appropriate therapy |
|--------|----------------|---------------|-----------|----------|---------------------|
| I | Pulmonary congestion | ≥ 2.5 | > 18 | > 100 | Diuretics, nitroglycerin |
| II | Pulmonary congestion Decreased perfusion | < 2.5 | > 18 | > 100 | Nitroprusside |
| III | Shock | < 2.5 | > 18 | < 90 | Dobutamine, Dopamine, (Norepinephrine) Intra-aortic balloon counterpulsation Vasodilators |

CI = cardiac index; PCWP = pulmonary capillary wedge pressure; SAP = systolic arterial pressure.
Source: Based on Gunnar, R.M. *et al. Am. J. Cardiol.* 50:393, 1982.

ally, monitoring changes in cardiac output, pulmonary capillary wedge pressure, arterial pressure, and systemic vascular resistance. If cardiac output increases along with a reduction in pulmonary capillary wedge pressure, the vasodilator therapy should be continued. If hypotension occurs before any significant change in cardiac output or pulmonary capillary wedge pressure, vasodilator therapy is unlikely to produce any benefit and, therefore, should be discontinued. In these patients, therapy can be initiated with the use of an inotropic agent such as dobutamine, and then vasodilators can be added. In occasional patients, a combination of dobutamine, nitroprusside, and nitroglycerin is needed to control hemodynamic abnormalities.

In patients in subset III, in addition to low cardiac output and elevated pulmonary capillary wedge pressure, hypotension is also present. Vasodilator agents cannot be used as initial therapy because of the potential risk of further hypotension. Vasopressor agents, dopamine, or norepinephrine are used to maintain arterial pressure until intra-aortic balloon counterpulsation can be inserted to maintain diastolic perfusion pressure. A vasodilator like nitroprusside and an inotropic agent like dobutamine can then be added to optimize the hemodynamic improvement. Once hemodynamic stability is achieved, left heart catheterization and coronary arteriography should be performed to determine whether surgical therapy is feasible. Without surgical intervention, the immediate prognosis in these patients is extremely poor (close to 100 percent mortality), despite intra-aortic balloon counterpulsation, vasodilator, and inotropic therapy.

## INTRA-AORTIC BALLOON COUNTERPULSATION

Intra-aortic balloon counterpulsation provides temporary support of circulation, and its use has gained widespread acceptance in the management of cardiogenic shock associated with low cardiac output and hypotension. With the advent of percutaneous techniques, intra-aortic balloon counterpulsation can be instituted rapidly without enhancing risks, and therefore its application should be considered in appropriate clinical circumstances.

With this device, several hemodynamic benefits can be anticipated. The balloon is inflated during diastole; thus, arterial diastolic pressure increases with this augmentation, which helps to maintain coronary artery perfusion pressure. The balloon is rapidly deflated at end-diastole; a decrease in intra-aortic volume and pressure results at the beginning of left ventricular systole, decreasing aortic impedance. This is associated with an increase in stroke volume and cardiac output. Decreased ejection impedance also causes a reduction in left ventricular end-diastolic pressure in most patients. Augmentation of diastolic pressure is expected to increase coronary blood flow; however, systolic unloading, which decreases left ventricular wall stress, also decreases myocardial oxygen requirements concomitantly. The net effect of intra-aortic balloon counterpulsation is usually a decrease in global coronary blood flow [185]. However, despite decreased global coronary blood flow, regional perfusion might improve during diastolic augmentation. Subendocardial perfusion is also likely to improve because of increased transmyocardial pressure gradient during diastole.

Use of intra-aortic balloon counterpulsation along with pharmacologic interventions without surgery do not appear to improve the immediate prognosis of patients with cardiogenic shock. In one study of 87 patients with cardiogenic shock receiving balloon counterpulsation, only 15 patients survived to leave the hospital [186].

How long the mechanical support should be continued in patients with acute myocardial infarction and cardiogenic shock also remains controversial. Short duration of support with early surgery (within 48 to 72 hours after infarction) in patients without mechanical defects has been associated with high mortality. The use of intra-aortic balloon counterpulsation for 10 to 14 days followed by corrective surgery has been shown to influence mortality favorably [187].

In patients with severe left ventricular failure without cardiogenic shock, the intra-aortic balloon counterpulsation has been shown to improve prognosis even when surgical treatment was not completed [188]. However, these studies were uncontrolled and the number of patients treated was too small. Thus, the value of the use of intra-aortic balloon counterpulsation for the treatment of left ventricular failure without hypotension or cardiogenic shock remains uncertain. It needs to be emphasized that the use of mechanical support devices is not without complications, especially in regard to peripheral arterial complications [189].

## MITRAL REGURGITATION AND VENTRICULAR SEPTAL RUPTURE

Severe mitral regurgitation due to papillary muscle infarction or fracture and left-to-right shunt due to ventricular septal rupture are infrequent but catastrophic complications of acute myocardial infarction. Sudden, excessive volume overload causes a marked and rapid deterioration of left ventricular performance associated with decreasing systemic output.

In patients with mitral regurgitation, vasodila-tor agents, like sodium nitroprusside and hydralazine, produce beneficial hemodynamic and clinical effects [190]. With decreased systemic vascular resistance, the regurgitant volume decreases and the forward stroke volume and cardiac output increases. Pulmonary capillary wedge pressure and the magnitude of the regurgitant V-wave decrease, along with decreased regurgitant fraction. Thus, the use of vasodilator agents in the initial management of acute severe mitral regurgitation complicating myocardial infarction is a rational therapeutic approach. In hypotensive patients, vasodilators should be avoided initially because of the risk of inducing further hypotension. Intra-aortic balloon counterpulsation also produces beneficial hemodynamic effects probably due to its systolic unloading effects, which decrease aortic impedance. Thus, in hypotensive patients, intra-aortic balloon counterpulsation therapy should be considered initially and then the vasodilators added. In patients with ventricular septal defect complicating acute myocardial infarction, the magnitude of the left-to-right shunt is primarily influenced by the ratio of the pulmonary to systemic vascular resistance [191], as the size of the ventricular septal defect is usually quite large and the defect itself offers little resistance to left-to-right shunt. Thus, a greater decrease in systemic vascular resistance than pulmonary vascular resistance is likely to be associated with increased systemic output and decreased left-to-right shunt. This is the rationale for vasodilator therapy for left-to-right shunt due to ventricular septal rupture. Indeed, in occasional patients, sodium nitroprusside and isosorbide dinitrate produced beneficial hemodynamic and clinical effects [192]. However, these vasodilator agents also decrease pulmonary vascular resistance; therefore, potential exists for increasing the magnitude of the left-to-right shunt if the ratio of pulmonary to systemic vascular resistance decreases. As intra-aortic balloon counterpulsation selectively decreases systemic vascular resistance by reducing aortic impedance, the magnitude of the left-to-right shunt is likely to decrease. The use of intra-aortic balloon counterpulsation is, therefore, the preferred initial therapy for the management of the left-to-right shunt resulting from ventricular septal rupture complicating myocardial infarction.

Although vasodilator therapy with or without the use of counterpulsation produces beneficial hemodynamic and clinical effects, such therapeutic approaches should be regarded as supportive rather than definitive treatment; surgical correction should be considered as soon as hemodynamic and clinical stabilization is achieved. It appears that earlier surgical intervention is associated with better prognosis in patients with severe mitral regurgitation or ventricular septal rupture.

## SURGERY

The most important indication of surgical therapy for the treatment of pump failure is the correction of mechanical defects, such as papillary muscle infarction or ventricular septal rupture. Surgical therapy should be considered as soon as the patient is stabilized. It has been reported previously that surgery for correction of a mechanical problem within the first 4 weeks of infarction was associated with a very high mortality [193]. Surgical mortality was lower if surgery could be deferred beyond this period. Most patients, however, do not survive 2 weeks of medical therapy. Thus, the recent trend has been to offer surgical therapy as soon as hemodynamic and clinical stabilization have been achieved with the use of pharmacologic interventions and, if necessary, with the use of intra-aortic balloon counterpulsation.

Experimental infarctectomy has been shown to improve cardiac performance, provided the extent of the resected myocardium does not exceed 30 percent of the left ventricular myocardium. With larger resection, mortality markedly increases [194]. Based on these experimental results, infarctectomy has been recommended in patients with cardiogenic shock unresponsive to medical therapy. Early intervention with intra-aortic balloon counterpulsation has been suggested. Following stabilization of the patient for 24 to 48 hours, an attempt to wean off mechanical support is warranted. In balloon-dependent patients, left ventriculography and coronary arteriography are performed to determine the feasibility for surgical intervention. Surgical mortality for the corrective surgery of mechanical defects appears to have declined, as evidenced in recent reports in surgical series [195–197]. A 20

to 30 percent mortality has been reported in patients with papillary muscle rupture undergoing surgical corrections. Both surgical and long-term mortality are related to residual left ventricular function and are inversely related to preoperative ejection fraction [196]. Controversy exists regarding indication of concomitant revascularization surgery. Some studies suggest that although revascularization surgery may not influence acute surgical mortality, long-term survival might improve [197].

Recently, important advances have been made in the surgical approach to the repair of ventricular septal rupture complicating myocardial infarction. The septal defect is closed with a Dacron or Teflon patch placed on the left ventricular side of the septum or on both sides of the septum (sandwich technique) after exposing the septum through the infarcted portion of the left ventricle. Surgical mortality for the repair of posterior septal rupture complicating diaphragmatic myocardial infarction is considerably higher. The overall surgical mortality in patients with ventricular septal rupture is approximately 40 percent when surgery is performed within 4 weeks of myocardial infarction. Early repair in hemodynamically stable patients is associated with less than 25 percent operative mortality [198]. Thus, early surgical intervention should be considered in these patients as soon as the hemodynamic stability is achieved. The role of concomitant revascularization surgery in improving either immediate or long-term prognosis of patients with ventricular septal rupture remains unknown. Most patients who survive surgical repair derive marked symptomatic improvement, and their long-term prognosis remains quite good. More than an 80 percent 5-year survival rate has been reported [199].

Cardiac rupture is another catastrophic complication of acute myocardial infarction until emergency surgical repair can be performed. Free wall rupture occurs in approximately 3 percent of patients with acute myocardial infarction and, after cardiogenic shock and primary dysrhythmias, is the third most common cause of early deaths, accounting for 10 to 20 percent of infarct related deaths [200]. Cardiac rupture involves the left ventricle in over 90 percent of the patients and usually appears as a tear or hemorrhagic dissection at the lateral border of the infarction, where shearing stress is maximal [201]. Approximately 85 percent of ruptures occur within the first week and not infrequently (approximately one third) within 24 hours of infarction. Cardiac rupture is more common in older patients, in women, and in patients with first transmural myocardial infarction [202]. Antemortum diagnosis is only infrequently made because of the rapidity with which hemopericardium, tamponade, and death occur.

Survival depends entirely on rapid diagnosis and surgical repair. With the acute onset of electromechanical dissociation, cardiopulmonary resuscitation and pericardiocentesis should be attempted. Emergency sternotomy and the institution of cardiopulmonary bypass may be life saving. However, the prospect of early diagnosis and surgical repair of cardiac rupture is extremely low in most patients.

## Factors Influencing Prognosis After Acute Myocardial Infarction

Several studies, both before and since the coronary care unit era, have demonstrated that the average annual mortality of patients surviving acute myocardial infarction is 5 to 8 percent, and this rate does not appear to have changed significantly during the last 20 years, despite improvements in patient monitoring and patient care and despite better understanding of the pathophysiology of acute myocardial infarction [203–209]. It is apparent, however, that among the survivors of acute infarction, certain subsets of patients are at higher risk of dying during the follow-up period. Generalization about prognosis without reference to the factors that influence prognosis does not, therefore, serve any useful clinical purpose.

### EFFECT OF LEFT VENTRICULAR DYSFUNCTION

Certain clinical variables present during the acute phase of myocardial infarction have an adverse influence on long-term prognosis. Clinical and radiologic evidence of left ventricular failure and cardiomegaly, ventricular conduction defects, advanced atrioventricular block, and previous myocardial infarction are associated

with a worse prognosis [210]. A higher mortality in such patients is likely related to more severe depression of cardiac function consequent to more extensive myocardial damage. In patients with ejection fractions of less than .40 percent as determined by radioisotopic techniques, a 1-year cumulative mortality of 30 percent has been reported; in contrast, an ejection fraction of more than 40 percent was associated with a more favorable prognosis [211]. Based on hemodynamic findings, the severity of depression of cardiac function can be determined, and the later prognosis can be estimated [212]. In patients with compensated left ventricular function (left ventricular filling pressure of less than 15 mmHg and a normal left ventricular stroke work index), 2-year mortality was only 10 percent, whereas in patients with a left ventricular stroke work index of 20 g-m/m$^2$ or less and a left ventricular filling pressure greater than 15 mmHg (indicating severe depression of cardiac function), the 2-year mortality exceeded 78 percent. The poor late prognosis in patients with severe left ventricular dysfunction does not appear to be influenced by vasodilator therapy during the acute phase. In patients with severe low output who are treated with vasodilators, the cumulative survival at 24 months was only 25 percent [213]. It appears, therefore, that the degree of left ventricular dysfunction is the major determinant of long-term prognosis in survivors of acute myocardial infarction.

### TYPE AND SITE OF THE INFARCTION

Controversy exists regarding the relation between the type of of infarct and the late prognosis. Some retrospective studies have indicated that patients with nontransmural (subendocardial) infarction have a poorer prognosis compared to those with transmural infarction [214–216]. Other prospective studies, however, have failed to show any difference in the immediate or late prognosis in these two subsets of patients [217]. Within the group of patients with transmural infarcts, however, regional cardiac dilatation demonstrated by two-dimensional echocardiography may be an ominous sign [218].

There is also considerable disagreement regarding the influence of the infarction site, whether anterior or inferior, on the late prognosis. The reason for such discrepancies in the results of various investigations is not easily apparent. It seems, however, that the extent and severity of the coronary artery disease, rather than the location of the infarction, is more likely to be of greater prognostic significance.

Only limited studies have been performed to evaluate the extent of coronary artery disease by selective coronary arteriography in patients with myocardial infarction [219, 220]. These studies indicate that the majority of such patients, irrespective of the type or location of the infarct, have significant double- and triple-vessel coronary artery disease. Even in patients with inferior wall myocardial infarction, particularly in those with moderate or severe postinfarction angina, the incidence of significant multivessel disease exceeds 50 percent [220]. The more extensive the coronary artery disease, the worse the long-term prognosis [221]. The identification of patients belonging to this high-risk group should be regarded as an important element in their postinfarction management. In patients with postinfarction angina or with persistent ST-T changes in the resting ECG that are indicative of myocardial ischemia, a higher incidence of severe coronary artery disease and higher late mortality have been reported [220, 222].

Angina recurring soon after myocardial infarction is associated with unfavorable prognosis [223]. Different studies have reported a mortality rate between 23 and 56 percent in patients with postinfarction angina [223, 224]. An inverse relation between the prognosis and the time of onset of postinfarction angina has been demonstrated. An early mortality rate (within 1 month) of 56 percent has been reported in patients who experience angina within 10 days of acute myocardial infarction. The location of new ischemia in relation to the area of infarction also influences the prognosis. Schuster and Bulkley [223] observed that patients with ischemia at a distance had a 44 percent mortality rate the first month and an overall mortality rate of 72 percent during a follow-up period of 6 months. Of the survivors, a vast majority of the patients had unstable angina or recurrent infarction or required coronary artery bypass surgery. In contrast, patients with ischemia in the infarct zone had a 1-month mortality of 15 percent and overall mortality of 33 percent. Of the survivors, recurrent infarction or need for coronary artery bypass surgery occurred in 39 percent of patients. Ischemia was diagnosed in these studies by the transient ST segment or T-wave changes in the electrocardiogram. In patients with ischemia at a distance, completed infarcts and a totally occluded coronary artery to the infarcted territory occurred more frequently. In patients with ischemia at the infarct zone, incomplete infarcts and patent but severely occluded coronary arteries were identified more frequently. The true incidence of postinfarction angina is difficult to estimate but an incidence as high as 64 percent and as low as 12 percent has been reported [225, 226]. This wide variation in the reported incidence in these studies reflects the variations in definitions and diagnostic difficulties. The pathogenesis of postinfarction angina also remains unknown. In patients who develop angina with limited activity, an increase in myocardial oxygen requirements precipitating the imbalance between myocardial oxygen supply and demand is likely to be the mechanism. However, an interruption of collateral flow to the noninfarcted myocardial segment or reduction in myocardial perfusion due to increased coronary vascular tone might also be the mechanism. Indeed, frank spasms of the epicardial coronary artery to the infarcted areas have been documented by angiographic studies [227]. Whatever the mechanism for the postinfarction angina, it is apparent that the prognosis of these patients remains unfavorable without appropriate therapy.

Aggressive medical therapy with the use of nitrates, beta-blockers, and calcium-channel blocking agents is frequently effective in controlling angina [228]. The use of intra-aortic balloon counterpulsation has also been found effective [229, 230] and has been used before cardiac catheterization and coronary artery bypass surgery. However, use of intra-aortic balloon counterpulsation is not required in the majority of patients unless hemodynamic instability exists [228].

That coronary artery bypass surgery can be performed relatively safely with low operative mortality in patients early after an acute myocardial infarction has been reported [228, 231]. Jones et al. [231] reported no hospital mortality in 116 patients undergoing revascularization surgery. Furthermore, actuarial survival in these patients was 97 percent at 18 months, and most patients had marked symptomatic improvement. Admittedly, these are uncontrolled studies and no definitive conclusion regarding the role of surgical therapy for the management of postinfarction angina can be reached. Nevertheless, a considerably better prognosis with surgical therapy compared to that with medical therapy seems probable. Thus, surgical therapy should be considered in appropriate patients with postinfarction angina.

Myocardial ischemia demonstrated by exercise stress testing, in the early postinfarction period, is also associated with unfavorable prognosis. Increased cardiac mortality and morbidity have been reported in patients who develop ST segment depression in the stress electrocardiogram during submaximal stress testing [232]. Stress thallium scintigraphy has also been found useful to detect myocardial ischemia in patients with recent myocardial infarction [233]. Although exercise stress testing can identify high-risk patients, the sensitivity of predischarge exercise testing is only 45 to 62 percent [234]. Myocardial thallium scintigraphy has been reported to be more sensitive than exercise stress testing in identifying high-risk patients with multi-vessel coronary artery disease. As only submaximal stress testing is performed in patients with recent myocardial infarction, the predictive value of the predischarge stress tests for determining high risk coronary artery disease is less than when maximal stress test is done. Dipyridamole-thallium-201 scintigraphy, performed in patients with acute myocardial infarction prior to discharge from the hospital, appears to have better predictive value in determining the risk of developing future cardiac events [234]. When thallium-201 is injected during the period of the peak effect of intravenous dipyridamole infusion, the results of myocardial perfusion scans are similar to those of maximal exercise study [235]. Leppo et al. [234] have demonstrated that serial myocardial imaging using dipyridamole in patients with myocardial infarction is a more sensitive predictor of subsequent cardiac events than stress thallium scintigraphy or a submaximal stress test. Whatever investigative technique is used, identification of the high-risk population in patients with recent myocardial infarction is helpful to prevent serious cardiac events in these patients.

## ARRHYTHMIAS AND CONDUCTION ABNORMALITIES
The relation between the incidence of postinfarction dysrhythmias and the long-term prognosis of survivors of acute myocardial infarction has been the subject of intensive investigations, and conflicting results have been reported. These are discussed in chapter 15. In brief, it has been suggested that potentially dangerous ventricular ectopic arrhythmias or conduction disturbances detected in the late-hospital phase of acute myocardial infarction are associated with a worse late prognosis [211, 222, 236–240]. A cumulative mortality of as high as 70 percent at 12 months has been reported in patients with late-hospital phase ventricular dysrhythmias. Similarly, the development of ventricular conduction disturbances with complete heart block and trifascicular and bifascicular block during the acute phase of myocardial infarction has been associated with a high late mortality [241]. Contrary to these previous reports, earlier studies indicated that ventricular tachycardia, when detected during the late-hospital phase of acute myocardial infarction, did not influence the late prognosis adversely [242]. It has been demonstrated, however, that an adverse long-term prognosis is to be expected if ventricular dysrhythmias accompany left ventricular dysfunction [243]. Life-threatening ventricular dysrhythmias are more prone to occur in patients with left ventricular failure. It seems, therefore, that the severity of depression of cardiac function, which in most instances reflects the extent of myocardial damage, is the major determinant of the long-term prognosis.

## MANAGEMENT AFTER DISCHARGE FROM THE HOSPITAL
Unfortunately, no definitive therapeutic intervention are yet available to modify an unfavorable prognosis. Control of risk factors for coronary artery disease, such as hypertension,

cigarette smoking, and hypercholesterolemia, has been advocated and is discussed in chapter 12, but the ability to modify an adverse long-term prognosis by controlling such factors remains uncertain. Rehabilitation of patients with exercise training is discussed at length in chapter 16.

The management of postinfarction angina has already been discussed. These patients, in general, initially need aggressive medical therapy, followed by delineation of coronary anatomy and left ventricular function. Revascularization surgery is indicated in appropriate patients.

Patients who demonstrate evidence of reversible ischemia either during submaximal stress testing with or without thallium-201 scintigraphy, or during dipyridamole serial thallium imaging, should undergo further evaluation by coronary arteriography. The best therapeutic approach for this patient population has not been determined by controlled studies. At the present time, therefore, the therapy should be individualized. If coronary arteriography and ventriculography demonstrate that large areas of myocardium are at risk, revascularization surgery should be considered. It is reasonable to continue medical therapy in the relatively low-risk patient.

The management of late congestive heart failure associated with low cardiac output depends on the severity of heart failure. Mild congestive heart failure responds satisfactorily to digitalis and diuretic therapy in most patients. Left ventriculography and coronary arteriography should be considered in patients with refractory failure to delineate coronary anatomy and to determine the feasibility of left ventricular aneurysmectomy.

Postmyocardial infarction syndrome *(Dressler's syndrome)* is an infrequent complication of myocardial infarction and occurs in less than 5 percent of patients. This clinical syndrome is characterized by pericardial pain, pleuritic chest pain, fever, and arthralgia. Pericardial rub, pleural effusion, and pulmonary infiltrates are frequently present. Large pericardial effusion is relatively uncommon and constrictive pericarditis rarely develops. Dressler's syndrome usually responds to therapy with aspirin or indomethacin, but recurrences are common.

Corticosteroid therapy may sometimes be necessary.

At the present time, perhaps the most promising approach to reducing mortality after recovery from an acute myocardial infarction is the use of $\beta$-adrenergic blocking agents. Some investigations [52–54] have indicated that the use of beta-blocking agents in uncomplicated patients can reduce the incidence of sudden death and the reinfarction rate. The mechanism for these beneficial effects is not clear. It is not related to the type of beta-blockers used, as both nonselective and cardioselective beta-blockers tend to produce reduction in mortality by very similar magnitudes. Furthermore, the time of institution of beta-blocker therapy after infarction does not appear to make any difference in reducing late mortality. Thus, beta-blocker therapy should be considered in patients with recent myocardial infarction provided there is no contraindication of beta-blocker therapy. The use of beta-blocking agents, particularly in larger doses, however, is contraindicated in patients with overt heart failure. In 1978, a significant reduction in deaths from a second myocardial infarction has been reported in patients treated with the drug sulfinpyrazone [244]. The duration of follow-up in this particular study, however, was short, and only the uncomplicated patients were treated. Further evaluation will therefore be needed to determine the ultimate place of this therapeutic approach. In patients with significant postinfarction left ventricular dysfunction, no therapy is as yet available that might be effective in improving their long-term prognosis. The role of surgical therapy such as aneurysmectomy and aortocoronary artery bypass surgery to improve left ventricular function and hence to improve the long-term prognosis in such patients has not been defined, and further investigations will be needed to evaluate its potential influence.

## Conclusions

The major therapeutic goals during the acute phase of myocardial infarction are (1) the early recognition and effective management of life-threatening arrhythmias (see chapter 15), (2) the reduction of the extent of myocardial ischemic injury at the onset of infarction, and (3) the precise diagnosis and rational treatment of the low output state.

Aside from arrhythmias, power failure is the major immediate cause of death in patients with acute myocardial infarction and is also the major determinant of the poor late prognosis in survivors of acute infarction. As the severity of power failure is related to the extent of myocardial damage, it seems logical that the reduction of infarct size should be an important therapeutic goal. In laboratory animals, many therapies based on the principle of reducing myocardial oxygen demand, increasing myocardial perfusion and oxygen supply, and reducing inflammatory reactions have been tested, and beneficial responses have been noted. Clinical evidence of the effectiveness of such therapeutic interventions in patients with acute myocardial infarction, however, is scanty and contradictory. Also, no sensitive and clinically applicable technique of measuring infarct size is as yet available. Until such methods are available, the evaluation of interventions to limit infarct size will remain empirical. Furthermore, carefully controlled studies on large numbers of patients will be needed to assess the results of interventions to limit myocardial ischemic injury, and without such knowledge such interventions cannot be recommended, particularly in patients with uncomplicated myocardial infarction.

Management of left ventricular dysfunction complicating myocardial infarction still remains a therapeutic challenge. Diuretics are useful to reduce pulmonary and systemic venous pressures; however, an increase in cardiac output is not usually observed with the use of diuretics. Inotropic agents, in general, do not produce any sustained beneficial hemodynamic response; furthermore, there is a potential risk of enhancing myocardial ischemia because of the increased myocardial oxygen demand. Therefore, the use of vasopressor agents is indicated only to maintain adequate perfusion pressure in severely hypotensive patients.

Vasodilator therapy improves cardiac performance in patients with low output complicating myocardial infarction. Of the various vasodilator drugs available, sodium nitroprus-

side and nitroglycerin or nitrates are the most commonly used agents. Nitroprusside, which has a balanced effect on both the arteriolar resistance bed and the venous capacitance bed, causes an increase in cardiac output along with a decrease in pulmonary and systemic venous pressures. Nitroglycerin or nitrates, on the other hand, because of their predominant effect on the venous bed, cause a significant reduction in pulmonary and systemic venous pressures with little or no increase in cardiac output. Therefore, the choice of vasodilator agent should be made according to the major hemodynamic deficits in individual patients. Although a beneficial hemodynamic response may be observed, there is a potential risk of enhancing myocardial ischemia by reducing coronary perfusion pressure; therefore, a significant decrease in arterial pressure must be avoided during vasodilator therapy. Controversy exists regarding the comparative effects of nitroprusside and nitroglycerin on myocardial metabolism and perfusion. Furthermore, the influence of vasodilator therapy on the immediate prognosis of patients with left ventricular failure has not been clearly defined.

In patients with cardiogenic shock, use of vasopressor agents, vasodilators, and intra-aortic balloon counterpulsation are frequently required to stabilize the patients before indications of corrective surgery are determined. Early corrective surgery is recommended for severe mitral regurgitation and ventricular septal defects.

As early postinfarction angina is associated with unfavorable late prognosis, revascularization surgery is recommended in appropriate patients. Often they are stabilized with medical therapy. Beta-blocker therapy appears to reduce the late mortality in patients with recent myocardial infarction; therefore, long-term beta-blocker therapy should be considered in the survivors if such therapy is not otherwise contraindicated.

## References

1. Alpert, J.S. and Francis, G.S. *Manual of Coronary Care.* Boston: Little, Brown, 1977.
2. Thompson, P.L. and Lown, B. Nitrous oxide as an analgesic in acute myocardial infarction. *JAMA* 235:924, 1976.

3. Goldberg, R.J., Gore, J.M., and Daley, J.E. The role of anticoagulant therapy in acute myocardial infarction. *Am. Heart J.* 108:1387, 1984.

4. McNeer, J.F., Wagner, G.S., Ginsburg, P.B., Wallace, A.G., McCants, C.B., Conley, M.J., and Rosati, R. Hospital discharge one week after acute myocardial infarction. *N. Engl. J. Med.* 298:229, 1978.

5. Liem, K.L., Lie, K.I., Schuilenberg, R.M., and Durrer, D. A five and a half year retro- and prospective study on early identification of candidates for development of late in-hospital ventricular fibrillation complicating acute myocardial infarction. *Circulation* 56 (Suppl. 3):148, 1977.

6. Page, D.L., Caulfield, J.B., Kastor, J.A., DeSanctis, R.W., and Sanders, C.A. Myocardial changes associated with cardiogenic shock. *N. Engl. J. Med.* 285:133, 1971.

7. DeWood, M.A., Spores, J., Notske, R.N., et al. Prevalence of total coronary occlusion during the early hours of transmural myocardial infarction. *N. Engl. J. Med.* 303:897, 1980.

8. Pardee, H.E.B. An electrocardiographic sign of coronary artery obstruction. *Arch. Intern. Med.* 26:244, 1920.

9. Maroko, P.R., Kjekshus, J.K., Sobel, B.E., Watanabe, T., Covell, J.W., Ross, J., Jr., and Braunwald, E. Factors influencing infarct size following experimental coronary artery occlusions. *Circulation* 43:66, 1971.

10. Muller, J.E., Maroko, P.R., and Braunwald, E. Precordial electrocardiographic mapping. A technique to assess the efficacy of interventions designed to limit infarct size. *Circulation* 57:1, 1978.

11. Maroko, P.R., Libby, P., Covell, J.W., Sobel, B.E., Ross, J., Jr., and Braunwald, E. Precordial S-T segment elevation mapping: An atraumatic method for assessing alterations in the extent of myocardial ischemic injury. *Am. J. Cardiol.* 29:223, 1972.

12. Becker, L.C., Ferreira, R., and Thomas, M. Mapping of left ventricular blood flow with radioactive microspheres in experimental coronary artery occlusion. *Cardiovasc. Res.* 7:391, 1973.

13. Wegria, R., Segers, M., Keating, R.P., and Ward, H.P. Relationship between the reduction in coronary flow and the appearance of electrocardiographic changes. *Am. Heart J.* 38:90, 1949.

14. Lekven, J., Ilebekk, A., Fonstelien, E., and Kil, F. Relationship between ST segment elevation and local tissue flow during myocardial ischemia in dogs. *Cardiovasc. Res.* 9:627, 1975.

15. Smith, J.H., Singh, B.N., Norris, R.M., John, M.B., and Hurley, P.J. Changes in myocardial blood flow and S-T segment elevation following coronary artery occlusion in dogs. *Circ. Res.* 36:697. 1975.

16. Scheuer, J. and Stezoski, S.W. Effects of high energy phosphate depletion and repletion on the dynamics and electrocardiogram of isolated rat hearts. *Circ. Res.* 23:519, 1968.

17. Karlsson, J., Templeton, G.H., and Willerson, J.T. Relationship between epicardial S-T segment changes and myocardial metabolism during acute coronary insufficiency. *Circ. Res.* 32:725, 1973.

18. Madias, J.E., Venkatraman, K., and Hood, W.B. Precordial ST segment mapping. I. Clinical studies in the coronary care unit. *Circulation* 52:799, 1975.

19. Haradarson, T., Henning, H., O'Rourke, R.A., Karliner, J.S., Ryan, W., and Ross, J., Jr. Variability, reproducibility and applications of precordial ST segment mapping following acute myocardial infarction. *Circulation* 57:1096, 1978.

20. Essen, R.V., Merx, W., and Effert, S. Spontaneous course of ST-segment elevation in acute anterior myocardial infarction. *Circulation* 59:105, 1979.

21. Hillis, L.D., Askenazi, J., Braunwald, E., Radvany, P., Muller, J.E., Fishbein, M.C., and Maroko, P.R. Use of changes in epicardial QRS complex to assess interventions which modify the extent of myocardial necrosis following coronary artery occlusion. *Circulation* 54:591, 1976.

22. Zmyslinski, R.W., Akiyama, T., Biddle, T.L., and Shah, P.M. Natural course of the S-T segment and QRS complex in patients with acute anterior myocardial infarction. *Am. J. Cardiol.* 43:29, 1979.

23. Lekven, J., Chatterjee, K., Tyberg, J.V., Stowe, D.F., Mathey, D.G., and Parmley, W.W. Pronounced dependence of ventricular endocardial QRS potentials on ventricular volume. *Br. Heart J.* 40:891, 1978.

24. Lekven, J., Chatterjee, K., Tyberg, J.V., and Parmley, W.W. Reduction in ventricular endocardial and epicardial potentials during acute increments in left ventricular dimensions. *Am. Heart J.* 30:891, 1978.

25. Kjekshus, J.K. and Sobel, B.E. Depressed myocardial creatine phosphokinase activity following experimental myocardial infarction in rabbit. *Circ. Res.* 27:403, 1970.

26. Kjekshus, J.K., Maroko, P.R., and Sobel, B.E. Distribution of myocardial injury and its relation to epicardial ST segment changes after coronary artery occlusion in the dog. *Cardiovasc. Res.* 6:490, 1972.

27. Henry, P.D., Sobel, B.E., and Braunwald, E. Protection of hypoxic guinea pig myocardium

with glucose and insulin. *Am. J. Physiol.* 226:-309, 1974.

28. Shell, W.E., Kjekshus, J.K., and Sobel, B.E. Quantitative assessment of the extent of myocardial infarction in the conscious dog by means of analysis of serial changes in serum creatine phosphokinase activity. *J. Clin. Invest.* 50:2614, 1971.

29. Shell, W.E., Lavell, J.F., Covell, J.W., and Sobel, B.E. Early estimation of myocardial damage in conscious dogs and patients with evolving acute myocardial infarction. *J. Clin. Invest.* 52:-2579, 1973.

30. Ross, J., Jr. General discussion. *Circulation* 53 (Suppl. 1):111, 1976.

31. Roe, C.R. and Starmer, C.F. A sensitivity analysis of enzymatic estimation of infarct size. *Circulation* 52:1, 1975.

32. Roe, C.R., Cobb, F.R., and Starmer, F. The relationship between enzymatic and histologic estimates of the extent of myocardial infarction in conscious dogs with permanent coronary occlusion. *Circulation* 55:438, 1977.

33. Thompson, P.L., Fletcher, E.E., and Katavatis, V. Enzymatic indices of myocardial necrosis: Influence on short- and long-term prognosis after myocardial infarction. *Circulation* 59:113, 1979.

34. Hackel, D.B., Reimer, K.A., Ideker, R.E. et al. Comparison of enzymatic and anatomic estimates of myocardial infarct size in man. *Circulation* 70:324, 1984.

35. Thygesen, K., Horder, M., Hyltoft Petersen, P., and Lyager Nielsen, B. Limitation of enzymatic models for predicting myocardial infarct size. *Br. Heart J.* 50:70, 1983.

36. Botvinick, E.H., Shames, D., Lappin, H., Tyberg, J.V., Townsend, R., and Parmley, W.W. Noninvasive quantification of myocardial infarction with technetium-99m pyrophosphate. *Circulation* 52:909, 1975.

37. Zaret, B.L., Lange, R.C., and Lee, J.C. Comparative assessment of infarct size with quantitative thallium-201 and technetium-99m pyrophosphate dual myocardial imaging in the dog. *Am. J. Cardiol.* 39:309, 1977.

38. Corbett, J.R., Lewis, S.E., Wolfe, C.L. et al. Measurement of myocardial infarct size by technetium pyrophosphate single-photon tomography. *Am. J. Cardiol.* 54:1231, 1984.

39. Sharpe, D.N., Botvinick, E.H., Shames, D.M., Norman, A., Chatterjee, K., and Parmley, W.W. The clinical estimation of acute myocardial infarct size with 99m technetium pyrophosphate scintigraphy. *Circulation* 57:307, 1978.

40. Braunwald, E. and Maroko, P.R. Limitation of Infarct Size. In Harvey, W.P. (ed.), *Current Problems in Cardiology.* Chicago: Year Book, 1978.

41. Braunwald, E. and Maroko, P.R. The reduction of infarct size—an idea whose time (for testing) has come. *Circulation* 50:206, 1974.

42. Nies, A.S. and Shand, P.G. Clinical pharmacology of propranolol. *Circulation* 52:6, 1975.

43. Becker, R.C., Fortuin, N.J., and Pitt, B. Effect of ischemia and antianginal drugs on the distribution of radioactive microspheres in the canine left ventricle. *Circ. Res.* 28:263, 1971.

44. Reimer, K.A., Rasmussen, M.M., and Jennings, R.B. On the nature of protection by propranolol against myocardial necrosis after temporary coronary occlusion in dogs. *Am. J. Cardiol.* 37:520, 1976.

45. Peter, T., Heng, M.K., Singh, B.N., Ambler, P., Nisbet, H., Elliot, R., and Norris, R.M. Failure of high doses of propranolol to reduce experimental myocardial ischemic damage. *Circulation* 57:534, 1978.

46. Mueller, H.S., Ayres, S.M., Religa, A., and Evans, R.G. Propranolol in the treatment of acute myocardial infarction. *Circulation* 49:-1078, 1974.

47. Pelides, L.J., Reid, D.W., Thomas, M., and Shillingford, J.P. Inhibition of beta blockade on the ST segment elevation after acute myocardial infarction. *Cardiovasc. Res.* 6:295, 1972.

48. Peter, T., Norris, R.M., Clarke, E.D., Heng, M.K., Singh, B.N., Williams, B., Howell, D.R., and Ambler, P.K. Reduction of enzyme levels by propranolol after acute myocardial infarction. *Circulation* 57:1091, 1978.

49. Herlitz, J., Elmfeldt, D., Hjalmarson, A., Holmberg, S., Malek, I., Nyberg, G., Ryden, L., Swedberg, K., Vedin, A., Waagstein, F., Waldenstrom, A., Waldenstrom, J., Wedel, H., Wilhelmsen, L., and Wilhelmsson, C. Effect of metoprolol on indirect signs of the size and severity of acute myocardial infarction. *Am. J. Cardiol.* 51:1282, 1983.

50. The International Collaborative Study Group. Reduction of infarct size with the early use of timolol in acute myocardial infarction. *N. Engl. J. Med.* 310:9, 1984.

51. Roberts, R. and the Mills Study Group. Effect of propranolol on myocardial infarct size in a randomized blinded multicenter trial. *N. Engl. J. Med.* 311:218, 1984.

52. Norwegian Multicentre Study Group. Timolol induced reduction in mortality and reinfarction in patients surviving acute myocardial infarction. *N. Engl. J. Med.* 304:801, 1981.

53. Hjalmarson, A., Elmfeldt, D., Herlitz, J., Holmberg, S., Malek, I., Nyberg, G., Ryden, L., Swedberg, K., Vedin, A., Waagstein, F., Walderstrom, A., Waldenstrom, J., Wedel, H., Wilhelmsen, L., and Wilhelmsson, C. Effect on mortality of metoprolol in acute myocardial infarction. *Lancet* 2:823, 1981.

54. Beta-blocker Heart Attack Trial Research Group. A randomized trial of propranolol in patients with acute myocardial infarction. I. Mortality results. *JAMA* 247:1707, 1982.

55. Forman, R., Kirk, E.S., Downey, J.M., and Sonnenblick, E.H. Nitroglycerin and heterogeneity of myocardial blood flow: Reduced subendocardial blood flow and ventricular contractile force. *J. Clin. Invest.* 52:905, 1973.

56. Hirshfeld, J.W., Jr., Borer, J.S., Goldstein, R.E., Barrett, M.J., and Epstein, S.E. Reduction in severity and extent of myocardial infarction when nitroglycerin and methoxamine are administered during coronary occlusion. *Circulation* 49:291, 1974.

57. Bussmann, W.D., Passek, D., Seidel, W., and Kaltenbach, M. Prospective randomized trial of intravenous nitroglycerin in acute myocardial infarction. *Circulation* 59 & 60 (Suppl. II):II-164, 1979 (Abstract).

58. Bowen, W.G., Branconi, J.M., Goldstein, R.A., Cain, M.E., Brodarick, S.M., Geltman, E.M., Jaffe, A.S., Ambos, H.D., and Roberts, R. A randomized prospective study of the effects of intravenous nitroglycerin in patients during myocardial infarction. *Circulation* 59 & 60 (Suppl. II):II-70, 1979 (Abstract).

59. Flaherty, J.T., Becker, L.C., Bulkley, B.H., Weiss, J.L., Gerstenblith, G., Kallman, C., Silverman, K.J., Wei, J.Y., Pitt, B., and Weisfeldt, M. A randomized prospective trial of intravenous nitroglycerin in patients with acute myocardial infarction. *Circulation* 68:576, 1983.

60. Gold, H.K., Chiariello, M., Leinbach, R.C., Davis, M.A., and Maroko, P.R. Deleterious effects of nitroprusside on myocardial injury during myocardial infarction. *Herz* 1:161, 1976.

61. Chiariello, M., Gold, H.K., Leinbach, R.C., Davis, M.A., and Maroko, P.R. Comparison between the effects of nitroprusside and nitroglycerin on ischemic injury during acute myocardial infarction. *Circulation* 54:766, 1976.

62. Magnusson, P., Shell, W.E., Forrester, J.S., Charuzi, Y., Singh, B.N., and Swan, H.J.C. Increased creatine phosphokinase release following blood pressure reduction in patients with acute infarction. *Circulation* 54(Suppl. 2):28, 1976.

63. Awan, N.A., Miller, R.R., Zakanddin, V., DeMaria, A.N., Amsterdam, E.A., and Mason, D.T. Reduction of ST segment elevation with infusion of nitroprusside in patients with acute myocardial infarction. *Am. J. Cardiol.* 38:435, 1976.

64. Durrer, J.D., Lie, K.I., Van Capelle, F.R.J., and Durrer, D. Effect of sodium nitroprusside on mortality in acute myocardial infarction. *N. Engl. J. Med.* 306:1121, 1982.

65. Cohn, J.N., Franciosa, J.A., Francis, C.S., et al. Effect of short-term infusion of sodium nitroprusside on mortality rate in acute myocardial infarction complicated by left ventricular failure. Results of Veterans Administration Cooperative Study. *N. Engl. J. Med.* 306:1129, 1982.

66. Mjos, O.D., Kjekshus, J.K., and Lekven, J. Importance of free fatty acids as a determinant of myocardial oxygen consumption and myocardial ischemic injury during norepinephrine infusion in dogs. *J. Clin. Invest.* 53:1290, 1974.

67. Opie, L.H., Bruyneal, K., and Owen, P. Effects of glucose, insulin, and potassium infusion on tissue metabolic changes within first hour of myocardial infarction. *Circulation* 52:49, 1975.

68. Prather, J.W., Russell, R.O., Mantle, J.O., McDaniel, H.G., and Rackley, C.E. Metabolic consequences of glucose-insulin-potassium infusion in the treatment of acute myocardial infarction. *Am. J. Cardiol.* 38:95, 1976.

69. Norris, R.M., Heng, M.K., Singh, B.N., and Barrat-Boyes, C. The effect of glucose, insulin and potassium on hemodynamics and infarct size after myocardial infarction. *Circulation* 52(Suppl. 2):107, 1975.

70. Rogers, W.J., Segall, P.H., McDaniel, H.G., et al. Prospective randomized trial of glucose-insulin-potassium in acute myocardial infarction. *Am. J. Cardiol.* 43:801, 1979.

71. Smullens, S.N., Weiner, L., Kasparian, H., Brest, A.N., Bacharach, B., Noble, P.H., and Templeton, J.Y., III. Evaluation and surgical management of acute evolving myocardial infarction. *J. Thorac. Cardiovasc. Surg.* 64:495, 1972.

72. Cheanvechai, C., Effler, D.B., Loop, F.D., Groves, L.K., Sheldon, W.C., Razavi, M., and Sones, F.M., Jr. Emergency myocardial revascularization. *Am. J. Cardiol.* 32:901, 1973.

73. Dawson, J.T., Hall, R.J., Hallman, G.L., and Cooley, D.A. Mortality in coronary artery bypass after previous myocardial infarction. *Am. J. Cardiol.* 31:128, 1973.

74. Gold, H.K., Leinbach, R.C., Sanders, C.A., Buckley, M.J., Mundth, E.D., and Austen, W.G. Intraaortic balloon pumping for control of recurrent myocardial ischemia. *Circulation* 47:1197, 1973.

75. Parmley, W.W., Chatterjee, K., Charuzi, Y., and Swan, H.J.C. Hemodynamic effects of noninvasive systolic unloading (nitroprusside) and diastolic augmentation (external counterpulsation) in patients with acute myocardial infarction. *Am. J. Cardiol.* 33:819, 1974.

76. Maroko, P.R., Davidson, D.M., Libby, P., DeLaria, G.A., Covell, J.W., Ross, J., Jr., and Braunwald, E. Effects of intraaortic balloon counterpulsation on the severity of myocardial

ischemic injury following acute coronary occlusion. *Circulation* 45:1150, 1972.

77. Sugg, W.L., Webb, W.R., and Echer, R.R. Reduction of extent of myocardial infarction by counterpulsation. *Ann. Thorac. Surg.* 7:310, 1969.

78. Leinbach, R.C., Gold, H.K., Harper, R.W., et al. Early intraaortic balloon pumping for anterior myocardial infarction without shock. *Circulation* 58:204, 1978.

79. Alpert, J., Bhaktan, E.K., Gielchinsky, I., Gilbert, L., Brener, B.J., Brief, D.K., and Parsonnet, V. Vascular complications of intraaortic balloon pumping. *Arch. Surg.* 111:1190, 1976.

80. Avmiger, L.C. and Gavin, J.B. Changes in the microvasculature of ischemic and infarcted myocardium. *Lab. Invest.* 33:51, 1975.

81. Willerson, J.T., Watson, J.T., Hutton, I., Fixler, D.E., Currey, G.C., and Templeton, G.H. The influence of hypertonic mannitol on regional myocardial flow during acute and chronic myocardial ischemia in anesthetized and awake intact dogs. *J. Clin. Invest.* 55:892, 1975.

82. Willerson, J.T., Powell, W.M., Jr., Guiney, T.E., Stark, J.J., Sanders, C.A., and Leaf, A. Improvement in myocardial function and coronary blood flow in ischemic myocardium after mannitol. *J. Clin. Invest.* 51:2989. 1972.

83. Powell, W.M.J., Jr., DiBona, D.R., Flores, J., and Leaf, A. The protective effect of hyperosmotic mannitol in myocardial ischemia and necrosis. *Circulation* 54:603, 1976.

84. Hirzel, H.O. and Kirk, E.S. The effect of mannitol following permanent coronary occlusion. *Circulation* 56:1006, 1977.

85. Maroko, P.R. and Braunwald, E. Modification of myocardial infarct size after coronary occlusion. *Ann. Intern. Med.* 79:720, 1973.

86. Maclean, D., Fishbein, M.C., Maroko, P.R., and Braunwald, E. Hyaluronidase induced reductions in myocardial infarct size. Direct quantification of infarction following coronary artery occlusion in the rat. *Science* 194:199, 1976.

87. Maroko, P.R., Hillis, L.D., Muller, J.E., Tavazzi, L., Heyndrick, G.R., et al. Favorable effects of hyaluronidase on electrocardiographic evidence of necrosis in patients with acute myocardial infarction. *N. Engl. J. Med.* 296:898, 1977.

88. Cairns, J.A., Holder, D.A., Tanser, P., and Missirlis, E. Intravenous hyaluronidase therapy for myocardial infarction in man: Double-blind trial to assess infarct size limitation. *Circulation* 65:764, 1982.

89. Maroko, P.R., Radvany, P., Braunwald, E., and Hale, S.L. Reduction of infarction size by oxygen inhalation following acute coronary occlusion. *Circulation* 52:360, 1975.

90. Madias, J.E., Madias, N.E., and Hood, W.B.

Precordial ST mapping. 2. Effects of oxygen inhalation on ischemic injury in patients with acute myocardial infarction. *Circulation* 53:411, 1976.

91. Ratliff, N.B., Hackel, P.V., and Mikat, E. Myocardial oxygen metabolism and myocardial blood flow in dogs with hemorrhagic shock. *Circ. Res.* 45:901, 1969.

92. Fox, A.C., Hoffstein, S., and Weissmann, G. Lysosomal mechanisms in production of tissue damage during myocardial ischemia and the effects of treatment with steroids. *Am. Heart J.* 91:394, 1976.

93. Spath, J.A., Lane, D.L., and Lefer, A.M. Protective action of methylprednisolone on the myocardium during experimental myocardial ischemia in the cat. *Circ. Res.* 35:44, 1974.

94. Vyden, J.K., Nagasawa, K., Rabinowitz, B., et al. Effect of methylprednisolone administration in acute myocardial infarction. *Am. J. Cardiol.* 34:677, 1974.

95. Hoffstein, S., Weissman, G., and Fox, A.C. Lysosomes in acute myocardial infarction: Studies by means of cytochemistry and subcellular fractionation, with observations on the effects of methylprednisolone. *Circulation* 53(Suppl. 1):-34, 1976.

96. Busuttil, R.W., George, W.J., and Hewitt, R.L. Protective effect of methylprednisolone on the heart during ischemic arrest. *J. Thorac. Cardiovasc. Surg.* 70:955, 1975.

97. Welman, E., Selwyn, A.P., and Fox, M.B. Lysosomal and cytosolic enzyme release in acute myocardial infarction: Effects of methylprednisolone. *Circulation* 59:730, 1979.

98. Johnson, A.S., Scheinberg, S.R., Gerisch, R.A., and Saltztein, H.C. Effects of cortisone on the size of experimentally produced myocardial infarcts. *Circulation* 7:224, 1953.

99. Libby, P., Maroko, P.R., Bloor, C.M., Covell, J.W., and Braunwald, E. Reduction of experimental myocardial infarct size, by corticosteroid administration. *J. Clin. Invest.* 52:599, 1973.

100. Opdyke, D.F., Lampert, A., Stoerk, H.C., Zanetti, M.E., and Kuna, S. Failure to reduce the size of experimentally produced myocardial infarcts by cortisone treatment. *Circulation* 8:-544, 1953.

101. Vogel, W.M., Zannoni, V.G., Abrams, G.D., and Lucchesi, B.R. Inability of methylprednisolone sodium succinate to decrease infarct size of preserved enzyme activity measured 24 hours after coronary occlusion in the dog. *Circulation* 55:588, 1977.

102. Morrison, J., Reduto, L., Pizzarello, R., Geller, K., Maley, T., and Gulotta, S. Modification of myocardial injury in man by corticosteroid administration. *Circulation* 53(Suppl. 1):200, 1976.

103. Roberts, R., DeMello, V., and Sobel, B.E. Deleterious effects of methylprednisolone in patients with myocardial infarction. *Circulation* 53(Suppl. 1):204, 1976.
104. Peters, R.W., Norman, A., Parmley, W.W., Emilson, B.B., Scheinman, M.M., and Cheitlin, M. Effect of therapy with methylprednisolone on the size of myocardial infarcts in man. *Chest* 73:483, 1978.
105. DeMello, V.R., Roberts, R., and Sobel, B.E. Deleterious effects of methylprednisolone in patients with evolving myocardial infarction. *Clin. Res.* 23:179A, 1975.
106. Kloner, R.A., Fishbein, M.C., Lew, H., Maroko, P.R., and Braunwald, E. Minimization of the infarcted myocardium by high dose corticosteroids. *Circulation* 57:56, 1978.
107. Bulkley, B.H. and Roberts, W.C. Steroid therapy during acute myocardial infarction. A cause of delayed healing and of ventricular aneurysm. *Am. J. Med.* 56:244, 1974.
108. Hammerman, H., Kloner, R.A., Hale, S., Schoen, F.J., and Braunwald, E. Dose dependent effects of short-term methylprednisolone on myocardial infarct extent, scar formation and ventricular function. *Circulation* 68:446, 1983.
109. Ebashi, S. and Endo, M. Calcium ion and muscle contraction. *Prog. Biophys. Mol. Biol.* 18:125, 1968.
110. Braunwald, E., Bloodwell, R.D., Goldberg, L.I., and Morrow, A.G. Studies on digitalis. IV. Observations in man on the effects of digitalis preparations on the contractility of the nonfailing heart and total vascular resistance. *J. Clin. Invest.* 50:52, 1961.
111. Mason, D.T. and Braunwald, E. Studies on digitalis. IX. Effects of ouabain on the nonfailing heart. *J. Clin. Invest.* 42:1105, 1963.
112. Sonnenblick, E.H., William, J.F., Jr., Glick, G., Mason, D.T., and Braunwald, E. Studies on digitalis. XV. Effects of cardiac glycosides on myocardial force-velocity relations in the nonfailing human heart. *Circulation* 34:532, 1966.
113. Braunwald, E. Editorial: On the difference between the heart's output and its contractile state. *Circulation* 43:171, 1971.
114. Bing, R.J., Maraist, F.M., Dammann, J.F., Jr., Draper, A., Jr., Heinbecker, R., Daley, R., Gerrard, R., and Colazel, P. Effect of strophanthus on coronary blood flow and cardiac oxygen consumption of normal and failing human hearts. *Circulation* 2:513, 1950.
115. Arnold, S.B., Byrd, R.C., Meister, W., Melmon, K., Cheitlin, M., Bristow, J.D., Parmley, W.W., and Chatterjee, K. Chronic digitalis therapy improves left ventricular function of patients with chronic heart failure. *N. Engl. J. Med.* 303:1443, 1980.
116. Cohn, K., Selzer, A., Kersh, E.S., Karpman, L.S., and Goldschlager, N. Variability of hemodynamic responses to acute digitalization in chronic cardiac failure due to cardiomyopathy and coronary artery disease. Am. J. Cardiol. 35:461, 1975.
117. Balcon, R., Hoy, J., and Sowton, E. Hemodynamic effects of rapid digitalization following acute myocardial infarction. *Br. Heart J.* 30:373, 1968.
118. Malmcrona, R., Schroder, G., and Werko, L. Hemodynamic effects of digitalis in acute myocardial infarction. *Acta Med. Scand.* 180:55, 1966.
119. Bezdeck, W., Forrester, J., Chatterjee, K., Ganz, W., Parmley, W., and Swan, H.J.C. Myocardial metabolic effect of ouabain in acute myocardial infarction (AMI). *Circulation* 46(Suppl. 2):113, 1972.
120. Hodges, M., Frilsinger, G.E., Riggins, R.C.K., and Dagenais, G.R. Effects of intravenously administered digoxin on mild left ventricular failure in acute myocardial infarction in man. *Am. J. Cardiol.* 29:749, 1972.
121. Rahimtoola, S.H., Sinno, M.Z., Chuquimia, R., Loeb, H.S., Rosen, K.M., and Gunnar, R.M. Effects of ouabain on impaired left ventricular function in acute myocardial infarction. *N. Engl. J. Med.* 253:527, 1972.
122. Forrester, J.S. and Chatterjee, K. Preservation of Ischemic Myocardium. In Vogel, J.H.K. (ed.), *Advances in Cardiology*. Vol. 11. *A Perspective on New Techniques in Congenital and Acquired Heart Disease.* Basel: Karger, 1974.
123. Rahimtoola, S.H., Loeb, H.S., and Gunnar, R. Digitalis in Acute Myocardial Infarction. In Gunnar, R.M., Loeb, H.S., and S.H. Rahimtoola (eds.), *Shock in Myocardial Infarction.* New York: Grune & Stratton, 1974.
124. Amsterdam, E.A., Huffaker, H.K., DeMaria, A., Vismara, L.A., Choquet, Y., Massumi, R., Zelis, R., and Mason, D.T. Hemodynamic effects of digitalis in acute myocardial infarction and comparison with furosemide. *Circulation* 46(Suppl. 2):113, 1972.
125. Kumar, R., Hood, W.B., Jr., Joison, J., Gilmour, D.P., Norman, J.C., and Abelman, W.H. Experimental myocardial infarction. VI. Efficacy and toxicity of digitalis in acute and healing phase in intact conscious dogs. *J. Clin. Invest.* 49:358, 1970.
126. Hood, W.B., Jr., McCarthy, B., and Lown, B. Myocardial infarction following coronary ligation in dogs. Hemodynamic effects of isoproterenol and acetyl stophanthidin. *Circ. Res.* 21:191, 1967.
127. Morris, J.J., Taft, C.V., Whalen, R.E., and McIntosh, H.D. Digitalis and experimental myocardial infarction. *Am. Heart J.* 77:342, 1969.

128. Schemm, F.R. Digitalis in cardiac disease without congestive heart failure or auricular fibrillation. *Postgrad. Med.* 7:385, 1950.

129. Askey, J.M. Digitalis in acute myocardial infarction. *JAMA* 146:1008, 1951.

130. Boyer, N. Digitalis in acute myocardial infarction. *N. Engl. J. Med.* 252:536, 1955.

131. Gunnar, R.M., Loeb, H.S., Pietras, R.J., and Tobin, J.R., Jr. Ineffectiveness of isoproterenol in shock due to acute myocardial infarction. *JAMA* 203:1124, 1967.

132. Mueller, H., Ayres, S.M., Giannelli, S., Jr., Conklin, E.F., Mazzara, J.T., and Grace, W.J. Effect of isoproterenol, L-norepinephrine and intra-aortic counterpulsation on hemodynamics and myocardial metabolism in shock following acute myocardial infarction. *Circulation* 45:335, 1972.

133. Morse, B.W., Danzig, R., and Swan, H.J.C. Effect of isoproterenol shock in shock associated with acute myocardial infarction. *Circulation* 36(Suppl. 2):192, 1967.

134. Loeb, H.S., Gunnar, R.M., and Rahimtoola, S.H. Pharmacologic Agents in Support of the Circulation. In Gunnar, R.M., Loeb, H.S., and Rahimtoola, S.H. (eds.), *Shock in Myocardial Infarction.* New York: Grune & Stratton, 1974.

135. Abrams, E., Forrester, J.S., Chatterjee, K., Danzig, R., and Swan, H.J.C. Variability in response to norepinephrine in acute myocardial infarction. *Am. J. Cardiol.* 32:919, 1973.

136. Mueller, H.S., Evans, R., and Ayers, S.M. Effect of dopamine on hemodynamics and myocardial metabolism in shock following acute myocardial infarction in man. *Circulation* 57:361, 1978.

137. Brendesky, R., Chatterjee, K., Parmley, W.W., Brundage, B.H., and Ports, T.A. Dobutamine in chronic ischemic heart failure: Alterations in left ventricular function and coronary hemodynamics. *Am. J. Cardiol.* 48:554, 1981.

138. Goldstein, R.A., Passamani, E.R., and Roberts, R. A comparison of digoxin and dobutamine in patients with acute infarction and cardiac failure. *N. Engl. J. Med.* 303:846, 1980.

139. Chatterjee, K. Digitalis versus newer inotropic agents. Which to use. Drug Therapy 12:83, 1982.

140. Lair, C.V., Heban, P.T., Huss, P., Bush, C.A., and Lewis, R.P. Comparative and systemic and regional hemodynamic effects of dopamine and dobutamine in patients with cardiomyopathic heart failure. *Circulation* 58:466, 1978.

141. Loeb, H.S., Bvedakis, J., and Gunner, R.M. Superiority of dobutamine over dopamine for augmentation of cardiac output in patients with low output cardiac failure. *Circulation* 55:375, 1977.

142. Milnor, W.R. Arterial impedance as ventricular afterload. *Circ. Res.* 36:565, 1975.

143. Mann, T., Cohn, P.F., Holman, B.L., Green, L.H., Markis, J.E., and Phillips, D.A. Effect of nitroprusside on regional myocardial blood flow in coronary artery disease: Results in 25 patients and comparison with nitroglycerin. *Circulation* 57:732, 1978.

144. Parmley, W.W. and Chatterjee, K. Vasodilator Therapy. In Harvey, W.P. (ed.), *Current Problems in Cardiology.* Chicago: Year Book, 1978.

145. Parmley, W.W., Chuck, L., Chatterjee, K., Swan, H.J.C., Klausner, S.C., Glantz, S.A., and Ratshin, R. Acute changes in the diastolic pressure volume relationship of the left ventricle. *Eur. J. Cardiol.* 4(Suppl.):105, 1976.

146. Chatterjee, K., Parmley, W.W., Ganz, W., Forrester, J., Walinsky, P., Crexells, C., and Swan, H.J.C. Hemodynamic and metabolic responses to vasodilator therapy in acute myocardial infarction. *Circulation* 48:1183, 1973.

147. Armstrong, P.W., Walker, D.C., Burton, J.R., and Parker, J.O. Vasodilator therapy in acute myocardial infarction. A comparison of sodium nitroprusside and nitroglycerin. *Circulation* 52:1118, 1975.

148. Walinsky, P.L., Chatterjee, K., Forrester, J., Parmley, W.W., and Swan, H.J.C. Enhanced left ventricular performance with phentolamine in acute myocardial infarction. *Am. J. Cardiol.* 33:37, 1974.

149. Chatterjee, K. and Parmley, W.W. The role of vasodilator therapy in heart failure. *Prog. Cardiovasc. Dis.* 19:301, 1977.

150. Kelly, D.T., Delgado, C.E., Taylor, D.R., Pitt, B., and Ross, R.S. Use of phentolamine in acute myocardial infarction associated with hypertension and left ventricular failure. *Circulation* 47:729, 1973.

151. Gould, L., Reddy, C.V.R., Kalanithi, P., Espina, L., and Gomprecht, R.F. Use of phentolamine in acute myocardial infarction. *Am. Heart J.* 88:144, 1974.

152. Perret, C.L., Gardaz, J.P., Reynaert, M., Grimbert, F., and Enrico, J.-F. Phentolamine for vasodilator therapy in left ventricular failure complicating acute myocardial infarction. Hemodynamic study. *Br. Heart J.* 37:640, 1975.

153. Gold, H.K., Leinbach, R.C., and Sanders, C.A. Use of sublingual nitroglycerin in congestive heart failure following acute myocardial infarction. *Circulation* 46:839, 1972.

154. Williams, D.O., Amsterdam, E.A., and Mason, D.T. Hemodynamic effects of nitroglycerin in acute myocardial infarction. Decrease in ventricular preload at the expense of cardiac output. *Circulation* 51:421, 1975.

155. Flaherty, J.T., Reid, P.R., Kelly, D.T., Taylor, D.R., Weisfeldt, M.L., and Pitt, B. Intravenous nitroglycerin in acute myocardial infarction. Circulation 51:132, 1975.

156. Come, P., Flaherty, J.T., Baird, M.C., Rouleau, J.R., Weisfeldt, M.L., Greene, H.L., Becker, L., and Pitt, B. Reversal by phenylephrine of the beneficial effects of intravenous nitroglycerin in patients with acute myocardial infarction. *N. Engl. J. Med.* 293:1003, 1975.

157. Borer, J.S., Redwood, D.R., Levitt, B., Cagin, N., Bianchi, C., Vallin, H., and Epstein, S.E. Reduction in myocardial ischemia with nitroglycerin plus phenylephrine administered during acute myocardial infarction. *N. Engl. J. Med.* 293:1008, 1975.

158. Armstrong, P.W., Mathew, M.T., Boroomand, K., and Parker, J.O. Hemodynamic effects of nitroglycerin ointment in acute myocardial infarction. *Circulation* 52(Suppl. 2):152, 1975.

159. Bussmann, W., Lohner, J., and Kaltenback, M. Orally administered isosorbide dinitrate in patients with and without left ventricular failure due to acute myocardial infarction. *Am. J. Cardiol.* 39:91, 1977.

160. Shell, W.E. and Sobel, B.E. Protection of jeopardized ischemic myocardium by reduction of ventricular afterload. *N. Engl. J. Med.* 291:481, 1974.

161. Rowe, G.G. and Henderson, R.H. Systemic and coronary hemodynamic effects of sodium nitroprusside. *Am. Heart J.* 87:83, 1974.

162. daLuz, P.L., Forrester, J. S., Wyatt, H.L., Tyberg, J.V., Chagrasulis, R., Parmley, W.W., and Swan, H.J.C. Hemodynamic and metabolic effects of sodium nitroprusside on the performance and metabolism of regional ischemic myocardium. *Circulation* 52:400, 1975.

163. LaJemtal, T.H., Nelson, R.G., Sonnenblick, E.H., and Kirk, E.S. Preload and afterload changes induced by nitroprusside: Beneficial and detrimental effects on ischemia. *Circulation* 54(Suppl. 2):69, 1976.

164. Lichtlen, P.R., Engel, H.J., and Hundeshagen, H. Regional myocardial blood flow in normal and poststenotic areas after nitroglycerin, beta blockade (atenolol), coronary dilatation (dipyridamole) and calcium antagonism (nifedipine). *Herz* 2:81, 1977.

165. Codini, M.A., Barfeld, P.A., and Spindola-Franco, H. Paradoxical effect of nitroglycerin on left ventricular wall motion in coronary artery disease. *Am. J. Cardiol.* 37:127, 1976.

166. Forrester, J.S., Ganz, W., Diamond, G., McHugh, T., Chonette, D., Swan, H.J.C. Thermodilution cardiac output determination with a single flow-directed catheter. *Am. Heart J.* 83:306, 1972.

167. Chatterjee, K. Bedside Hemodynamic Monitoring. In, Hooshang Bolooki (ed.), *Clinical Applications of Intra-Aortic Balloon Pump.* Mt. Kisco, N.Y.: Futura, 1977, pp. 197–220.

168. Chastre, J., Corrud, F., Bouchama, A., Viau, F., Benacerraj, R., and Gilbert, C. Thrombosis as a complication of pulmonary-artery catheterization via the internal jugular vein. Prospective evaluation by phlebography. *N. Engl. J. Med.* 306:278, 1982.

169. Russell, R.O., Jr., Rackley, C.E., Pombo, J., Hung, D., Potanin, C., and Dodge, H.T. Effects of increasing left ventricular filling pressure in patients with acute myocardial infarction. *J. Clin. Invest.* 49:1539, 1970.

170. Crexells, C., Chatterjee, K., Forrester, J.S., Dikshit, K., and Swan, H.J.C. Optimal level of left heart filling pressures in acute myocardial infarction. *N. Engl. J. Med.* 289:1263, 1973.

171. Cohn, J.N., Guicha, N.H., Broder, M.I., and Constantinos, J.L. Right ventricular infarction: Clinical and hemodynamic features. *Am. J. Cardiol.* 33:209, 1974.

172. Lorell, B., Leinbach, R.C., Pohost, A.M., Gold, H.K., Dinsmore, R.E., Hutter, A.M., Pastore, J.O., and Desanctis, R.W. Right ventricular infarction: Clinical diagnosis and differentiation from cardiac tamponade and pericardial constriction. *Am. J. Cardiol.* 43:465, 1979.

173. Goldstein, A.J., Vlahakes, G.J., Verrier, E.D., Schiller, N.B., Tyberg, J.V., Ports, T.A., Parmley, W.W., and Chatterjee, K. The role of right ventricular systolic dysfunction and elevated intrapericardial pressure in the genesis of low output in experimental right ventricular infarction. *Circulation* 65:513, 1982.

174. Candell-Riera, J., Figueras, J., Valle, V., Alvarez, A., Gutierrez, L., Cortadellas, J., Cinca, J., Salas, A., and Rios, A. Right ventricular infarction and relationships between ST segment elevation in V4R and hemodynamic, scintigraphic and electrocardiographic findings in patients with acute inferior myocardial infarction. *Am. Heart J.* 101:281, 1981.

175. Sharpe, D.N., Botvinick, E.H., Shames, D.M., Schiller, N.B., Massie, B.M., Chatterjee, K., and Parmley, W.W. The noninvasive diagnosis of right ventricular infarction. *Circulation* 57:483, 1978.

176. Wackers, F.J.T., Lie, K.I., Sokote, E.B., Res, J., Van Der Schoot, J.B., and Durrer, D. Prevalence of right ventricular involvement in inferior wall infarction assessed with myocardial imaging with thallium-201 and technetium-99m pyrophosphate. *Am. J. Cardiol.* 42:358, 1978.

177. Tobinick, E.H., Schelbert, H.R., Henning, H., LeWinter, M., Taylor, A., Ashburn, W.L., and Karliner, J.S. Right ventricular ejection fraction in patients with acute anterior and inferior myocardial infarction assessed by radionuclide angiography. *Circulation* 57:1078, 1978.

178. Holt, J.P., Rhose, E.A., and Kuies, H. Pericardial and ventricular pressure. *Circ. Res.* 8:1171, 1960.

179. Goldstein, J.A., Vlahakes, G.J., Verrier, E.D., Schiller, N.B., Botvinick, E., Tyberg, J.V., Parmley, W.W., and Chatterjee, K. Volume loading improves low cardiac output in experimental right ventricular infarction. *J. Am. Col. Cardiol.* 2:270, 1983.

180. Lloyd, E.A., Gersh, B.J., and Kennelly, B.M. Hemodynamic spectrum of dominant right ventricular infarction in 19 patients. *Am. J. Cardiol.* 48:1016, 1981.

181. Topol, E.J., Goldschlager, N., Ports, T.A., DiCarlo, L.A., Jr., Schiller, N.B., Botvinick, E.H., and Chatterjee, K. Hemodynamic benefit of atrial pacing in right ventricular myocardial infarction. *Ann. Intern. Med.* 96:594, 1982.

182. Dikshit, K., Vyden, J.K., Forrester, J.S., Chatterjee, K., Prakash, R., and Swan, H.J.C. Renal and extrarenal hemodynamic effects of furosemide in congestive heart failure after acute myocardial infarction. *N. Engl. J. Med.* 288:1087, 1973.

183. Chatterjee, K. and Parmley, W.W. Vasodilator therapy for acute myocardial infarction and chronic congestive heart failure. *J. Am. Col. Cardiol.* 1:133, 1983.

184. Gunnar, R.M., Lambrew, C.T., Abrams, W., Adolph, R.J., Chatterjee, K., Cohn, J.N., Derryberry J.S., Horowitz, L.N., Martin, W.B., Siciliano, E.G., Temple, R., and Tuckman, J. Task Force IV: Pharmacologic interventions. *Am. J. Cardiol.* 50:393, 1982.

185. Port, S.C., Patel, S., and Schmidt, D.H. Effects of intraaortic balloon counterpulsation on myocardial blood flow in patients with severe coronary artery disease. *J. Am. Col. Cardiol.* 3:1367, 1984.

186. Scheidt, S., Wilner, G., Mueller, H., Summers, D., Lesch, M., Wolff, G., Krakauer, J., Rubenfire, M., Fleming, P., Noon, G., Oldham, N., Killip, T., and Kantrowitz, A. Intra-aortic balloon counterpulsation in cardiogenic shock. Report of a cooperative clinical trial. *N. Engl. J. Med.* 288:979, 1973.

187. Johnson, S.A., Scanlon, P.J., Loeb, H.S., Moran, J.M., Pifarre, R., and Gunnar, R.M. Treatment of cardiogenic shock in myocardial infarction by intraaortic balloon counterpulsation and surgery. *Am. J. Med.* 62:687, 1977.

188. Hagemeijer, F., Laird, J.D., Haalebos, M.M.P., and Hugenholtz, P.G. Effectiveness of intraaortic balloon pumping without cardiac surgery for patients with severe heart failure secondary to a recent myocardial infarction. *Am. J. Cardiol.* 40:951, 1977.

189. McCabe, J.C., Abel, R.M., Subramanian, V.A., and Gay, W.A., Jr. Complications of intra-aortic balloon insertion and counterpulsation. *Circulation* 57:769, 1978.

190. Chatterjee, K., Parmley, W.W., Swan, H.J.C., Berman, G., Forrester, J., and Marcus, H.S. Beneficial effects of vasodilator agents in severe mitral regurgitation due to subvalvular apparatus. *Circulation* 48:684, 1973.

191. Synhorst, D.P., Lauer, R.M., Doty, D.B., and Brody, M.J. Hemodynamic effects of vasodilator agents in dogs with experimental ventricular septal defects. *Circulation* 54:472, 1976.

192. Tecklenberg, P.L., Fitzgerald, J., Allaire, B.I., Alderman, E.L., and Harrison, D.C. Afterload reduction in the management of postinfarction ventricular septal defect. *Am. J. Cardiol.* 38:956, 1976.

193. Austen, W.G., Sokol, D.M., DeSanctis, R.W., and Sanders, C.A. Surgical treatment of papillary muscle rupture complicating myocardial infarction. *N. Engl. J. Med.* 278:1137, 1968.

194. Jude, J.R. Surgical treatment of experimental myocardial infarction. *JAMA* 203:451, 1968.

195. Gula, G. and Yacouv, M.H. Surgical correction of complete rupture of the anterior papillary muscle. *Ann. Thorac. Surg.* 32:88, 1981.

196. Kay, J.H., Zubiate, P., Mendez, M.A., et al. Surgical treatment of mitral insufficiency secondary to coronary artery disease. *J. Thorac. Cardiovasc. Surg.* 79:12, 1980.

197. Merin, G., Giuliani, E., Pluth, J., et al. Surgery for mitral valve incompetence after myocardial infarction. *Am. J. Cardiol.* 32:322, 1973.

198. Thomas, C.S., Alford, W.C., Burrus, G.R., et al. Urgent operation for acquired ventricular septal defect. *Ann. Surg.* 195:706, 1982.

199. Guadiani, V.A., Miller, D.C., Stinson, E.B., et al. Postinfarction ventricular septal defect: An argument for early operation. *Surgery* 89:48, 1981.

200. Kouchoukos, N.T. Surgical treatment of acute complications of myocardial infarction. *Cardiovasc. Clin.* 11:141, 1981.

201. Bates, R.J., Beutler, S., Resnekov, L., and Anagnostopoulos, C.E. Cardiac rupture—challenge in diagnosis and management. *Am. J. Cardiol.* 40:429, 1977.

202. Rasmussen, S., Leth, A., Kjoller, E., and Pedersen, A. Cardiac rupture in acute myocardial infarction. *Acta Med. Scand.* 205:11, 1979.

203. Cole, D.R., Singian, E.G., and Katz, L.N. Long-term prognosis following myocardial infarction and some facts which affect it. *Circulation* 9:321, 1954.

204. Honey, G.E. and Truelove, S.C. Prognostic factors in myocardial infarction. *Lancet* 1:1213, 1957.

205. Pell, S. and D'Alonzo, C.A. Immediate mortality and five year survival of employed men with a first myocardial infarction. *N. Engl. J. Med.* 270:915, 1964.

206. Beard, O.W., Hipp, H.R., Robbins, M., and Verzolini, V.R. Initial myocardial infarction

among veterans. Ten-year survival. *Am. Heart J.* 73:317, 1967.

207. Norris, R.M., Caughey, D.E., Mercer, C.J., Deeming, L.W., and Scott, P.J. Coronary prognostic index for predicting survival after recovery from acute myocardial infarction. *Lancet* 2:-485, 1970.

208. Norris, R.M., Caughey, D.E., Mercer, C.J., and Scott, P.J. Prognosis after myocardial infarction: Six year follow-up. *Br. Heart J.* 36:786, 1974.

209. Helmers, C. Assessment of three year prognosis in survivors of acute myocardial infarction. *Br. Heart J.* 37:593, 1975.

210. Greeberg, H., McMaster, P., Dwyer, E.M., Jr. et al.: Left ventricular dysfunction after acute myocardial infarction: Results of a prospective multicenter study. *J. Am Coll. Cardiol.* 4:867, 1984.

211. Schulze, R.A., Strauss, H.W., and Pitt, B. Sudden death in the year following myocardial infarction. Relation to ventricular premature contractions in the last hospital phase and left ventricular ejection fraction. *Am. J. Med.* 62:-192, 1976.

212. Chatterjee, K. and Brundage, B. Prognostic factors in acute myocardial infarction. *Practical Cardiol.* 4:23, 1978.

213. Chatterjee, K., Swan, H.J.C., Kaushik, V.S., Jobin, G., Magnusson, P., and Forrester, J.S. Effects of vasodilator therapy for severe pump failure in acute myocardial infarction on short term and late prognosis. *Circulation* 53:797, 1976.

214. Hollander, G., Ozick, H., Greengert, A., Shan, J., and Lichstein, E. High mortality and early reinfarction with first nontransmural infarction. *Am. Heart J.* 108:1412, 1984.

215. Kennedy, H.L., Szklo, M., and Tonascia, J. Short and long term prognosis of transmural and subendocardial infarction. *Am. J. Cardiol.* 41:398, 1978.

216. Hutter, A.M., Jr., Yeatman, L.A., Flynn, T., and DeSanctis, R.W. Long-term course of subendocardial myocardial infarction compared to that of anterior and inferior transmural infarction. A controlled study. *Am. J. Cardiol.* 41:398, 1978.

217. Mahoney, C., Aronin, N., and Wagner, C. The excellent short and long term prognosis of patients with subendocardial infarction. *Am. J. Cardiol.* 41:407, 1978.

218. Eaton, L.W., Weiss, J.L., Buckley, B.H., Garrison, J.B., and Weisfeldt, M. Regional cardiac dilatation after acute myocardial infarction. *N. Engl. J. Med.* 300:57, 1979.

219. Hamby, R.I., Hoffman, I., Hilsenrath, J., Aintabilan, A., Shaniso, S., and Pamanabhan, V.S. Clinical, hemodynamic and angiographic aspects of inferior and anterior myocardial infarc-

tions in patients with angina pectoris. *Am. J. Cardiol.* 34:513, 1974.

220. Chaitman, B.R., Waters, D.D., Corbara, F., and Bourassa, M.G. Prediction of multivessel disease after inferior myocardial infarction. *Circulation* 57:1085, 1978.

221. Bruschke, A.V.G., Proudfit, W.L., and Sones, F.M.J. Progress study of 590 consecutive nonsurgical cases of coronary disease followed 5-9 years. I. Arteriographic correlations. *Circulation* 47:1147, 1973.

222. The Coronary Drug Project Research Group. The prognostic importance of the electrocardiogram after myocardial infarction. Experience in the coronary drug project. *Ann. Intern. Med.* 77:677, 1972.

223. Schuster, E.H. and Bulkley, B. Early postinfarction angina. Ischemia at a distance and ischemia in the infarct zone. *N. Engl. J. Med.* 305:1101, 1981.

224. McQuay, N.W., Edwards, J.E., and Burchell, H.B. Types of death in acute myocardial infarction. *Arch. Int. Med.* 96:1, 1955.

225. Taylor, G.J., Humphries, J.O., Mellits, E.D., Pitt, B., Schulze, R.A., Griffith, L.S.C., and Achuff, S.C. Predictors of clinical course, coronary anatomy, and left ventricular function after recovery from acute myocardial infarction. *Circulation* 62:960, 1980.

226. Lofmark, R. T wave changes and postinfarction angina pectoris predictive of recurrent myocardial infarction. *Br. Heart J.* 45:512, 1981.

227. Koiwaya, Y., Tori, S., Takeshita, A., Nakagaki, O., and Nakamura, M. Postinfarction angina caused by coronary arterial spasm. *Circulation* 65:275, 1982.

228. Brundage, B.H., Ullyot, D.J., Winokur, S., et al. The role of aortic balloon pumping in postinfarction angina: A different perspective. *Circulation* 62(Suppl. 1):I-119, 1980.

229. Gold, H.K., Leinbach, R.C., Sanders, C.A., Buckley, M.J., Mundth, E.D., and Austen, W.G. Intra-aortic balloon pumping for control of recurrent myocardial ischemia. *Circulation* 47:1197, 1973.

230. Bardet, J., Rigand, M., Kahn, J.C., Huret, J.F., Gandjbakhch, I., and Bourdarias, J.P. Treatment of postmyocardial infarction angina by intra-aortic balloon pumping and emergency revascularization. *J. Thorac. Cardiovasc. Surgery* 74:299, 1977.

231. Jones, E.L., Waites, T.F., Craver, J.M., Bradford, J.M., Douglas, J.S., King, S.B., Bone, D.K., Dorney, E.R., Clements, S.D., Thompkins, T., and Hatcher, C.R. Coronary bypass for relief of persistent pain following acute myocardial infarction. *Annals Thorac. Surg.* 32:33, 1981.

232. Theroux, P., Waters, D.D., Halphen, C.,

Debaisieux, J-C, and Mizgala, H.F. Prognostic value of exercise testing soon after myocardial infarction. *N. Engl. J. Med.* 301:341, 1979.

233. Gibson, R.S., Taylor, G.J., Watson, D.D., et al. Predicting the extent and location of coronary artery disease during the early postinfarction period by quantitative thallium-201 scintigraphy. *Am. J. Cardiol.* 47:1010, 1981.

234. Leppo, J.A., O'Brien, J., Rotendler, J.A., Getchell, J.D., and Lee, V.W. Dipyridamole-thallium 201 scintigraphy in the prediction of future cardiac events after acute myocardial infarction. *N. Engl. J. Med.* 310:1014, 1984.

235. Josephson, M.A., Brown, B.G., Hecht, H.S., Hopkins, J., Pierce, C.D., and Peterson, R.B. Noninvasive detection and localization of coronary stenoses in patients: Comparison of resting dipyridamole and exercise-thallium 201 myocardial perfusion imaging. *Am. Heart J.* 103:1008, 1982.

236. Vismara, L.A., Amsterdam, E.A., and Mason, D.T. Relation of ventricular arrhythmias in the late hospital phase of acute myocardial infarction to sudden death after hospital discharge. *Am. J. Med.* 59:6, 1975.

237. Ruberman, W., Weinblatt, E., Frank, C.W., Goldberg, J.D., Shapiro, S., and Feldman, C.L. Ventricular premature beats and mortality of men with coronary heart disease. *Circulation* 52(Suppl. 3):199, 1975.

238. Kofler, M.N., Tabatznik, B.M Mower, M.M., and Tominaga, S. Prognostic significance of ventricular ectopic beats with respect to sudden death in the late post-infarction period. *Circulation* 47:959, 1973.

239. Moss, A.J., DeCamilla, J.J., Davis, H.P., and Bayer, L. Clinical significance of ventricular ectopic beats in the early post-hospital phase of myocardial infarction. *Am. J. Cardiol.* 39:635, 1977.

240. Bornheimer, J., Guzman, M.D., and Haywood, L.J. Analysis of in-hospital deaths from myocardial infarction after coronary care unit discharge. *Arch. Intern. Med.* 135:1035, 1975.

241. Anderson, K.P., DeCamilla, J., and Moss, A.J. Clinical significance of ventricular tachycardia (3 beats or longer) detected during ambulatory monitoring after myocardial infarction. *Circulation* 57:890, 1978.

242. Koch-Weser, J., Klein, S.W., Foo-Canto, L.L., Kastor, J.A., and DeSanctis, R.W. Antiarrhythmic prophylaxis with procainamide in acute myocardial infarction. *N. Engl. J. Med.* 281:1253, 1969.

243. Olson, H.G., Lyons, K.P., Troop, P., Butman, S., and Piters, K.M. The high-risk acute myocardial infarction patient at 1-year followup: Identification at hosptial discharge by ambulatory electrocardiography and radionuclide ventriculography. *A. Heart J.* 107:358, 1984.

244. The Anturane Reinfarction Trial Research Group. Sulfinpyrazone in the prevention of cardiac death after myocardial infarction. *N. Engl. J. Med.* 298:289, 1978.

# 14. SURGICAL TREATMENT OF CORONARY ARTERY DISEASE

John J. Collins, Jr.

Lawrence H. Cohn

Richard J. Shemin

The concept of surgical myocardial revascularization was initially explored by Beck [1], who observed large collateral vessels between the pericardium and the epicardium in persons who had had pericarditis in association with coronary obstructive disease. Beck reasoned that production of a pericardial inflammatory reaction might produce anastomoses between the pericardial vessels and the coronary arteries, which would provide an extraneous source of arterial blood to supply the ischemic myocardium. A variety of techniques for producing epicardial scarring and inflammation were introduced, and although some persons appeared to have symptomatic relief, it was never adequately demonstrated that the improvement of myocardial blood supply was significant in terms of relief of angina, improvement in longevity, or other criteria. The earliest attempts at direct relief of coronary arterial obstruction involved endarterectomy [2].

In 1962, Sones and Shirey [3] reported that angiography through a mammary implant pedicle in a patient who had been operated on several months previously by Vineberg [4] showed dye filling the native coronary arterial tree. On the basis of this information, the operation of mammary artery implantation rose quickly in popularity and soon became fairly widespread, at least in the United States. There were still many doubters, however, and as noted in chapter 12, a number of experimental observations

either failed to show improvement in overall myocardial blood supply or showed a lack of improvement in perfusion within the native coronary arterial system to account for the apparent improvement in symptoms of angina. It was never successfully demonstrated that internal mammary artery implantation prolonged life or reduced the subsequent incidence of myocardial infarction. DeBakey and associates [5] in 1964 and, on a large scale, Favaloro and others [7, 8] at the Cleveland Clinic had shown limited success with a variety of venous patch techniques and interposition grafts. With the introduction of the saphenous vein bypass graft operation, however, relief of angina was immediate, and the operation proved safe and effective in skilled hands and had a low mortality rate for patients with good ventricular function suffering from angina pectoris.

The utilization of saphenous vein bypass grafting for amelioration of angina pectoris and for a variety of other clinical syndromes associated with myocardial ischemia has increased greatly since the introduction of this technique. In fact, there has been some concern that the widespread utilization of revascularization surgery is inappropriate or, at least, inordinately expensive [9]. In this chapter, some of the concepts, techniques, and controversies surrounding the modern era of myocardial revascularization and the management of mechanical complications of myocardial infarction will be reviewed. Points of controversy include not only the indications for surgical therapy, discussed at length from a "medical" point of view in chapters 12 and 13, but also the methods of myocardial preservation during cardiopulmonary bypass, types of grafts used for revascularization procedures, improvement in longevity following myocardial revascularization, and additional problems of revascularization when combined with valvular surgery.

## Rationale for Myocardial Revascularization

The course of medically treated coronary obstructive disease has become a matter of great controversy. Since the initial description of angina pectoris by Heberden in 1772 [10] and the subsequent demonstration by Osler [11] and Herrick [12] of the correlation among symptoms of angina pectoris, the occurrence of myocardial infarction, and obstruction of major coronary arteries, a number of medical interventions have been aimed at alleviating discomfort and prolonging life. There is no satisfactory clinical study of any group of patients in whom no treatment was used. There is, however, remarkable uniformity in the results of medical management of patients with angina pectoris up until the introduction of $\beta$-adrenergic blocking agents, long-acting nitrates, and calcium-channel blockers. The studies of Richards et al. [13], Oberman et al. [14], Kannel and Feinlieb [15], Block et al. [16], Zukel et al. [17] showed an expected mortality of approximately 4 percent per year in patients having the clinical syndrome of angina pectoris.

Subsequent observations revealed that the mortality rate expected in persons with angiographically demonstrated coronary obstructive disease as well as the angina syndrome was approximately 6 percent per year [18–21]. These observations appear to indicate that not all patients with clinical angina pectoris have coronary obstructive disease. In most cardiac catheterization laboratories, the incidence of normal coronary anatomy in patients undergoing angiography for investigation of chest pain ranges from 15 to 35 percent [22], while about 90 percent of patients with "typical" angina have at least one coronary artery with significant obstruction. Since as many as 35 percent of patients with atypical angina may show normal coronary arter-

ies [22], a fair estimate would be that the average clinical population of patients with the anginal syndrome has an 85 percent incidence of some degree of coronary obstruction. Noninvasive studies including the utilization of exercise testing may help to identify persons with coronary obstructive disease in a population unstudied by angiography, but there still will remain a number of persons with angina who actually do not have a significant risk of death from coronary artery disease.

The effectiveness of surgical intervention can be ascertained in a reasonable manner only by comparison of surgical results with results of medical management. If general agreement does not exist regarding the prognosis with medical management in patients with various degrees of coronary obstruction, improvement with surgical management will be impossible to demonstrate. One of the great problems at the present time is achieving agreement among cardiologists as to the prognosis of medically treated patients in various categories, despite the aforementioned angiographically documented "natural history" studies [18–21]. Nevertheless, coronary bypass surgery is effective in relieving angina [23, 24], increasing exercise capacity [25, 26], and improving ventricular function at rest in some patients and with exercise in others [27, 28].

Recent publication of the Coronary Artery Surgery Study (CASS), sponsored by the National Heart, Lung and Blood Institute, provides data that may perhaps clarify the role of surgery in the management of patients with mild chronic angina pectoris and coronary artery obstruction [29]. In this prospective, randomized, controlled clinical trial, comparable patients were assigned to surgical or nonsurgical treatment and followed thereafter for 5 years. While survival was slightly more favorable for patients with single-, double-, and triple-vessel disease in the surgical group, the numbers were insufficient for this trial to be statistically significant. Among patients assigned to medical therapy, 4.7 percent per year underwent revascularization surgery. The indication for this change in therapeutic program was worsening symptoms. These patients were continued in the "medical" group. The investigators concluded "that patients similar to those enrolled in this trial can safely defer bypass surgery until symptoms worsen to the point that surgical palliation is required." While this conclusion is precisely and accurately stated, interpretation of the study has been somewhat different. The public information media especially have interpreted the study as showing that medical and surgical management produce equivalent results. This is neither the result of the study nor the stated conclusion of the investigators.

A second publication concerning the same CASS group showed that patients assigned to surgical management had significant improvement in the quality of life (relief of chest pain, improvement in subjective and objective functional status, and a diminished requirement for drug therapy) [30]. No significant effect on employment or status of recreational activities was observed.

Patients in the CASS group who had severe left ventricular dysfunction (mean ejection fraction .36) showed substantial benefit from revascularization surgery with or without myocardial resection when presenting symptoms were predominantly angina pectoris. No significant relief of symptoms caused primarily by heart failure was shown in these patients. The observed operative mortality was 6.9 percent in this high-risk group, and the investigators hastened to point out that the conclusions of the study are applicable to other centers only if the operative mortality equals or betters this figure.

## Indications for Myocardial Revascularization

The indications for utilization of myocardial revascularization surgery depend to a considerable extent on the results obtained in any individual center. If myocardial revascularization can be demonstrated to offer significant improvement in prognosis, including particularly a low operative mortality, over what may be obtained by other means, then the operation should be made available. At the present time, the indications for myocardial revascularization at the Brigham and Women's Hospital include (1) the various subsets of angina pectoris; (2) congestive heart failure (in selected patients); (3) ancil-

lary revascularization in patients with other types of cardiovascular disease, especially valvular disease; (4) prophylactic restoration of blood supply in asymptomatic patients at risk of developing new or additional complications of ischemic heart disease; (5) acute myocardial infarction with shock (left ventricular power failure); and (6) uncomplicated acute myocardial infarction in selected cases.

Patients having angina pectoris with coronary artery obstructive disease may be classified as having stable, unstable, or Prinzmetal's angina. Stable angina pectoris implies that symptoms have been present for 6 or more months, occur with exertion or other predictable excitatory stimuli, and are relieved by rest or short-acting vasodilator drugs. Angina of brief duration, changing pattern of severity, duration, or causation, occurring at rest or during sleep, is considered unstable. Similarly, angina continuing after myocardial infarction or failing to respond to in-hospital maximum medication is considered unstable. Patients with congestive heart failure secondary to myocardial ischemia may have acute intermittent failure from global ischemia, intermittent or chronic failure on the basis of valvular dysfunction, or failure due to a mechanical complication of myocardial infarction such as septal defect or left ventricular aneurysm. Patients with valvular heart disease or failure from other types of mechanical cardiac dysfunction may have significant coronary artery obstructive disease, either with or without symptoms of angina pectoris. In such instances, most surgeons recommend the performance of coronary bypass surgery, even though symptoms may be more directly related to heart failure than to coronary obstruction. Because complications of myocardial ischemia account for the majority of early deaths after surgery for peripheral vascular complications of arteriosclerosis, many surgeons now require exercise testing before resection of abdominal aneurysms or other peripheral arterial reconstructions. Patients with previous symptoms or positive stress tests are subjected to coronary angiography for either preliminary elective myocardial revascularization or, in emergencies, for simultaneous coronary bypass and peripheral vascular reconstruction.

Certain asymptomatic patients have a high risk

of ischemic complications of coronary obstructive disease. In young patients following myocardial infarction, in patients with a strongly positive exercise test, in patients with a strong family history of ischemic heart disease, and in patients with certain metabolic risk factors, there may be sufficient indication to justify coronary arteriography. Under these circumstances, the finding of significant coronary obstructions may constitute an indication for revascularization surgery. As might be expected, revascularization for asymptomatic persons is an area of even greater controversy in this already controversial choice of therapy [31, 32]. In our experience, patients who have suffered myocardial infarction without preceding angina pectoris are likely to do so again. If patients have a defective anginal warning system, surgery, or at least angiography, may be justified in the absence of angina. Results of the CASS study indicate that in patients with stable, mild angina pectoris, sudden catastrophic worsening is unlikely to occur without worsening of angina symptoms. This is an important consideration because (except for left main coronary artery obstruction) patients with severe coronary obstruction and mild angina were formerly often operated on to prevent "sudden death." The CASS study suggests that persons with stable mild angina may be safely followed until symptoms worsen, then operated on with little or no increased surgical risk.

The syndrome of cardiogenic shock or left ventricular power failure following acute myocardial infarction has been associated with such a dismal prognosis when conservative therapy is used that the effect of myocardial revascularization is of great interest. Myocardial revascularization surgery with balloon counterpulsation for circulatory assistance has been investigated in a number of centers [33–35]. There seems little doubt that the mortality from cardiogenic shock can thereby be improved, but it still remains high. The criteria that have evolved for the selection of patients with cardiogenic shock for acute surgical intervention have been carefully outlined [36]. These include adequate residual left ventricular function and collateral visualization of the obstructed artery distally. Recently, improved medical therapy and more aggressive use of balloon counterpulsation have improved

the nonoperative results in left ventricular power failure so that greater selectivity for surgical therapy should be possible.

Myocardial revascularization during or shortly after uncomplicated acute myocardial infarction has been practiced in only a few centers. Results reported by Berg and co-workers [38] did not sufficiently document an improvement in prognosis with this operation over that which might be expected in the absence of surgery to justify widespread utilization of routine angiography and operation for persons with acute evolving infarction. Certain patients, however, may well benefit from immediate operation, even occasionally without coronary angiography. For example, a young person with no previous symptoms and living an active life-style presents within an hour of the onset of pain with severe widespread anterior and lateral ECG changes of ischemia. Involvement of the anterior descending or main left coronary artery is certain. Equally certain is the inadequacy of collaterals from other areas. The possibility of an inoperable left anterior descending coronary artery is very low, probably zero, if there have been no previous symptoms at all. Prompt revascularization of the left anterior descending coronary artery and principal posterior circulation may well be the most effective means for significant myocardial preservation in those units where selective intracoronary clot lysis is not immediately available. Operation should be undertaken if obstruction of a coronary artery occurs during angiography or if the patient, after catheterization, develops infarction while awaiting surgery [39–40].

## Techniques for Revascularization Surgery

Myocardial revascularization operations provide a new source of blood supply from the proximal aorta to the native coronary artery beyond arteriosclerotic obstructions. Indirect techniques of revascularization, including mammary artery implanatation and venovenous grafts, cause blood supply to the myocardium to increase via collateral pathways.

Revascularization operations should be done with cardiopulmonary bypass and a motionless heart. Some have advocated operating on the anterior descending or right coronary artery without bypass [41], but there is little justification for this approach in most instances, since the efficacy of revascularization procedures depends on precise suturing of 1.5 to 2.0 mm vessels and the safety of cardiopulmonary bypass is excellent. Myocardial preservation during cardiopulmonary bypass surgery has been a subject of great debate in recent years. Three basic myocardial protection techniques are available for performance of the distal coronary anastomoses:

1. Segmental occlusion of the coronary artery with a perfused, fibrillated heart.
2. Intermittent aortic cross-clamping with intermittent reperfusion.
3. Continuous aortic cross-clamping with local cardiac hypothermia and cardioplegia.

Experimentally, the third technique is superior in the dog or in isolated heart preparations [42–44], but clinically, no significant difference has been noted in centers where more than one technique was used by expert surgeons [45–47].

Some surgeons perform the proximal aortovenous anastomoses first, believing pump time is decreased. We believe the distal anastomoses should be done first, because maximum flexibility and exposure for the most important anastomoses should be the rule.

SAPHENOUS VEIN GRAFTS

By far the most common technique for myocardial revascularization involves the utilization of autogenous saphenous vein grafts. In most instances, these vein grafts provide a single conduit to each artery through a proximal aortic anastomosis and a distal end-to-side coronary artery anastomosis. We use continuous monofilament suture, although some surgeons utilize interrupted sutures (figure 14–1). The difference in results of these techniques in the hands of surgeons of comparable skill appears to be negligible.

More recently introduced is the technique of side-to-side anastomosis between saphenous vein segments and the native coronary arteries (figure 14–2). Use of this technique enables revascularization of several coronary artery branches with a single saphenous vein graft segment, thereby ob-

viating multiple individual aortic anastomoses [48–49]. The usual technique involves selection of a coronary artery branch in which high flow is expected for the distal end-to-side anastomosis. The vein graft is then led in a gently looping fashion over the surface of the heart, and as it crosses the site of other obstructed coronary artery branches, side-to-side anatomoses are constructed in a sequential fashion. The vein is eventually led to the ascending aorta, where an anastomosis is made. Three or four or more anastomoses to a single vein segment may be constructed. The advantages of such a configuration include a higher flow through the proximal anastomosis, which should contribute to the maintenance of patency in the proximal portion of the vein. The possibility of revascularization of multiple coronary arterial branches is also more easily realized than it would be with a greater number of individual end-to-side grafts, each requiring a separate aortic anastomosis. In addition, it is possible that the side-to-side anastomosis may tend to stay open more reliably when the flow through the graft as a whole is higher than would be obtained if an individual graft were used to a low runoff branch. Excellent patency rates with multiple sequential anastomoses have been reported [50, 51]. One cautionary note in the utilization of sequential anastomoses is that the vein may easily be kinked at the site of an anastomosis. It is desirable to avoid twists and transverse venous incisions of more than half the diameter of the vein.

For patients in whom the greater saphenous vein is not usable as an autogenous graft, the cephalic or brachial veins from the arms may be utilized. The lesser saphenous vein, which might not have been removed in previous vein strippings, is often excellent. The arm veins have a considerably thinner wall than the saphenous vein and are more difficult to work with in general. Patency rates following utilization of arm veins are not available, although the clinical course of patients with such grafts appears to be satisfactory.

INTERNAL MAMMARY ARTERY AND OTHER ARTERIAL GRAFTS

The most commonly used alternative to the saphenous vein for revascularization of the ante-

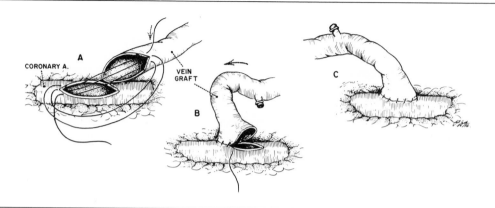

rior descending coronary artery is the left internal mammary artery. Green [52] and associates popularized direct mammary anastomosis to the native coronary circulation, and such grafts provide excellent revascularization of the anterior descending and diagonal branches of the anterior descending coronary artery with excellent long-term patency [53–55]. The mammary artery can also be utilized for marginal branches of the circumflex system. The right coronary artery is not easily revascularized by the right internal mammary because the length of the mammary on that side is often not sufficient to achieve an

FIGURE 14-1. Distal end-to-side venoarterial coronary bypass anastomosis using continuous suture. (From Cohn, L.H., Surgical Techniques of Emergency Coronary Revascularization. In Cohn, L.H. (ed.), *The Treatment of Acute Myocardial Ischemia: An Integrated Medical-Surgical Approach.* Mt. Kisco, N.Y.: Futura, 1979.)

anastomosis distal to all atheromatous plaques. The indications for use of the internal mammary artery as a coronary bypass vessel have undergone modifications, as experience and follow-up with this procedure have grown [56]. Multiple sequential anastomoses using the internal mammary have sometimes been used, and in selected patients this technique may offer a significant alternative to multiple vein grafts [57]. The mammary artery should be equal to or greater in size than the native coronary to which it is attached, and the free flow should be more than 100 ml/min. It should not be used in patients with diffuse fibrotic ventricles, where there is poor distal runoff, or where there is left ventricular hypertrophy. Long-term patency of internal mammary artery grafts has been excellent, with relative freedom from the intimal hyperplasia and accelerated atherosclerosis so often observed in vein grafts [58]. Mammary artery grafts have remained patent even when connected to small, diffusely diseased coronary arteries with limited runoff where vein grafts have proved very disappointing.

The right internal mammary artery has also been removed from its origin and reanastomosed to the ascending aorta in some patients [59]. This is a technically difficult operation. Other systemic arteries have also been used

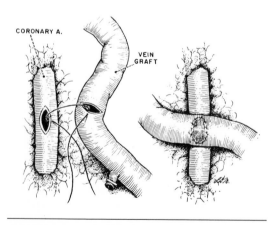

FIGURE 14-2. Side-to-side venoarterial coronary bypass anastomosis using continuous suture. (From Cohn, L.H., Surgical Techniques of Emergency Coronary Revascularization. In Cohn, L.H. (ed.), *The Treatment of Acute Myocardial Ischemia: An Integrated Medical-Surgical Approach.* Mt. Kisco, N.Y.: Futura, 1979.)

from time to time for aortocoronary conduits, the most common of which has been the radial artery [60]. The operation to remove the radial artery, however, produces a considerable amount of scarring in the forearm and is not a generally useful procedure because of poor long-term patency [61].

## OTHER SOURCES OF GRAFTS
Some surgeons have utilized homograft veins for bypass conduits. These appear to have a higher failure rate than that which is expected with autogenous saphenous veins [62]. In the absence of any other useful conduit, such an operation may be justifiable. A few operations have been done using prosthetic materials for tubular grafts between the aorta and native coronary arteries [63]. We have utilized polytetrafluoroethylene (Gore-Tex) for such grafts in five patients and had acceptable clinical results in three [64]. Although the Gore-Tex grafts may offer a measurable advantage over woven cloth grafts in small-diameter vascular bypasses, the tendency to early closure is sufficiently great that all other possibilities should be explored and exhausted before prosthetic grafts are used.

## INDIRECT MYOCARDIAL REVASCULARIZATION TECHNIQUES
The indirect techniques of myocardial revascularization are no longer widely used. Mammary artery implantation of a vascularized pedicle into the ventricular myocardium enjoyed an era of popularity from about 1962 through 1969, but then more direct methods of revascularization became available. That some persons were considerably benefited by mammary artery implantation is of little doubt, and in a number of isolated instances a patient's life was demonstrated to be dependent on the mammary implant [65]. In some patients with diffuse coronary artery disease, mammary implantation may still be useful, particularly in the area of distribution of the circumflex coronary artery, to supplement other more direct methods of myocardial revascularization.

The utilization of grafts into the coronary venous system from the aorta has undergone occasional clinical trial [66]. Although some success has been reported with this method of revascularization, it has not been widely utilized. The early experience of Beck and Leighninger [67] in the employment of venous revascularization suggested that arterialization of the coronary venous system was likely to be followed by early closure.

## CORONARY ARTERY DILATATION
The concept of arterial dilatation, which was originally proposed by Dotter and Judkins [68], has had a renaissance with the development by Gruntzig and colleagues [69] of balloon catheters for percutaneous transluminal angioplasty. The technique is discussed fully in chapter 9. The characteristics of lesions likely to be benefited by dilatation include absence of calcification, smooth contours of the arterial wall, absence of distal obstruction, and, preferably, adequate blood supply by other uninvolved arteries to make the possibility of acute complications unlikely in the event of dilatation failure. Nevertheless, cardiac surgery must be available on a "standby" basis in case such emergencies do arise. The morphology of atherosclerotic coronary arteries after balloon dilatation suggests that the intima is disrupted with splitting of the plaque. In some patients serial angiograms have shown progressive increase in lumen diameter over several months after dilatation. For this reason, intraoperative balloon angioplasty has been used to extend the benefits of coronary bypass surgery [70–71]. Some success has also been reported in dilatation of anastamotic stenosis or lesions occurring in vein bypass conduits [72].

## Results of Myocardial Revascularization Surgery
The results of operations for myocardial revascularization may be expressed in terms of angina relief, improved longevity, lessening of ventricular arrhythmias, improvement of life-style, improvement in exercise capacity, and reduction of overall cost of medical treatment of arteriosclerotic heart disease.

### RELIEF OF PAIN
The relief of angina pectoris may be expected as an initial operative benefit in approximately 90 percent of persons undergoing revascularization

for chronic or acute anginal syndromes [23, 24]. Over the subsequent years, angina will recur in some patients and in most instances will not be as severe as that prior to surgery. This is to be expected in a progressive metabolic disease, the basic defect of which is not altered by mechanical introduction of a new blood supply. Return of angina can be due to progression of disease in nonoperated vessels or distal to the anastomosis in operated vessels, as well as to graft closure [73–75]. Graft closure within the first year after operation (about 10 percent of total grafts) is usually related to technical factors such as vein size and quality, adequacy of anastomosis, recipient vessel size, and runoff. Grafts patent at 1 year are likely to be patent at 5 years. Late graft closure is related to intimal hyperplasia or atherosclerosis in vein conduits or to progression of atherosclerosis in recipient arteries.

Figure 14–3 shows the pattern of recurrence of angina pectoris following revascularization in 637 patients with acute or chronic angina operated on between July 1970 and June 1976 at the Peter Bent Brigham Hospital. The number of patients at each annual interval in the 6 years following surgery is indicated. The incidence of death, severe angina, moderate angina, mild angina, or absence of angina for each group represents a cumulative total for that group of patients. Patients with mild angina are those who have occasional discomfort but take no medication. Those with moderate angina take medication on an occasional or moderately frequent basis, but they take no

medication or only a small amount of $\beta$-blockers on a regular basis. Patients with severe angina pectoris are those whose life-styles are severely altered or who take large amounts of medication for control of angina pectoris. Figure 14–3 clearly shows that angina tends to recur following coronary bypass surgery, but that more than 60 percent of patients are still significantly relieved 6 years after surgery. Reoperation has become increasingly common. Earlier data suggested that the best results for reoperation would be obtained in patients with a new or previously not bypassed critical lesion [76]. Increased experience and technical improvements in reoperation surgery have led to lower operative risk (2 to 5 percent), more complete revascularization, better symptomatic relief, and improved long-term survival [77].

## Improved Longevity

Longevity following coronary bypass surgery has been generally regarded as significantly improved over medical treatment in those patients with left main coronary artery disease and angina pectoris [78, 79]. Longevity improvement in patients with other types of coronary obstructive disease, however, has not been conclusively determined, although a number of surgical reports have indicated strikingly good long-term results compared with unmatched controls or with those expected from United States life expectancy tables [80–82]. The Veterans Administration National Cooperative Study published in 1977 [84] indicated no difference in medical versus surgical long-term mortality in patients with stable angina, probably because operative mortality of surgical patients was too high and the follow-up period too short. However, in other groups of patients with more severe coronary obstructive disease and less adequate ventricular function who were operated on by us as well as by others, an encouraging improvement in longevity compared to that of the Veterans Administration medical group can be demonstrated in various reports. Our own results in patients with three-vessel, two-vessel, and one-vessel coronary obstructive disease (figures 14–4, 14–5, 14–6) indicate a high probability that life is

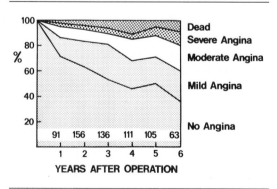

FIGURE 14–3. Pattern of cumulative angina recurrence observed after coronary bypass surgery during 1970 to 1976.

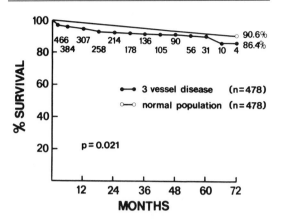

FIGURE 14–4. Actuarial analysis of survival in patients with three-vessel coronary obstruction compared with that of age- and sex-matched normal population. (From Collins, J.J., Jr. et al. In Mason, D.T. (ed.), *Advances In Heart Disease,* Vol. 3. New York: Grune & Stratton, 1980.)

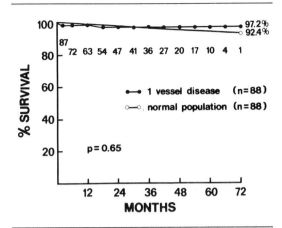

FIGURE 14–6. Actuarial analysis of survival in patients with single-vessel coronary obstruction compared with that of age- and sex-matched normal population. (From Collins, J.J., Jr., et al. In Mason, D.T. (ed.), *Advances in Heart Disease,* Vol.3. New York: Grune & Stratton, 1980.)

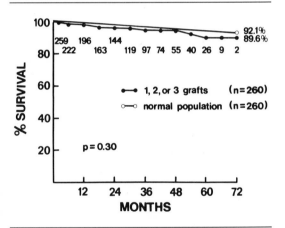

FIGURE 14–5. Actuarial analysis of survival in patients with two-vessel coronary obstruction compared with that of age- and sex-matched normal population. (From Collins, J.J., Jr., et al. In Mason, D.T. (ed.), *Advances in Heart Disease,* Vol. 3. New York: Grune & Stratton, 1980.)

prolonged in both three-vessel and two-vessel coronary artery disease[85].

The Coronary Artery Surgery Study (CASS) cited earlier analyzed 780 patients randomized between medical and surgical therapy and has helped to clarify the approach to patients with mild to moderate angina and to angina-free survivors of myocardial infarction with surgically operable single-, two-, or three-vessel coronary artery disease [29]. This group also includes patients with good ventricular function. The annual risk was 1.1 percent for surgical patients and 1.6 percent for medical patients. A small subgroup of patients with ejection fractions of less than 50 percent but greater than 35 percent revealed a statistically nonsignificant advantage for patients assigned to surgical therapy. The decision to proceed to bypass surgery in these patients was based upon the level of symptoms. Medical management was continued until symptoms worsened, and then coronary artery bypass grafting was performed. The excellent survival in the medical group at 5 years included 23 percent of medical patients who crossed over to the surgical therapy group.

The European Collaborative Study of three-vessel-disease patients having ejection fractions greater than 50 percent demonstrated an improved survival for surgical patients versus medical patients. In addition, there appeared to be an advantage for patients with two-vessel disease treated surgically if there was a high grade left anterior descending coronary occlusion [86]. The incidence of further infarction was the same in the medical and surgical groups, but the incidence of fatal infarction was significantly lower in surgically treated patients.

IMPROVED LIFE-STYLE

One of the major questions that has arisen relative to the results of coronary surgery is the impact of such operations on the life-style of patients following surgery. This question is complex, since the interpretation of "life-style" varies greatly from person to person. In an admittedly limited approach, we recently asked 637 patients by personal interview what they considered their life-style to be; the results are shown in fig. 14–7. The data clearly show that most patients found their life-style generally satisfactory, even at 6 years following coronary surgery, although limitation of life-style did increase somewhat as time passed following surgery. Improvement in quality of life as measured by relief of angina, improved subjective and objective assessment of functional status, and reduced requirement for drug therapy were found in surgical patients in the CASS study as well, although no apparent significant effect was shown on employment or recreational status [87].

ARRHYTHMIAS

Evidence presently shows that the absolute incidence of ventricular premature beats as well as the pattern of occurrence of ventricular ectopic activity do not seem to be altered by coronary bypass surgery in most patients [88]. This is an interesting observation in view of the fact that the incidence of sudden death in patients with coronary obstructive disease has been correlated with the occurrence of ventricular ectopic rhythm. The incidence of sudden death in patients who have undergone coronary bypass surgery appears to be lower than that of medically managed patients with similar degrees of coronary obstruction [89].

"COST-BENEFIT" ESTIMATES TO SOCIETY

Finally, the point has been made that even if coronary bypass surgery were shown to improve longevity as well as promote relief of angina and improve life-style, the enormous costs of such operations simply could not be borne by society [90]. This argument has been expanded in scope to include various theoretical calculations of costs based upon the large numbers of operations that might be done considering the size of the population having angina pectoris. Conversely, no data are readily available to indicate what the cost of management of such persons might be without surgery. An attempt to derive some information comparing the cost of surgery to the cost of medical management in similar patients has been reported from our institution [91]. In 100 consecutive patients operated on for chronic angina pectoris, hospitalization postoperatively was found to be significantly less frequent and less costly. The expense of surgery could be amortized over a 4-year period by the amount saved from a decreased hospitalization rate after surgery. Attempts to assess the probability of return to gainful employment have not shown a positive influence of coronary bypass surgery as compared to medical management. Significant nonmedical variables appear to influence substantially the likelihood of return to work after coronary surgery. These include preoperative work status, nonwork income, occupation, age, and education. While relief of symptoms is also a significant factor, the number and importance of variables unrelated to health are sufficiently confounding that, despite better symptom relief, surgical patients are, overall, probably less likely to return to work [92, 93].

## Combined Valvular Disease and Coronary Artery Obstruction

Development of the technique for coronary artery bypass has brought about a major improvement in surgical risk for those patients afflicted with both significant valve dysfunction and coronary artery obstruction. The majority

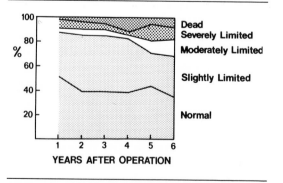

FIGURE 14–7. Responses of 637 postoperative patients to the question, "How is your life-style?"

of such patients have valvular disease of rheumatic or congenital origin, and the presence of significant coronary obstruction is incidental, though often important. Angina pectoris may occur with or without significant coronary obstructive disease, and significant coronary obstruction may exist in the absence of angina. In a group of patients from the Peter Bent Brigham Hospital with aortic valve disease, angina was a symptom in approximately 60 percent, regardless of whether the lesion produced stenosis, insufficiency, or both [94]. Significant coronary obstruction according to angiographic criteria was found in 21 percent of patients with aortic stenosis (33 percent of those with angina), 28 percent of patients with mixed lesions (42 percent of those with angina), and 14 percent with aortic insufficiency (22 percent of those with angina). These data are at variance with our general impression that angina is less common in aortic regurgitation and is more likely to be associated with coronary artery obstruction when present.

A remarkable diversity of opinion supported by studies on relatively small patient populations has appeared in the literature [95–97], from all of which one may eventually conclude that (1) the probability of coronary artery lesions in patients with valvular heart disease increases with age and the presence of angina pectoris (or history of myocardial infarction), and it is higher in association with isolated aortic valve disease than with other lesions; and (2) in the absence of angina pectoris, significant coronary obstructive disease is unlikely, though possible, in patients with rheumatic valve lesions.

The question of whether "routine" coronary angiography should be performed before valve replacement surgery is easy to answer; in our opinion, it need not be done. When a combination of youth, rheumatic lesions, and absence of angina is present, coronary arteriography is unnecessary. All older patients with isolated aortic valve disease and a history of angina pectoris should have coronary angiography. For patients with various combinations other than these, individual judgment will be necessary. The risk of angiography as well as the factors already mentioned must be considered.

Significant obstructions in coronary arteries supplying substantial portions of myocardium should be bypassed at the time of valve replacement surgery. It is neither necessary nor advisable to place a graft on every small obstructed tributary, but the anterior descending artery and dominant posterior vessels should be well perfused if there is to be a high incidence of satisfactory surgical results. The safety of combined valve replacement and coronary bypass surgery has been well documented, although the late survival of patients with extensive coronary obstructive disease is likely to be poorer than what is usually observed after valve replacement [98–101]. However, one large series has been recently reported with comparable survival [102].

Valvular dysfunction due to myocardial ischemia is seen only with the mitral valve. Intermittent mitral insufficiency may occur with papillary muscle ischemia to the point of producing pulmonary edema in the absence of papillary muscle infarction. Such patients may experience long-term improvement by revascularization alone. More commonly, significant mitral valve dysfunction is associated with papillary muscle rupture or fibrosis. The prognosis for most patients with mitral insufficiency following myocardial infarction is often poor when progressive congestive heart failure is also present—if the acute episode itself does not prove fatal [103]. The risk of valve replacement in such patients is higher than usual, and the long-term outlook is less optimistic than in patients with rheumatic disease [104].

It has become our practice to perform the indicated coronary bypasses before proceeding to valve replacement, because manipulation of the heart is easier and the attached grafts may be used for infusion of iced cardioplegic solution during the valve replacement. The heart is cooled additionally by constant external and intermittent internal application of iced saline solution (4°C) with the patient on cardiopulmonary bypass at 28 or 30°C. A single period of aortic clamping is customary. The grafts are anastomosed to the ascending aorta during rewarming using a partially occluding clamp to allow flow through the native coronary arterial bed throughout the warming phase.

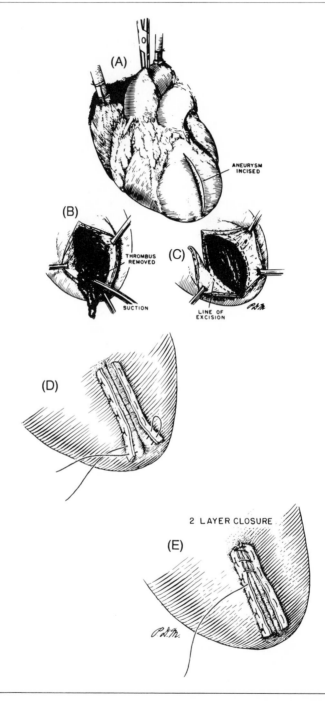

FIGURE 14–8. Surgical technique for excision of left ventricular aneurysm and repair of resulting defect. (From Collins, J.J., Jr. et al., Surgical Management of Mechanical Complications of Myocardial Infarction. In Cohn, L.H. (ed.), *The Treatment of Acute Myocardial Ischemia: An Integrated Medical-Surgical Approach.* Mt. Kisco, N.Y.: Futura, 1979.)

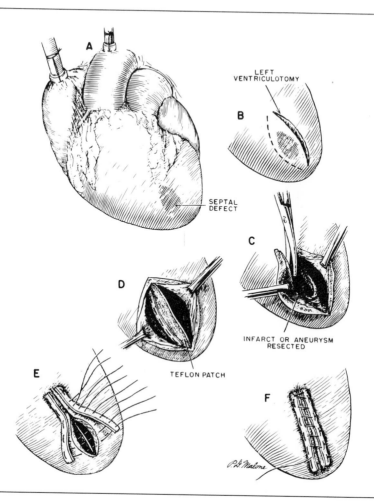

FIGURE 14–9. Repair of postinfarction ventricular septal defect. (From Collins, J.J., Jr. et al., Surgical Management of Mechanical Complications of Myocardial Infarction. In Cohn, L.H. (ed.), *The Treatment of Acute Myocardial Ischemia: An Integrated Medical-Surgical Approach.* Mt. Kisco, N.Y.: Futura, 1979.)

## Surgery for Mechanical Complications of Myocardial Infarction

Mechanical complications of myocardial infarction include diffuse myocardial contractility disturbances resulting in shock or heart failure, discrete left ventricular aneurysms, mitral regurgitation secondary to papillary muscle dysfunction (discussed previously), and myocardial rupture.

Diffuse myocardial contractility disturbances resulting in pump failure may be seen in patients with infarction or severe ischemia of 40 percent or more of the left ventricular mass. Acute loss of large areas of myocardium results in cardiogenic shock, whereas progressive loss by multiple, smaller infarctions may result in progressive congestive heart failure with ventricular dilation and eventual death due to low cardiac output.

The likelihood of substantial functional improvement in left ventricular performance with revascularization surgery is even less in patients with chronic, inexorable heart failure than in patients with cardiogenic shock. We do not advocate operating on persons with congestive heart failure of a chronic sort to improve left ventricular function when the cause of left ventricular failure appears to be diffuse hypokinesis. If such patients have severe angina pectoris, surgery can often be performed successfully to

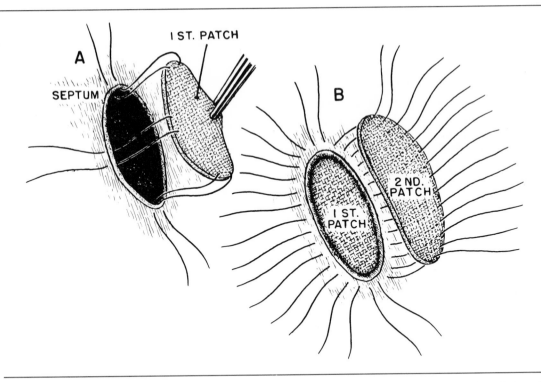

FIGURE 14-10. Double patch ("sandwich") technique for repair of early postinfarction ventricular septal defect. (From Collins, J.J., Jr. et al., Surgical Management of Mechanical Complications of Myocardial Infarction. In Cohn, L.H. (ed.), *The Treatment of Acute Myocardial Ischemia: An Integrated Medical-Surgical Approach.* Mt. Kisco, N.Y.: Futura, 1979.)

relieve angina, but functional improvement in left ventricular mechanics is not likely to be great.

Left ventricular aneurysm developing as a complication of myocardial infarction tends to be a progressive problem and is manifested by congestive heart failure in most patients. One may also see the occurrence of arrhythmias or, on occasion, embolism. The major functional impairment is congestive heart failure, and resection of left ventricular aneurysm for treatment of congestive heart failure can be expected to meet with a high degree of success (figure 14–8). Long-term follow-up of large numbers of such patients has not been carried out. Some patients really do quite well, while others appear to deteriorate within a year or two after surgery. The key to prognosis appears to be integrity of the residual myocardium and sufficiency of blood supply as provided by either intact native coronary circulation or functioning bypass grafts to the remaining viable myocardium. The functional result is likely to be best when the aneurysm has a quite localized origin and there is normally contractile muscle in other areas [105,

106]. The result will be less beneficial if the remainder of the myocardium is already diffusely scarred or if there is diffuse obstruction in the coronary arteries to the remaining myocardium.

Myocardial rupture may cause acute cardiogenic shock with early demise, or it may be tolerated for some period of time after its onset. A considerable literature has described occasional surgical success in the repair of a ventricular septal defect early after myocardial infarction, although this is a technically more difficult operation with a less certain outcome than the operation for repair of such defects in patients who have managed to survive for a few weeks or months (Figure 14–9 and 14–10). Rupture of the free wall of the left ventricle into the pericardium may, in some instances, occur with enough warning so that surgical repair should be possible. In many instances, however, the occurrence of rupture is not recognized until fatal tamponade supervenes.

## Conclusions

There seems to be little doubt that myocardial dysfunction manifested by angina pectoris and myocardial infarction is primarily a result of mechanical impediment to blood supply caused by arteriosclerotic narrowing of the coronary arteries. In many instances, the coronary arteries beyond the obstruction are sufficiently large to be amenable to bypass operations utilizing saphenous veins or mammary arteries as conduits. If patients are treated by bypass operations at a stage of development of coronary obstructive disease when the distal vessels are still relatively normal and before diffuse myocardial damage occurs, the relief of symptoms of myocardial ischemia as well as protection from myocardial infarction and improvement of longevity may be expected. The inexorable tendency to progression of arteriosclerosis continues to influence long-term results, however. Surgery for complications of myocardial infarction appears to be helpful only when certain mechanical defects (such as a ruptured ventricular septum) can be corrected.

## References

1. Beck, C.S. The development of a new blood supply to the heart by operation. *Ann. Surg.* 102:801, 1935.
2. Bailey, C.P., May, A., and Levinson, W.M. Survival after coronary and endarterectomy in man. *JAMA* 164:641, 1957.
3. Sones, F.M., Jr. and Shirey, E.K. Cine coronary angiography. *Mod. Concepts Cardiovasc. Dis.* 31:735, 1962.
4. Vineberg, A. Development of anastomoses between the coronary vessels and a transplanted internal mammary artery. *Can. Med. Assoc. J.* 55:117, 1946.
5. DeBakey, M., Garrett, H.E., and Dennis, E.W. Aorto-coronary bypass with saphenous vein graft. Seven-year followup. *JAMA* 233:792, 1973.
6. Favaloro, R.G. Saphenous vein graft in the surgical treatment of coronary artery disease. *J. Thorac. Cardiovasc. Surg.* 58:178, 1969.
7. Effler, D.P., Sones, F.M., Jr., Favaloro, R., and Groves, L.K. Coronary endarterectomy with patch graft reconstruction. *Ann. Surg.* 162:590, 1965.
8. Favaloro, R.G. Saphenous vein autograph replacement of severe segmental coronary artery occlusion. *Ann. Thorac. Surg.* 5:334, 1968.
9. Braunwald, E.B. Coronary artery surgery at the crossroads. *N. Engl. J. Med.* 297:661, 1977.
10. Heberden, W. Some account of a disorder in the breast. *Med. Trans. Coll. Physicians* (London) 2:59, 1772.
11. Osler, W. *Lectures on Angina Pectoris and Allied States.* Edinburgh and London: Pentland, 1897, and New York: D. Appleton, 1897.
12. Herrick, J.B. Clinical features of sudden obstruction of the coronary arteries. *JAMA* 59:2015, 1912.
13. Richards, D.W., Bland, E.F., and White, P.D. A completed twenty-five year follow-up study of 456 patients with angina pectoris. *J. Chronic Dis.* 4:423, 1956.
14. Oberman, A., Jones, W.B., Riley, C.P., Reeves, T.J., Sheffield, L.T., and Turner, M.E. Natural history of coronary artery disease. *Bull. N.Y. Acad. Med.* 48:1109, 1972.
15. Kannel, W.B. and Feinlieb, M. Natural history of angina pectoris in the Framingham study: Prognosis and survival. *Am. J. Cardiol.* 29:154, 1972.
16. Block, W.J., Jr., Crumpacker, E.L., Dry, I. J., and Gage, R.P. Prognosis of angina pectoris. Observations in 6,882 cases. *JAMA* 150:259, 1952.
17. Zukel, W.J., Cohen, B.M., Mattingly, T.W., and Hrubec, Z. Survival following first diagnosis of coronary heart disease. *Am. Heart J.* 78:159, 1969.
18. Reeves, T.J., Oberman, A., Jones, W.B., and Sheffield, L.T. Natural history of angina pectoris. *Am. J. Cardiol.* 33:423, 1974.
19. Proudfit, W.J., Bruschke, A.V.G., MacMillan, J.P., Williams, G.W., and Sones, F.M., Jr. Fifteen year survival study of patients with obstructive coronary artery disease. *Circulation* 68:986, 1983.
20. Webster, J.A., Moberg, C., and Rincon, G. Natural history of severe proximal coronary artery disease documented by coronary cine angiography. *Am. J. Cardiol.* 33:195, 1974.
21. Bruggraf, G.W. and Parker, J.O. Prognosis in coronary artery disease. Angiographic, hemodynamic and clinical factors. *Circulation* 51:146, 1975.
22. Kemp, H.G., Vokonas, P.S., Cohn, P.F., and Gorlin, R. The anginal syndrome associated with normal coronary angiograms. *Am. J. Med.* 54:735, 1973.
23. Barboriak, J.J., Hughes, C.V., Anderson, A.J., and Rimm, A.A. Effect of aortocoronary bypass

operation on factors precipitating angina. *J. Thorac. Cardiovasc. Surg.* 75:47, 1978.

24. Chatterjee, K., Matloff, J.M., and Swan, H.J.C. Improved angina threshold and coronary reserve following direct revascularization. *Circulation* 51 (Suppl. 1):81, 1975.

25. Barry, W.H., Pfeifer, J.F., Lipton, J.J., Tikian, A.G., and Hultgren, H.V. Effects of coronary artery bypass grafting on resting and exercise hemodynamics in patients with unstable angina. *Am. J. Cardiol.* 37:823, 1976.

26. Siegel, W., Lim, L.S., Proudfit, W.L., Sheldon, W.C., and Loop, F.D. The spectrum of exercise testing and angiographic correlations in myocardial revascularization surgery. *Circulation* 51 (Suppl. 1):156, 1975.

27. Kent, K.M., Borer, J.S., Green, M.V., Bacharach, S.L., McIntosh, C.L., Conkle, D.M., and Epstein, S.E. Effects of coronary artery bypass on global and regional left ventricular function during exercise. *N. Engl. J. Med.* 298:-1434, 1978.

28. Brundage, B.H., Massie, B.M., and Botvinick, E.H. Improved regional ventricular function after successful surgical revascularization. *J. Am. Coll. Cardiol.* 3:902, 1984.

29. CASS principal investigators and their associates. Coronary Artery Surgery Study (CASS): A randomized trial of coronary artery bypass surgery. Survival Data. *Circulation* 68:939, 1983.

30. Alderman, E.L., Fisher, L.D., Litwin, P., Kaiser, G.C., Myers, W.O., Maynard, C., Levine, F., and Schloss, M. Results of coronary artery surgery in patients with poor left ventricular function (CASS). *Circulation* 68:785, 1983.

31. Wynne, J., Cohn, L.H., Collins, J.J., Jr., and Cohn, P.F. Myocardial revascularization in patients with multivessel coronary artery disease and minimal angina pectoris. *Circulation* 58(Suppl. 1):92, 1978.

32. Johnson, W.D., Hoffman, J.F., Jr., and Shore, R.T. Myocardial revascularization in the absence of cardiac symptoms. *Am. J. Cardiol.* 39:-268, 1977.

33. McEnany, W.T., Kayn, H.R., Buckley, M.J., Daggett, W.M., Erdmann, A.J., Mundth, E.D., Rao, R.S., Detoeuf, J., and Austen, W.G. Clinical experience with intra-aortic balloon pump support in 728 patients. *Circulation* 58 (Suppl. 1):124, 1978.

34. Lamberti, J.J., Cohn, L.H., Lesch, M., and Collins, J.J. Intra-aortic balloon counterpulsation for postoperative left ventricular power failure: Indications and long-term results. *Arch. Surg.* 109:766, 1974.

35. Weintraub, R.M., Voukydis, P.C., Aroesty, J.M., Cohen, S.I., Ford, P., Kurland, G.S., LaRaia, P.J., Morkin, E., and Paulin, S. Treatment of preinfarction angina with intra-aortic balloon counterpulsation and surgery. *Am. J. Cardiol.* 34:809, 1974.

36. Hutter, A.M., Jr., Gold, A.K., Leinbach, R.C., Buckley, M.J., and Austen, W.G. Various Uses of Intra-aortic Balloon Pump in Acute Myocardial Infarction. In Kaindl, F., (ed.), *The First 24 Hours in Myocardial Infarction.* New York: Verlag Gerhard Witzrock, 1977, p. 169.

37. Hageimeijer, F., Laird, J.D., Haalebos, M.M.P., and Hugenholtz, P.G. Effectiveness of intra-aortic balloon pumping without cardiac surgery for patients with severe heart failure secondary to a recent myocardial infarction. *Am. J. Cardiol.* 40:951, 1977.

38. Berg, R., Kendall, R.W., Duvoisin, L., Ganji, J.H., Rudy, L.W., and Everhart, F.J. Acute myocardial infarction—a surgical emergency. *J. Thorac. Cardiovasc. Surg.* 70:432, 1975.

39. Cohn, L.H., Gorlin, R., Herman, M.V., and Collins, J.J., Jr. Aortocoronary bypass for acute coronary occlusion. *J. Thorac. Cardiovasc. Surg.* 64:503, 1972.

40. Pifarre, R., Spinazzola, A., Nemickas, H., Scanlon, P.J., and Tobin, J.R. Emergency aortocoronary bypass for acute myocardial infarction. *Arch. Surg.* 103:525, 1971.

41. Ankeney, J.L. To use or not to use the pump oxygenator in coronary bypass operations. *Ann. Thorac. Surg.* 19:108, 1975.

42. Gay, W.A. and Ebert, P.A. Functional metabolic and morphologic effects of potassium-induced cardioplegia. *Surgery* 74:284, 1973.

43. Kappelman, M.D. and Hewitt, R.L. Protection of the ischemic heart with energy substrate and potassium during cardiopulmonary bypass. *Surg. Forum* 25:153, 1974.

44. Mundth, E.D., Goel, I.P., Morgan, R.J., McEnany, M.T., and Austen, W.G. Effect of potassium cardioplegia and hypothermia on left ventricular function in hypertrophied and nonhypertrophied hearts. *Surg. Forum* 26:257, 1975.

45. Koster, J.K., Jr., Cohn, L.H., Collins, J.J., Jr., Sanders, J.H., Muller, J.E., and Young, E. Continuous hypothermic arrest versus intermittent ischemia for myocardial protection during coronary revascularization. *Ann. Thorac. Surg.* 24:330, 1977.

46. Adams, P.X., Cunningham, J.N., Jr., Brazier, J., Pappis, M., Trehan, N., and Spencer, F.C. Technique and experience using potassium cardioplegia during myocardial revascularization for pre-infarction angina. *Surgery* 83:12, 1978.

47. Adappa, M.G., Jacobson, L.B., Hetzer, R., Hill, J.D., Kamm, B., and Kerth, W.J. Cold hyperkalemic cardiac arrest versus intermittent aortic crossclamping and topical hypothermia for coronary bypass surgery. *J. Thorac. Cardiovasc. Surg.* 75:171, 1978.

48. Flemma, R.J., Johnson, W.D., and Lepley, D., Jr. Triple aorto-coronary vein bypass for coronary insufficiency. *Arch. Surg.* 103:82, 1971.

49. Bartley, T.D., Bigelow, J.C., and Page, U.S. Aorto-coronary bypass grafting with multiple sequential anastomoses to a single vein. *Arch. Surg.* 105:915, 1972.

50. Grondin, C.M. and Linet, R. Sequential anastomoses in coronary artery grafting: Technical aspects and early and late angiographic results. *Ann. Thorac. Surg.* 23:1, 1977.

51. Bigelow, J.C., Bartley, T.D., Page, U.D., and Krause, A.H. Long-term follow-up of sequential aortocoronary venous grafts. *Ann. Thorac. Surg.* 22:507, 1976.

52. Green, G.E. Internal mammary artery to coronary artery anastomosis. *Ann. Thorac. Surg.* 14:260, 1972.

53. Loop, F.D., Irarrazaval, M.J., Bredee, J.J., Siegel, W., Taylor, P.C., and Sheldon, W.C. Internal mammary artery graft for ischemic heart disease. Effect of revascularization on clinical status and survival. *Am. J. Cardiol.* 39:516, 1977.

54. Kay, E.B., Naraghipour, H., Beg, R.A., DeManey, M., Tambe, A., and Zimmerman, H.A. Internal mammary artery bypass graft. *Ann. Thorac. Surg.* 18:269, 1974.

55. Tector, A.J., Davis, L., Gabriel, R., Gale, H., Singh, H., and Flemma, R. Experience with internal mammary artery grafts in 298 patients. *Ann. Thorac. Surg.* 22:515, 1976.

56. Barner, H.B., Swartz, M.T., Mudd, J.G., and Tyras, D.H. Late patency of internal mammary artery as a coronary artery bypass conduit. *Ann. Thorac. Surg.* 34:408, 1982.

57. Lytle, B.W., Cosgrove, D.M., Saltus, G.L., Taylor, P.C., and Loop, F.D. Multivessel coronary revascularization without saphenous vein: Long term results of bilateral internal mammary artery grafting. *Ann. Thorac. Surg.* 36:540, 1983.

58. Okies, J.E., Page, U.S., Bigelow, J.C., Krause, A.H., and Salomon, N.W. The left internal mammary artery: the graft of choice. *Circulation* 70(suppl. I):213, 1984.

59. Loop, F.D., Spampinato, N., Cheanverchai, C., and Effler, D.B. Free internal mammary artery bypass grafts: The use of the IMA in the aorto-coronary position. *Ann. Thorac. Surg.* 15:50, 1973.

60. Carpentier, A., Guermonprez, J.L., DeLoche, A., Frechette, C., and DuBost, C. The aorto-to-coronary radial artery bypass graft: A technique avoiding pathological changes in grafts. *Ann. Thorac. Surg.* 16:111, 1973.

61. Chiu, C. Why do radial artery grafts for aorto-coronary bypass fail? A reappraisal. *Ann. Thorac. Surg.* 22:520, 1976.

62. Tice, D.A., Zerbino, V.R., Isom, O.W., Cunningham, J.N., and Engelman, R.M. Coronary artery bypass with freeze-preserved saphenous vein allografts. *J. Thorac. Cardiovasc. Surg.* 71:378, 1976.

63. Schloemer, R.L. and Logan, G. Successful Use of the USCI-Sauvage Filamentous Vascular Prosthesis in the Right Coronary Artery of Man. In Sawyer, P. and Kaplitt, M.J. (eds.), *Vascular Grafts.* New York: Appleton-Century-Crofts, 1978, p. 378.

64. Cohn, L.H. and Collins, J.J., Jr. The Use of Polytetrafluoroethylene (PTFE) as an Aorto-Coronary Bypass Graft in Vascular Grafts. In Sawyer, P. and Kapli-t, M.J. (eds.), *Vascular Grafts.* New York: Appleton-Century-Crofts, 1978, p. 398.

65. Gorlin, R. and Taylor, W.J. Myocardial revascularization with internal mammary artery implantation. JAMA 207:907, 1969.

66. Bhayana, J.H., Olsen, D.B., Byrne, J.P., and Kolff, W.J. Reversal of Myocardial ischemia by arterialization of the coronary vein. *J. Thorac. Cardiovasc. Surg.* 67:125, 1974.

67. Beck, C.S. and Leighninger, D.S. Scientific basis for the surgical treatment of coronary artery disease. *JAMA* 159:1264, 1955.

68. Dotter, C.T. and Judkins, M.P. Transluminal treatment of arteriosclerotic obstruction. Description of a technique and a preliminary report of its application. *Circulation* 30:654, 1964.

69. Gruntzig, A.R., Myler, R.K., Hanna, E.S., and Turina, M.I. Coronary transluminal angioplasty. *Circulation* 56(Suppl. 3):84, 1977.

70. Block, P.C., Cowley, M.J., Kaltenbach, M., Kent, K.M., and Simpson, J. Percutaneous angioplasty of stenoses of bypass grafts or of bypass graft anastomotic sites. *Am. J. Cardiol.* 53:666, 1984.

71. Jones, E.L. and King, S.B. Intraoperative angioplasty in the treatment of coronary artery disease. *J. Am. Coll. Cardiol.* 1:970, 1983.

72. Jones, E.L., Douglas, J.S., Gruntzig, A.R., Graver, J.M., King, S.B., Guyton, R.A., and Hatcher, C.R. Percutaneous saphenous vein angioplasty to avoid reoperative bypass surgery. *Ann. Thorac. Surg.* 36:389, 1983.

73. Gould, B.L., Clayton, P.D., Jensen, R.L., and Liddle, H.V. Association between early graft patency and late outcome for patients undergoing artery bypass graft surgery. *Circulation* 69:569, 1984.

74. Frey, R.R., Bruschke, A.V.G., and Vermeulen, F.E.E. Serial angiographic evaluation 1 year and 9 years after aorta-coronary bypass. *J. Thorac. Cardiovasc. Surg.* 87:167, 1984.

75. Campeau, L., Enjalhert, M., Lesperance, J., and Bourassa, M.E. Arteriosclerosis and late closure of aorto-coronary saphenous vein grafts. Se-

quential angiographic studies at 1 year, 5–7 years, and 10–12 years after surgery. *Circulation* 68(Suppl. 2):1, 1983.

76. Norwood, W.I., Cohn, L.H., and Collins, J.J., Jr. Surgical management of recurrent angina pectoris following coronary artery bypass surgery. *Ann. Thorac. Surg.* 23:9, 1977.

77. Laird-Meeter, K., VanDen Brand, M.J.B.M., Serruys, P.W., Penn, O.C.K.M., Haalebos, M.M.P., Bos, E., and Hugenholtz, P.G. Reoperation after aortocoronary bypass procedure. Results in 53 patients in a group of 1041 with consecutive first operations. *Br. Heart J.* 50:157, 1983.

78. Cohn, L.H., Koster, J.K., Jr., Mee, R.B.B., and Collins, J.J., Jr. Surgical treatment of left main coronary stenosis. *World J. Surg.* 2:998, 1978.

79. Takaro, T., Hultgren, H.N., Lipton, J., and Detre, K.M. The VA cooperative randomized study of surgery for coronary arterial occlusive disease. II. Subgroup with significant left main lesions. *Circulation* 54 (Suppl. 3):107, 1976.

80. Cohn, L.H., Boyden, C.M., and Collins, J.J., Jr. Improved longevity after aorto-coronary bypass for advanced coronary artery disease. *Am. J. Surg.* 129:380, 1975.

81. Isom, O.W., Spencer, F.G., Glassman, E., et al. Does coronary bypass increase longevity? *J. Thorac. Cardiovasc. Surg.* 75:28, 1978.

82. Hammermeister, K.E. The effect of coronary bypass surgery on survival. *Prog. Cardiovasc. Dis.* 25:297, 1983.

83. Ullyot, D.J., Wisneski, J., Sullivan, R.W., and Gertz, E.W. Improved survival after coronary artery surgery in patients with extensive coronary artery disease. *J. Thorac. Cardiovasc. Surg.* 70:405, 1975.

84. Murphy, M.L., Hultgren, H.N., Detre, K., Thomson, J., and Takaro, T. Treatment of chronic stable angina: A preliminary report of survival data of the randomized Veterans Administration Cooperative study. *N. Engl. J. Med.* 297:621, 1977.

85. Collins, J.J., Jr., Cohn, L.H., and Koster, J.K., Jr. Elective and Emergency Coronary Bypass Surgery: Myocardial Revascularization Prolongs Life in Chronic Disease and in Unstable Angina Pectoris. In Mason, D.T. (ed.), *Advances in Heart Disease* (vol. 3). New York: Grune & Stratton, 1980.

86. European Coronary Artery Study Group: Long Term Results of a prospective randomized study of coronary bypass surgery in stable angina pectoris. *Lancet* 2:1173, 1982.

87. CASS Principal Investigators and their associates. Coronary Artery Surgery Study (CASS): A randomized trial of coronary artery bypass surgery. Quality of life in patients randomly assigned to treatment groups.*Circulation* 68:951, 1983.

88. Graboys, T.B., Lown, B., Collins, J.J., Jr., and Cohn, L.H. Does coronary revascularization reduce the prevalence of ventricular ectopic activity? *Am. J. Cardiol.* 41:401, 1978.

89. Vismara, L.A., Miller, R.R., Price, J.E., Karen, R., DeMaria, A.N., and Mason, D.T. Improved longevity due to reduction of sudden death by aorto-coronary bypass in coronary atherosclerosis. *Am. J. Cardiol.* 39:919, 1977.

90. McIntosh, H.D. and Garcia, J.A. The first decade of aorto-coronary bypass grafting. *Circulation* 57:405, 1978.

91. Collins, J.J., Jr., Kopf, G., Tucker, W.Y., Koster, J.K., Jr., Mee, R.B.B., and Cohn, L.H. The impact of revascularization surgery upon hospital costs in patients with angina pectoris (abstract). *Am. J. Cardiol.* 41:447, 1978.

92. Oberman, A., Wayne, J.B., Kouchoukos, N.T., Charles, E.D., Russell, R.O., and Rogers, W.J. Employment status after coronary bypass surgery. *Circulation* 65(Suppl. 2):115, 1982.

93. Smith, H.C., Hammes, L.N., Gupta, S., Vlietstra, R.E., and Elveback, L. Employment status after coronary artery bypass surgery. *Circulation* 65(Suppl. 2):120, 1982.

94. Graboys, T.B. and Cohn, P.F. The prevalence of angina pectoris and abnormal coronary arteriograms in severe aortic valvular disease. *Am. Heart J.* 93:683, 1977.

95. Bonchek, L.I., Anderson, R.P., and Rosch, J. Should coronary arteriography be performed routinely before valve replacement? *Am. J. Cardiol.* 31:462, 1973.

96. Goldschlager, N., Pfeifer, J., Cohn, K., Popper, R., and Selzer, A. The natural history of aortic regurgitation. *Am. J. Med.* 54:577, 1973.

97. Exadactylos, N., Sugrue, D.D., and Oakley, C.M. Prevalence of coronary artery disease in patients with isolated aortic valve stenosis. *Br. Heart J.* 41:121, 1984.

98. Lytle, B.W., Cosgrove, D.M., Loop, F.D., Taylor, P.C., Gill, C.C., Golding, L.A.R., Goormastic, M., and Groves, L.K. Replacement of aortic valve combined with myocardial revascularization: Determinants of early and late risk for 500 patients, 1967–1981. *Circulation* 68:1149, 1983.

99. Ciaravella, J.M., Oschsner, J.L., and Mills, N.L. Combined procedure of coronary artery bypass grafting and valve repair. *Ann. Thorac. Surg.* 23:20, 1977.

100. Loop, F.D., Phillips, D.F., Roy, M., Taylor, P.C., Graves, L.K., and Effler, D.B. Aortic valve replacement combined with myocardial revascularization. Late clinical results and survival of surgically-treated aortic valve patients with and

without coronary artery disease. *Circulation* 55:-169, 1977.

101. Miller, D.C., Stinson, E.B., Dyer, P.E., Rossiter, S.J., Reitz, B.A., and Shumway, N.E. Surgical implications and results of combined aortic valve replacement and myocardial revascularization. *Am. J. Cardiol.* 43:494, 1979.

102. Richardson, J.V., Louchoukos, N.T., Wright, S.O., III, and Karp, R.B. Combined aortic valve replacement and myocardial revascularization. Results in 220 patients. *Circulation* 59:75, 1979.

103. Vlodaver, Z. and Edwards, J.E. Rupture of ventricular septum or papillary muscle complicating myocardial infarction. *Circulation* 55:815, 1977.

104. Salomon, N.W., Stinson, E.B., Griepp, R.B., and Shumway, N.E. Patient-related risk factors as predictors of results following isolated mitral valve replacement. *Ann. Thorac. Surg.* 24:519, 1977.

105. Kapelanski, D.P., Al-Sadir, J., Lamberti, J.J., and Anagnastopoulous, C.E. Ventriculographic features predictive of surgical outcome for left ventricular aneurysm. *Circulation* 58:1167, 1978.

106. Cohen, M., Packer, M., and Gorlin, R. Indications for left ventricular aneurysmectomy. *Circulation* 67:717, 1983.

# 15. THERAPY OF CARDIAC ARRHYTHMIAS AND CONDUCTION ABNORMALITIES IN CORONARY ARTERY DISEASE

J. Thomas Bigger, Jr.

James A. Reiffel

Edward B. Leahey, Jr.

Two of the most important treatable causes of death in patients with coronary artery disease are the cardiac arrhythmias and conduction abnormalities. They may be associated with acute myocardial infarction (AMI) or chronic ischemia. Detection of such rhythm and conduction abnormalities has been discussed in chapter 5, and their pathophysiology was commented on in chapter 2. For the purpose of discussing therapeutic approaches, AMI can be divided into four phases: (1) the prehospital phase, (2) the CCU phase, (3) the post-CCU phase, and (4) the posthospital phase. The cardiac arrhythmias and conduction defects encountered in each of these phases will be discussed, as will their therapy. The management of arrhythmias encountered in the setting of chronic ischemic heart disease will also be discussed.

Areas of controversy include the treatment of bradyarrhythmias in the prehospital phase; the use of lidocaine for antiarrhythmic prophylaxis in the prehospital phase as well as in the CCU phase; the significance of warning ventricular premature depolarizations, or VPD we prefer this term, rather than ventricular premature beats [VPBs]) prior to ventricular fibrillation in the CCU; the role of prophylaxis for ventricular arrhythmias, especially as it pertains to lidocaine treatment; the role of the intermediate coronary care unit (ICCU); the question of who should have long-term in-hospital monitoring following AMI; the selection of patients with ischemic heart disease for temporary or permanent pacing or both; the harbingers of sudden death and who should have long-term treatment to reduce mortality in ischemic heart disease; the pros and cons of acute drug testing; and finally, the treatment of VPD in the chronic setting.

## The Prehospital Phase of Acute Myocardial Infarction

More deaths occur in the first 6 hours following acute myocardial infarction than in the subsequent 6 months. A substantial body of information on the arrhythmias that occur in the early hours of infarction is available from mobile coronary care units, fixed life-support stations, and early admissions to coronary care units (CCU). Two major categories of arrhythmias frequently occur in the first hours of AMI: the bradyarrhythmias and ventricular arrhythmias. Table 15–1 lists the frequency of various arrhythmias

This study was supported in part by NIH Grant HL-22982 and HL-70204 from the National Heart, Lung and Blood Institute, Bethesda, Maryland; by Grant RR-00645 from the Research Resources Administration, Bethesda, MD; by a Grant-in-Aid from the American Heart Association, Dallas, Texas; and by grants from the Winthrop and Chernow Foundations, New York. Address for reprints: J. T. Bigger, Jr., M.D., The Arrhythmia Control Unit, The Columbia-Presbyterian Medical Center, 622 West 168th Street, New York, N.Y. 10032.

found by Pantridge et al. [1] during the first 4 hours of AMI.

## BRADYARRHYTHMIAS

In the very first hours of AMI, bradyarrhythmias —sinus or nodal bradycardias, and atrioventricular (AV) block—are much more common than in the CCU phase. The incidence of sinus bradycardia during the first 4 hours of AMI is estimated in different reports to be from 8 to 38 percent; its occurrence is highest in the very earliest moments following AMI [1–5]. Pantridge et al. [1] (see also table 15–1) observed 240 patients in the first hour of AMI and found that 28 percent had sinus bradycardia; only 6 percent more developed sinus bradycardia in hours 2 through 4. Patients with inferior myocardial infarction are significantly more likely to develop sinus bradycardia than are those with anterior infarction [6–7]. In Adgey's study [6] of 284 patients seen in the first hour of AMI, the site of infarction was inferior in 134 and anterior in 135. The frequency of sinus or nodal bradycardia was 36 percent in inferior infarction, compared to 18 percent in anterior infarction (z= 3.19, P < 0.01). Similarly, bradycardia due to second-degree or third-degree AV block is more common very early in AMI and in inferior infarction. The frequency of AV block in the first hour of infarction is in the range of 5 to 12 percent; the incidence in the first hour almost equals the incidence in the remainder of the hospital course [1, 4, 6].

A controversy has arisen about treatment of the bradyarrhythmias associated with AMI. Atropine therapy has been judged both helpful [7–9] and harmful [10–13]. In experimental infarction in dogs, atropine therapy can increase spontaneous ventricular arrhythmias [14–16] and decrease the electrical ventricular fibrillation threshold [17]. Other experiments suggest that either marked bradycardia or tachycardia promote ventricular arrhythmias [18]. Such results have led to circumspection in applying atropine therapy to the bradyarrhythmias in AMI.

Bradyarrhythmias (either sinus bradycardia or AV block) in the prehospital phase of AMI are commonly associated with significant hypotension [7, 8, 19–20], which is due not only to low heart rate, but also to cholinergically mediated peripheral vasodilation. In 89 patients seen within 30 minutes of the onset of symptoms, Pantridge and associates [1] found that 28 of the patients (32 percent) had both bradyarrhythmias and hypotension. Left untreated, bradycardia and hypotension are associated with increased mortality [21].

The hypotension and bradycardia of AMI usually respond to atropine therapy [1, 7, 8, 19]. Whether atropine treatment will reduce mortality has not been studied in a controlled trial and is not likely to be. Warren and Lewis [9] found that the mortality associated with bradycardia and hypotension was 27 percent (6 of 22) when treated with atropine and 75 percent (3 of 4) when untreated; this result is not statistically significant, but it should encourage further study. Pending further information, we recommend

TABLE 15–1. Incidence of arrhythmias within 4 hours among patients seen within the first hour of acute myocardial infarction

| Arrhythmia | Total patients assessed | Number (percentage) of patients who developed arrhythmias | | | |
|---|---|---|---|---|---|
| | | 0–1 hour | 1–2 hours | 2–4 hours | Total 0–4 hours |
| Bradyarrhythmias | 248 | 84 (34%) | 9 (4%) | 7 (3%) | 100 (40%) |
| Ventricular premature depolarizations | 294 | 171 (58%) | 80 (27%) | 24 (8%) | 275 (94%) |
| Ventricular tachycardia | 294 | 6 (2%) | 4 (1%) | 1 (0.3%) | 11 (4%) |
| Ventricular fibrillation | 294 | 28 (10%) | 13 (4%) | 5 (2%) | 46 (16%) |
| Supraventricular arrhythmias | 266 | 4 (2%) | 7 (3%) | 5 (2%) | 16 (6%) |

Modified from Pantridge, J.F. et al. *The Acute Coronary Attack.* New York: Grune & Stratton, 1975.

that atropine be used to treat the combination of bradycardia and hypotension. A dose of 0.5 mg can be given intravenously and repeated every 5 minutes until the heart rate and blood pressure respond adequately; one dose may be sufficient, but several may be required. It has been shown that intramuscular atropine is also effective, and this route may be simpler to use under adverse circumstances in the early moments of infarction.

Excessive heart rates should be avoided, and clinical experiments with sotalol and practolol showed that $\beta$-adrenergic blocking drugs can be used to prevent or reverse the excessive tachycardia induced by atropine [22, 23]. Some evidence suggests that propranolol is more likely to produce adverse effects than practolol in the setting of AMI. Jewitt and co-workers [24] found that 25 mg of practolol had less adverse hemodynamic effects than 5 mg of propranolol; both drugs were given intravenously to patients hospitalized for AMI. Sotalol and practolol, however, are not available in the United States, and no clinical trials have been done to demonstrate that small intravenous doses of propranolol are useful and safe for reducing excessive sinus tachycardial due to atropine treatment. Awaiting further information, we advise that the atropine doses be carefully titrated to avoid excess tachycardia (particularly if the site of infarction is anterior); the use of intravenous propranolol for excessive tachycardia should be considered experimental. However, if propranolol is used for this purpose, 1 mg intravenous doses every 3 to 5 minutes is the preferred method of administration.

VENTRICULAR ARRHYTHMIAS

Although about 75 percent of patients with AMI have some VPD within the first 4 to 6 hours [1, 25–27], frequent VPD are uncommon in the prehospital phase of AMI [1, 25, 28]. Five to 10 percent will have ventricular tachycardia (VT) [1–3, 25, 28], and about 15 percent will have ventricular fibrillation (VF) [2, 3–5, 25–28]. VF is more likely to occur during the first 6 hours of infarction than in the CCU and the late hospital phases of AMI put together.

Adgey et al. [28] analyzed the factors that may predispose to VF in 48 patients who de-

veloped VF outside hospital after continuous ECG recording had been established by a mobile coronary care unit team. In this group of 48 patients, the mean age was 56 years, 83 percent were men, 27 percent had had a previous myocardial infarction, and 63 percent had anterior infarction. The median time between onset of chest pain and arrival of the mobile coronary care unit in Adgey's study was 68 minutes; 22 patients were seen within 1 hour [28]. The mean duration of ECG recording before VF occurred was 25 minutes. The rhythm on arrival of the mobile team was sinus rhythm in 25 patients, sinus bradycardia in 10, sinus tachycardia in 10, atrial fibrillation in 2, and second-degree A-V block in 1. On arrival of the team the mean heart rate was $84 \pm 4$ per minute, the range being 47 to 175 per minute. The average heart rate increased significantly between the time of arrival and onset of VF; at the latter time the heart rate averaged $98 \pm 5$ per minute ($p < 0.01$). A careful analysis was made of the ventricular arrhythmias seen during the recording period prior to VF. Frequent or repetitive VPD were uncommon. Nearly all episodes of VF began either with an R-on-T VPD (69 percent) or by degeneration of ventricular tachycardia (19 percent). Of the 48 patients, 29 (60 percent) had a single episode of VF and 19 (40 percent) had more than one. Ultimately, 35 of the patients (73 percent) who developed VF under observation in the first hour of myocardial infarction survived to be discharged from hospital.

Because of the high incidence of VF in the prehospital phase of AMI, antiarrhythmic prophylaxis has been recommended. One approach is to begin therapy immediately before the patient is moved to the hospital. Lidocaine therapy should be started as a 1 mg/kg intravenous injection and a 2 to 4 mg/min infusion. A second injection of .5 mg/kg should be given 15 to 20 minutes after the initial injection. Additional doses may have to be given if ventricular arrhythmias emerge. The intravenous infusion rate can be readjusted upon arrival at hospital. The intramuscular route may be more convenient in emergencies; doses of 4 mg/kg given in the deltoid muscle rapidly produce therapeutic plasma concentrations that usually persist for more than 2 to 3 hours [29–31]. In 1974 Valentine and co-workers [32] reported results of a randomized, double-blind trial of intramuscular lidocaine in the prehospital phase of AMI. The median time of injection was 70 to 75 minutes after onset of symptoms; 156 patients received 300 mg of lidocaine (10 percent solution) in the deltoid muscle, and 113 received a placebo. The death rate in the lidocaine group in the 2 hours following injection was significantly lower (three deaths versus eight in the control group; p < 0.05). The salvage was mainly in younger age groups. No significant difference was seen in late death rates between the two groups, which suggests that the treatment group held its early advantage.

The effectiveness of lidocaine therapy in the first hour or two of AMI has been questioned. Some workers believe that lidocaine is much less effective in this phase of AMI [6, 32]; others contest this assertion [2]. Because of this question and the acknowledged role of the sympathetic nervous system in rendering the ischemic ventricle more susceptible to fibrillation, Mulholland and Pantridge [22] and Allen et. al. [23], in Ireland, have used sotalol or practolol as therapy for ventricular arrhythmias in the prehospital phase of AMI, particularly when the heart rate is increased or when lidocaine is ineffective. Experimental studies in dogs show that $\beta$-adrenergic blocking drugs are effective for the ventricular arrhythmias that occur in the hour after acute coronary occlusion [33, 34]. Also, $\beta$-adrenergic blocking drugs can elevate VF threshold and prevent electrically induced VT 4 to 6 days after experimental AMI in the dog [35]. These clinical and experimental results are encouraging, but this approach is not recommended for widespread use in the United States until the British results are confirmed in trials conducted with one of the $\beta$-adrenergic blocking drugs available in the United States.

Even with appropriate drug therapy, many instances of VF are likely to occur in the prehospital phase of AMI. Prompt defibrillation is the mainstay of therapy. The energy available from light, easily portable defibrillators is almost always efficacious if applied promptly [36].

## The Coronary Care Unit Phase of Acute Myocardial Infarction

The arrhythmias seen in the coronary care unit (CCU) phase of AMI are significantly different from those seen in the prehospital phase. The therapeutic approach, therefore, is different in the CCU phase of AMI.

### BRADYARRHYTHMIAS

*Sinus Bradycardia.* About 20 percent of patients in the CCU will have a sinus rate less than 60 beats/min. Persistent bradycardia, S-A arrest, and S-A exit block, however, are much less frequent [37]. About 35 percent of patients with inferior infarction and about 10 percent of those with anterior infarction have some degree of sinus bradycardia [38–41]. The higher incidence with inferior MI reflects in part the right coronary origin of both the sinus node artery and the inferior wall vasculature in approximately 65 percent of patients. Sinus bradycardia in the CCU phase is usually not associated with hypotension or other significant hemodynamic abnormalities. Evidence accumulated from a number of studies indicates that the in-hospital mortality from AMI among those who have sinus bradycardia in the CCU is less than half the overall mortality [38–45]; this may be expected from the strong association between inferior myocardial infarction and sinus bradycardia in the CCU. If chamber dilatation is absent, the decrease in $M\dot{V}O_2$ associated with bradycardia may be an additional factor. Sinus bradycardia in the CCU infrequently requires therapy; however, when bradycardia is associated with hypotension or refractory ventricular arrhythmias, therapy is indicated. When therapy is required, the heart rate may be increased to the desired range by sequential doses of atropine (.5 mg intravenously). Repeated or large atropine dosing may be attended by blurred vision, dry mouth, urinary retention, and in the elderly patient, severe confusion. Glaucoma and prostatism are contraindications to atropine. Therefore if the need for therapy persists, pacemaker therapy is usually more effective and is associated with fewer undesirable effects than long-term atropine therapy. The heart rate can be selected precisely to avoid ischemia during pacing, and pacing can be terminated immediately when no longer required.

*Atrioventricular Block.* First-degree atrioventricular (AV) block occurs in 6 to 20 percent of patients with AMI during the early hospital phase [39, 43, 44, 46–52]. It occurs in about 25 percent of patients with inferior infarction, in which it is three to four times more common than in anterior infarction [39, 46, 53]. About half the patients who develop first-degree AV block during AMI subsequently develop second-or third-degree block [46, 54–58]. Although first-degree AV block is not an indication for pacing, it does mandate continued monitoring because of the high likelihood of progression. First-degree AV block usually resolves spontaneously, and monitoring may be discontinued following resolution.

Second-degree AV block occurs in about 5 percent of patients with AMI during their CCU stay [39, 43, 44, 46–52, 59], being most common in inferior infarction [54–56, 60, 61], where impaired conduction is usually the result of ischemia, autonomic and humoral influences, or both on the AV node or upper bundle branches [60–63]. Moreover the anatomic location of the infarct has significant bearing on ECG pattern, prognosis, and treatment of second-degree AV block (see below). Approximately two-thirds of those with second-degree AV block develop complete heart block [39, 46, 59, 60].

Patients with *inferior* AMI often progress through first- and second-degree AV block (or vice versa) during the development or resolution of complete heart block [54, 56, 60, 62, 64–67]. The escape rhythm usually is reasonably rapid, and on the electrocardiogram the QRS is narrow, which suggests an origin in or above the bundle of His. In those patients with inferior MI who developed high-grade AV block, it will be present on admission in as many as half and will be present in 92 percent by 72 hours; rarely will it appear later than the fifth day [68]. High-grade but transient AV block with inferior MI usually lasts ½ hour to 16 days [68] but can rarely last up to a month and still resolve. In 37

percent it will last less than 24 hours; in 47 percent it will last more than 3 days [68]. The development of Wenckebach or Mobitz type 1 second-degree AV block is not an indication for the insertion of a temporary pacemaker if the heart rate is adequate to maintain cardiac output. If AV block is thought to contribute to left ventricular dysfunction, this possibility can be confirmed by hemodynamic studies. If pacing decreases the pulmonary arterial diastolic (or pulmonary capillary wedge) pressure, increases the cardiac output, or both, temporary pacing should then be utilized until the conduction disturbance resolves. Pacing is apt to improve power failure if the ventricular rate is less than 50 but has been reported to be infrequently helpful with ventricular rate greater than 50 [68]. Temporary VVI pacing is also advisable when antiarrhythmic drugs are given, since these may suppress the escape rhythm as well as the arrhythmia. In inferior MI, high-grade AV block is associated with more extensive damage and a higher mortality rate then occurs in its absence [68].

AV block in acute *anterior* AMI usually indicates extensive involvement of the interventricular septum and damage to the conduction system below the bundle of His. Complete heart block often develops abruptly from a sinus rhythm with a normal PR interval [59, 60, 62, 69, 70]. Usually unifascicular or bifascicular block patterns appear first; occasionally, Mobitz type 2 second-degree AV block is also seen as an intermediate state [60]. When complete AV block occurs, subsidiary pacemakers are often slow and the QRS is wide and aberrant, which suggests an origin below the bundle of His or a conduction impairment in the bundle branches. The development of even transient Mobitz type 2 AV block should be considered an indication for temporary pacing [46, 52, 57, 64, 67, 71]. Central station monitoring of both leads I and II simultaneously is advisable so as to optimize detection of any evolving fascicular block pattern.

Mortality is very high in patients who develop complete heart block during AMI because of the concomitant extensive myocardial damage and severe left ventricular failure. This is particularly true with anterior infarctions [68]. In-hospital mortality of patients with complete heart block is approximately 35 percent in inferior infarction and 80 percent in anterior infarction [53, 55, 63, 64, 69–76].

Extensive infarction and high mortality rates are also associated with bundle branch block that appears during acute infarction even in the absence of progression to Mobitz type 2 or complete heart block. Of 852 patients who developed new left or right bundle branch block during AMI, 58 percent died during hospitalization, mainly as a result of left ventricular failure and shock [39, 43, 46, 49, 58, 76–84]. There is no significant difference in survival between patients who acutely develop RBBB and those who develop left bundle branch block [76, 77, 80, 83, 84]. Isolated hemiblock, however, does not appear to pose much risk [85, 86]. To identify patients at particularly high risk of developing complete AV block, Lie and co-workers [76] performed His bundle recordings on 25 patients who developed new bundle branch block during anteroseptal infarction; 11 of 15 with prolonged H-V intervals eventually developed complete AV block, while only 1 of 10 with a normal H-V interval progressed to complete AV block (p < 0.05). Furthermore, they showed that the PR interval was a poor predictor of complete heart block. Seven of 15 patients with increased H-V intervals had a normal PR interval, and four of these seven eventually progressed to complete heart block.

Because of the extremely poor prognosis of high-degree AV block or new bundle branch block during AMI, several authors have questioned the value of aggressive management [73–76]. In 14 patients with anteroseptal infarction and complete heart block, Lie and associates [76] were able to demonstrate temporary benefit from pacing in 10, and eventually restoration of 1:1 AV conduction occurred in each. However, all died of severe left ventricular dysfunction [76]. However, there is little or no margin for error in patients with extensive infarction. A period of severe bradycardia or asystole can adversely affect outcome. If aggressive management of the hemodynamic consequences of infarction is undertaken, then we believe an equally aggressive approach should be taken in

the management of conduction defects [87–92]. Recent data from a multicenter study group indicate the high risk for many patients with bundle branch block in this setting [93]. We believe, as do others [90–93], that temporary pacing is indicated in any patient who develops a new bundle branch block during AMI. If bundle branch block is present upon admission, it should be presumed to be acute if no records exist to establish its duration. Properly performed electrode catheter insertion should not increase morbidity, and individual patients may benefit even though the overall mortality is little affected. There are two advantages to early, semielective insertion of a temporary pacemaker: (1) abrupt, marked bradycardia and its serious sequelae, including hypotension and infarct extension, are prevented, and (2) the delays and increased morbidity of hurried pacemaker insertion are avoided. Pacemaker insertion also relieves the concerns about suppression of ventricular escape foci or enhancement of bundle branch or AV block by antiarrhythmic medications, which are frequently required because of concomitant ventricular arrhythmias in patients with extensive MI. Antiarrhythmic drug worsening of A-V block does occur infrequently [94]. Pacemaker insertion, however, does not alleviate the consequences of poor ventricular function present in most of these patients or lessen the risk of lethal ventricular arrhythmias to which they are prone. For the latter, protracted (6 weeks) monitoring has been advised [68].

## SUPRAVENTRICULAR TACHYARRHYTHMIAS

About 40 percent of patients with AMI will have atrial premature depolarizations (APD) in the CCU [39, 40, 44, 45, 50]. APD usually indicate left ventricular dysfunction with associated atrial hypertension or arterial hypoxemia, although they may be caused by atrial infarction or pericarditis. APD are associated with increased hospital mortality (about twofold), but specific treatment of the APD probably does not alter prognosis [40]. APD usually require no specific treatment in AMI unless they trigger atrial tachyarrhythmias, and APD often decrease in frequency when left ventricular function improves (e.g., with vasodilator therapy).

About 10 percent of patients will have atrial flutter or fibrillation in the CCU [40, 95, 96]. Mortality is increased fivefold in patients with these rhythms, probably due to the strong association with left ventricular dysfunction. These arrhythmias usually should be treated with digitalis. Atrial flutter or fibrillation is often transient, but it may be recurrent, with paroxysms lasting from minutes to a few hours [95, 96]. This pattern makes cardioversion inappropriate unless acute hemodynamic deterioration or severe ischemia is precipitated by rapid ventricular response. Intravenous propranolol or verapamil, when ventricular function is adequate, offers temporary but immediate means of achieving rate control prior to achieving digitalis-induced slowing. Doses are guided by heart rate and blood pressure responses.

A .5 mg intravenous dose of digoxin can be given immediately, and .25 to .50 mg may be repeated orally or intravenously at 1- to 6-hour intervals to a total of 1 to 1.5 mg as indicated for rate control. A maintenance dose, generally .125 to .25 mg, should be based on judgments about absorption, renal function, and cardiac response [97–99]. Care should be used during digitalization because ischemic myocardium can show increased sensitivity to digitalis [100–102]. Determinations of serum digoxin concentration can be useful in monitoring therapy, providing the samples are drawn at least 8 hours after the most recent dose. Within 24 hours of its appearance, atrial flutter or fibrillation usually resolves [95, 96]. If APD, atrial fibrillation, or both persist after digitalization and require treatment, quinidine or procainamide should be used. Quinidine sulfate 300 to 400 mg orally every 6 hours or procainamide 500 to 2,000 mg orally every 4 to 6 hours is usually effective. If digoxin is inadequate for rate control, oral propranolol or verapamil may be added. Caution must be used with drug combinations, however, as quinidine in most patients and verapamil in 50 percent will result in elevations of digoxin levels and possibly digitalis effect and/or toxicity.

VENTRICULAR ARRHYTHMIAS
Careful analysis of the electrocardiogram (ECG) during the CCU phase will reveal VPD in almost 90 percent of patients [39, 44, 45, 50,

103]. Frequent VPD and ECG characteristics such as R-on-T, multiple configurations, and pairs of runs of VPD are associated with higher CCU mortality [39, 43, 104]. Severe ventricular arrhythmias are common: VT, 30 to 40 percent; VF, 6 percent; and primary VF, 3 percent [39, 43, 44, 105–108].

An important issue that is currently being clarified is how often primary VF is preceded by "warning arrhythmias," that is, by frequent or complex ventricular arrhythmias. Until recently, the strategy in most CCUs was to treat frequent or complex ventricular arrhythmias with lidocaine or other drugs; this approach was based on the assumption that primary VF is usually preceded by warning arrhythmias [47, 55, 109, 110]. However, table 15–2 lists reports from four different groups [106–108, 111] who found that only about half of the patients show warning arrhythmias prior to primary VF. Also, the incidence of warning arrhythmias was about as high in patients who did not develop primary VF as in those who did. One of the best studies of primary VF early in the CCU course was done by Campbell et al. [112] at Newcastle-upon-Tyne. These workers analyzed continuous ECGs recorded in the CCU from 38 selected patients during the first 12 hours of acute myocardial infarction. Seventeen patients were selected because they developed primary VF; the rest did not develop VF and served as a control group. None of the 17 patients with primary VF had received antiarrhythmic drugs, digitalis, or $\beta$-adrenergic blocking drugs during the 72 hours prior to the myocardial infarction. The two groups were similar with respect to age, sex, history of previous infarction, site of AMI, and peak SGOT level. Continuous ECG recordings were available during most of the first 12 hours of infarction. Some interesting information was obtained on the mode of onset of primary VF. In 16 of the 17 patients (94 percent) in the VF group, primary VF began with an R-on-T VPD $(R-V/QT < 0.85)$; in the remaining patient, artifact prevented analysis of the mode of onset. Also, the frequency of R-on-T VPD often increased significantly in the 10-minute period just before primary VF occurred. In contrast to VF, VT usually began with late-cycle VPD. Although this study importantly advanced our

TABLE 15–2. Warning arrhythmias in patients with ventricular fibrillation (VF)*

| Series | Number of patients with primary VF | Number of patients with warning arrhythmias | Percent |
|---|---|---|---|
| Dhurandhar et al. [106] | 20 | 12 | 60 |
| Wyman and Hammersmith [107] | 12 | 5 | 42 |
| Saunamaki and Pederson [111] | 21 | 12 | 57 |
| Lie et al. [108] | 20 | 12 | 60 |
| Total | 73 | 41 | 56 |

*VF occurring in the absence of cardiogenic shock or acute heart failure.

knowledge about the initiation of primary VF, it did not show how to identify and manage patients at risk. Interestingly, there were no differences between the two groups with respect to ventricular arrhythmias aside from primary VF. Paired VPD, ventricular tachycardia, and R-on-T VPD were recorded with equal frequency in the two groups when the ECG data were adjusted for duration of recording. Thus, there were no reliable "warning arrhythmias" that predicted the occurrence of primary VF.

Lack of warning arrhythmias prior to primary VF has led to the suggestion that routine antiarrhythmic drug prophylaxis should be used in the CCU to prevent primary VF [113]. Many trials of antiarrhythmic prophylaxis have been conducted in CCU patients. Of these, only one controlled trial has shown a significant reduction in primary VF in the CCU. Lie and his colleagues in Amsterdam [114] enrolled 105 patients into a control group and 107 into a group treated with high-dose lidocaine. To be eligible for the study, patients had to be admitted within 6 hours of the onset of symptoms, be less than 70 years of age, and have definite evidence of AMI. The treatment group received a 100 mg intravenous dose of lidocaine on admission and a continuous infusion of 3 mg/min for 48 hours. The mean plasma level 6 hours after beginning therapy was 3.5 ug/ml and showed a wide range. Adverse effects were seen in 16 of the lidocaine-treated patients; adverse effects were three times more common in patients age 60 or older than in younger patients. VT occurred in six control patients and in two treated patients (this difference is not statistically significant); primary VF occurred in nine control patients and in none

of the treated patients (p < 0.01). No difference in overall mortality was found between the two groups; 10 control patients and eight treated patients died. It should be pointed out that the incidence of primary VF in the control group was unusually high and that if one episode of VF had occurred in the lidocaine treated group, the difference between groups would not be significant. Several other trials in which lower doses were used also did not show benefit from lidocaine prophylaxis nor was benefit shown from intramuscular injections of the drug [115].

In contrast, the hypothesis that high-dose lidocaine prevents primary VF is supported by a large, uncontrolled study by Wyman and Hammersmith [107]. Ideally, this conclusion should be confirmed by several additional controlled studies, but these will be difficult to conduct in the prevailing climate. In our present state of knowledge, antiarrhythmic prophylaxis for 48 hours after AMI to prevent primary VF is a matter of choice. Several agents could be used for this purpose, but the evidence of efficacy is strongest for lidocaine. Infusion of lidocaine (3 mg/min) should be very carefully controlled (e.g., with an infusion pump), and lower doses should be used in patients with left ventricular failure or hypotension. A high incidence of adverse effects will be encountered on this regimen, so early signs of toxicity should be sought frequently. (Because the incidence of adverse effects is very high in patients older than 60 years and primary VF is rare, one should consider withholding prophylaxis in this group.)

If lidocaine is ineffective or toxic or if the physician prefers, procainamide prophylaxis can be utilized. A loading dose of 750 mg can be infused intravenously over 35 minutes, and then infusion at 2 to 4 mg/min may be maintained continuously over the next 48 hours [116].

## The Late In-Hospital Phase of Acute Myocardial Infarction

Although the introduction of the CCU has reduced mortality among patients admitted to hospital with AMI, about half of all hospital deaths occur in patients after leaving the CCU [117–120]. Approximately one-half of these deaths are sudden [117, 118, 121]. In one series [118], 23 of 273 AMI patients experienced cardiac arrest or died suddenly after leaving the CCU. VF was the terminal event in 13 of the 20 cases where rhythm was identified. Several series have shown that late in-hospital deaths occur with almost equal frequency during the 6 weeks after leaving the CCU [118, 120].

### THE INTERMEDIATE CORONARY CARE UNIT

In an attempt to extend the benefits derived from CCUs to those patients who leave them, Grace and Yarvote [119] proposed the establishment of an intermediate coronary care unit (ICCU) to provide extended ECG monitoring and the capability of cardiac resuscitation without the more elaborate features of a CCU. Their early experience with the ICCU [119, 122] as well as the experience of others [118, 120, 123] demonstrated increased immediate survival from cardiac arrest [118, 124–126]. Several series, however, showed little reduction in overall mortality through use of the ICCU. Weinberg [124] reported no difference in the number of late hospital deaths between the 2 years prior to establishment of an ICCU (4 percent) and the 2 years subsequent (5 percent). Reynell [125] randomized 1,000 patients leaving the CCU either to the ICCU or to general medical ward care. The patients in the ICCU were much more likely to be resuscitated (46 versus 21 percent), but overall late hospital mortality rates were about the same: 8.5 percent (44 of 520 patients) in the ICCU and 9.0 percent (43 of 480 patients) in the general medical ward.

Although overall mortality has not been greatly reduced, other benefits have followed the establishment of ICCUs. Freiden and Cooper [123] studied the impact of an ICCU on hospital utlization of CCU beds. All patients with proved myocardial infarction were transferred to the ICCU when stable. Of 1,917 patients, 27 (1.4 percent) sustained cardiac arrest in the ICCU, from which 18 (67 percent) were successfully resuscitated, a figure comparable to those reported from other ICCUs [117, 119, 120, 126]. Moreover, there was a 15 percent increase in CCU admissions because the monitored beds in the ICCU permitted earlier discharge of patients with uncomplicated AMI. Direct admission to the ICCU of patients for whom monitored beds would otherwise have been unavailable resulted in an additional 37 percent increase in total cardiac admissions. Early ambulation using ECG monitoring to ensure patient safety and confidence reduced the average hospitalization for AMI by 3 days. Increased efficiency in the utilization of beds, equipment, and trained personnel, combined with a decrease in the average length of stay, all acted to reduce the costs to the hospital and to patients. The ICCU also permits antiarrhythmic drugs to be begun under monitored conditions so that efficacy and adverse effects can be evaluated carefully.

### IN-HOSPITAL MONITORING

Because of the high cost of monitoring all patients for their entire hospitalization, efforts have been made to identify a high-risk group of patients and to monitor such patients selectively. Arrhythmias in the CCU, even VT and primary VF, do not correlate well with ventricular arrhythmias later in the hospital course [127–130]. Left ventricular failure, anterior wall infarction, infarct size, and persistent sinus tachycardia have all been shown to be predictors of late in-hospital death [117, 118, 120, 121, 126]. Lie and co-workers [126] studied 966 patients discharged from the CCU 3 to 7 days following AMI; of the 30 patients with left ventricular failure in the CCU, 20 had recurrent VF (67 percent), and the mortality was 65 percent. Lie et al. [129] found that patients with new bundle branch block during infarction had a very high risk of primary VF in the 6 weeks following CCU discharge. Because the episodes of VF were evenly distributed over the 6 weeks, they recommended that monitoring be continued for 6 weeks in these patients. Wilson and Pantridge [130] found that the presence of 2 mm ST segment elevation 48 to 72 hours after AMI was associated strongly with the occurrence of VT or VF between CCU discharge and hospital discharge. The association between 2 mm ST elevation and late VT or VF persisted when adjusted for left ventricular failure.

The presence and severity of ventricular arrhythmias as well as the severity of left ventricular dysfunction should be considered in assessing the need for monitoring. We believe that prolonged monitoring is indicated in patients who develop new bundle branch block, patients with transient complete heart block, and patients awaiting permanent pacemaker implantation. Available evidence suggests that patients with severe left ventricular dysfunction, as manifested by persistent sinus tachycardia, hypotension, oliguria, or pulmonary edema, and patients with persistent ST elevation are also at high risk of developing late VF, whether or not ventricular arrhythmias are present in the CCU. We believe that such patients should also be monitored, particularly during the period of early ambulation.

PERMANENT PACEMAKER INSERTION
Permanent pacemaker insertion prior to hospital discharge should be used to treat several conditions: a heart rate that is too slow to maintain cardiac output; bifascicular block with persistent or intermittent second-degree AV block; evidence of trifascicular conduction system disease, especially if confirmed by His bundle recordings; alternating bundle branch block; or intermittent complete heart block beyond the acute stage of myocardial infarction.

Ritter and associates [131], for example, found a greater length of survival (mean survival 18 months) in 12 patients with bifascicular block and transient trifascicular block who received permanent pacemakers than in six comparable patients who were not paced (mean survival 2.4 months). Five of these six patients who did not receive permanent pacemakers died (one was lost to follow-up). Only one of these six deaths, however, resulted from complete heart block. Occasionally, persistent, symptomatic post-MI

sinus node dysfunction will require permanent pacing [37].

Despite the lack of clear evidence of benefit, permanent pacing has also been advocated for all patients who have developed any of the following during the *CCU phase* of acute anterior MI: bifascicular block, transient complete heart block, or bifascicular block with prolongation of the PR interval [46, 78, 81–83, 89]. Mullins [132] reviewed the survival of patients who developed bifascicular block during their AMI and strongly advocated pacing as a possible means of reducing the 67 percent mortality (16 of 24) in this group. Many others concur with these conclusions [89, 90, 93].

If late deaths in patients who developed new *bifascicular block* during AMI were due to conduction disturbances, pacing would have an excellent rationale, but the majority of such patients seem to die as a result of left ventricular failure and/or ventricular arrhythmias [129]. Lichstein et al. [133] monitored 24 patients with acute bifascicular block throughout their entire hospitalization. Although seven (50 percent) died before discharge, only one death resulted from heart block. Five of the seven deaths resulted from left ventricular failure. Similar results were noted by Hauer et al. [134], who also reported that adverse outcome in 18 patients usually was not the result of high-grade block and concluded that permanent pacers usually were not required. Rahimtoola and McAnulty [91] and McAnulty et al. [135] agree that the data mandating permanent pacing for patients with bundle branch block or transient complete heart block are not conclusive. Moreover, as described previously, Lie and associates [76] have demonstrated that prolongation of the H-V interval predicts those patients who are likely to develop complete heart block during the acute phase of AMI, but one cannot extrapolate their results to include permanent pacing. Lichstein et al. [136] performed sequential His bundle recordings on six survivors of a group of 23 patients with prolonged H-V intervals during AMI; in four of the six, the H-V interval returned to normal within 3 weeks of the acute infarction, which suggests a reduction of the risk of complete heart block.

To resolve the issue of permanent pacing for

survivors of AMI who have acutely developed bifascicular block, randomization into "paced" and "not paced" groups is necessary to obtain firm evidence upon which to base recommendations for patients who develop bifascicular block during AMI. In the absence of clear evidence but because of the benefit from permanent pacing suggested by some studies [89, 90, 92, 93, 131, 132], we believe that those patients who develop bifascicular block during AMI and survive should have His bundle recordings performed prior to discharge. Right atrial pacing in addition to His bundle electrograms are necessary for optimal evaluation. Those with prolonged H-V intervals and inducible sub-Hisian block should receive permanent pacemakers. Noninvasive identification of intermittent conduction defects beyond the acute phase of myocardial infarction may also be useful. A 24-hour ECG recording prior to discharge is an excellent way to identify transient high-grade AV block, and it should be performed in all patients who developed bundle branch block or high-grade AV block during AMI independent of whether it is applied for ventricular arrhythmia assessment and subsequent risk stratification in all patients post-MI. Similarly, exercise testing may expose conduction defects that either are rate related or occur only during ischemia.

Soon after AMI, the ventricular wall near the infarct is susceptible to perforation by a catheter. Therefore, permanent pacemaker insertion should be deferred for at least 3 weeks after AMI to minimize the risk of perforation of the ventricle. During this interval, the patient should have continuous ECG monitoring and a flexible, temporary pacemaker left in place.

## The PostHospital Phase

The mortality rate from AMI is three- to fivefold greater over that expected in chronic ischemic heart disease for a period up to 6 months following hospital discharge [128, 137–139]. Of patients surviving at least 24 hours after AMI, about 6 percent die a cardiac death in the following month, and about 8 percent die in the subsequent 5 months [139]. After 6 months the incidence of cardiac mortality drops to between 3 and 4 percent per year, which is comparable to

the mortality rate in chronic ischemic heart disease [128, 142, 144].

Since the excess mortality following AMI is highest during the 6 months immediately following hospital discharge, any intervention designed to decrease postinfarction mortality should be applied early. Furthermore, discontinuing some interventions after 6 months may be reasonable. Since diagnostic and therapeutic approaches have their own mortality and morbidity, it is worthwhile to identify a low-risk group in order to spare such patients the cost and adverse effects of unnecessary therapy, as well as the anxiety of a poorly defined prognosis. Although arrhythmias recorded in the CCU do not identify those at high risk of dying in the posthospital phase of AMI [143, 145–147], those found 2 weeks after infarction do [128, 142–144, 148–151]. Hence, careful evaluation just prior to discharge is essential.

### 24-HOUR ECG RECORDING

Information obtained from analysis of ventricular arrhythmias in a predischarge 24-hour Holter ECG recording is valuable in identifying groups at high and low risk during the year following AMI. Table 15–3 lists the prevalence of ventricular arrhythmias 2 weeks after AMI. As discussed in chapter 5, VPD are nearly ubiquitous following AMI [152–154], and a search has been made for characteristics that are strongly associated with sudden death or reinfarction. Recently, Bigger et al. [141] have shown that frequent VPD and repetitive VPD are independently associated with mortality occurring in the 2-year period following myocardial infarction.

A low frequency of VPD 2 weeks following AMI is associated with a good prognosis. Thus, Bigger and co-workers [141] found that patients with less than 1 VPD per hour had a 2-year mortality of 6 percent, a value 2.5 times less than those with a higher frequency of VPD. Conversely, frequent VPD 2 weeks after AMI identify a high-risk group. The odds of cardiac death within 2 years after AMI increase from 2- to 12-fold if 10 or more VPD per hour are present [128, 140, 141, 143, 151, 155, 156]. Comparison of data from several other studies [126, 131] is limited by the authors' use of the Lown classifi-

TABLE 15-3. Prevalence and character of ventricular arrhythmias 2 weeks after acute myocardial infarction

| Institution | Duration of recording (hours) | Number of patients | Frequency of VPD (%) | | | VPD characteristics (%) | | | |
|---|---|---|---|---|---|---|---|---|---|
| | | | 0 | ≥1/hour | ≥10/hour | Multi-form | Pairs | VT | R-on-T |
| Stanford University | 10 | 95 | 24 | 76 | 30 | 43 | 16 | 17 | — |
| University of Rochester | 6 | 500 | 47 | — | 5 | 10 | 3 | 1 | 10[a] |
| University of Ghent | 6–8 | 150 | 41 | 58 | 23 | 24 | 24 | 15 | 2[b] |
| Washington University | 10 | 238 | 26 | 43 | 17 | 45 | 15 | 2 | 18[a] |
| Columbia University | 24 | 616 | 16 | 50 | 25 | 54 | 31 | 12 | 27[a] |
| MPIP | 24 | 819 | 14 | 41 | 20 | 64 | 17 | 11 | 24[a] |

[a]R-V/QT < 1.00.
[b]R-V/QT < 0.85.

MPIP = Multicenter Post Infarction Program; VPD = ventricular premature depolarizations; VT = ventricular tachycardia.

cation of ventricular arrhythmias [157], which obscures the frequency of VPD [155, 158].

Particularly impressive is the association between VT recorded 2 weeks after AMI and subsequent death. Early studies with small numbers of patients indicated that the odds of cardiac death 1 to 2 years after AMI if VT is present are 3 to 42 times greater (weighted average 19) than when this characteristic is absent [128, 143, 155, 156, 159].

More recently, several sizable postinfarction studies have found that VT (runs of three or more consecutive VPD) has the strongest association with mortality of any ventricular arrhythmia variable. Table 15–4 summarizes four

major studies of nonsustained VT in patients with recent myocardial infarction [141, 160–162]. The prevalence of VT in a population at the time of hospital discharge varies with (1) the overall mortality rate, (2) the recording duration, (3) the sensitivity and specificity of the analysis method, and (4) the definition of VT. If predischarge 24-hour recordings are done in a representative sample of the U.S. postinfarction population with a 10 percent 1-year mortality and are analyzed by sensitive digital computer methods, the prevalence of VT is about 10 percent [141]. Table 15–4 shows that the mortality influence of VT is large and the odds ratio for mortality given VT is similar across these four

TABLE 15-4. Studies of nonsustained ventricular tachycardia (VT) recorded about 2 weeks after myocardial infarction

| | Anderson | Bigger | Kleiger | Bigger |
|---|---|---|---|---|
| Number of patients | 915 | 430 | 289 | 819 |
| Age limit | <66 | <76 | <71 | <70 |
| 1-year mortality | 4% | 13% | 9% | 9% |
| Duration of ECG recording (hours) | 6 | 24 | 10 | 24 |
| DEFINITION OF VT | | | | |
|   Consecutive complexes | ≥3 | ≥3 | ≥3 | ≥3 |
|   Rate | ≥100/min | Any | Any | Any |
| Prevalence of VT | 1.1% | 11.6% | 3.4% | 11.2% |
| Follow-up time (months) | 48 | 36 | 12 | 24 |
| MORTALITY | | | | |
|   With VT | 25% | 38% | 14% | 25% |
|   Without VT | 13% | 12% | 7% | 9% |
| Odds ratio | 4.8 | 4.7 | 2.1 | 3.0 |

major studies. In patients with VT, no relationship has been found between the number of episodes of VT or the length of VT runs and mortality in a year or more of follow-up [160, 161]. However, the studies that have addressed this question so far have been small and therefore have had limited power to detect such relationships should they exist. Nearly all episodes of VT detected in predischarge 24-hour ECG recordings are brief, infrequent, and asymptomatic [160, 161]. Half of the patients have only three VPD in the longest run, and 30 percent have but a single run of VT in the 24-hour ECG recording. Considering these facts, it is remarkable that patients with nonsustained VT have such a high mortality during follow-up after myocardial infarction. The current working hypothesis is that patients who have nonsustained VT are much more likely to develop sustained VT or VF.

## RELATIONSHIP BETWEEN VENTRICULAR ARRHYTHMIAS AND LEFT VENTRICULAR DYSFUNCTION

The relationship among left ventricular dysfunction, ventricular arrhythmias, and death in patients who have just had myocardial infarction is a key to secondary preventive measures for postinfarction arrhythmic death. There are two conflicting currents views on this issue: (1) ventricular arrhythmias contribute independent mortality force after adjusting for the effects of left ventricular dysfunction; and (2) ventricular arrhythmias are so strongly associated with left ventricular dysfunction that ventricular arrhythmias do not contribute independently to mortality after adjusting for left ventricular dysfunction. The major studies that address these conflicting views are summarized in table 15–5.

Ruberman et al. [153] and Moss et al. [154] sought a relationship between "complex" ventricular arrhythmias (bigeminy, multiform, pairs, runs or R-on-T) and post infarction mortality, adjusting for left ventricular dysfunction using the clinical diagnosis of heart failure. Both of these studies were large—1,739 and 940 patients, respectively—and used fairly brief ECG recordings—1 hour and 6 hours, respectively.

Both analyses yielded similar results: complex ventricular arrhythmias were significantly associated with follow-up mortality after adjusting for clinical left ventricular failure.

In a more recent study of 395 coronary heart disease patients referred for cardiac catheterization, Califf et al. [163] addressed the same question. This was not a postinfarction study; only 53 percent of the study group had a previous myocardial infarction, most of them in the remote past. Angiographic left ventricular ejection fraction (LVEF) was used to adjust for left ventricular dysfunction. Arrhythmias detected in 24-hour ECG recordings were graded with a hierarchical scoring system that used frequency, multiformity, pairs, and runs. R-on-T was not used in their analysis. Unadjusted for LV dysfunction, the ventricular arrhythmia score had a very strong association with mortality during follow-up. When Califf et al. [163] used the *clinical* diagnosis of heart failure to adjust for left ventricular dysfunction, the relationship between ventricular arrhythmias and mortality remained significant. However, after adjusting for left ventricular dysfunction with angiographic LVEF, no significant relationship was found between ventricular arrhythmias and mortality. Thus, Califf et al. concluded that the adjustment procedure of Ruberman and Moss failed because they used an inadequate variable, i.e., clinical heart failure, to represent left ventricular dysfunction [163]. Even though the findings of Califf et al. were not obtained in patients with recent myocardial infarction (47 percent had no infarction at all), they nevertheless seriously challenge the conclusions of Ruberman and Moss.

Even more recently, other groups [141, 164, 165] have studied the relationships among left ventricular dysfunction, ventricular arrhythmias, and mortality after myocardial infarction. The Multicenter Investigation of the Limitation of Infarct Size (MILIS) reported their findings in 388 patients [164] and the Multicenter Post Infarction Program (MPIP) reported an analysis of 766 patients [141]. Radionuclide LVEF and 24-hour ECG recordings were obtained prior to hospital discharge. Both of these studies used sensitive and specific computer

TABLE 15–5. Independent relationship between ventricular arrhythmias or left ventricular dysfunction and mortality in coronary heart disease

|  | Ruberman | Moss | Califf | MILIS | MPIP |
|---|---|---|---|---|---|
| Number of patients | 1739 | 940 | 395 | 388 | 766 |
| Time of enrollment (weeks after infarction) | 12 | 2–3 | —* | 1–2 | 1–2 |
| Measure of LV dysfunction | Clinical | Clinical | Angio EF | RNEF | RNEF |
| Duration of ECG recording (hours) | 1 | 6 | 24 | 24 | 24 |
| Ventricular arrhythmia variable | Complex | Complex | Score | Repetitive | Frequent VPD, Repetitive VPD |
| Duration of follow-up (years) | 3 | 4 | 3 | 1 | 2 |
| Number of deaths | 208 | 115 | 58 | 25 | 86 |
| Ventricular arrhythmias and LV dysfunction found to be independent | Yes | Yes | No | Yes | Yes |

*Not a postinfarction study.

MILIS = Multicenter Investigation of the Limitation of Infarct Size; MPIP = Multicenter Post-Infarction Program.

Angio EF = angiographic ejection fraction; LV = left ventricular; Complex ventricular arrhythmias = R-on-T VPD, $\geq 2$ consecutive VPD, multiform VPD, bigeminy; Repetitive VPD = $\geq 2$ consecutive ventricular premature depolarizations; RNEF = radionuclide ejection fraction.

Ventricular arrhythmia score = 0 - no VPD; 1 - < 30 VPD/hour; 2 - $\geq$ 30 VPD/hour; 3 - multiform VPD; 4 - paired VPD; 5 - $\geq$ 3 consecutive VPD.

methods to analyze the 24-hour ECG recordings and cross-validated radionuclide methods to measure LVEF. The cross-tabulation of repetitive VPD, LVEF < 40 percent, and 1-year mortality for the MILIS and MPIP studies is shown in table 15–6. The MILIS study showed a much stronger unadjusted univariate relationship between repetitive VPD and mortality than did the MPIP. The odds ratio for dying during follow-up for patients with repetitive VPD versus those without repetitive VPD was 5.6 for MILIS and only 2.3 for MPIP. The unadjusted univariate relationship between LVEF < 40 percent and mortality was more comparable between the two studies: odds ratio 5.2 for MILIS and 3.4 for MPIP. Within the studies, repetitive VPD and LVEF < 40 percent contributed almost equally to mortality risk in the MILIS study, whereas LVEF < 40 percent was a much stronger risk factor than repetitive VPD in the MPIP study. In MILIS, repetitive VPD was strongly related to mortality after adjusting for left ventricular dysfunction with LVEF < 40 percent. No data on the mortality effect of VPD frequency have been published by MILIS. In MPIP, Bigger et al. [141] applied multivariate survivorship tech-

TABLE 15–6. Mortality one year after infarction as a function of left ventricular ejection fraction and repetitive VPD

| Ejection fraction | Repetitive VPD | Number of patients | | Mortality | | Odds ratio | |
|---|---|---|---|---|---|---|---|
|  |  | MILIS | MPIP | MILIS | MPIP | MILIS | MPIP |
| $\geq$ 40% | No | 199 | 391 | 2% | 5% | 4.9 | 2.4 |
|  | Yes | 55 | 119 | 7% | 12% |  |  |
| < 40% | No | 87 | 157 | 7% | 17% | 4.4 | 1.7 |
|  | Yes | 47 | 99 | 25% | 25% |  |  |
| Total |  | 388 | 766 | 6% | 11% |  |  |

VPD = ventricular premature depolarization; MILIS = Multicenter Investigation of the Limitation of Infarct Size; MPIP = Multicenter Post-Infarction Program.

niques and found that VPD frequency, repetitive VPD, and LVEF were each independently associated with mortality. Since the risk of dying in the year after myocardial infarction is independently increased by LV dysfunction and ventricular arrhythmias, these two risks multiply to give an overall risk factor. For example, if the odds ratio for dying with arrhythmias is 3 and the odds ratio for dying with LVEF under 30 percent is 4, the odds of dying for a group of patients with both is increased 12-fold greater than a group with neither.

### EXERCISE TESTING

Until recently, AMI was considered a contraindication for exercise testing. Several studies, however, have shown that exercise testing at low levels can be performed safely 2 weeks after AMI [166, 167]. As discussed in chapter 5, several groups [155, 168–172] have recently shown that arrhythmias found during exercise in some patients were not found on a 24-hour ECG [155, 169, 170, 172]. Exercise may provoke arrhythmias by one or more of the following actions: decreased vagal tone, increased sympathetic tone, increased ischemia, and increased heart rate. Weld et al. [172] evaluated the significance of cardiac arrhythmias that occurred during a predischarge exercise test after myocardial infarction. Exercise arrhythmias had a strong and significant relationship with death during a year of follow-up. Mortality rate was increased fourfold in patients with positive exercise VPD over the rate in patients who did not have exercise VPD (table 15–7). Exercise capacity and ST segment depression were also significantly related to mortality during follow-up, but there were no significant interactions between exercise arrhythmias and exercise capacity or ST depression with respect to postinfarction mortality [172]. Further study with long-term follow-up will be required before exercise testing can be definitely established as a source of additional valuable information about cardiac arrhythmias. Exercise testing does, however, provide additional quantitative information that may be used to guide rehabilitation, evaluate postinfarction angina, determine the need for coronary angiography, or determine prognosis.

TABLE 15–7. Exercise test VPD and one-year cardiac mortality

| Exercise test VPD | Cardiac death within 1 year | | Totals | Mortality |
|---|---|---|---|---|
| | Yes | No | | |
| None | 6 | 154 | 160 | 4% |
| Either exercise or rest | 7 | 70 | 77 | 9% |
| Rest only | (1) | (27) | | 4% |
| Exercise only | (6) | (43) | | 12% |
| Both exercise and rest | 14 | 74 | 88 | 16% |
| Totals | 27 | 298 | 325 | 8% |

VPD = ventricular premature depolarization.

### POSTINFARCTION ELECTROPHYSIOLOGICAL TESTS

Electrophysiological testing is a new approach for evaluating postinfarction risk. This approach is an outgrowth of the now well established observation that electrophysiological studies are valuable in evaluating patients with known ventricular tachyarrhythmias and in guiding their therapy.

*Repetitive Ventricular Responses.* Only a few electrophysiological studies have been conducted in patients with recent myocardial infarction. In 1978 Greene et al. [173] published the first study. Using A1V2 stimulation, they found that the presence of repetitive ventricular responses (RVR) was associated with increased risk for the occurrence of VT or cardiac death in the first year after infarction (table 15–8). Fifteen of 19 patients (79 percent) who suffered cardiac death or VT had RVR, while only four of 29 patients (14 percent) without VT or cardiac death had RVR. These results await confirmation in other centers. Using A1V2 stimulation, we studied 24 patients 10 to 24 days following myocardial infarction and found a 4 percent prevalence of intraventricular RVR; this contrasts sharply with the 40 percent reported by Greene et al. [173].

TABLE 15-8. Programmed ventricular stimulation to assess risk early after myocardial infarction

|  | Greene et al. [173] | Hamer et al. [174] | Richards et al. [175] |
|---|---|---|---|
| Number of patients | 48 | 37 | 165 |
| PROGRAMMED VENTRICULAR STIMULATION |  |  |  |
| Endpoint | RVR | > 5 VPD | > 10 sec VT |
| Positive | 40% | 34% | 23% |
| MORTALITY RATE |  |  |  |
| Negative Test | 14% | 4% | 6% |
| Positive Test | 42% | 42% | 26% |
| Odds Ratio | 4.1 | 12.0 | 5.9 |

RVR = repetitive ventricular response; VPD = ventricular premature depolarization; VT = ventricular tachycardia.

*Ventricular Tachycardia and Fibrillation.*
More recently, two Australian groups have used more aggressive programmed ventricular stimulation to evaluate patients in the first month after myocardial infarction [174, 175]. Hamer et al. [174] studied 70 patients whose infarction was complicated by heart failure or arrhythmias. Programmed stimulation was performed 7 to 20 days after infarction. In each patient, electrophysiologic studies were performed off of antiarrhythmic drugs. The electrophysiological studies included stimulation of the right ventricular apex in all 70 patients, V2 during A1 pacing (at paced cycle lengths of 500 and 600 msec) in 35 patients, V2 during V1 pacing (at paced cycle lengths of 500 and 400 msec) in all 70 patients, high current V2 and V2V3 in 33 patients, and V1V2 stimulation at a second right ventricular site in 50 patients. Of the 37 patients who underwent the entire protocol, 12 had either sustained VT (8 patients) or nonsustained VT of > 5 complexes (4 patients). The mortality rate during a year of follow-up was 42 percent in patients with inducible sustained VT or nonsustained VT of 5 or more complexes compared to a 4 percent 1-year mortality in the 25 patients with a negative response to programmed ventricular stimulation. The authors concluded that the mechanism of sudden death is usually a ventricular tachyarrhythmia and that programmed ventricular stimulation provides a useful direct method for evaluating ventricular electrical instability.

Richards et al. [175] studied 165 "hemodynamically stable" patients 6 to 28 days after myocardial infarction. V1V2 and V1V2V3 stimulation were applied at the right ventricular apex and right ventricular outflow tract at both low and high (10 mA) current intensities. They called inducible VF or VT that lasted more than 10 seconds electrically unstable. The 10 mA stimulus amplitude significantly increased the number of positive responses in postinfarction patients but not in other groups, e.g., normal subjects or patients with chronic coronary heart disease [176]. The 23 percent of infarct survivors who were unstable did not differ in age or clinical status from stable patients. The 1-year mortality was 26 percent in unstable patients and 6 percent in stable patients (p < 0.001). In the unstable patients 80 percent of the deaths were instantaneous and ventricular tachyarrhythmias were documented in 63 percent, while none of the deaths in stable patients was instantaneous. Thus, Richards et al. concluded that a positive response to programmed ventricular stimulation 6 to 28 days after myocardial infarction indicates a high risk of sudden cardiac death during the subsequent year. Spielman et al. [177] and Buxton et al. [178] studied patients longer after myocardial infarction and concluded that patients with LVEF < 40 percent and nonsustained VT in a 24-hour ECG recording were at very high risk of lethal ventricular arrhythmias. Almost half of this group had a positive response to programmed ventricular stimulation, and their mortality is very high during follow-up. An unanswered question is whether the positive response to programmed ventricular stimulation is just as high in patients with LVEF < 40 percent who do not have nonsustained VT.

*Comparison of Programmed Ventricular Stimulation with Noninvasive Testing.* There are very little data comparing programmed ventricular stimulation to 24-hour ECG or exercise to detect ventricular arrhythmias after myocardial infarction. Hamer et al. [174] did 24-hour ECG recordings in all of their patients and reported that only 5 of the 12 patients with more than five extra responses to programmed ventricular stimulation had spontaneous ventricular arrhythmias in a 24-hour ECG that "suggested a need for treatment." We have found that VT or VF can be elicited during programmed ventricular stimulation in patients who have very few or no spontaneous VPD in a 24-hour ECG recording.

Richards et al. [175] did not compare electrophysiological studies to ambulatory ECG recordings, but they did compare electrophysiological studies to exercise tests in 74 patients. They found that programmed ventricular stimulation is a more potent identifier of sudden cardiac death risk in the year following myocardial infarction than is exercise testing, but that both together identified all first year mortality.

Although the specific role for programmed ventricular stimulation after myocardial infarction awaits further delineation, several small series suggest that electrophysiological studies may be more sensitive indicators of arrhythmic risk following myocardial infarction than either ambulatory ECG recording or exercise testing. Currently, we recommend electrophysiologic studies prior to discharge in patients who have nonsustained VT detected in 24-hour ECG recordings and in patients who have radionuclide LVEF < 40 percent. We find that more than 25 percent of patients with these characteristics have a positive response to programmed ventricular stimulation and that the mortality is high in these groups. However, the impact of electrophysiologically guided antiarrhythmic drug treatment in this group is yet to be defined.

## DRUG THERAPY

*β-adrenergic Blocking Drugs.* Although unproved, many physicians assume that the control of ventricular arrhythmias in the posthospital phase of AMI will improve the chances of the patient's surviving this critical period. However, only the β-adrenergic blocking drugs have been shown to be effective in reducing postinfarction mortality. Several smaller, double-blind, placebo-controlled studies ( < 1,000 patients) showed a trend toward improved survivorship in the beta-blocker-treated groups [179–186]. These small studies tended to show most effect in retrospective subgroup analyses, e.g., efficacy in younger patients, anterior myocardial infarction, or in Q-wave infarcts. Three large-scale, long-term, randomized, double-blind, placebo-controlled trials have been reported [187–190] (table 15–9). In these three trials, the doses of β-adrenergic blocking drugs were relatively high, and in the Beta-Blocker Heart Attack Trial doses were adjusted to a target plasma concentration. All of these large studies show a reduction in total mortality that varies from 23 to 39 percent. The reduction in sudden cardiac death was larger in each study, from 28 to 45 percent. The Norwegian timolol study and the Beta-Blocker Heart Attack Trial showed a decrease in mortality in older patients and in patients with inferior myocardial infarction. The timolol study showed improved survivorship in patients who had non-Q-wave infarcts as well. The ability of larger studies to show benefit of treatment in various subgroup analyses probably relates to their better sampling distributions and greater statistical power.

A short-term (90-day), large-scale, randomized, double-blind, placebo-controlled trial was conducted with metoprolol in several Swedish centers (see table 15–9) [191]. Metoprolol treatment was begun with a 15 mg intravenous injection and continued with 100 mg oral doses every 12 hours. Mortality was reduced by 36 percent in this study (p < 0.05). Also, preliminary results suggest that infarct size, judged by area under creatine kinase curves, was significantly reduced [191]. As a result of these studies, we recommend that β-adrenergic blocking drugs be given to all patients who can tolerate them. The drugs should be started around day 5 to 7 and given in the following doses: timolol, 10 to 20 mg bid; or propranolol, 80 mg tid. If patients cannot tolerate a nonspecific β-adrenergic blocking drug, then metoprolol, 100 mg bid,

TABLE 15–9. Large-scale, randomized, placebo-controlled, double-blind trials with β-adrenergic blocking drugs after myocardial infarction

|  | International multicenter study | Norwegian multicenter study | Beta-blocker heart attack trial | Multicenter metoprolol study |
|---|---|---|---|---|
| Beta-blocker | Practolol | Timolol | Propranolol | Metoprolol |
| Dose (mg/day) | 400 | 20 | 180–240 | 200 |
| No. of patients | 3,053 | 1,884 | 3,837 | 1,395 |
| Time of enrollment (days) | 7–30 | 7–30 | 5–21 | 1–2 |
| Follow-up (months) | 14 | 17 | 25 | 3 |
| NO. OF DEATHS |  |  |  |  |
| Controls | 124 | 152 | 188 | 62 |
| Treated | 96 | 98 | 138 | 40 |
| Reduction in mortality | 23% | 39% | 26% | 36% |

should be used. Treatment should be continued for 1 to 2 years.

How much of the increased postinfarction survivorship with antiarrhythmic drug treatment is due to an antiarrhythmic effect is not known. Data from the Beta-Blocker Heart Attack Trial and Norwegian Multicenter Study indicate that β-adrenergic blocking drugs decrease the prevalence of frequent VPD in the early posthospital phase by about 40 to 50 percent. The Swedish metoprolol trial showed a significant reduction in CCU lidocaine usage in patients treated with metoprolol within 12 hours of the onset of infarction pain (70 percent of the treated group). Woosley et al. [192] showed that high but not low doses of propranolol reduced VPD frequency in patients with chronic coronary heart disease. Experimental studies in dogs have shown that both timolol and propranolol reduce the incidence of sustained VT and VF after acute coronary occlusion [193]. Also, timolol and propranolol normalize the electrical VF threshold and prevent the induction of sustained VT by programmed ventricular stimulation in dogs with large subacute anterior myocardial infarction [35]. Thus, moderate doses of β-adrenergic blocking drugs have a moderate effect on VPD frequency and a more marked antifibrillatory effect.

*Conventional Antiarrhythmic Drugs.* A number of feasibility studies have been conducted with conventional antiarrhythmic drugs [194, 195]. Only a few of these studies selected pa-

tients with arrhythmias for treatment, used plasma drug concentrations to adjust dosing, or used 24-hour ECG recordings to establish antiarrhythmic efficacy [195]. Moreover, none of the trials had had a sample size large enough to permit detection of a 25 to 40 percent reduction in mortality. At present, the National Heart, Lung and Blood Institute is conducting a feasibility study, the Cardiac Arrhythmia Pilot Study (CAPS), to determine if a strategy can be found that would permit a 70 percent or greater reduction in VPD frequency for a year after infarction in patients who have 10 or more VPD per hour or multiple runs of VPD in a qualifying 24-hour ECG recording. If such a strategy can be found, a full-scale trial may be conducted to determine whether reducing ventricular arrhythmias effectively will improve survival in postinfarction patients who have frequent or repetitive VPD.

Until such studies are completed, we recommend that one of the following approaches be used to manage patients at high risk to lethal arrhythmias. One rational approach is to enroll patients with antiarrhythmias into controlled trials. This approach gives the maximum likelihood of taking the correct action in the absence of definitive information and will produce the critical information needed for managing future patients. When patients are to be treated individually, we recommend that treatment be restricted to patients who have 10 or more VPD per hour or those with VT. Antiarrhythmic drugs should be used in doses that significantly reduce the frequency and complexity of ventricular arrhythmias (70 percent or greater reduction in frequency and eradication of VT). To achieve this goal, careful evaluation of therapy with repeated analysis of 24-hour ECG recordings is required.

Table 15–10 lists the oral antiarrhythmic agents available in the United States and some of their kinetic properties. An ideal drug would control arrhythmias without adverse effects. Currently available agents are not effective for all patients and have a relatively high incidence of adverse effects. If a drug is ineffective at the initial dose chosen, it should be increased with careful monitoring of its effect. Measurement of plasma drug concentration may identify patients in whom ineffectiveness results from poor absorption or rapid elimination; in such cases, either the dose administered or the dosing interval may be adjusted accord-

ingly. More than one drug may be required for rhythm control.

*Acute Drug Testing.* Unless therapy is individualized and efficacy is assessed with ample ECG samples, rhythm control is, often as not, inadequate. At best, whether changes in ventricular rhythm are due to the drug employed or to spontaneous variation in rhythm is difficult to judge [196]. Thus, determination of efficacy can be a difficult and time-consuming process. Gaughan et al. [197] have proposed a method of acute drug testing that requires only 72 hours and the analysis of one 24-hour ECG recording to evaluate efficacy. The initial judgment of efficacy is made on the basis of a 5-½-hour test period. Control data are taken for 30 minutes; then a single large dose of drug is given. The ECG is sampled every third minute and recorded in

TABLE 15–10. Administration of antiarrhythmic drugs

| | Quinidine | Procainamide | Propranolol | Diphenylhydantoin | Disopyramide |
|---|---|---|---|---|---|
| Effective concentration (ug/ml) | 2–6 | 4–20 | 0.1–1.0 | 5–18 | 2–4 |
| KINETIC DATA | | | | | |
| Volume of distribution (liters/kg body weight) | 2.2 | 2.0 | 1.8 | 1.0 | 1.0–2.0 |
| Half-life (hours) | 6–7 | 3–4 | 2–3 | 20–30 | 5–6 |
| Protein binding | 60% | 15% | 90% | 90% | 30–40% |
| Hepatic metabolism | Hydroxylation | Acetylation | Hydroxylation | p-Hydroxylation glucuronide conjugation | N-Dealkylation |
| Renal excretion of unchanged drug | 20–50% | 30–60% | 1% | 5% | 65–70% |
| ORAL ADMINISTRATION | | | | | |
| Total daily dose (mg) | 1,200–2,400 | 2,000–8,000 | 160–1,000 | 300–800 | 600–1,200 |
| Frequency | q4–8 hr | q3–6 hr | q3–6 hr | o.d. to q.i.d. | q.i.d. |
| Time to peak plasma conconcentration (single dose) | 1.5–2 hr | 1–1.5 hr | 2–4 hr | 6–12 hr | 0.5–3.0 hr |
| Time to plateau plasma concentration (multiple oral dosage) | 1–2 days | 1–2 days | 1–2 days | 6–7 days | 1–2 days |

compressed form to permit on-line review of efficacy and toxicity. A "response" is defined as at least 50 percent reduction in VPD frequency and complete absence of either pairs of VPD or VT for at least 30 minutes. If evidence of efficacy is not obtained within 3 hours, the test is terminated. If the single test dose shows efficacy, the patient is placed on maintenance doses. After 48 hours an exercise test is performed, and during the third day a 24-hour ECG is performed. If all goes well, the patient who responds in the initial acute test will be on satisfactory maintenance by the third day.

*Conventional Dose Ranging.* There is a major difference between acute drug testing and the usual protocols for determining dose range. In the latter, the initial dose is moderate and efficacy is evaluated on a steady-state dose. Often, one or two dose changes are made before antiarrhythmic efficacy is achieved. This method establishes the relationship between steady-state plasma concentrations and antiarrhythmic response. Also, dose-related undesirable effects are detected while they are minimal.

In our opinion, traditional dose-ranging protocols are more informative and safer in the early stages of investigation of a new antiarrhythmic drug. Once a body of knowledge accumulates about the kinetics, effective concentration range, and toxic concentration range, acute drug testing has much to recommend it. Previously acquired knowledge can be used to select a large test dose likely to be efficacious and safe. If the acute drug testing method as proposed by Gaughan et al. is extended to include measurement of pharmacokinetic constants, then the selection of the maintenance regimen for responders will be much more accurate and take less time. A note of caution about the interpretation of the acute drug test has been raised by Winkle [196], who simulated this procedure in individuals who had frequent ventricular arrhythmias. He counted VPD frequency for 5 ½ hours as though a drug dose were given, even though none was. In 13 of 20 patients, responses were observed that would have been interpreted as showing drug efficacy, and in several others, "toxic" responses were observed. This simulation underscores the need for large

samples of ECG data to assess antiarrhythmic drug efficacy or toxicity.

Once adequate control is reached, the steady-state plasma level of antiarrhythmic drug can be measured; this value may be useful for dealing with problems that subsequently arise during therapy. There is still a real need for additional antiarrhythmic drugs that can be used orally and chronically for prophylaxis in the posthospital phase of AMI. An ideal drug would be (1) effective in preventing ventricular arrhythmias and arrhythmic death, (2) relatively free of undesirable effects, (3) suitable for once or twice daily dosing, and (4) free of interactions with other drugs. A number of promising new drugs are undergoing clinical trials in the United States. Several—for example, mexiletine, tocainide, ethmozin, and amiodarone—have been used successfully in Europe and are nearing their review by the Food and Drug Administration (Tocainide was recently approved by the FDA) [198–200]. Recent reports suggest that tricyclic antidepressants are excellent type IA antiarrhythmic agents [201]. Recently, a new class of antiarrhythmic drugs, the type IC drugs, such as flecainide or encainide have been shown to have marked effects on cardiac conduction and to be extremely potent against ventricular arrhythmias [202–204]. One or several of these latter agents may prove useful for prophylaxis of ventricular arrhythmias in the posthospital phase.

## Therapy of Arrhythmias in Chronic Coronary Heart Disease

A large percentage of patients with chronic coronary heart disease and rhythm disturbances are first seen by a physician in the office or emergency room setting when the patient has an arrhythmia but does not have myocardial infarction.

### SUPRAVENTRICULAR TACHYARRHYTHMIAS

Left atrial enlargement is frequently found in association with left ventricular enlargement in ischemic heart disease because of previous hypertension or left ventricular failure. Atrial fibrillation may occur after long-standing atrial dilatation as well as during AMI. Atrial fibrillation reduces cardiac output in patients with ischemic heart disease, particularly if ventricular compliance is reduced, by decreasing ventricular filling during diastole, as well as by contributing to increased left ventricular dysfunction at rapid heart rates. The major risk of atrial flutter or fibrillation in patients with ischemic heart disease is that the ventricular response may be so rapid that coronary blood supply is insufficient, resulting in ischemia, angina, hypotension, or a combination of these. When atrial fibrillation develops, the clinical status of the patient determines appropriate therapy. If acute atrial fibrillation is associated with severe angina, hypotension, or pulmonary edema, immediate electrical cardioversion is indicated. Mild sedation may be given with intravenous morphine or diazepam and is immediately followed by application of synchronized DC shock; we recommend beginning with 100 joules.

When angina, hypotension, and pulmonary edema are absent but the ventricular rate is rapid, digitalization should be accomplished expeditiously. Therapy may be begun with .5 mg intravenous digoxin, and additional intravenous doses of 0.125 or 0.25 mg may be given at 1- to 6-hour intervals until the ventricular response has slowed to 80 to 100 beats/min or until the atrial fibrillation reverts to sinus rhythm. If the clinical situation is not acute, the patient can be digitalized orally over a period of time. If digoxin fails to maintain sinus rhythm, either quinidine or procainamide may be used for this purpose (see discussion on supraventricular arrhythmia during the CCU phase of AMI). If atrial fibrillation is associated with mild angina or dyspnea without hypotension, intravenous verapamil or propranolol may be used to quickly achieve ventricular rate control in the interval before digitalis effect is achieved.

SVT, rather than atrial fibrillation or flutter, is a much less common sequelae of myocardial infarction. When it occurs in the stage of chronic ischemic heart disease, it is more apt to follow inferior than anterior infarction. Digitalis is the drug of choice.

When patients abruptly develop atrial arrhythmias, AMI should be excluded. It is worth noting that electrical cardioversion does not usually obscure the laboratory diagnosis of AMI

[205]. If elevation of cardiac isoenzymes (creatine phosphokinase or lactate dehydrogenase) is found after cardioversion, myocardial ischemia or infarction must be presumed to be the cause, not the cardioversion itself [205]. Myocardial damage may cause the arrhythmia or vice versa.

## VENTRICULAR ARRHYTHMIAS

*Medical Therapy.* Ventricular arrhythmias pose a problem in coronary heart disease when they occur remote from myocardial infarction or in patients with angina pectoris who have never had myocardial infarction. For the purpose of selecting management strategies, ventricular arrhythmias in this setting can be classified as malignant, potentially malignant, or benign [152]. The approach to management of each of these categories is quite different.

MALIGNANT VENTRICULAR ARRHYTHMIAS. Two forms of malignant ventricular arrhythmias are recognized in coronary heart disease: (1) out-of-hospital cardiac arrest and (2) recurrent, sustained VT. Out-of-hospital cardiac arrest usually is caused by VT that degenerates into VF or by ventricular ischemia that triggers VF. Other mechanisms occur more rarely, e.g., drug-induced torsades des pointes. Survivors of out-of-hospital cardiac arrest are usually those with VT that degenerates into VF. This selective survival is accounted for by a period of VT that is a viable, if tenuous, rhythm. This gives the patient a chance to call or reach help. Ischemic VF, on the other hand, tends to occur abruptly without prior VT, killing the patient before he has any opportunity to seek help. Less than one-third of the out-of-hospital cardiac arrest survivors have myocardial infarction as judged by Q-waves in the 12-lead ECG [207, 208]. Patients with recurrent, sustained VT usually have ventricular scarring due to previous myocardial infarction or, more rarely, cardiomyopathy or valvular heart disease. Patients with these malignant ventricular arrhythmias should be managed aggressively because of their high mortality rate of 25 to 40 percent per year. Two approaches have been advocated for management of malignant ventricular arrhythmias: (1) a noninvasive approach and (2) an electrophysiologic approach with programmed ventricular stimulation [209–212]. The noninvasive approach has been discussed in detail in chapter 5. One report suggests very strongly that this method gives excellent results [213]. The electrophysiologic approach, outlined in table 15–11, has been shown by several authors to be effective in identifying successful drug treatment [209–212]. Neither approach has proven that drug treatment is responsible for the improved outcome in patients who respond to treatment. It may be that drug responsiveness is an epiphenomenon and not causally related to outcome. Controlled trials will be required to answer this question. Even so, these two methods do identify the groups that do well or badly on medical treatment. Patients who are nonresponders to medical treatment should be treated surgically or by implantation of the automatic defibrillator [214, 215]. Since no head-to-head comparison has been made between the noninvasive approach and electrophysiologically guided therapy, the two must be regarded as more or less equivalent for the management of malignant ventricular arrhythmias.

POTENTIALLY MALIGNANT VENTRICULAR ARRHYTHMIAS. Potentially malignant ventricular arrhythmias in coronary heart disease are the repetitive ventricular arrhythmias in the presence of significant left ventricular dysfunction. Patients with repetitive ventricular arrhythmias should be evaluated for left ventricular dysfunction using radionuclide ventriculography. Patients with nonsustained VT and LVEF < 40 percent have a high mortality in follow-up and should be considered for treatment. Electrophysiologic studies in such patients show that about half will have sustained VT and that those with positive responses to programmed ventricular stimulation have a very high mortality during follow-up [177, 178]. There have been no studies yet to show the relative merits of electrophysiologically guided treatment and the noninvasive approach in the potentially malignant arrhythmias. We recommend that physicians use the same approach for these arrhythmias that they use for malignant ventricular arrhythmias.

BENIGN VENTRICULAR ARRHYTHMIAS. Frequent ventricular arrhythmias seen without repetitive forms or left ventricular dysfunction are usually benign. These do not require treatment unless they are symptomatic. If such rhythms cause palpitations, they can be treated with reassurance and by removing any provocative influences identified by a careful history and by diaries kept during 24-hour ECG recording. Occasionally, symptoms will be sufficient cause for treatment with an antiarrhythmic drug. We recommend that β-adrenergic blocking drugs be tried first in this situation if the patient has no contraindication to beta-blocker treatment. Beta-blockers may decrease VPD frequency substantially, or they may diminish palpitations even though VPD frequency is minimally affected. The control of symptoms without control of ventricular arrhythmias is considered adequate for management of benign ventricular arrhythmias. If the physician judges that more VPD reduction is needed than β-adrenergic blocking drugs provide, a type IB drug, e.g., tocainide or mexiletine, should be added to the beta-blocker. The combination of one of the type IB drugs and a beta-blocker gives very high efficacy and low toxicity [216].

*Surgical Therapy.* Surgery may also be used in the treatment of ventricular arrhythmias in ischemic heart disease, though some aspects of the surgical approach must still be considered investigational. Candidates for surgical approaches to arrhythmia control are those with recurrent ventricular tachycardia or those who have been resuscitated from ventricular fibrillation espe-

TABLE 15–11. Electrophysiologic approach to malignant ventricular arrhythmias

1. Stabilize patient; treat complications of arrest
2. Continuous ECG monitoring in intensive care or telemetry unit
3. Withdraw antiarrhythmic drugs
4. Determine inducibility using programmed ventricular stimulation
5. Therapy
    * Antiarrhythmic drug
    * Arrhythmia surgery
    * Antitachycardia pacemaker
    * Automatic implanted defibrillator
    * Stop antiarrhythmic drug
6. Determine inducibility using programmed ventricular stimulation

cially if drug resistant or if surgery is independently needed for angina (coronary artery bypass grafting, CABG) or pump failure (aneurysmectomy). The greatest and longest experience of surgery for arrhythmias is with resection of ventricular aneurysm alone or combined with myocardial revascularization [217–229]. Aneurysmectomy will improve or abolish ventricular arrhythmias in about 50 percent of cases.

Initially, resections of aneurysms for ventricular arrhythmia were done without coronary artery bypass grafting. Subsequently, aneurysmectomy and coronary artery bypass grafting were performed together. Although the combination probably does not improve the success of aneurysmectomy as an arrhythmia control procedure, it may decrease overall mortality and surgical risk. Waxman et al. [230] used combined myocardial resection and revascularization to treat eight patients who had ventricular tachycardia that persisted after AMI. Although the mortality within the first year was at least 50 percent, it was an improvement over the mortality of six comparable patients (100 percent mortality within 1 month) who were treated medically. Each of these 14 patients had extensive AMI with significant left ventricular dysfunction.

In general, the mortality associated with resection of ventricular aneurysms depends on the proximity of the operation to the occurrence of previous AMI and on the severity of coexisting left ventricular failure. Operations performed within 4 to 6 weeks following AMI carry a prohibitive mortality, whereas operations performed later carry an operative mortality of about 10 to 15 percent.

Several reports are available on the results of coronary artery bypass grafting alone in treating ventricular arrhythmias [231–237]. Some success has been experienced, although the failure rate is high and the mortality significant. Early studies suggested that as a general rule, the frequency of sporadic ventricular arrhythmias or of ventricular tachyarrhythmias does not change after coronary artery bypass grafts [238, 239]; most subsequent studies confirm these conclusions.

Because CABG and simple aneurysmectomy, alone or in combination, are not highly effective antiarrhythmic modalities, additional approaches have been sought. For example, Spurrell et al. [240, 241] attempted to interrupt reentrant ventricular tachycardia in ischemic heart disease by division of the anterior radiation of the left bundle branch in four patients, with success in two. Others have not pursued this approach; experience with this procedure, therefore, is too meager to warrant conclusions.

Fontaine et al. [242], in Paris, have reported considerable success with ventriculotomy for drug-resistant ventricular tachycardia in nonischemic heart diseases. After detailed epicardial mapping during electrically induced ventricular tachycardia, a linear transmural incision is made at sites of early epicardial breakthrough. The early results of simple ventriculotomy, however, have been very disappointing in ischemic heart disease [242, 243].

Significantly greater success has been achieved with two additional approaches. In one, developed by Guiraudon et al. [244], an endocardial incision is made that encircles the entire infarct and is almost epicardial in depth. The extensive incision is then repaired and the ventricle closed. This encircling endocardial ventriculotomy electrically isolates the presumed arrhythmic focus, though ischemic destruction of the arrhythmic site by microvascular interruption also appears to be a factor in its success. This approach, though often effective, has been associated with a significant degree of ventricular dysfunction and probably isolates a larger area of tissue than is actually necessary.

The second and more sophisticated approach is ablative surgery guided by electrophysiological mapping. By electrically defining areas of prolonged, delayed, or impaired myocardial depolarization, possible substrate areas for reentrant circuits, or by defining areas of initial activation during spontaneous or induced ventricular tachycardia, limited and discrete areas for ablative surgery may be defined. Such electrophysiological mapping is initially performed via catheterization preoperatively; then more refined epicardial, endocardial, and sometimes transmyocardial mapping is performed in the operating room. Antiarrhythmic drug slowing of the ventricular tachycardias is often required for mapping, and intraoperative induction of the tachycardia to be mapped is not always possible under the influence of anesthesia, myocardial cooling, or ventricular decompression following ventriculotomy; hence, the need for the preoperative study. Generally, the foci of origin are found in areas adjacent to, but not within, aneurysms or infarct scars. Once mapping has defined the region felt to be responsive for the tachycardia, ablative surgery is performed. This may take the form of a limited encircling endocardial incision analogous to that discussed above or, more often, an endocardial resection or peel as described by Horowitz et al. [245] is carried out. In this latter approach, the scarred areas of endocardium and subendocardial His-Purkinje tissue of the area of origin is resected. Cryoablation may also be used. These mapping–guided endocardial ablations thus limit the amount of tissue destruction or resection required and thereby prevent needless damage to widespread regions, including the papillary muscle sacrifice or ventricular septal perforation that can be associated with total scar encircling or excision. Mapping–guided surgery also enhances the likelihood of success. Mason et al. [229], for example, showed that arrhythmia recurrence was only 17 percent at 3 months and 29 percent at 24 months with mapping–guided resection compared to 56 percent with blind aneurysmectomy. Additionally, we have found that even if the arrhythmia is not abolished, it is often converted to a drug responsive form. For the interested reader, additional, more extensive details of arrhythmia mapping and of the surgical approaches to ventricular arrhythmias can be found in several excellent recent reports [239, 245–249].

It should be emphasized that the surgical procedures require extensive technological resources. Preoperative and intraoperative studies are required and detailed excitation maps must be made expeditiously during catheterization and/or operation. Personnel and equipment are expensive, and relatively few centers can adequately mount such an effort. The development of the automatic implantable defibrillator [214, 215] now in clinical trials and the development of more automated and rapid mapping systems, however, may shortly and quickly expand the utility and geographic breadth of arrhythmia surgery.

## Conclusions

Therapy of arrhythmias and conduction disturbances in ischemic heart disease can be divided into five phases, four of which relate to AMI. The first of these is the prehospital phase of an acute infarction, the second the CCU phase, the third the late in-hospital phase. The fourth the posthospital phase. The fifth and final phase is chronic ischemic heart disease.

In the first hours of an AMI, bradyarrhythmias and VF are the most frequent rhythm disturbances. The treatment of bradyarrhythmias is controversial, but at present, atropine is recommended primarily for the hypotension that accompanies the bradyarrhythmias; the dose of atropine must be titrated to avoid excessive heart rate. To prevent VF the mainstay of therapy is still early response and ready availability of DC defibrillation. Intravenous or intramuscular lidocaine can be used as prophylaxis.

In the CCU, sinus bradycardia, junctional bradycardia, or second-degree AV block in inferior myocardial infarction should be treated by temporary transvenous pacing when hypotension due to inadequate heart rate is present. Second-degree AV block in anterior infarction is usually Mobitz type 2; either Mobitz type 2 block or any acute bundle branch block is an indication for a temporary VVI pacemaker. In the CCU, there is some evidence that high doses of lidocaine given prophylactically can prevent primary VF, but this therapy frequently produces undesirable effects.

During the late hospital course, patients with new bundle branch block, transient complete heart block, persistent ST elevation, and severe left ventricular dysfunction are at high risk. Such patients should be monitored throughout their hospital course. A permanent pacemaker should be implanted before discharge in those patients whose heart rate is too slow to maintain cardiac output or in patients who develop bundle branch block during AMI and have persistent trifascicular conduction system disease.

Arrhythmias found 2 weeks after AMI identify patients with a high risk of dying in the posthospital phase of AMI. A 24-hour ECG should be performed on all patients with AMI about 1 to 2 weeks after the infarction. Treatment with oral antiarrhythmic agents should be considered for patients with nonsustained VT and those with more than 10 VPD per hour. Repeat 24-hour ECG recording should be used to determine antiarrhythmic drug efficacy.

In chronic ischemic heart disease, ventricular arrhythmias again provide a major source of controversy regarding the value of treatment, since there is currently no ideal drug for long-term oral therapy of ventricular arrhythmias. It is clear that recurrent sustained VT or out-of-hospital cardiac arrest without AMI should be treated. It has been shown that effective therapy judged either by electrophysiologic testing or by 24-hour ECG recordings and exercise testing is associated with a much improved long-term survival. Recent evidence suggests that patients with nonsustained VT and LVEF < 40 percent are at high risk and should be treated. The final group that should be treated is patients whose VPD are symptomatic. New drugs are actively being developed, and the results of current work may alter future recommendations.

## References

1. Pantridge, J.F., Adgey, A.A.J., Geddes, J.S., and Webb, S.W. *The Acute Coronary Attack.* New York: Grune & Stratton, 1975, pp. 27–42.

2. Goldreyer, B.N. and Wyman, M.G. The effect of first hour hospitalization in myocardial infarction. *Circulation* 50(Suppl. 3):121, 1974.

3. Grace, W.J. and Chadbourn, J.A. The first hour in acute myocardial infarction (AMI): Observation in 50 patients. *Circulation* 42(Suppl. 3):-160, 1970.

4. Rose, R.M., Lewis, A.J., Fewkes, J., Clifton, J.F., and Criley, J.M. Occurrence of arrhythmias during the first hour of acute myocardial infarction. *Circulation* 50(Suppl. 3):121, 1974.

5. Skjaggestad, O. and Berstad, S. Arrhythmias in the earliest phase of acute myocardial infarction. *Acta Med. Scand.* 196:271, 1974.

6. Adgey, A.A.J., Geddes, J.S., Mulholland, H.C., Keegan, D.A.J., and Pantridge, J.F. Incidence, significance and management of early bradyarrhythmia complicating acute myocardial infarction. *Lancet* 2:1097, 1968.

7. Webb, S.W., Adgey, A.A.J., and Pantridge, J.F. Autonomic disturbance at onset of acute myocardial infarction. *Br. Med. J.* 3:89, 1972.

8. Pantridge, J.F., Geddes, J.S., Webb, S.W., and Adgey, A.A.J. Atropine and infarction bradycardia. *Ann. Intern. Med.* 81:126, 1974.

9. Warren, J.V. and Lewis, R.P. Beneficial effects of atropine in the pre-hospital phase of coronary care. *Am. J. Cardiol.* 37:68, 1976.

10. Massumi, R.A., Mason, D.T., Amsterdam, E.A., DeMaria, A., Miller, R.R., Scheinman, M.M., and Zelis, R. Ventricular fibrillation and tachycardia after intravenous atropine for treatment of bradycardias. *N. Engl. J. Med.* 287:336, 1972.

11. Zipes, D.P. and Knoebel, S.B. Rapid rate-dependent ventricular ectopy. Adverse responses to atropine-induced rate increase. *Chest* 62:255, 1972.

12. Richman, S. Adverse effect of atropine during myocardial infarction. Enhancement of ischemia following intravenously administered atropine. *JAMA* 228:1414, 1974.

13. Epstein, S.E., Goldstein, R.E., Redwood, D.R., Kent, K.M., and Smith, E.R. The early phase of acute myocardial infarction: Pharmacologic aspects of therapy. *Ann. Intern. Med.* 78:918, 1973.

14. Kent, K.M., Smith, E.R., Redwood, B.R., and Epstein, S.E. The deleterious electrophysiological effects produced by increasing heart rate during experimental coronary occlusion. *Clin. Res.* 20:379, 1972.

15. Redwood, D.R., Smith, E.R., and Epstein, S.E. Coronary artery occlusion in the conscious dog. Effects of alterations in heart rate and arterial pressure on the degree of myocardial ischemia. *Circulation* 46:323, 1972.

16. Epstein, S.E., Redwood, D.R., and Smith, E.R. Atropine and acute myocardial infarction. *Circulation* 45:1273, 1972.

17. Kent, K.M., Smith, E.R., Redwood, D.R., and Epstein, S.E. Electrical stability of acutely ischemic myocardium. *Circulation* 47:291, 1973.

18. Chadda, D.D., Banka, V.S., and Helfant, R.H. Rate dependent ventricular ectopia following acute coronary occlusion. The concept of an optimal antiarrhythmic heart rate. *Circulation* 49:-654, 1974.

19. Scheinman, M.M., Thornburn, D., and Abbot, J.A. Use of atropine in patients with acute myocardial infarction and sinus bradycardia. *Circulation* 52:627, 1975.

20. Shillingford, J. and Thomas, M. Treatment of bradycardia and hypotension syndrome in patients with acute myocardial infarction. *Am Heart J.* 75:843, 1968.

21. Myerburg, R.J., Estes, D., Zaman, L. et al. Outcome of resuscitation from bradyarrhythmic or asystolic prehospital cardiac arrest. *J. Am. Coll. Cardiol.* 4:1118, 1984.

22. Mulholland, H.C. and Pantridge, J.F. Heart rate changes during movement of patients with acute myocardial infarction. *Lancet* 1:1244, 1974.

23. Allen, J.D., Pantridge, J.F., and Shanks, R.G. The effects of practolol on the dysrhythmias complicating acute ischemic disease. *Am. J. Med.* 58:199, 1975.

24. Jewitt, D.E., Burgess, P.A., and Shillingford, J.P. The circulatory effects of practolol (ICI-50172) in patients with acute myocardial infarction. *Cardiovasc. Res.* 1:188, 1970.

25. Moss, A.J., Goldstein, S., Green, W., and DeCamilla, J. Prehospital precursors of ventricular arrhythmias in acute myocardial infarction. *Arch. Intern. Med.* 129:756, 1972.

26. Lawrie, D.M., Higgins, M.R., Godman, M.J., Julian, D.G., and Donald, K.W. Ventricular fibrillation complicating acute myocardial infarction. *Lancet* 2:523, 1968.

27. Lewis, R.P. and Warren, J.V. Factors determining mortality in the prehospital phase of acute myocardial infarction. *Am. J. Cardiol.* 33:152, 1974.

28. Adgey, A.A.J., Devlin, J.E., Webb, S.W., and Mulholland, H.C. Initiation of ventricular fibrillation outside hospital in patients with acute ischemic heart disease. *Br. Heart J.* 47:55, 1982.

29. Fehmers, M.C.O. and Dunning, A.J. Intramuscularly and orally administered lidocaine in the treatment of ventricular arrhythmias in acute myocardial infarction. *Am. J. Cardiol.* 29:514, 1972.

30. Bernstein, V., Bernstein, M., Griffiths, J., and Peretz, D.I. Lidocaine intramuscularly in acute myocardial infarction. *JAMA* 219:1077, 1972.

31. Sloman, G., Isaac, P., Harper, R., and Penington, C. Plasma levels of lidocaine after intramuscular injection. *Heart Lung* 2:669, 1973.

32. Valentine, P.A., Frew, J.L., Mashford, M.L., and Sloman, G. Lidocaine in the prevention of sudden death in the pre-hospital phase of acute infarction. *N. Engl. J. Med.* 291:1327, 1974.

33. Pentecost, B.L. and Austen, W.G. Beta-adrenergic blockade in experimental myocardial infarction. *Am. Heart J.* 72:790, 1966.

34. Khan, M.I., Hamilton, J.T., and Manning, G.W. Early arrhythmias following coronary occlusion in conscious dogs and their modification by beta-adrenoreceptor blocking drugs. *Am. Heart J.* 86:347, 1973.

35. Gang, E.S., Bigger, J.T., Jr., and Uhl, E.W. The effects of timolol and propranolol on inducible sustained ventricular tachyarrhythmias in dogs with subacute myocardial infarction. *Am. J. Cardiol.* 53:275, 1984.

36. Stults, K.R., Brown, D.D., Schuf, V.L., and Bean, J.A. Prehospital defibrillation performed by emergency medical technicians in rural communities. *N. Engl. J. Med.* 310:219, 1984.

37. Simonsen, E., Nielsen, B.L., and Nielsen, J.S. Sinus node dysfunction in acute myocardial infarction. *Acta Med. Scand.* 208:463, 1980.

38. Imperial, E.S., Carballo, R., and Zimmerman, H.A. Disturbances in rate, rhythm and conduction in acute myocardial infarction. A statistical study of 153 cases. *Am. J. Cardiol.* 5:24, 1960.

39. Julian, D.T., Valentine, P.A., and Miller, G.G. Disturbances of rate, rhythm and conduction in acute myocardial infarction. A prospective study of 100 consecutive unselected patients with the aide of electrocardiographic monitoring. *Am. J. Med.* 37:915, 1964.

40. Cristal, N., Szwarcberg, J., and Gueron, M. Supraventricular arrhythmias in acute myocardial infarction. Prognostic importance of clinical setting; mechanism of production. *Ann. Intern. Med.* 83:35, 1975.

41. George, M. and Greenwood, T.W. Relation between bradycardia and the site of myocardial infarction. *Lancet* 2:739, 1967.

42. Norris, R.M. Bradyarrhythmia after myocardial infarction. *Lancet* 1:313, 1969.

43. Lawrie, M., Greenwood, T.W., Goddard, M., Harvey, A.C., Donald, K.W., Julian, D.G., and Oliver, M.F. A coronary-care unit in the routine management of acute myocardial infarction. *Lancet* 2:109, 1967.

44. Wyman, M.G. and Hammersmith, L. Coronary care in the small community hospital. *Dis. Chest* 53:584, 1968.

45. Jewitt, D.E., Balcon, R., Raftery, E.B., and Oram, S. Incidence and management of supraventricular arrhythmias after acute myocardial infarction. *Lancet* 2:734, 1967.

46. Haft, J. I. Clinical implications of atrioventricular and intraventricular conduction abnormalities. II. Acute myocardial infarction. *Cardiovasc. Clin.* 8:65, 1977.

47. Lown, B., Fakhro, A.M., Hood, W.B., Jr., and Thorn, G.W. The coronary care unit. New perspectives and directions. *JAMA* 199:188, 1967.

48. Lown, B., Vassaux, C., Hood, W.B., Jr., Fakhro, A.M., Kaplinsky, E., and Roberge, G. Unresolved problems in coronary care. *Am. J. Cardiol.* 20:494, 1967.

49. Medias, J.E., Chahine, R.A., Gorlin, R., and Blacklow, D.J. A comparison of transmural and nontransmural acute myocardial infarction. *Circulation* 49:498, 1974.

50. Meltzer, L.E. and Kitchell, J.B. The incidence of arrhythmias associated with acute myocardial infarction. *Prog. Cardiovasc. Dis.* 9:50, 1966.

51. Stock, E., Gobel, A., and Sloman, G. Assessment of arrhythmias in myocardial infarction. *Br. Med. J.* 2:719, 1973.

52. Furman, S. Cardiac pacing and pacemakers. I. Indications for pacing bradyarrhythmias. *Am. Heart J.* 93:523, 1977.

53. Thanavaro, S., Kleiger, R.E., Province, M.A., Hubert, J.W., Miller, J.P., Krone, R.J., and Oliver, G.C. Effect of infarct location on the in-

hospital prognosis of patients with first transmural infarction. *Circulation* 66:742, 1982.

54. Stock, R.J. and Macken, D.L. Observations on heart block during continuous electrocardiographic monitoring in myocardial infarction. *Circulation* 38:993, 1968.

55. Norris, R.M. and Mercer, C.J. Significance of idioventricular rhythms in acute myocardial infarction. *Prog. Cardiovasc. Dis.* 16:455, 1974.

56. Brown, R.W., Hunt, D., and Sloman, J.G. The natural history of atrioventricular conduction defects in acute myocardial infarction. *Am. Heart J.* 78:460, 1969.

57. Kitchen, J.G. and Kastor, J.A. Pacing in acute myocardial infarction—indications, methods, hazards and results. *Cardiovasc. Clin.* 7:219, 1975.

58. Col, J.J. and Weinberg, S.L. The incidence and mortality of intraventricular conduction defects in acute myocardial infarction. *Am. J. Cardiol.* 29:344, 1972.

59. Hurwitz, M. and Eliot, R.S. Arrhythmias in acute myocardial infarction. *Dis. Chest* 45:616, 1964.

60. Dhringra, R.C., Denes, P., Wu, D., Chuquimia, R., and Rosen, K.M. The significance of second-degree atrioventricular block and bundle branch block: Observations regarding site and type of block. *Circulation* 49:638, 1974.

61. Norris, R.M. Heart block in posterior and anterior myocardial infarction. *Br. Heart J.* 31:352, 1969.

62. Scheinman, M. and Brenman, B.A. Clinical and anatomical implications of intraventricular conduction blocks in acute myocardial infarction. *Circulation* 46:753, 1972.

63. Friedberg, C.K., Cohen, H., and Donoso, E. Advanced heart block as a complication of acute myocardial infarction. Role of pacemaker therapy. *Prog. Cardiovasc. Dis.* 10:466, 1968.

64. Paulk, E.A. and Hurst, J.W. Complete heart block in acute myocardial infarction. A clinical evaluation of the intracardiac bipolar catheter pacemaker. *Am. J. Cardiol.* 17:695, 1966.

65. Jackson, A.E. and Bashour, F.A. Cardiac arrhythmias in acute myocardial infarction. I. Complete heart block and its natural history. *Dis. Chest* 51:31, 1967.

66. Zipes, D.P. The clinical significance of bradycardiac rhythms in acute myocardial infarction. *Am. J. Cardiol.* 24:814, 1969.

67. Leth, A., Hansen, J.F., and Meibom, J. Acute myocardial infarction complicated by third degree atrioventricular block treated with temporary pacing. *Acta Med. Scand.* 195:391, 1975.

68. Tans, A.C., Lie, K.I., and Durrer, D. Clinical setting and prognostic significance of high degree atrioventricular block in acute inferior myocardial infarction: A study of 144 patients. *Am. Heart J.* 99:44, 1980.

69. Scott, M.E., Geddes, J.S., Patterson, G.C., Adgey, A.A.J., and Pantridge, J.F. Management of complete heart block complicating acute myocardial infarction. *Lancet* 1:1382, 1967.

70. Kostuck, W.J. and Beanlands, D.S. Complete heart block associated with acute myocardial infarction. *Am. J. Cardiol.* 26:380, 1970.

71. Beregovich, J., Fenig, S., Lasser, J., and Allen, D. Management of acute myocardial infarction complicated by advanced atrioventricular block. Role of artificial pacing. *Am. J. Cardiol.* 23:54, 1969.

72. Biddle, T.L., Ehrich, D.A., Yu, P.N., and Hodges, M. Relation of heart block and left ventricular dysfunction in acute myocardial infarction. *Am. J. Cardiol.* 39:961, 1977.

73. Hatee, L. and Rokseth, R. Conservative treatment of A-V block in acute myocardial infarction. *Br. Heart J.* 33:595, 1971.

74. Chatterjee, K., Harris, A., and Leatham, A. The risk of pacing after infarction and current recommendations. *Lancet* 2:1061, 1969.

75. Lie, K.I., Wellens, H.J., Schuilenburg, R.M., and Durrer, D. Observations on acquired and chronic bundle branch block in myocardial infarction. *Circulation* 52(Suppl. 2):113, 1975.

76. Lie, K.I., Wellens, H.J., Schuilenburg, R.M., Becker, A.E., and Durrer, D. Factors influencing prognosis of bundle branch block complicating antero-septal infarction. The value of His bundle recordings. *Circulation* 50:935, 1974.

77. Norris, R.M. and Croxson, M.S. Bundle branch block in acute myocardial infarction. *Am. Heart J.* 79:728, 1970.

78. Waugh, R.A., Wagner, G.S., Haney, T.L., Rosati, R.A., and Morris, J.J., Jr. Immediate and remote prognostic significance of fascicular block during acute myocardial infarction. *Circulation* 47:765, 1973.

79. Gould, L., Ramana, G.V., and Gomprecht, R.F. Left bundle branch block: Prognosis in acute myocardial infarction. *JAMA* 225:626, 1973.

80. Scheidt, S. and Killip, T. Bundle branch block complicating acute myocardial infarction. *JAMA* 222:919, 1972.

81. Lasser, R.P., Haft, J.I., and Friedberg, C.K. Relationship of right bundle branch block and marked left axis deviation (with left parietal or peri-infarction block) to complete heart block and syncope. *Circulation* 37:429, 1968.

82. Lichstein, E., Gupta, P.K., Chadda, K.D., Liu, H.M., and Sayeed, M. Findings of prognostic value in patients with incomplete bilateral branch block complicating acute myocardial infarction. *Am. J. Cardiol.* 39:913, 1973.

83. Godman, M.J., Lassers, B.W., and Julian, D.G. Complete bundle branch block complicating

acute myocardial infarction. *N. Engl. J. Med.* 282:237, 1970.

84. Hunt, D. and Sloman, G. Bundle branch block in acute myocardial infarction. *Br. Med. J.* 1:85, 1969.

85. Jones, M.E., Terry, G., and Kenmure, A.C. Frequency and significance of conduction defects in acute myocardial infarction. *Am. Heart J.* 94:163, 1977.

86. Otterstad, J.E., Gundersen, S., and Anderssen, N. Left anterior hemi-block in acute myocardial infarction. Incidence and clinical significance in relation to the presence of bundle branch block and to the absence of intraventricular conduction defects. *Acta Med. Scand.* 203:529, 1978.

87. Bruce, R.A., Blackmon, J.R., Cobb, L.A., and Dodge, H.T. Treatment of asystole or heart blocking during acute myocardial infarction with electrode catheter pacing. *Am. Heart J.* 69:460, 1965.

88. Romero, C.A. Cardiac pacing in acute myocardial infarction. *Am. J. Cardiol.* 36:412, 1975.

89. Escher, D.J. Use of cardiac pacemakers. *Hosp. Pract.* 16(9):49, 1981.

90. Hindman, M.C., Wagner, G.S., Jaro, M., Atkins, J.M., Scheinman, M.M., DeSanctis, R.W., Hutter, A.H., Jr., Yeatman, L., Rubenfire, M., Pujura, C., Rubin, M., and Morris, J.J. The clinical significance of bundle branch block complicating acute myocardial infarction. 1. Clinical characteristics, hospital mortality, 1 year follow-up. *Circulation* 58:679, 1978.

91. Rahimtoola, S.H. and McAnulty, J.N. High risk bundle branch block. *Hosp. Pract.* 16(1):73, 1981.

92. Fisch, G.R., Zipes, D.P., and Fisch, C. Bundle branch block and sudden death. *Prog. Cardiovas. Dis.* 23:187, 1981.

93. Hindman, M.C., Wagner, G.S., Jaro, M., Atkins, J.M., Scheinman, M.M., DeSanctis, R.W., Hutter, A.H., Jr., Yeatman, L., Rubenfire, M., Pujura, C., Rubin, M., and Morris, J.J. The clinical significance of bundle branch block complicating acute myocardial infarction. 2. Indications for temporary and permanent pacemaker insertion. *Circulation* 58:689, 1978.

94. Scheinman, M.M., Remedios, P., Cheitlin, M.D., Peters, R.W., Holford, N., Desai, J., and Abbott, J.A. Effects of antiarrhythmic drugs on antrioventricular conduction in patients with acute myocardial infarction. *Circulation* 62:20, 1980.

95. Helmers, C., Lundman, T., Mogensen, L., Orinius, E., Sjogren, A. and Wester, P.O. Atrial fibrillation in acute myocardial infarction. *Acta Med. Scand.* 193:39, 1973.

96. Klass, M. and Haywood, L.H. Atrial fibrillation associated with acute myocardial infarction. *Am. Heart J.* 79:752, 1970.

97. Smith, T.W. and Haber, E. Digitalis. *N. Engl. J. Med.* 289:1010, 1973.

98. Marcus, F.I. Digitalis pharmacokinetics and metabolism. *Am. J. Med.* 68:452, 1975.

99. Doherty, J.E. and Kane, J.J. Clinical and pharmacology of digitalis glycosides. *Ann. Rev. Med.* 26:159, 1975.

100. Lown, B., Klein, M.D., Barr, L., Hagemeijer, F., Kosowsky, B.D., and Garison, H. Sensitivity to digitalis drugs in acute myocardial infarction. *Am. J. Cardiol.* 30:388, 1972.

101. Rahimtoola, S.H. and Gunnar, R.M. Digitalis in acute myocardial infarction: Help or hazard? *Ann. Intern. Med.* 82:234, 1975.

102. Beller, G.A., Smith, T.W., and Hood, W.B., Jr. Effects of ischemia and coronary reperfusion on myocardial digoxin uptake. *Am. J. Cardiol.* 36:902, 1975.

103. Mogensen, L. A controlled trial of lignocaine prophylaxis in the prevention of ventricular tachyarrhythmias in acute myocardial infarction. *Acta Med. Scand.* 513:1, 1971.

104. Ambos, H.D., Roberts, R., Oliver, G.C., Cox, J.R., Jr., and Sobel, B.E. Infarct size: A determinant of persistence of severe ventricular arrhythmias. *Am. J. Cardiol.* 37:116, 1976.

105. Lawrie, D.M., Higgins, M.R., Godman, M.J., Julian, D.G., and Donald, K.W. Ventricular fibrillation complicating acute myocardial infarction. *Lancet* 2:523, 1968.

106. Dhurandhar, R.W., MacMillan, R.L., and Brown, W.G. Primary ventricular fibrillation complicating acute myocardial infarction. *Am. J. Cardiol.* 27:347, 1971.

107. Wyman, M.G. and Hammersmith, S. Comprehensive treatment plan for the prevention of primary ventricular fibrillation in acute myocardial infarction. *Am. J. Cardiol.* 33:661, 1974.

108. Lie, K.I., Wellens, H.J., Downar, E., and Durrer, D. Observations on patients with primary ventricular fibrillation complicating acute myocardial infarction. *Circulation* 52:755, 1975.

109. Kimball, J.T. and Killip, T. Aggressive treatment of arrhythmias in acute myocardial infarction. Procedures and results. *Prog. Cardiovasc. Dis.* 19:483, 1968.

110. Lown, B., Klein, M.D., and Hirshberg, P.I. Coronary and precoronary care. *Am. J. Med.* 46:705, 1969.

111. Saunamaki, K.I. and Pederson, A. Significance of cardiac arrhythmias preceding first cardiac arrest in patients with acute myocardial infarction. *Acta Med. Scand.* 199:461, 1976.

112. Campbell, R.W.F., Murray, A., and Julian, D.G. Ventricular arrhythmias in the first 12 hours of acute myocardial infarction. Natural history study. *Br. Heart J.* 46:351, 1981.

113. Harrison, D.C. Should lidocaine be adminis-

tered routinely to all patients after acute myocardial infarction? *Circulation* 58:581, 1978.

114. Lie, K.I., Wellens, H.J., Van Capelle, F.J., and Durrer, D. Lidocaine in the prevention of primary ventricular fibrillation. *N. Engl. J. Med.* 291:1324, 1974.

115. Lie, K.I., Liem, K.L., Lourditz, W.J., Janse, M.J., Willebrands, A.F., and Durrer, D. Efficacy of lidocaine in preventing primary ventricular fibrillation within 1 hour after a 300 mg intramuscular injection. *Am. J. Cardiol.* 42:486, 1978.

116. Bigger J.T., Jr. Pharmacologic and clinical control of antiarrhythmic drugs. *Am. J. Med.* 58:479, 1975.

117. Bornheimer, J., deGuzman, M., and Haywood, L.J. Analysis of in-hospital deaths from myocardial infarction after coronary care unit discharge. *Arch. Intern. Med.* 135;1035, 1975.

118. Thompson, P. and Sloman, G. Sudden death in-hospital after discharge from coronary care unit. *Br. Med. J.* 4:136, 1971.

119. Grace, W.J. and Yarvote, P.M. Acute myocardial infarction: The course of the illness following discharge from the coronary care unit. *Chest* 59:15, 1971.

120. Resnekov, L. The intermediate coronary care unit. A stage in continued coronary care. *Br. Heart J.* 39:357, 1977.

121. Graboys, T.B. In-hospital sudden death after coronary care unit discharge. *Arch. Intern. Med.* 135:512, 1975.

122. Grace, W.J. Intermediate coronary care units revisited. *Chest* 67:510, 1975.

123. Freiden, J. and Cooper, J.A. The role of the intermediate cardiac care unit. *JAMA* 245:816, 1976.

124. Weinberg, S.L. Intermediate coronary care: The failure of a concept. *Am. J. Cardiol.* 37:181, 1976.

125. Reynell, P.C. Intermediate coronary care. A controlled trial. *Br. Heart J.* 37:166, 1975.

126. Lie, K.I., Wellens, H.J.J., Downar, E., and Durrer, D. Early identification of patients developing late in-hospital ventricular fibrillation after discharge from CCU. *Am. J. Cardiol.* 37:152, 1976.

127. Lindsay, J., Jr. and Gorfinkel, H.J. Arrhythmias in the post-CCU phase of myocardial infarction: Their correlation with the acute illness. *Chest* 72:571, 1977.

128. Bigger, J.T., Jr., Heller, C.A., Wenger, T.L., and Weld, F.M. Risk stratification after acute myocardial infarction. *Am. J. Cardiol.* 42:202, 1978.

129. Lie, K.I., Liem, K.L., Schuilenberg, R.N., David, G.K., and Durrer, D. Early identification of patients developing late in-hospital ventricular fibrillation after discharge from the coronary care unit. A 5 ½ year retrospective and prospective study of 1897 patients. *Am. J. Cardiol.* 41:674, 1978.

130. Wilson, C. and Pantridge, J.F. ST segment displacement and early hospital discharge in acute myocardial infarction. *Lancet* 2:1284, 1973.

131. Ritter, W.S., Atkins, J.M. Blomqvist, C.G., and Mullins, C.B. Permanent pacing in patients with transient trifascicular block during acute myocardial infarction. *Am. J. Cardiol.* 38:205, 1975.

132. Mullins, C.B. Indications for pacing after acute myocardial infarction in patients with fascicular block. *J. Electrocardiol.* 8:297, 1975.

133. Lichstein, E., Letafati, A., Gupta, P.K., and Chadda, K.D. Continuous Holter monitoring with bifascicular block complicating anterior wall myocardial infarction. *Am. J. Cardiol.* 40:860, 1977.

134. Hauer, R.N.W., Lie, K.I., Liem, K.L., and Durrer, D. Long term prognosis in patients with bundle branch block complicating acute anteroseptal infarction. *Am. J. Cardiol.* 49:1581, 1982.

135. McAnulty, J.H., Rahimtoola, S.H., Murphy, E., DeMots, H., Ritzmann, L., Kanarek, P.E., and Kauffman, S. Natural history of "high risk" bundle branch block. Final report of a prospective study. *N. Engl. J. Med.* 307:137, 1982.

136. Lichstein, E., Grupta, P.K., and Chadda, K.D. Long term survival of patients with incomplete bundle-branch block complicating acute myocardial infarction. *Br. Heart J.* 37:924, 1975.

137. Helmers, C. Short and long term prognostic indices in acute myocardial infarction. A study of 606 patients initially treated in a coronary care unit. *Acta Med. Scand.* 555(Suppl.):54, 1973.

138. Pell, S. and DÁlonzo, C.A. Immediate mortality and five year survival of employed men with a first myocardial infarction. *N. Engl. J. Med.* 270:915, 1964.

139. Weinblatt, E., Shapiro, S., Frank, C.W., and Sager, R.V. Prognosis of men after first myocardial infarction: Mortality and first recurrence in relation to selected parameters. *Am. J. Public Health* 58:1329, 1968.

140. The Multicenter Postinfarction Research Group. Risk stratification and survival after myocardial infarction. *N. Engl. J. Med.* 309:331, 1983.

141. Bigger, J.T., Jr., Fleiss, J.L., Kleiger, R., Miller, J.P., Rolnitzky, L.M., and the Multicenter Post-Infarction Group. The relationship between ventricular arrhythmias, left ventricular dysfunction, and mortality in the two years after myocardial infarction. *Circulation* 69:250, 1984.

142. Moss, A.J., DeCamilla, J.J., Davis, H.P., and Bayer, L. Clinical significance of ventricular ec-

topic beats in the early post-hospital phase of myocardial infarction. *Am. J. Cardiol.* 39:635, 1977.

143. Vismara, L.A., Hughes, J.AhL., Kraus, J., Borhani, N.O., Zelis, R., Mason, D.T., and Amsterdam, E.A. Relation of ventricular arrhythmias in the late hospital phase of acute myocardial infarction to posthospital sudden death. *Am. J. Cardiol.* 33:175, 1975.

144. Norris, R.M., Crughey, D.E., Mercer, C.J., Deeming, L.W., and Scott, P.J. Coronary prognostic index for predicting survival after recovery from acute myocardial infarction. *Lancet* 2:485, 1970.

145. Bigger, J.T., Jr., Weld, F.M., Coromilas, J., Rolnitzky, L.M., and DeTurk, W.E. Prevalence and Significance of Arrhythmias in 24-Hour ECG Recordings Made Within One Month of Acute Myocardial Infarction. In Kulbertus, H. and Wellens, H.J.J. (eds.), *The First Year after a Myocardial Infarction*. Boston: Martinus Nijhoff, 1983, p. 161.

146. DeSoyza, N., Kane, J., Bisset, J., and O'Murphy, M. Correlation of ventricular arrhythmia during acute and late phases of myocardial infarction. *Am. J. Med.* 64:377, 1978.

147. Moss, A.J., Schnitzler, R., Green, R., and DeCamilla, J. Ventricular arrhythmias three weeks after acute myocardial infarction. *Ann. Intern. Med.* 75:837, 1971.

148. Kotler, M.N., Tabatznik, B., Mower, M.M., and Tominaga, S. Prognostic significance of ventricular ectopic beats with respect to sudden death in the late post infarction period. *Circulation* 47:959, 1973.

149. Moss, A.J., DeCamilla, J., and Davis, H. Cardiac death in the first six months after myocardial infarction: Potential for mortality reduction in the early post hospital period. *Am. J. Cardiol.* 39:816, 1977.

150. Oliver, G.C., Nolle, F.M., and Tiefenbrunn, J. Ventricular arrhythmias associated with sudden death in survivors of acute myocardial infarction. *Am. J. Cardiol.* 33:160, 1974.

151. Schulze, R.A., Jr., Reau, J., Rigo, P., Bowers, S., Strauss, H.W., and Pitt, B. Ventricular arrhythmias in the late hospital phase of acute myocardial infarction. Relation to left ventricular function detected by gated cardiac blood pool scanning. *Circulation* 52:1006, 1975.

152. Ryden, L., Waldenstrom, A., and Holnberg, S. The reliability of intermittent ECG sampling in arrhythmia detection. *Circulation* 52:540, 1975.

153. Ruberman, W., Weinblatt, E., Goldberg, J.D., Frank, C.W., and Shapiro, S. Ventricular premature beats and mortality after myocardial infarction. *N. Engl. J. Med.* 297:750, 1977.

154. Moss, A.J., Davis, H.T., DeCamilla, J., and Bayer, L.W. Ventricular ectopic beats and their relation to sudden and nonsudden cardiac death after myocardial infarction. *Circulation* 60:998, 1978.

155. Bigger, J.T., Jr., and Weld, F.M. Analysis of prognostic significance of ventricular arrhythmias after myocardial infarction: Shortcomings of Lown grading system. *Br. Heart J.* 45:717, 1981.

156. Van Durme, J.P. and Pannier, R.H. Prognostic significance of ventricular dysrhythmias one year after myocardial infarction. *Am. J. Cardiol.* 37:178, 1976.

157. Lown, B. and Wolf, M. Approaches to sudden death from coronary disease. *Circulation* 44:130, 1971.

158. Bigger, J.T., Jr., Wenger, T.L., and Heissenbuttel, R.H. Limitations of the Lown grading system for the study of human ventricular arrhythmias. *Am. Heart J.* 93:727, 1977.

159. Bigger, J.T., Jr., Dresdale, R.J., Heissenbuttel, R.H., Weld, F.M., and Wit, A.L. Ventricular arrhythmias in ischemic heart disease: Mechanism, prevalence, significance and management. *Prog. Cardiovasc. Dis.* 19:255, 1977.

160. Anderson, K.P., DeCamilla, J., and Moss, A.J. Clinical significance of ventricular tachycardia (3 beats or longer) detected during ambulatory monitoring after myocardial infarction. *Circulation* 57:890, 1978.

161. Bigger, J.T., Jr., Weld, F.M., and Rolnitzky, L.M. Prevalence, characteristics and significance of ventricular tachycardia (three or more complexes) detected with ambulatory electrocardiographic recording in the late hospital phase of acute myocardial infarction. *Am. J. Cardiol.* 48:815, 1981.

162. Kleiger, R.E., Miller, J.P., Thanavaro, S., Marin, T.F., Province, M.A., and Oliver, G.C. Relationship between clinical features of acute myocardial infarction and ventricular runs two weeks to one year following infarction. *Circulation* 63:64, 1981.

163. Califf, R.M., McKinnis, R.A., Burks, J., Lee, K.L., Harrell, F.E., Behar, V.S., Pryor, D.B., Wagner, G.S., and Rosati, R.A. Prognostic implications of ventricular arrhythmias during 24-hour ambulatory monitoring in patients undergoing cardiac catheterization for coronary artery disease. *Am. J. Cardiol.* 50:23, 1982.

164. Mukharji, J., Rude, R.E., Poole, K., Croft, C., Thomas, L.J., Jr., Strauss, H.W., Roberts, R., Raabe, D.S., Jr., Braunwald, E., Willerson, J.T., and cooperating investigators Multicenter Investigation of the Limitation of Infarct Size (MILIS). Late sudden death following acute myocardial infarction, importance of combined presence of repetitive ventricular ectopy and left ventricular dysfunction. *Clin. Res.* 30:108A, 1982 (abstract).

165. Olson, H.G., Lyons, K.P., Troop, P., Butman, S., and Piters, K.M. The high-risk acute myocardial infarction patient at 1-year follow-up: Identification at hospital discharge by ambulatory electrocardiography and radionuclide ventriculography. *Am. Heart. J.* 107:358, 1984.

166. Ericson, M., Granath, A., Ohlsen, P., Sodermark, T., and Volpe, U. Arrhythmia and symptoms during treadmill testing three weeks after myocardial infarction in 100 patients. *Br. Heart J.* 35:707, 1973.

167. Ibsen, H., Kjoller, E., Styperek, J., and Pederson, A. Routine exercise ECG three weeks after acute myocardial infarction. *Acta Med. Scand.* 198:463, 1975.

168. Sami, M., Kraemer, H., and DeBusk, R.F. The prognostic significance of serial exercise testing after myocardial infarction. *Circulation* 60:1238, 1979.

169. Smith, J.W., Dennis, C.A., Gassman, A., Gaines, J.A., Staman, M., Phibbs, B. and Marcus, F.I. Exercise testing three weeks after myocardial infarction. *Chest* 75:12, 1979.

170. Sivertssen, E., Bay, G., Hansen, G., Leren, P., Lippestad, C., Saltvedt, E., and Skjaeggestad, O. The prognostic value of arrhythmias at rest and in connection with an exercise stress test in the late hospital phase of acute myocardial infarction. *J. Oslo City Hosp.* 28:23, 1978.

171. Theroux, P., Waters, D.D., Halphen, C., Debaisieux, J.C., and Mizgala, H.F. Prognostic value of exercise testing soon after myocardial infarction. *N. Engl. J. Med.* 301:341, 1979.

172. Weld, F.M., Chu, K-L., Bigger, J.T., Jr., and Rolnitzky, L.M. Risk stratification with low level exercise testing two weeks after acute myocardial infarction. *Circulation* 64:306, 1981.

173. Greene, H.L., Reid, P.R., and Schaeffer, A.H. The repetitive ventricular response in man: A predictor of sudden death. *N. Engl. J. Med.* 299:729, 1978.

174. Hamer, A., Vohra, J., Hunt, D., and Sloman, G. Prediction of sudden death by electrophysiologic studies in high risk patients surviving acute myocardial infarction. *Am. J. Cardiol.* 50:223, 1982.

175. Richards, D.A., Cody, D.V., Denniss, A.R., Russell, P.A., Young, A.A., and Uther, J.B. Ventricular electrical instability during the first year following myocardial infarction. *Am. J. Cardiol.* 51:75, 1983.

176. Richards, D.A., Denniss, A.R., Cameron, M., and Uther, J.B. What is the incidence of nonstimulated ventricular beating after programmed stimulation? *Circulation* 68(III):243, 1983 (abstract).

177. Spielman, S.R., Yacone, L.A., Greenspan, A.M., Webb, C.R., and Horowitz, L.N. Electro-physiologic testing in high-risk patients with nonsustained ventricular tachycardia and abnormal ventricular function. *Circulation* 68(III):56, 1983 (abstract).

178. Buxton, A.E., Waxman, H.L., Marchlinski, F.E., and Josephson, M.E. Predictors of sudden death in nonsustained ventricular tachycardia. *Circulation* 68(III):108, 1983 (abstract).

179. Wilhelmsson, C., Vedin, J.A., Wilhelmsen, L., Tibblin, G., and Werko, L. Reduction of sudden deaths after myocardial infarction by treatment with alprenolol. *Lancet* 2:1157, 1974.

180. Vedin, A., Wilhelmsson, C., and Werko, L. Chronic alprenolol treatment of patients with acute myocardial infarction after discharge from hospital: Effects on mortality and morbidity. *Acta Med. Scand.* (Suppl.)575:3, 1975.

181. Ahlmark, G., Saetre, H., and Korsgren, M. Reduction of sudden death after myocardial infarction. *Lancet* 2:1563, 1974.

182. Ahlmark G. and Saetre, H. Long term treatment with beta-blockers after myocardial infarction. *Eur. J. Clin. Pharmacol.* 10:77, 1976.

183. Andersen MP, Bechsgaard P, Frederiksen J, Hansen DA, Jurgensen HJ, Nielsen B, Pedersen F, Pedersen-Bjergaard O, and Rasmussen SL. Effect of alprenolol on mortality among patients with definite or suspected acute myocardial infarction: Preliminary results. *Lancet* 2:865, 1979.

184. Barber, J.M., Boyle, D.M., Chaturvedin, C., Singh, N., and Walsh, M.J. Practolol in acute myocardial infarction. *Acta Med. Scan.* (Supp)587:213, 1976.

185. Wilcox, R.G., Roland, J.M., Banks, D.C., Hampton, J.R., and Mitchell, J.R.A. Randomized trial comparing propranolol with atenolol in immediate treatment of suspected myocardial infarction. *Br. Med. J.* 280:885, 1980.

186. Baber, N.S., Evans, D.W., Howitt, G., Thomas, M., Wilson, C., Lewis, J.A., Dawes, P.M., Handler, K., and Tuson, R. Multicentre post-infarction trial of propranolol in 49 hospitals in the United Kingdom, Italy and Yugoslavia. *Br. Heart J.* 44:96, 1980.

187. Multicenter International Study. Improvement in prognosis of myocardial infarction by long term beta-adrenoreceptor blockade using practolol. *Br. Med. J.* 3:735, 1975.

188. Multicenter International Study Group. Reduction in mortality with long-term beta-adrenoreceptor blockade: A multicentre international study. *Br. Med. J.* 2:49, 1977.

189. The Norwegian Multicenter Study Group. Timolol-induced reduction in mortality and reinfarction in patients surviving acute myocardial infarction. *N. Engl. J. Med.* 1981; 304: 801–807.

190. Beta-blocker Heart Attack Trial Research

Group. A randomized trial of propranolol in patients with acute myocardial infarction. *JAMA* 247:1707, 1982.

191. Hjalmarson, A., Elmfeldt, D., Herlitz, J., Holmberg, S., Malek, I., Nyberg, G., Ryden, L., Swedberg, K., Vedin, A., Waagstein, F., Waldenstrom, A., Waldenstrom, J., Wedel, H., Wilhelmsen, L., and Wilhelmsson, C. Effect on mortality of metroprolol in acute myocardial infarction. A double-blind randomized trial. *Lancet* 4:823, 1981.

192. Woosley, R.L., Kornhauser, D., Smith, R., Reele, S., Higgins, S.B., Nies, A.S., Shand, D.G., and Oates, J.A. Suppression of chronic ventricular arrhythmias with propranolol. *Circulation* 60:819, 1979.

193. Warner, N.J. and Bigger, J.T., Jr. Timolol, but not propranolol, decreases ventricular arrhythmias after coronary occlusion in the dog. *Clin. Res.* 30:229A, 1982.

194. Koch-Weser, J. Antiarrhythmia prophylaxis in ambulatory patients with coronary heart disease. *Arch. Intern. Med.* 129:763, 1972.

195. May, G.S., Eberlein, K.A., Furberg, C.D., Passamani, E.R., DeMets, D.L. Secondary prevention after myocardial infarction: A review of long-term trials. *Prog. Cardiovasc. Dis.* 24:331, 1982.

196. Winkle, R.A. Antiarrhythmic drug effect mimicked by spontaneous variation of ventricular ectopy. *Circulation* 57:1116, 1978.

197. Gaughan, C.E., Lown, B., Lanigan, J., Voukydis, P., and Bessen, H.W. Acute oral testing for determining antiarrhythmic drug efficacy. I. Quinidine. *Am. J. Cardiol.* 38:677, 1976.

198. Pratt, C.M., Young, J.B., Francis, M.J., Taylor, A.A., Norton, H.J., English, L., Mann, D.E., Kopelen, H., Quinones, M.A., and Roberts, R. Comparative effect of disopyramide and ethmozine in suppressing complex ventricular arrhythmias by use of a double-blind, placebo-controlled, longitudinal crossover design. *Circulation* 69:288, 1984.

199. Singh, J.B., Rasul, A.M., Shah, A., Adams, E., Flessas, A., and Kocot, S.L. Efficacy of mexiletine in chronic ventricular arrhythmias compared with quinidine: A single-blind, randomized trial. *Am. J. Cardiol.* 53:84, 1984.

200. Zipes, D.P., Prystowsky, E.N., and Heger, J.J. Amiodarone: Electrophysiologic actions, pharmacokinetics and clinical effects. *J. Am. Coll. Cardiol.* 3:1059, 1984.

201. Giardina, E.G.V. and Bigger, J.T., Jr. Antiarrhythmic effect of imipramine hydrochloride in patients with ventricular premature complexes without psychological depression. *Am. J. Cardiol.* 50:172, 1982.

202. Flecainide research study group. Flecainide versus quinidine for treatment of chronic ventricular arrhythmias. A multicenter clinical trial. *Circulation* 67:1117, 1983.

203. Roden, D.M., Reele, S.B., Higgins, S.B., Mayol, R.F., Gammans, R.E., Oates, J.A., and Woosley, R.L. Total suppression of ventricular arrhythmias by encainide. *N. Engl. J. Med.* 302:877, 1980.

204. Mason, J.W. and Peters, F.A.. Antiarrhythmic efficacy of encainide in patients with refractory recurrent ventricular tachycardia. *Circulation* 63:670, 1981.

205. Reiffel, J.A., Gambino, S.R., McCarthy, D.A., and Leahey, E.B., Jr. Effect of direct current cardioversion on CK, LDH and their myocardial isoenzymes. *JAMA* 239:122, 1978.

206. Bigger, J.T., Jr. Antiarrhythmic treatment: An overview. *Am. J. Cardiol.* 53:8B, 1984.

207. Cobb, L.A., Werner, J.A., and Trobaugh, G.B. Sudden cardiac death. I.A. decade's experience with out-of-hospital resuscitation. *Modern Concepts Cardiovasc. Dis.* 49:31, 1980.

208. Cobb, L.A., Werner, J.A., and Trobaugh, G.B. Sudden cardiac death. II. Outcome of resuscitation, management and future directions. *Modern Concepts Cardiovasc. Dis.* 49:37, 1980.

209. Josephson, M.E. and Horowitz, L.N. Electrophysiologic approach to therapy of recurrent sustained ventricular tachycardia. *Am. J. Cardiol.* 43:631, 1979.

210. Mason, J.W. and Winkle, R.A. Accuracy of the ventricular tachycardia-induction study for predicting long-term efficacy and inefficacy of antiarrhythmic drugs. *N. Engl. J. Med.* 303:1077, 1980.

211. Kowley, P.R., Friehling, T., Mesiter, S.G., and Engel, T.R. Late induction of tachycardia in patients with ventricular fibrillation associated with acute myocardial infarction. *J. Am. Coll. Cardiol.* 3:690, 1984.

212. Swerdlow, C.D., Winkle, R.A., and Mason, J.W.. Determinants of survival in patients with ventricular tachyarrhythmias. *N. Engl. J. Med.* 308:1436, 1983.

213. Graboys, T.B., Lown, B., Podrid, P.J., and DeSilva, R. Long-term survival of patients with ventricular arrhythmia treated with antiarrhythmic drugs. *Am. J. Cardiol.* 50:437, 1982.

214. Reid, P.R., Mirowski, M., Mower, M.M., Platia, E.V., Griffith, L.S.C., Watkins, L., Jr., Bach, S.M., Jr., Imran, M., and Thomas, A. Clinical evaluation of the internal automatic cardioverter-defibrillator in survivors of sudden cardiac death. *Am. J. Cardiol.* 51:1608, 1983.

215. Winkle, R.A. The implantable defibrillator in ventricular arrhythmias. *Hosp. Pract.* 18:149, 1983.

216. Leahey, E.B., Jr., Heissenbuttel, R.H., Giardina, E.G.V., and Bigger, J.T., Jr. Combined mexiletine and propranolol treatment of refrac-

tory ventricular tachycardia. *Br. Med. J.* 281:-357, 1980.

217. Cough, D.A. Cardiac aneurysm with ventricular tachycardia and subsequent excision of aneurysm. *Circulation* 20:251, 1959.

218. Hunt, D., Sloman, G., and Westlake, G. Ventricular aneurysmectomy for recurrent tachycardia. *Br. Heart J.* 31:264, 1969.

219. Favaloro, R.G., Effler, D.B., Groves, L.K., Wescott, R.N., Suarez, E., and Lozada, J. Ventricular aneurysm. Clinical experience. *Ann. Thorac. Surg.* 6:227, 1968.

220. Kremer, R., Chalant, C., Ponlot, R., and Lavenne, F. Recurrent ventricular tachycardia cured by resection of a parietal aneurysm of the left ventricle. *Acta Cardiol.* (Brux.) 24:523, 1969.

221. Magidson, O. Resection of post myocardial infarction ventricular aneurysm for cardiac arrhythmia. *Dis. Chest* 56:211, 1969.

222. Schlesinger, Z., Lieberman, Y., and Neufeld, H.N. Ventricular aneurysmectomy for severe rhythm disturbances. *J. Thorac. Cardiovasc. Surg.* 61:602, 1971.

223. Thind, G.S., Blakemore, W.S., and Ainsser, H.F. Ventricular aneurysmectomy for the treatment of recurrent ventricular tachyarrhythmia. *Am. J. Cardiol.* 27:690, 1971.

224. Welch, T.G., Fontana, M.E., and Vasko, J.S. Aneurysmectomy for recurrent ventricular tachyarrhythmias. *Am. Heart J.* 85:685, 1973.

225. Ricks, W.B., Winkle, R.A., Shumway, N.E., and Harrison, D.C. Surgical management of life-threatening ventricular arrhythmias in patients with coronary artery disease. *Circulation* 56:38, 1977.

226. Liotta, D., Ferrari, H., Pisanu, A., Pujadas, G., Oliveri, R., and Donato, O. Medically uncontrollable recurrent ventricular tachyarrhythmia in association with ventricular aneurysm. *Am. J. Cardiol.* 33:693, 1974.

227. Gallagher, J.J., Oldham, H.N., Wallace, A.G., Peter, R.H., and Cassell, J. Ventricular aneurysm with ventricular tachycardia. Report of a case with epicardial mapping and successful resection. *Am. J. Cardiol.* 35:696, 1975.

228. Sami, M., Chaitman, B.R., Bourassa, M.G., Charpin, D., and Chabot, M. Long-term follow-up of aneurysmectomy for recurrent ventricular tachycardia or fibrillation. *Am. Heart J.* 96:303, 1978.

229. Mason, J.W., Stinson, E.B., Winkle, R.A., Griffin, J.C., Oyer, P.E., Ross, D.L., and Derby, G. Surgery for ventricular tachycardia: Efficacy of LV aneurysm resection compared with operation guided by electrical activation mapping. *Circulation* 65:1148, 1982.

230. Waxman, M.B., Wald, R.B., Goldman, B.S., and Gunstensen, J. Intractable ventricular ta-

chyarrhythmia post myocardial infarction. *Circulation* 52(Suppl.2):109, 1975.

231. Ecker, R.R., Mullins, C.B., Grammer, J.C., Rea, W.J., and Atkins, J. Control of intractable ventricular tachycardia by coronary revascularization. *Circulation* 44(Suppl.2):66, 1971.

232. Lambert, C.J., Adam, M., Geisler, G.F., Verzosa, E., Nazarian, M., and Mitchell, B.F. Emergency myocardial revascularization for impending infarctions and arrhythmias. *J. Thorac. Cardiovasc. Surg.* 62:522, 1971.

233. Hutchinson, J.E., III, Kemp, H.G., and Schwartz, M.J. Emergency treatment of cardiac arrest in coronary heart disease with coronary bypass graft. *JAMA* 216:1645, 1971.

234. Nakhjavan, F.K., Morse, D.P., Nichols, H.T., and Goldgerg, H. Emergency aortocoronary bypass. Treatment of ventricular tachycardia due to ischemic heart disease. *JAMA* 216:2128, 1971.

235. Mundth, E.D., Buckley, M.J., DeSanctis, R.W., Daggett, W.M., and Austen, W.G. Surgical treatment of ventricular irritability. *J. Thorac. Cardiovasc. Surg.* 66:943, 1973.

236. Byson, A.L., Parisi, A.F., Schechter, E., and Wolfson, S. Life-threatening ventricular arrhythmias induced by exercise. Cessation after coronary bypass surgery. *Am. J. Cardiol.* 32:995, 1973.

237. Alexander, S., Makar, Y., and Ellis, F.H. Recurrent ventricular fibrillation. Threatment by emergency aortocoronary saphenous vein bypass. *JAMA* 228:70, 1974.

238. Boineau, J.P. and Cox, J.L. Rationale for a direct surgical approach to control ventricular arrhythmias. Relation of specific intraoperative techniques to mechanism and location of arrhythmia circuit. *Am. J. Cardiol.* 49:381, 1982.

239. deSoyza, N., Murphy, M.L., Bissett, J.K., Kane, J.J., and Doherty, J.E., III. Ventricular arrhythmia in chronic stable angina pectoris with surgical or medical treatment. *Ann. Intern. Med.* 39:10, 1978.

240. Spurrell, R.A.J., Sowton, E., and Deuchar, D.C. Ventricular tachycardia in 4 patients evaluated by electrical stimulation of the heart and treated in 2 patients by surgical division of anterior radiation of left bundle branch. *Br. Heart J.* 33:-1014, 1973.

241. Spurrell, R.A.J., Yates, S.K., Thornburn, C.W., Sowton, G.E., and Deuchar, D.C. Surgical treatment of ventricular tachycardia after epicardial mapping studies. *Br. Heart J.* 37:115, 1975.

242. Fontaine, G., Guiraudon, G., Frank, R., Vedel, J., Grosgogeat, Y., Cabrol, C., and Facquet, J. Stimulation Studies and Epicardial Mapping in Ventricular Tachycardia: Study of Mechanisms and Selection for Surgery. In Kulbertus, H.E.

(ed.), *Reentrant Arrhythmias.* Lancaster, England: MTP Press, 1977, pp. 334–350.

243. Guiraudon, G., Fontaine, G., Frank, R., Escande, G., Etivent, P., Vignes, R., Mattee, C., Cabrol, A., and Cabrol, C. Traitment de la tachycardie ventriculaire orientee par cartographie epicardiaque. A propos de 22 cas. *Arch. Mal. coeur* 71:1255, 1978.

244. Guiraudon, G., Fontaine, G., Frank, R., Escande, G., Etivent, P., and Cabrol, C. Encircling endocardial ventriculotomy. A new surgical treatment for life-threatening ventricular tachycardias resistant to medical treatment following myocardial infarction. *Ann. Thorac. Surg.* 26:438, 1975.

245. Horowitz, L.N., Harken, A.L., Josephson, M.E., and Kastor, J.A. Surgical treatment of ventricular arrhythmias in coronary artery disease. *Ann. Int. Med.* 95:88, 1981.

246. Garan, H., Ruskin, J.N., DiMarco, J.P., McGovern, B., Levine, F.H., and Buckley, M.J. Refractory ventricular tachycardia complicating recovery from acute myocardial infarction: Treatment with map-guided infarctectomy. *Am. Heart J.* 107:571, 1984.

247. Klein, H., Karp, R.B., Kouchoukos, N.T., Zorn, G.L., James, T.N., and Waldo, A.L. Intraoperative electrophysiological mapping of the ventricles during sinus rhythm in patients with a previous myocardial infarction. *Circulation* 66:847, 1982.

248. Miller, J.M., Kienzle, M.G., Harken, A.H., and Josephson, M.E. Morphologically distinct sustained ventricular tachycardia in coronary artery disease. Significance and surgical results. *J. Am. Coll. Cardiol.* 4:1073, 1984.

249. Cox, J.L. Surgery for cardiac arrhythmias. *Current Problems Cardiol.* 8(4):1, 1983.

# 16. REHABILITATION FOLLOWING MYOCARDIAL INFARCTION

Herman K. Hellerstein

That more liberal attitudes toward the management of myocardial infarction prevail today than existed a generation ago and even in the past decade is obvious [1]. The period of confinement to bed is as brief as possible; patients are permitted to resume at least mild activity early in the course of illness unless significant complication supervenes. As noted in chapter 13, for uncomplicated cases the total hospital stay has been reduced to 10 to 14 days, and in selected cases it has been recommended that discharge be as early as 4 or 5 days. From all evidence, patients managed on such a regimen come to no harm, provided they are properly selected [1, 2]. The combination of early mobilization and resumption of activity as an important stage in the active rehabilitation of the uncomplicated postinfarction patient is considered more often than it was a decade ago. Furthermore, there is a growing realization that a planned program featuring early exercise testing and training accompanied by other measures will markedly enhance the success of rehabilitation of the postinfarction patient.

By definition, *rehabilitation* is the process by which a patient is returned realistically to his or her optimal physiologic, mental, psychologic, emotional, social, vocational, and economic usefulness and, if employable, is provided an opportunity for gainful employment in a competitive world [3]. Rehabilitation in the contemporary sense also includes vigorous efforts to reverse or to prevent the progression of the underlying disease process. The reality of this expectation may be close at hand (4). Thus, successful rehabilitation is not restricted to economic or vocational rehabilitation alone; rather, it is the *complete* development of a pattern of living that will enable the individual to enjoy the fullest physical and mental capacities, with due allowances for disabilities.

Traditionally, the principles of rehabilitation have been applied chiefly to disorders of the musculoskeletal and nervous systems. They also have a valid and necessary place in the management of the patient with myocardial infarction or other manifestations of coronary artery disease. Exercise training and physical conditioning have been shown to play an important role in the rehabilitation of selected coronary patients [5]. In our studies begun 18 years ago and subsequently confirmed by others, emphasis was placed on the enhancement of physical fitness of coronary patients [6], but physical conditioning was only *part* of a comprehensive program that also involved weight control, diet therapy, cessation of smoking, regular performance of prescribed supervised exercise, continuation of gainful employment and of a normal social mode of life, adequate recreation, and rest.

In this chapter, the progress made in the past decade will be considered from the standpoint of new facts, new attitudes, new concepts, and unresolved questions and controversies. These controversies include the problem of how soon

This study was supported in part by grants from the United States Department of Health, Education, and Welfare, Office of Human Development Services, Rehabilitation Services Administration, Grant 13-P 55917, and grants from Mr. and Mrs. Leo Demsey, Mr. and Mrs. Harry E. Figgie, Jr., Mr. and Mrs. Donald Krush, Mrs. William Lipman, and Mr. and Mrs. Harry Mann.

after the myocardial infarction to begin exercise conditioning, how to determine whether the patient should pursue a "standard" job or one markedly restricted in activities, how to best enhance functional activity (at home and at work) by physical training, the importance of the specificity of training responses in relation to the skeletal muscles being conditioned, mechanisms of benefit from exercise conditioning, limitations of standard exercise tests for occupational "prescriptions," the role of coronary bypass surgery (and percutaneous transluminal angioplasty) as bonafide rehabilitation measures, and the influence of psychosocial factors following myocardial infarction. These topics will be addressed in the course of the chapter.

## Historical Background and Current Concepts

### BEFORE 1950: QUESTIONS ABOUT THE WISDOM OF ENFORCED BED REST

Physical conditioning in reference to heart disease is actually far from new. Over 160 years ago, Heberden wrote, "I know one who set himself a task of sawing wood for half an hour every day and was nearly cured" [7]. Although that was long before the first mention of acute myocardial infarction in the medical literature, no doubt some of Heberden's patients with angina pectoris had sustained an infarct. Needless to say, his counsel was all but forgotten following Herrick's original clinical description in 1912 [8]. The worry lest physical exertion heighten the risk of ventricular aneurysm or rupture or aggravate arterial hypoxemia kept patients virtually immobilized in bed for 6 to 8 weeks. This restriction was based in part on the pathologic findings in experimental myocardial infarctions described by Mallory et al. [9]. They found that 3 to 4 weeks were required until the major portion of the necrotic myocardium is removed and organized.

The prolonged bed rest concept of 6 weeks, twice the healing time, developed with support from impressive authorities. Sir Thomas Lewis, for example, felt that every effort should be made to avoid physical activities [10]. Upon discharge, anything as strenuous as stair climbing

was forbidden for at least a year. A few patients returned to work many months after hospital discharge; for most, all chances of a normal life were past. In 1944 the abuse and ill-effects of bed rest were recognized and highlighted by clinical observations and experimental studies of World War II conscientious objectors [11–13]. Similar studies approximately three decades later showed a deterioration of cardiovascular functions with 2 to 3 weeks of bed rest that simulated the effects found in illness [14]. Credit is due to Drs. Samuel Levine and Bernard Lown [15] of the Peter Bent Brigham Hospital for probably being the first to question the wisdom of enforced bed rest and inactivity for a prolonged period following the onset of infarction. They recommended, largely on an empirical basis, the "chair" treatment of acute coronary thrombosis to avoid thromboembolic or respiratory complications.

Increased physical activity *after* discharge from the hospital had been encouraged a decade before the "chair" treatment. In 1940 the New York State Employment Service asked the New York Heart Association to assist in evaluating workers with cardiac disease in order to determine the level of activity the cardiac patient could perform safely [16]. This led to the establishment in 1944 of the Work Classification Clinic at Bellevue Hospital by Dr. Leonard Goldwater. Without doubt, extenuating circumstances at that time (i.e., manpower needs during World War II) spurred efforts to shorten the period of hospitalization and invalidism of postinfarction patients. Goldwater and associates also helped to change attitudes among physicians as well as patients as to the feasibility of returning at least some heart attack victims to work after the healing process was completed. Many were surprised that fully 60 to 70 percent of the patients, mostly indigent, could return to work, although not necessarily at the same job as before.

Our experience at the Cleveland Work Classification Clinic, the second to be established (in 1950), indicated that an even higher proportion of heart attack victims—80 to 85 percent—could resume working [17, 18]. Moreover, it became clear that patients with coronary disease could work productively in a great variety of gainful occupations without hazard to themselves, fellow workers, or employees. Many of the jobs required relatively high energy levels. This was established in a series of studies with techniques developed by work physiologists who measured the energy cost of on-the-job activity [19]. In essence, the energy costs of most jobs in the industrial world and in urban society proved to be relatively small [20, 21]. For sedentary workers, often the maximal effort required by the jobs proved to be less than that imposed by walking or by most recreational activities. In any case, patients with coronary artery disease could perform most tasks with no more evidence of "strain" than their healthy co-workers [20, 21].

## 1950–1960: THE ERA OF WORK CLASSIFICATION AND THE UTILIZATION OF RESIDUAL CAPACITY OF THE CARDIAC PATIENT

This new philosophy placed greatest emphasis on *selective job placement,* which was preceded by a comprehensive, multidisciplinary evaluation of cardiovascular structure and function, emotional and social needs, and vocational aptitudes and abilities. The work classification experience invalidated the previously held concepts of "cardiac" jobs and "standard" jobs. Multiple factors other than the cardiac state were also found to influence the employability of the cardiac patient, such as emotions, skills, and job opportunities [17, 18, 22].

Following the establishment in 1950 of the Cleveland Area Heart Association Work Classification Clinic and its large experience representing a cross section of urban society, work classification clinics proliferated, leading to the establishment of 50 such centers, not only in the United States, but also in Europe, New Zealand, Australia, and elsewhere. The myth of cardiac unemployability was dispelled. Thus, the work classification clinic approach reversed *vocational death.* On-the-job studies *(Arbeitesphysiologie)* proved that not only in light manufacturing but also in heavy industry such as the steel mill, the energy requirements of most jobs were far lower than anticipated [20, 21]. Indeed, in every area of the mill except the open hearth and blast furnace, there were jobs requiring no greater energy expenditure than in the manufacturing plant. The average energy cost per work shift was generally less than 2.5 calories per minute, and the energy cost rarely attained a sustained level of 4 or 5 calories per minute.

The physiologic cost of work can be expressed in several ways: in terms of calories, in terms of oxygen cost (milliliters of oxygen per kilogram of body weight per minute, or ml $O_2$/kg/min) for an average subject, or in METs (metabolic units), a MET being defined as the $O_2$ uptake per kilogram of body weight per minute when the subject is sitting quietly in a chair or at supine rest. Generally, the oxygen uptake is 3.5 to 4 ml $O_2$/kg/min [23].

As might be expected, the capacity for energy expenditure above the basal level varies both with health status and previous physical conditioning. Among champion athletes, the aerobic capacity is likely to approach or exceed 20 METs whereas in healthy but untrained young men it is likely to be closer to 12 METs. On the other hand, a middle-aged man who has recovered from an uncomplicated myocardial infarction has a capacity in the range of 7 to 9 METs. If less than ordinary activity produces signs or symptoms, the capacity is probably closer to 4 METs per minute. The relation between the physiologic costs attainable by postinfarction patients to the energy costs of typical job and recreational activities makes it all the more evident that the capacity of most, even before healing is completed, is well above their occupational needs.

## 1960-PRESENT: ENHANCEMENT OF PHYSICAL FITNESS AND WORK CAPACITY AND SECONDARY PREVENTION OF CORONARY HEART DISEASE

In previous decades the emphasis was on restoring the levels of function in daily activities to where they had been before the patient was stricken. Recently, however, the concept developed that the functional capacity of the cardiac patient at home or at work can be *enhanced* by active physical conditioning and that it should be developed because doing so may be protective. In this era, coronary care units became widely available and flourished [24]. The coronary care units expanded their scope from the control of cardiac rhythms, with a resultant decrease in deaths due to arrhythmias, to initiating secondary prevention programs. The latter included early mobilization, systematic exercise testing, dietary counseling, and so on. During this period, various methods of exercise testing were developed and applied prior to the patients' discharge from the hospital [25–31].

In 1961, Cain and associates [25] monitored the electrocardiograms during activities of daily living at 10 progressively increasing intensities (levels). The higher levels involved walking down ramps and up and down flights of stairs (18 six-inch steps) when the patient had been hospitalized usually between 18 to 30 days. In the past decade, the period of bed rest after acute myocardial infarction has been shortened, ambulation has been instituted earlier, and the hospital stay has been reduced from 6 to 2 or 3 weeks, or even 1 week. The pace of physical activity in the intensive care and step-down areas can be based on clinical observations of the patient's tolerance to low-level activities, such as dangling, self-care, and ambulation. The guidelines are based on the development of symptoms (e.g., weakness, chest pain, dizziness, or diaphoresis), circulatory signs (e.g., new murmurs, gallops, dyspnea, or hypotension), excessive tachycardia for the low levels of effort (i.e., above 115 to 120 beats/min), and dysrhythmias (i.e., multiform ventricular premature beats, salvos, tachycardia) or marked ST-T displacement [27].

*Low-level Exercise Tests.* Low-level ergometric tests for the convalescent, ambulatory, uncomplicated, infarction patient prior to discharge have been developed [25–31]. They have been shown to be safe and valuable. They provide objective and quantitative information regarding the patient's functional status, therapeutic needs, and degree of recovery, as well as guidelines for clinical management at the home of the individual patient and, ultimately, during the return to work.

Davidson and DeBusk [32] have presented data regarding the *prognostic* significance of the type of responses observed during exercise testing. Freedom from cardiac events in a 3-year follow-up was found in 83 percent of subjects who developed neither ventricular ectopic activity (VEA) nor ST-T displacement in predischarge exercise tests; this percentage was in contrast to the 64 percent in the subjects who developed VEA but no ST-T displacement and the 43 percent in subjects who developed ST-T displacement with or without VEA. Thus, the prognosis was best in the subjects who had neither ST-T changes nor VEA and worst in subjects who had ST-T displacement with exercise [32]. Generally, the low-level exercise tests are conducted after the self-care stage, and the ill effects of bed rest will have been minimal. The subjects usually are ambulatory within the confines of the hospital room before being eligible for discharge from the hospital 10 to 14 days after acute infarction.

The purpose of the low-level in-hospital exercise tests is to determine the tolerance of the patient to activities comparable to those performed at home during convalescence, generally those requiring less than 3 to 4 METs. For this reason, the low-level exercise tests have been designed to impose comparable workloads of less than 3 to 3.5 METs, equal to 10 to 14 ml $O_2$/kg/min. In the absence of signs or symptoms, occasional patients can be tested to higher levels of 4 to 5 METs. Figure 16–1 presents several exercise protocols for low-level testing. The treadmill test consists of walking continuously on a treadmill at a speed of 1.2 miles per hour (1.9 kilometers per hour) for 3 minutes each at 0, 3, and 6 percent gradients [31]. Bicycle ergometer tests consist of pedaling 60 turns per minute for 4 minutes at each of two work levels that are adjusted for body weight to impose peak loads of 3 METs. A 2-minute rest period is recommended between each workload. The criteria for stopping the low-level exercise test are more rigorous than those for stopping peak or maximal performance tests (table 16–1). Delaying their discharge from the hospital or retesting them after administration of antiarrhythmic drugs or nitrates may be indicated for those patients who show significant arrhythmias, ST-T displacement, or hypotension during

In the past several years, several investigators have increased the level of predischarge exercise tests from low-level to symptom-limited peak performance [30, 33]. The validity and necessity of such testing are currently being evaluated as well as disputed. Markiewicz et al. [30]

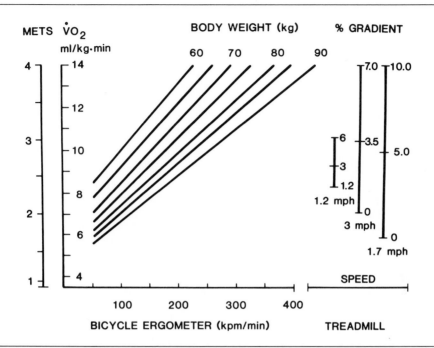

FIGURE 16–1. Estimated oxygen and MET requirements of four low-level exercise protocols suitable for testing patients with acute myocardial infarction before discharge from the hospital. Comparable workloads can be obtained from stages 2 and 3 of the National Exercise and Heart Disease Project [42], Sivarajan et al. [31], and bicycle ergometer load corrected for body weight.

started test 1 of treadmill exercise at 2 mph and a 3.5 percent grade (3 METs), and they increased the workload by one stage (1 MET) every third minute until either an arbitrary "target" heart rate of 130 beats/min was attained (heart-rate-limited test), end-points of symptoms appeared, systolic blood pressure decreased, or ventricular tachycardia occurred. At the fifth and seventh weeks, the target heart rate was increased to 140 and 150 beats/min, respectively. Tests at 9 and 11 weeks were sign, or symptom, limited [30].

Wohl et al. [33] used bicycle ergometry to evaluate cardiovascular function during early recovery (at 3, 6, 12, and 18 weeks) from acute myocardial infarction. In asymptomatic patients, the test performed one day prior to hospital discharge was terminated at a heart rate of 130 beats/min. The target of subsequent tests was a

TABLE 16–1. Guidelines for stopping low-level in-hospital exercise tests of acute myocardial infarction patients prior to discharge

SIGNS AND SYMPTOMS
Chest pain, discomfort
Severe dyspnea, extreme fatigue
Dizziness, faintness, light-headedness
Apprehension, cyanosis, confusion
Incoordination, ataxia
Heart rate above 115 beats/min
Decrease or failure to increase the heart rate and systolic blood pressure
New murmurs or gallops

ECG SIGNS
Frequent ventricular ectopic beats, salvos, bigeminy, multiform, R-on-T phenomenon, tachycardia
Paroxysmal atrial or supraventricular tachycardia or fibrillation
Second- or third-degree AV block
Displacement of the ST-T segment more than 2 mm from the preexercise level

symptom-limited maximal level [33]. The finding that within 2 to 3 weeks after myocardial infarction, most subjects with uncomplicated infarcts can increase their heart rate and systolic blood pressure products showed that they can increase the rate of myocardial oxygen uptake ($M\dot{V}o_2$) to meet the metabolic demand imposed by the exercise tests. Later in convalescence (from 3 to 5 weeks and 12 to 24 weeks), cardiovascular healing and function improved as demonstrated by an increase of cardiac output during exercise, stroke volume, and work capacity [33].

Earlier activation and supervised ambulation reduces the deconditioning effects of bed rest and accounts in part for the lower occurrence of subjective complaints of weakness, depression, anxiety, and low self-esteem than what was recorded in previous decades [14]. In their classic work, Saltin and associates [14] demonstrated the ill effects of prolonged inactivity (21 days of bed rest in five healthy young men). All five subjects showed a decrease in maximal oxygen uptake (which was reduced 20 to 46 percent) after the extended rest. The decrease correlated closely with a drop in maximal cardiac output and stroke volume. After the end of the bed-rest phase, the young men undertook vigorous physical training for 55 days. In the habitually sedentary and unfit subjects, the oxygen uptake after training almost doubled. Interestingly, the sedentary subjects took less time to return to their prebed-rest levels (8 to 13 days) than did the habitually active subjects (20 to 43 days). The authors concluded: "A long history of a high level of activity associated with a high maximal oxygen uptake offers little or no protection against loss of performance capacity following a drastic reduction of physical activity. Correspondingly, a long history of restricted physical activity and extremely low maximal oxygen uptake does not preclude rapid improvement following physical training" [14].

*Beneficial Effects of Physical Training.* In the last decade, numerous carefully supervised and prescribed comprehensive exercise training programs for postinfarction patients consistently produced improvement in 75 to 85 percent of the subjects [5, 34]. As noted in several studies [35–39], the beneficial effects may include (1) improvement of subjective well-being and decrease of psychologic depression; (2) decreased tension-time index and variable effects on the

stroke volume, ejection fraction, dP/dt, and the like; (3) decreased lactate production for the same workload; (4) reduction of hypertensive blood pressure values during exercise and of peripheral resistance; (5) diminution of the heart rate at rest, during sleep, and during exercise; (6) quantitative lessening of ST-T displacement; (7) lowering of serum catecholamines and of serum lipid levels, especially in type IV hyperlipoproteinemia, and an increased ratio of high-density lipoprotein cholesterol to total cholesterol; (8) reduction of adipose tissue and increase of lean body mass; (9) enhancement of sexual activity; (10) reduction of the serum insulin level and the insulin-glucagon ratio; and (11) beneficial effects on blood coagulation and fibrinolysis. Enhancement of intercoronary collateral vessel formation, however, has rarely been demonstrated by pre- and posttraining angiograms [5, 40]. The improvement in the "quality of living" was unequivocal, and this was more convincing than the suggestive reduction of mortality rates in the nonrandomized studies to date. Ventricular fibrillation occurring in supervised monitored training areas has been uncommon, and with rare exceptions it has been reversible, with complete recovery following [41].

The value of exercise training in ischemic (coronary) heart disease has been assessed in three studies, including the National Exercise and Heart Disease Project [42], of patients who participated in randomized clinical trials of the effects of prescribed, supervised exercise. A cumulative analysis showed a consistent reduction of mortality ranging from 35 percent within the first two years to 24 percent at four years (43).

## Methods for Quantitating Exercise Testing and Exercise Training

The characterization of the response to exercise tests can be expressed in quantitative terms (chronotropic, aerobic, myocardial aerobic capacities, changes in electrical functions, radioisotopic myocardial perfusion, and hemodynamics), which have been found to be useful in evaluating cardiac function as well as the responses to various types of interventions (e.g., drug administration surgery or physical conditioning) [37, 44, 45]. These methods have been described in chapter 6 and will be commented on only briefly in this chapter.

## CHRONOTROPIC RESERVE AND IMPAIRMENT

One of the major adaptive mechanisms of the heart is to increase the heart rate in order to increase the cardiac output to meet the increasing demands of the body during exercise. Peak or maximal effort assesses the age-related reduction of chronotropic capacity and the threshold at which dysrhythmias occur, and it provides information about myocardial oxygen capacity ($M\dot{V}_{O_2}$). The age-predicted maximal heart rate can be estimated by subtracting the age in years from 220 or .66 times the age in years from 215. The maximal heart rate decreases not only with age, but also even more with heart disease. Quantitative impairment of chronotropic capacity due to heart disease can be calculated by the formula

$$\% \text{ chronotropic impairment} = \frac{A - B}{A} \times 100,$$

where $A$ is the age-predicted maximal heart rate and $B$ is heart rate attained at peak or maximal effort [44].

## TOTAL BODY AEROBIC CAPACITY ($\dot{V}_{O_2}$) AND IMPAIRMENT

The oxygen cost of peak or maximal effort is a measure of the functional aerobic capacity of the body ($\dot{V}_{O_2}$). To determine the degree of *functional* aerobic impairment (FAI), the subject's performance must be compared to values of healthy individuals of the same age, sex, and habitual physical activity status. Subjects can be classified as "sedentary" if they do not exert themselves sufficiently to develop sweating at least once a week. The FAI percentage can be calculated from the following formula:

$$\text{FAI\%} = \frac{\dot{V}_{O_2} \text{ max (age- and sex-predicted)} - \text{attained } \dot{V}_{O_2}}{\dot{V}_{O_2} \text{ max (age- and sex-predicted)}} \times 100.$$

The severity of the FAI can be categorized as mild, moderate, or marked, which represent 15 to 25 percent, 26 to 40 percent, and 41 to 51

percent FAI, respectively. The concept of FAI is particularly useful in making serial evaluations of individuals in comparison with appropriate peers [44, 45].

## MYOCARDIAL AEROBIC CAPACITY ($M\dot{V}_{O_2}$) AND IMPAIRMENT

Several investigators have shown that an excellent correlation exists between measured myocardial oxygen consumption (ml $O_2$/100g of left ventricle/min) and two of its major determinants, heart rate (HR) and systolic blood pressure (SBP) [46, 47]:

$$M\dot{V}_{O_2} = 0.28HR - 14 \ (r = .88).$$

$M\dot{V}_{O_2}$ can be calculated from the HR and SBP product:

$$M\dot{V}_{O_2} = (0.14HR \times SBP \times 10^{-2}) - 6.3 \ (r - .92).$$

Our studies on the job [17, 18, 20, 21] and in the laboratory [48] have demonstrated that upper extremity effort elicits greater responses than those of lower extremity effort of equal magnitude in terms of heart rate, blood pressure, minute ventilation, oxygen uptake, respiratory exchange ratio, and ST-T changes. In other words, for the same effort, the myocardial oxygen cost is greater for upper extremity than lower extremity effort.

The response of an individual to physical or occupational stresses can be expressed in terms of heart rate, percentage of chronotropic capacity, chronotropic reserve, the HR-SBP product, or the estimated $M\dot{V}_{O_2}$. An increase of the HR-SBP product after training or any intervention indicates a greater ability to increase the myocardial oxygen consumption to meet the metabolic demands imposed by the given level of activity. The maximal HR-SBP product can be considered to be a measure of cardiovascular adequacy, that is, of myocardial aerobic capacity. The maximal HR-SBP or calculated $M\dot{V}_{O_2}$ decreases with age, mainly because of the decrease of the HR, and it declines even more with the advent of heart disease. In the latter case, symptoms or ECG changes during exercise tests may preclude the attainment of the maximal HR-SBP product.

The relative changes in the oxygen consumption of the heart and of the body at rest and at peak effort can be expressed by either (1) the ratio of the calculated $M\dot{V}O_2$ to the estimated or measured oxygen uptake of the body ($M\dot{V}O_2$ /$\dot{V}O_2$) or (2) by the ratio of the HR-SBP product to the estimated oxygen uptake of the body. The $M\dot{V}O_2/\dot{V}O_2$ ratio provides insight into the relative cardiac "efficiency"; the higher the ratio, the greater is the ratio of the energy input to output (or cost-to-benefit ratio) and the lower the efficiency.

*Myocardial aerobic impairment* (MAI) can be calculated by relating the individual HR-SBP product at peak effort to its value for healthy individuals of the same sex and age [45].

CHANGES IN ELECTRICAL FUNCTION
Although the ST-T displacement is causally non-specific, it can be considered to be electrophysiologically specific, since it represents an imbalance between myocardial oxygen supply and demand elicited by effort. New insight has been obtained in the importance of ST-T displacement in coronary patients [45, 49, 50]. As discussed in chapter 6, exercise ST-T segment responses have greater value when quantitated and related to the development of chest discomfort or pain, the level of effort at which it occurs, the duration of its persistence after completion of the exercise test, and the heart rate and blood pressure at the onset of pain or ST-T displacement.

In our experience, changes in exercise ECG responses have been related to changes of physical fitness, especially in the subjects with initial borderline or abnormal exercise ECGs [49]. Improvement in the exercise ECG occurred in 79 percent of coronary subjects with initial borderline or abnormal exercise tests whose fitness improved. There was a decrease in the ST-T point displacement and an increase in the slope of the 80-msec ST segment. Opposite changes in the ST-J point displacement and ST slope occurred in subjects who showed deterioration of the exercise ECG and physical fitness.

New techniques of ECG recording have improved the yield of abnormal responses in exercise tests [51, 52]. As noted in chapter 6, multiple leads (reflecting X, Y, and Z components) are often helpful, since the ST-T changes during exercise in some patients occur in all spatial di-

rections and therefore may be missed by a single lead. Thus, the use of a single unipolar or bipolar $V_5$ lead is associated with a large number (approximately 11 percent) of false-negative (normal) responses; that is, 11 percent of subjects who show abnormal responses when monitored with multiple leads will show normal responses with a unipolar or bipolar $V_5$ lead.

Exercise-induced arrhythmias must always be considered as potentially dangerous and may merit termination of the test unless they subside as the test proceeds.

## The Exercise Prescription

The underlying principles of conditioning apply equally to normal or abnormal subjects. The conditioning program must provide for progressive yet gradual increase in the exercise level. Overload on the heart as well as on skeletal muscle is required. Unless functional aerobic capacity is taxed, conditioning is not likely to succeed. "Overload" is defined as being greater than customary activity and does not imply exceeding the individual's maximal capacity.

In evaluating patients with coronary artery disease, exercise testing is a prerequisite. The exercise training recommendation should be approached with the same respect and caution as when any potent pharmacologic agent is prescribed. Consideration must be given to numerous factors, including the patient's age, sex, health status, current medication, orthopedic and musculoskeletal integrity, degree of motivation, individual recreational preferences, and, most importantly, diagnostic and functional evaluation as obtained from exercise tolerance tests. The following information derived from a multistage exercise test is vital to the exercise prescription: estimated or measured peak oxygen uptake, peak attained heart rate, limiting symptoms and their physiologic accompaniments, occurrence of symptomatic or asymptomatic ischemic ECG changes, dysrhythmias, or excessive blood pressure responses. The prescribed intensity should be above the threshold level needed to demonstrate a conditioning response, yet below the intensity that evokes significant clinical symptoms or significant ECG abnormalities.

The physical sessions should include a warm-up period, an endurance phase, and a cool-down period with an optional recreational activity [35, 45]. The endurance phase should be prescribed in terms of intensity, duration, frequency, and type of activity.

WARM-UP PERIOD

The warm-up period provides adaptation for the transition from rest to exercise. Physiologically, it facilitates a gradual circulatory adjustment; minimizes the oxygen deficit and the formation of lactic acid; increases muscle and core temperature, which enhances muscular efficiency and oxygen dissociation; decreases total pulmonary vascular resistance and increases pulmonary circulation; increases the rate of nerve conduction; decreases muscular viscosity; decreases the tendency toward injury; and decreases the occurrence of ischemic ECG changes and arrhythmias following sudden exertion. Warming up, therefore, has preventive value and enhances performance.

THE ENDURANCE PHASE

The endurance phase serves to stimulate directly the oxygen transport system. Some of the dynamic activities that improve endurance include walking, jogging in place or moving, running, stationary or mobile cycling, skiing, swimming, rope skipping, ice skating, rowing, and bench or stair climbing. Because of the relative consistency of energy expenditure found among these activities, they lend themselves particularly well to exercise prescription. Recent studies have shown them to be equally efficient modes of training [45].

The three critical elements of the endurance phase—intensity, duration, and frequency—have been quantified. The interrelations among these three factors permit a modification in one to be partially or totally compensated for by an appropriate change in one or both of the other factors. Proper adjustment of these factors plays a major role in providing an effective yet safe exercise dosage. The optimal intensity of exercise should be in the range of 57 to 78 percent of $\dot{V}o_2$ max, which corresponds to 70 to 85 percent of peak attained heart rate [35]. At this relative range, several key physiological and bio-chemical changes occur that indicate that the individual's aerobic metabolism is being stressed: the respiratory exchange ratio approaches unity; increases occur in the blood lactate levels, fibrinolytic activity, urinary catecholamine excretion, the capacity to oxidize fatty acids, the release of fatty acids from adipose tissue, the capacity to regenerate high-energy phosphate compounds by oxidative phosphorylation, and the protein content of the mitochondrial fraction of skeletal muscle, and so on. These are desirable changes and are associated with favorable adaptation and improvement [35]. High-intensity training (95 to 100 percent of $\dot{V}o_2$ max) is not desirable for most subjects, not only because it cannot be sustained long enough to develop endurance, but, more importantly, it also increases the risk of cardiovascular complications. Targets for training include not only heart rate, but signs or symptoms, arrhythmias, and changes of blood pressure as well.

*Duration.* In order to achieve the desired cardiovascular effects, the subject should perform dynamic exercise for a period long enough to stimulate energy production predominantly through aerobic, rather than anaerobic, energy pathways. The duration of exercise necessary to produce a significant conditioning response varies *inversely* with the intensity: the lower the intensity, the longer the duration needed. Conversely, the greater the intensity (up to about 80 percent $\dot{V}o_2$ max), the shorter is the duration necessary to achieve the same benefits. Exercise training at 75 percent $\dot{V}o_2$ max for 10 to 15 minutes improves the $\dot{V}o_2$ max, for example, but 30-minute sessions are even more effective. However, 45-minute sessions do not produce a greater increase in $\dot{V}o_2$ max, and moreover, they increase the risk of orthopedic complications [45].

*Continuous Versus Intermittent Exercise Training.* Both continuous and intermittent exercise training possess certain advantages [23]. The continuous method enhances endurance, and the intermittent, with its rest-work pauses, increases strength. In conditioning a cardiac patient, interval training has several advantages. The patient can achieve a larger total workload per session with less fatigue, the severely limited angina patient can accomplish a larger total workload prior to increasing symptoms, and a larger number of training stimuli are presented to the heart during each session through the repeated increases of stroke volume, venous return, and intracardiac pressure. Intermittent exercise incorporating a variety of upper and lower extremity exercises is better suited to the enhancement of total fitness that is necessary for the patient's return to occupational and leisure activities. Work capacity can be enhanced through increasing dynamic aerobic capacity, which involves sustained movement of the large muscle groups of the upper extremities and torso, as well as of the lower extremities. Walking, jogging, swimming, bicycling, rowing, cross-country skiing, and running games (tennis, handball, squash, and basketball) are included in this category.

*Frequency.* Once-a-week conditioning is *not* enough to elicit an increase in $\dot{V}o_2$ max. Older normal subjects or cardiac patients who have a low initial $\dot{V}o_2$ max may respond to slightly less than twice-weekly exercise. A twofold increase in $\dot{V}o_2$ max occurs when the exercise frequency increases from two to four times per week. Additional benefits of more frequent training (five or more sessions per week) appear minimal, while the occurrence of orthopedic injury increases markedly. Thus, three or four evenly spaced workouts per week appear to represent the most practical and cost-effective training frequency.

Our experiences with 254 subjects with coronary artery disease who participated in three 1-hour training sessions per week revealed that significantly more subjects who trained with an average of 2.2 to 3 or more sessions per week showed greater improvement in aerobic capacity and ECG responses to exercise than did their counterparts who averaged 1 to 2 sessions per week. Surprisingly, the subjects who attended 3.5 to 5 sessions per week showed no greater improvement than the subjects who attended 2.2 to 3 times per week [34].

*Training Specificity.* Numerous investigations have shown that cardiovascular-respiratory conditioning responses are best demonstrated when the subjects activate the specific muscles that

were trained. Swimming or one-leg training, for example, does not improve the $\dot{V}o_2$ max for running [53, 54]. Similar findings were reported by Clausen and associates [55], who trained two groups of men: one group exercised using their arms and the other, using their legs. In tests after training, both groups alternated between arm and leg exercises, using the same exercise protocol. Training of arm muscles affected the heart rate response only during arm exercise, and a similar finding was reported regarding the leg muscles. The lack of cross-adaptation is a cogent reason for including arm and torso exercise, as in calisthenics, and not restricting training to jogging alone. Clausen and associates [55] and other investigators [53] suggested that an extracardiac or peripheral drive regulates the exercise heart rate following arm training alone or leg training alone. A substantial portion of the relative bradycardia in exercise (i.e., the reduction of exercise heart rate for the same effort) is secondary to primary changes in the trained skeletal muscles. Presumably, the afferent nervous discharges from the working muscle produce the sympathetic drive from cerebral centers.

Other studies have shown that a substantial portion of the increase in $\dot{V}o_2$ max is due to local adaptation in the skeletal muscles trained and to more effective distribution of cardiac output. Redistribution of cardiac output and blood flow in regional vascular beds were measured in patients with coronary heart disease before and after physical training (two levels of submaximal exercise were used during 4 to 10 weeks) [55]. After training at a "moderate" workload, the cardiac output was reduced largely because of a decreased heart rate. Increasing to a higher workload produced a small increment in cardiac output, which reflected a small increase in stroke volume. Significantly, hepatic blood flow, which is normally reduced by exercise in the untrained subject, was less reduced after training than before; this suggested that a greater fraction of left ventricular output was being directed to tissues not directly involved in exercise. Indeed, when changes in quadriceps muscle blood flow were estimated after submaximal exercise training from the clearance rate of locally injected xenon-133, blood flow was shown to be lower after training than before. Thus, skeletal muscles seemed able to perform the same submaximal workload with less perfusion; presumably some factor had increased oxygen extraction by the muscle.

Various changes in skeletal muscle have been associated with adaptation, among them lower lactate levels and slower glycogen depletion in response to exercise, which are possibly mediated by biochemical changes within the muscles themselves. Holloszy and co-workers at Washington University [56] reported intriguing findings in rats trained to run on a treadmill to increase endurance. On visual examination, the animals' leg muscles and homogenates thereof manifested a deep red color, which was accounted for by increased myoglobin concentration. In fact, the myoglobin level in the muscles increased by 80 percent, and all the increase was confined to exercised muscles. Holloszy [56] suggested that whatever accounted for the increased myoglobin, its presence might facilitate oxygen utilization in tissues by enhancing its transport. Increases in enzymatic and oxidative capacity of these muscles were also observed in response to training.

Investigations into training specificity have clarified some aspects of the lack of crossover effects [57, 58]. Studies of effects or running training on $Vo_2$ max and of heart rate changes during running and swimming have shown that the increase in treadmill running was significantly greater ($p < .01$) than the increase during swimming ($p < .05$). It appears that exercise of relatively large muscle masses modifies local changes and either cardiac or extracardiac central circulatory factors. On the other hand, the smaller muscle masses of the upper extremities may be more adaptable to local changes with training. The possibility, however, cannot be excluded that the small albeit significant (at the $p < .05$ level) increase in aerobic power in swimming after leg training may "actually reflect the specificities of leg training, as the legs are used to some degree in tethered swimming at heavy work levels" [57].

*Implications of Training Specificity.* The lack of significant cardiovascular benefits of training of upper extremity muscles crossing over to lower extremity efforts and vice versa implies that a substantial portion of the conditioning response derives from peripheral events (e.g., increased arteriovenous oxygen extraction) in the exercising muscle. Training specificity has significant implications for the design of cardiac exercise training programs. Since few recreational and occupational activities require sustained lowered extremity exertion, the rationale of the prevalent practice of restricting exercise training to the lower extremities (walking-jogging format) appears questionable.

The principle of specificity of training has largely been ignored in the planning of most adult fitness and cardiac exercise training programs. Many cardiac reconditioning programs, with the exception of the ongoing National Exercise and Heart Disease Project [42], are based on lower extremity training, such as walking, jogging, or stationary bicycling. Such programs are limited in scope; ignore the small group of patients (approximately 8 percent) who, because of orthopedic problems, arthritis, or peripheral vascular disease, have significant limitations in performing lower extremity activities; and neglect to consider that daily living activities employ all major muscle groups. An individual whose occupation requires arm movements needs to be concerned with training these muscle groups. Since one of the primary objectives of cardiac rehabilitation is to prepare an individual for return to occupational and leisure-time physical activities, a physical conditioning program should include exercise for the arms as well as for the legs and torso. Examples of upper body exercise programs to be used in conjunction with jogging, walking, or cycling are sports (e.g., volley ball, paddle ball, or basketball) and specific calisthenic exercises aimed at arm, shoulder, and trunk movements. Additional recommended exercises include rowing, arm ergometry, use of wall pulleys and shoulder wheels, gardening, raking, and wood sawing.

COOL-DOWN PERIOD
Disregard for the cool-down period may represent the single most common cause of cardiovascular complications after exercise. Upon suddenly stopping exercise, the free flow of blood into the limbs continues despite inactivation of the skeletal muscle pump. Compensatory adjust-

ments in peripheral resistance secondary to the fall in cardiac output after cessation of exercise may not occur instantaneously. Consequently, blood may accumulate or pool in the lower extremities until normal vasoconstriction is reestablished. The best way to prevent the pooling of blood in the limbs is to maintain a massaging action of the muscles through continued movement. A 5- to 10-minute cool-down period involving walking or low-intensity exercise usually permits an appropriate circulatory readjustment and a return of heart rate and blood pressure to near preexercise values, allows dissipation of the heat load, and promotes a more rapid removal of lactic acid than does resting recovery [45].

## ADHERENCE

The attendance and adherence to long-term exercise programs range from poor to excellent [34, 59, 60]. The more successful programs have recognized and incorporated the following important features: organization of the program design, preliminary and follow-up evaluations (retesting) with feedback of results, exclusion of subjects with specific contraindications, supervision, recreational aspects, group camaraderie stimulus, regularity of the sessions, positive attitude of the spouse to the program, freedom from injury, reward system of recognition, and symbols of participation.

## REVISION OF EXERCISE PRESCRIPTION

Fitness tests should be performed prior to and at approximately 3- to 6-month intervals throughout the conditioning program in order to assess the cardiac responses or lack of responses to the exercise stimuli. Signs of favorable cardiovascular adaptation to the physical conditioning program include decreased heart rate and systolic blood pressure at rest and at submaximal workloads, decreased myocardial oxygen requirements for comparable levels of submaximal work, increased working capacity, and decreased evidence of cardiac arrhythmias, particularly ventricular premature beats. Medication and dosage adjustments should be modified at the time of reevaluation and also during the training period. Antiarrhythmic agents and nitroglycerin may be administered prophylactically to patients who develop ventricular ar-

rhythmias, angina, or ST-T changes without symptoms during the exercise training period. Also, antihypertensive drugs may be required if excessive blood pressure responses occur during submaximal effort. The intensity of training effort should be reduced when the environment changes adversely, that is, when cold, heat, or high humidity cause water loss, excessive sweating, or other adverse effects.

## FAILURE TO RESPOND TO TRAINING

Primary determinants of response to the training program are the severity of the underlying disease process, the program design, and participation [45, 61]. Patients who are unable to perform at 2 METs (equivalent to 2 mph on zero gradient or 250 to 350 kilopond-meters per minute) are considered to be ineligible for participation in exercise training programs [59]. Candidates with a poor rehabilitation potential often show severely reduced inotropic or chronotropic reserve; severe angina pectoris; myocardial dyskinesia, aneurysms, or both; frequent unifocal R-on-T or multiform ventricular ectopic beats; or pronounced ST-T displacement during or after exercise.

Our experience indicates that approximately 15 percent of post-infarction patients showed minimal or no improvement despite faithful attendance and active participation in the exercise program [61]. In some of these patients, coronary arteriograms demonstrated severe involvement of three major coronary arteries and 90 percent or more stenosis of two major arteries. Thus, *the degree of severity and progression of the underlying coronary disease* represents a major obstacle to improvement [61]. In such patients, consideration should be given earlier to surgical intervention. Coronary arteriograms may be necessary to exclude patients who are unlikely to profit from a conditioning program. Other factors accounting for a lack of improvement include intercurrent injury or illness, inadequate adherence to the exercise prescription, exercise below the threshold necessary for improvement, failure of supervision, poor motivation, and indifference of the spouse.

Once training is underway, adequate supervision is mandatory. In our facility, a physician or physical educator trained in basic cardiopulmonary resuscitation (CPR) and advanced life-support is always immediately available. Physical therapists and other health professional personnel are trained in CPR and defibrillation equipment, and medications are always on hand. Sudden mechanism "death" associated with physical effort has proved to be completely reversible without fatality if promptly treated [43].

MECHANISMS OF BENEFIT

As noted in chapters 11 and 12, the beneficial effects of exercise conditioning are easier to identify and to quantitate than to explain in toto. The local changes in the peripheral skeletal musculature readily account for the increased arteriovenous oxygen extraction. The myocardium in humans has not yet been shown to develop increased levels of myofibrillar adenosinetriphosphatase. This has been shown to occur in the rat, but not in the dog [62]. However, the reduction of plasma catecholamines at rest and after peak effort and of myocardial epinephrine uptake may account for the reduced heart rate and blood pressure observed after physical and sexual effort, as well as for the decreased myocardial oxygen requirements for a given workload [34, 39]. Several studies have shown no increase of intercoronary collateral vessel formation or reversal of atherosclerosis occurring as a result of physical training [40].

The improvement in oral glucose tolerance in bed-rested exercising subjects has been documented but not adequately explained. Dolkas and Greenleaf [38] attribute this effect to the release of an insulin inhibitor during bed rest that is reduced or blocked during effort. Physical training modifies not only the aerobic power, but also the fasting triglyceride and insulin levels; it increases the sensitivity of adipose tissue to catecholamines, leading to greater mobilization of fatty acids and the capacity to oxidize them, and it decreases the decrement of blood glucose as well as plasma insulin during prolonged exertion. The nature of the increase in the ratio of HDL to total cholesterol is obscure.

The improvement in mood and emotions may be the result of the summation of the above changes, which restore, in large part, physical strength, cardiovascular reserve, sexual performance, and self-esteem. Such improvement provides evidence of recovery from the "infarct of the ego" that accompanies the myocardial insult. The psychologic effects of physical training have been amply demonstrated. In addition to objective evidence of improvement in physical capacity, there is also statistically significant psychological improvement: decreased anxiety, depression, fatigue levels, aggression, and anxiety levels, and increase in motivation to adjust. Exercise training contributes to psychological well-being by improving life patterns, promoting more restful sleep and better sexual adjustment, decreasing tension at work and at home, and reducing the feeling of being treated as an invalid [63].

## Realistic Exercise Testing After Hospital Discharge

Physical fitness tests are valuable in many areas of medical practice and research. Although commonly used to "diagnose" ischemic heart disease, they have a greater application: to evaluate the responses to various types of therapy and, as stated by a WHO Expert Committee on Rehabilitation, "to determine the response of the individual to efforts at given levels, and from this information to estimate probable performance in specific life and occupational situations" [64].

LIMITATIONS OF STANDARD EXERCISE TESTS IN FORMULATING WORK PRESCRIPTIONS

This newer application requires recognition of the limitations of clinical exercise tests and the need to make modifications for rehabilitation purposes. Contemporary exercise tests rarely simulate real-life situations. Our on-the-job studies have revealed many shortcomings in the design and application of the results of standardized exercise tests that were originally intended to diagnose myocardial ischemia [20, 21, 65, 66]. Debusk and associates [67] have approached this problem by comparing bicycle to arm ergometry as a guide to occupational work assessment. Regardless of the apparatus used (treadmill, bicycle, steps, or arm ergometers), exercise tests are designed to be performed under standard conditions (e.g., involving gym clothes, privacy, room temperature, meals, rest, sleep, and the like) with measurable physical workloads that are increased stepwise and advanced to predetermined end-points of heart rate, blood pressure, ECG changes, or symptoms [65, 66]. Despite their limitations (which will be described later), standard exercise test conditions have the advantage of providing reproducibility and quantitative assessment of cardiovascular functions.

Studies of a large number of subjects, while engaged in the pursuit of their customary occupations, have indicated that the cardiovascular responses to the stresses of exercise in the controlled environment of a clinical testing laboratory differ from those in the world of work [19–22, 68]. *These marked differences challenge the usefulness of standard exercise tests in formulating work prescriptions, unless certain modifications are introduced.*

Occupational stresses are different in type and magnitude from those of exercise tests. The aerobic stresses of exercise tests exceed those of most occupations and fail to account for most of the important determinations of successful performance of work. The stress of standardized tests is mainly muscular (almost always of the lower extremities), occurs at high submaximal or maximal peak levels, and takes place in a controlled physical environment as described above. The physical stresses of occupational energy expenditure usually are low, submaximal muscular effort of brief duration and are rarely sustained at high levels for more than 2 or 3 minutes; that is, they are intermittent, not continuous. In addition, a significant portion of each work shift (30 to 45 percent) is expended at levels of rest with numerous pauses [3, 20, 21]. The subjects at work perform muscular effort fully clad, often after the ingestion of meals, coffee, or prescribed medications and after smoking tobacco. The physical and emotional factors are rarely as well controlled as in the exercise laboratory. The majority of occupations entail other stresses that are carefully avoided or minimized in exercise testing: upper extremity efforts that produce greater cardiovascular responses than those from equal efforts of the legs, manual skills, emotional and intellectual demands (e.g., cognition, mentation, decision

making, competitions, interpersonal relationships, distractions, and supervision), and environmental stresses (e.g., dangers of physical trauma, extremes of heat, noises, fumes, dust, and additive effects of meals and tobacco). Aerobic expenditure rarely constitutes the major occupational stress in most societies.

Cardiovascular responses to muscular effort at work differ from those seen in exercise testing. In the latter, heart rate and blood pressure increase linearly with effort and $\dot{V}o_2$. In contrast, this effect does not occur in the majority of occupations, in large part because of the combined effects of emotions, heat stress, or both during periods of low caloric expenditure in sedentary or standing activities [20, 21, 68]. The method of equivalence by which the heart rate response at work is equated to the energy expenditure of an equal heart rate during exercise testing has been shown to be invalid in subjects whose oxygen uptake rarely approaches one liter of $O_2$ per minute (5 calories) [68]. Above this level, Poulsen and Asmussen [69] have shown excellent correlations between heart rate and oxygen uptake. Few occupations in modern Western society, however, require such high energy expenditures. The method of equivalence can be used with reasonable accuracy when the work design and workload of both exercise tests and occupational work are comparable, but such application is misleading in work or recreational situations that are associated with other stresses.

INDIVIDUAL CHARACTERISTICS
MEDIATING STRESSFUL EXPERIENCES
Exercise tests fail to take into account the individual's *perception of stresses* other than the muscular effort of the lower extremities and of the laboratory testing per se. In fact, every effort is customarily made to reduce the emotional stresses of the test procedure. On-the-job observations point out the importance of the individual's perception of stresses, which are usually intellectual, cognitive, or mentative. Numerous examples have demonstrated great differences in responsiveness to the same stresses, whether in low- or high-energy occupations or in a standardized quiz test conducted in a laboratory. As Rabkin and Struening state, "Such perception depends on personal characteristics determining

the appraisal of the significance of potentially harmful, challenging, or real or perceived threatening events" [70]. The great variations seen among firefighters exposed to the same heat, dusts, fumes, noises, and hazards provide good examples of the importance of perception.

## SUGGESTED MODIFICATIONS OF EXERCISE PERFORMANCE TESTS TO ENHANCE APPLICATION IN PRESCRIPTION FOR WORK OR OTHER ACTIVITIES

The question logically may be raised as to whether the above-cited limitations of exercise tests negate their usefulness in estimating probable performance in specific life and occupational situations.

Although few occupations require as much as 50 percent of the aerobic capacity (which explains why cardiac patients can perform safely in most occupations in industry), other information obtained from exercise testing does have relevance to work performance. The occurrence of ventricular arrhythmias and of ST-T displacement during exercise testing has been found to be predictive of similar changes at work [68]. Exercise tests may be more sensitive than on-the-job observations in detecting ST-T displacements (84.2 compared to 36.8 percent) and premature ventricular beats (79.2 compared to 45.8 percent, respectively) [68]. This difference suggests that the combined stresses of the job may be less than that of the single stress of muscular effort in the exercise laboratory. In a few subjects (16 to 21 percent), however, ST-T displacement, premature ventricular beats, or both may occur at work but not during peak or maximal testing. This implies that stresses other than muscular effort are operative [20, 21, 68].

The objective of the stress test and the type of subjects being evaluated should determine its design. Table 16–2 summarizes the types, equipment, and purposes of various types of tests used for cardiac rehabilitation. Performance tests that simulate reality (reality stress tests) should also consider past or present skills, the type and duration of skeletal muscle contraction used to stress the cardiovascular system, and the application of the test results to the anticipated vocational, recreational, or training activities of the individual. In addition to isotonic "steady-state" exercise of the lower extremities, non-steady-state exercise, isometric exercise, hyperventilation, Valsalva maneuver (Flack test), and carotid sinus reflex evaluation are frequently indicated. A subject with a hypersensitive carotid sinus reflex, for example, may be able to perform dynamic isotonic exercises such as in walking, jogging, or cycling, but would be more appropriately evaluated by the addition of static isometric contractions, such as hand-grip or weight-lifting exercises or carrying either alone or in combination with isotonic effort [45].

The magnitude of most effort tests is generally unrealistic; that is, it is excessive from the standpoint of the energy requirements of most occupations. For the few subjects who are exposed to multiple stresses of high-level effort and of adverse environment, however, *supermaximal* testing may be indicated. In 8 percent of subjects working under such circumstances, their heart rate exceeded not only their peak exercise performance, but also all published maximal heart rates for subjects of their age and sex [68]. In such subjects, the use of an arbitrary heart rate end-point, such as 85 percent of the age-predicted maximal heart rate, should be discouraged; this constitutes *undertesting*. The inadequacy of using a heart rate end-point of 85 percent of the age-predicted maximal value is indicated by our finding that on the job, 33 of 105 firefighters exceeded more than 85 percent of the age-predicted maximal heart rate [68].

Most subjects, however, are *overtested*. The observations made on normal subjects and cardiac patients in a great variety of occupations indicated that the aerobic capacity was rarely taxed more than 50 percent of the load of high submaximal or maximal peak exercise tests [20, 21, 68]. Furthermore, the peak heart rate responses during highly emotional, cognitive, or decision-making moments usually occur during low-level efforts (i.e., at 2 or 3 METs), which are equivalent to the lowest stages of treadmill or bicycle ergometric tests. In selected cases, submaximal tests at 85 percent of maximal heart rate or higher may be indicated, not because of the relation between heart rate and oxygen uptake, but rather for determining the heart rhythm and ST-T responses of individuals whose work en-

TABLE 16–2. Indications for various types of exercise and other stress tests in cardiac rehabilitation

| Type of test | Equipment | Objectives, evaluations, and applications |
|---|---|---|
| **RHYTHMIC, ISOTONIC**<br>Lower extremities | Bicycle, steps, treadmill | To determine submaximal, maximal, or peak aerobic capacity and $Vo_2$ max for leg exercise<br><br>*Occupations:* mail carriers, police officers, supervisors, field workers<br><br>*Recreation and training:* walking, jogging, running, climbing, soccer, golf |
| Upper extremities | Arm cycle ergometer, wall pulley, wheel arm crank | Submaximal, maximal, or peak aerobic capacity and $Vo_2$ max for upper extremity exercise<br><br>*Occupations:* sawing, manufacture, machine operation, typing, pianist, dentist, surgeon, music conductor<br><br>*Recreation and training:* swimming, canoeing, games, volley ball, pool, billiards |
| Upper and lower extremities | (See above) | Performance of activities involving entire body<br><br>*Occupations:* manual labor, ditch digging, shoveling, gardening, ladder climbing<br><br>*Recreation and training:* basketball, handball, mountain climbing, cross-country skiing, tennis, football, fencing, squash, paddle ball, horseback riding, dancing |
| **ISOMETRIC**<br>Hand-grip | Hand dynamometer, sphygmomanometer, weights, handbag filled with weights | Cardiovascular responses to isometric activities (heart rate, blood pressure, ECG)<br><br>*Occupations:* hand and arm effort, saw, levers, portage, jack hammer operator, controls operator, steel mill, factory, fire fighter, control of fire hose<br><br>*Recreation and training:* weight lifting and water skiing |
| **ORTHOSTATIC:**<br>Postural | Changes from supine and upright postures | Changes in HR, BP, and ECG with postural changes<br><br>*Occupations:* mechanics, plumbers<br><br>*Training:* floor exercises |
| Hyperventilation | Sphygmomanometer, electrocardiograph | To distinguish effects of increased minute-ventilation due to muscular effort, respiratory effort per se, or hypocapnia |

TABLE 16–2. (Continued)

| Type of test | Equipment | Objectives, evaluations, and applications |
|---|---|---|
| Valsalva maneuver (Flack test) | Mouthpiece attached to sphygmomanometer | Cardiovascular responses to increased intrathoracic pressure may reveal syncope in patients with chronic lung disease or hypersensitive carotid sinus reflex in cardiac patients<br>*Closed glottis activities:* occupations requiring sustained or near isometric activity (e.g., use of wrenches, levers, or wind instruments)<br>*Recreation and training:* push-ups, leg raising, body contact sports such as wrestling or line football |

tails low levels of energy expenditure and significant emotional or environmental stresses.

In addition to standardized effort testing to establish functional capacity and clinical diagnosis, performance tests should take into consideration the demands of the anticipated work or occupation. Although it is not possible to anticipate or to reproduce faithfully in the laboratory all the stresses encountered at work, some of the most common and important ones can be reproduced or simulated. These include effort involving the upper and lower extremities that is performed in work clothes after meals and emotionally and intellectually stressful quizzes or problem-solving tests that allow for or purposely tax the subject's education and knowledge. These and other modifications attempt to *simulate* the reality of the work environment. The validity of the work prescription can be determined either directly by on-the-job observations or, more practically, indirectly by continuous monitoring of the heart rate, blood pressure, or both with newly developed, automatic recording devices.

To summarize, modifications of present exercise testing techniques can enhance their value in vocational counseling of both normal subjects and cardiac patients. Stress testing may be expanded to include (1) *standardized effort* for diagnostic and quantitative purposes, (2) *reality stress testing* with one or more stresses in various combinations to simulate the anticipated work situation, and (3) *situational testing* performed directly by on-the-job evaluations or indirectly with automated portable equipment to record both the ECG and blood pressure.

## Comprehensive Therapy After Discharge From the Hospital

Comprehensive treatment is essential for the successful rehabilitation of the postinfarction patient. It includes not only treatment of coronary heart disease and its complications and management of the associated cardiac and noncardiac conditions, but also the identification and modification of modifiable coronary risk factors.

### RATIONALE FOR PREVENTIVE PRACTICE

Many of the important risk factors that are related to the appearance of the first coronary event have been shown to exert a significant influence on subsequent risk among the survivors of a myocardial infarction. Table 16–3 presents 16 prognostically important entry factors for the occurrence of death in 3 years among myocardial infarction survivors studied by the Coronary Drug Project Research Group [71].

*The nonmodifiable risk factors* were found to be mainly electrocardiographic. An ECG that reverted to normal following infarction was associated with a favorable prognostic status, about 1 percent mortality per year, in comparison to the over 4 percent mortality in subjects

TABLE 16-3. Entry prognostic factors for death in 3 years among myocardial infarction survivors (2,789 placebo-treated men, ages 35–64)

ST segment depression (rest ECG)
Cardiomegaly (chest roentgenogram)
NYHA functional class
Ventricular conduction defect (rest ECG)
Diuretic therapy
Intermittent claudication
Serum total cholesterol
Frequent ventricular premature beats (10 percent or more of beats, rest ECG)
Physical inactivity
Q-QS waves (rest ECG)
Heart rate (rest ECG)
Number of prior infarctions
Systolic blood pressure
Diastolic blood pressure
Oral hypoglycemic therapy
Number of cigarettes smoked

Adapted from Coronary Drug Project Research Group. *J. Chronic Dis.* 27:267, 1974.

with any ECG residua [72]. Unfavorable prognosis was associated with nonspecific ST-T changes, left ventricular hypertrophy, intraventricular block, complete left bundle branch block, and Q-QS waves. Unlike ST depression at rest, exercise-induced ST depression is modifiable by exercise training or by augmenting coronary blood flow through bypass surgery [5].

Fortunately, *the major postinfarction risk factors* —hypercholesterolemia, cigarette smoking, hypertension, and physical unfitness—are modifiable. The beneficial effects of combined therapy of diet and cholestyramine on the progression of coronary arteriosclerosis in patients with Type II hyperlipoproteinemia and coronary artery disease included significant reduction of rate of progression in the cholestyramine-treated patients, especially of lesions causing 50 percent or greater stenosis. Cardiovascular end-points, death, and nonfatal myocardial infarction favored the cholestyramine-treated group [73]. The persistence of a significant relation between these factors and the recurrence rates in coronary patients is sound evidence that they not only affect long-term atherogenesis, but also that their influence remains active *after* the first

event. To many cardiologists, this relation provides a sound rationale for preventive measures. It must be recognized, however, that in the postinfarction patient, the coronary disease and myocardial involvement are well established. As discussed in chapters 11 and 12, the later in the course of the disease that corrective measures are undertaken, the less likely that substantial benefits will be produced; yet Blackburn has emphasized that it "seems inappropriate and inconsistent to reject safe and reasonable interventions on health habits such as overeating, cigarette smoking, and sedentary life-style. Strong associations and logical mechanisms exist to justify attempts at risk factor reduction" [74].

MODIFYING HEALTH BEHAVIOR
The success of the multidisciplinary exercise conditioning programs has provided a model for systematic efforts to modify *other* risk-related health behavior. Stunkard [75] has described various techniques of modifying behavior. These include self-observation and record-keeping to involve the patient directly and to get feedback on his or her progress, environmental (stimulus) control to reduce temptation by removing it, modeling to demonstrate the desired behavior, guided practice to train in shaping skills to introduce new preferences, and reinforcement by praise, rewards, and other inducements [75]. Such approaches have been employed in modifying eating and smoking habits and aggressive behavior patterns. Impressive evidence has accumulated that "information, motivation and skills for change can be more effectively imparted to groups of individuals and to communities than in the traditional prescription oriented medical practices by the private physician alone" [76].

PSYCHOSOCIAL "RISK" FACTORS
Although certain psychosocial emotional and personality factors have been reported to be related to coronary heart disease end-points such as myocardial infarction and angina pectoris, there is little evidence showing an influence of behavior, personality, or life stress on the recurrence or mortality rates *after* myocardial infarction [77]. Similarly, there are few data on the effectiveness of modifying such characteristics in

an attempt to reduce the risk of reinfarction [78]. As Jenkins has pointed out, "our present knowledge of social and psychological factors of coronary disease . . . is still too rudimentary to permit comments on the implications of these findings for control programs" [79].

There is considerable evidence of the importance of psychosocial adaptations following an acute myocardial infarction (as discussed in chapter 17). For this reason, the importance of group therapy in selected patients cannot be overemphasized. A recent study reported that death from recurrent myocardial infarction was significantly higher in control groups who received no counseling than in groups that received either cardiologic counseling and in groups that received advice and instruction designed to modify other behavior [63]. At the end of the first year of a 5-year study, the rates of infarction and cardiovascular deaths were significantly lower among the subjects who received cardiologic counseling and those who received behavioral counseling compared to a control group. However, the mechanism by which the mortality rate was reduced has not been clarified.

## PHYSICIAN'S ATTITUDES TOWARD PREVENTIVE MEASURES
In a recent survey, few physicians thought it necessary to employ exercise testing in evaluating a patient's status; some felt this because they considered their clinical judgment would be equally helpful, when in fact it could not substitute for objective evaluations [1]. Others were concerned for their patients' safety during exercise testing, although a relative lack of risk has been demonstrated. To some extent, the excessive caution and concern about acute myocardial infarction that prevailed in previous decades still seem to persist, despite the changes that have taken place. Most physicians were and still are cautious in allowing such activities as stair climbing until 30 days after the acute myocardial infarction.

Just as private physicians should not remain complacent about the patients who have successfully stopped smoking but who have gained weight and have suffered an associated rise in blood pressure and serum lipid values, they should also be aware that patients who fail to adhere to a physical activity program would benefit by reinforcement by the physician and other health professionals involved in exercise training [77].

## VOCATIONAL GUIDANCE
Return to work is of major psychological importance to the previously employed individual recovering from an infarct, as it represents a combination of physical recovery and successful emotional adjustment. Because many patients have problems in returning to work [80], vocational guidance is an important aspect of care. All patients who were working prior to the illness will benefit from discussion with their doctor about their perception of their physical and emotional capability to meet the requirements of their job. If the employer is unwilling to take the patient back, the vocational expert can help the patient seek and find a similar job elsewhere or obtain retraining for a suitable new job. Evaluation of the previous work, educational level, former training, skills, interests, achievements, and intelligence using clinical interviews and appropriate psychological tests provides the necessary background. As a result it is usually possible to specify any suitable type of job that takes into account the patient's physical and emotional limitations, special interests, and ability. The reduction of the energy demands of many jobs enables many patients with limited physical capacity, but with intelligence and appropriate interest, to be retrained to meet the cognitive and skill requirements of newly developed jobs. Where change is indicated, vocational retraining will be necessary [63]. A major determinant of employment in both medically and surgically treated patients appears to be the recent work status; the longer the patient had been unemployed, the less likely the return to work.

## SURGERY (AND TRANSLUMINAL CORONARY DILATATION) AS VALID REHABILITATIVE MEASURES
Eighty to 85 percent of patients with patent bypass grafts obtain partial or complete relief of angina pectoris after coronary bypass surgery, and many of these objectively demon-

strate improved functional status as a result of the procedure. Extremely good results have been found in the young as well as in older subjects [81]. Despite the improvement of functional capacity, the vocational results have been less than optimal because of socioeconomic factors, the severity of the disease, and the symptomatic relief offered by surgery. The major factors in determining whether the patient will return to work after surgery include the level of education, the hours worked before surgery, the degree of relief of angina 1 year after surgery, absence of congestive heart failure symptoms after surgery, presence of angina before surgery, the number of vessels diseased, and the number of grafts placed [79, 80]. Physical or mental demands of the job may preclude some individuals from returning to work. Also, the fear that stress will precipitate cardiovascular problems may deter productive occupational activities. Some subjects cannot return to work because of company or union policies concerning cardiac patients. The physician may use an overly restrictive approach in the management of such patients, especially with regard to physical activity and return to work. Sometimes the family may adopt an overly protective role toward the patient. Clearly, more emphasis must be placed on the rehabilitation of coronary bypass patients after surgery if return to work is a desirable goal, for these procedures, which, though effective, are costly. Thus, bypass surgery does not bypass the need for rehabilitation measures [80]. Postoperative patients may benefit from group therapy and by participation in postoperative groups such as the "Mended Heart," just as postmyocardial infarction patients benefit from sharing of experiences. The benefits of prescribed, supervised exercise in the postoperative patients are similar [82] but greater than those after myocardial infarction. The training levels are considerably higher in the former because of the improved myocardial perfusion.

It can be expected that transluminal coronary angioplasty (described in chapters 9 and 12) will also be seen as a rehabilitative measure, as more and more cases are done. Return-to-work figures for this procedure are still fragmentary, however.

*Return to Sexual Activity.* A coronary patient's return to sexual activity after coronary bypass surgery depends on the patient's status before the illness, the direct and indirect effects of heart disease, and changes in cardiovascular functions. The changes in the frequency and quality of sexual activity after coronary bypass surgery are comparable to those produced by systemic physical training in unoperated coronary patients [5, 83]. Coronary bypass surgery is associated with significant improvement of physical fitness, aerobic capacity, highest attained peak heart rate, and improved heart rate–systolic blood pressure (HR-SBP) product during exercise.

A large majority of patients report substantial postoperative improvement, which is confirmed by performance of exercise tests, myocardial imaging, echocardiograms, etc. However, sexual functioning may not improve as much as physical fitness. Impotence, diminished satisfactory sexual activity, and other sexual impairments independent of physical status may occur in over half of the subjects. However, over 70 percent of patients who have been limited sexually because of angina pectoris return to their preillness levels of sexual functioning following successful coronary artery bypass surgery and relief of angina pectoris [63].

In addition, the frequency and quality of sexual activity improve. Fifty-six percent of the subjects who showed improvement in cardiovascular function on the basis of multistage exercise testing also indicated better quality and increased frequency of sexual activity. None of the subjects who showed deterioration of cardiovascular function after surgery showed improvement in the quality of sexual activity [83].

In counseling the postoperative patient who wishes to return to an active sexual life, the physician must take into account the many factors that influence the return to sexual activity and modify them if possible. The sexual activity of the postoperative coronary patient depends of age, sexual drive, performance in earlier life, the spouse's health and attitudes, psychologic factors, cardiovascular functional status prior to the illness, the degree of improvement after bypass surgery, the response to medical management and treatment, and, particularly, the effects of drugs, alcohol, and other illnesses such as diabetes mellitus, prostatectomy, and certain neurological diseases.

## Unresolved Questions and Future Challenges

Deficiencies and unmet needs are numerous despite the above-cited substantial attainments. A few will be cited in regard to (1) training (methods, effectiveness, facilities, and cost), (2) research, and (3) society, attitudes, and perspective.

### TRAINING

A plethora of needs exists. Some remaining problems are to determine an optimal intensity of training and the number of years required to demonstrate substantial long-term training effects; to enhance adherence to training programs by identifying susceptible dropouts; to avoid the danger of therapeutic "nihilism," that is, false-negative conclusions on ineffectiveness of physical conditioning based on inadequate intensity of training, poor compliance, and faulty project management; to reduce the economic cost and to determine the cost-effectiveness of various rehabilitation procedures; and to consider changing criteria of successful rehabilitation by including "quality of life" as well as morbidity and mortality.

### RESEARCH

There are needs for better understanding of the adaptation of individuals to intervention at the cellular, organic, and individual levels; for evaluation of methods of exercise testing and training and their relation to specific occupations; for more research on the impact of illness and of health maintenance on society at large; and for more basic research on the pathogenic factors of health disease and especially on the progression of arteriosclerosis after a myocardial infarction.

### SOCIETY

The role of physical training should be placed in proper perspective to incorporate it into the fabric of a long lifetime. "Faddism" and the establishment of new unsubstantiated dogma and ritualization of care must be avoided. There is a need to improve life-style alternatives as technology increases and thereby diminishes human energy expenditures; that is, opportunities must be developed for vigorous living off the job. Running addiction, the current fad and popularization of marathon running (for which only a small percentage of myocardial infarction patients are eligible) [84, 85], and the current pursuit of physical fitness as a new religion are hazardous, however, when intellectual, social, vocational, emotional, and nutritional aspects are slighted.

Overpublicized marathon running by a few subjects has aroused unrealistic expectations in the majority of coronary heart disease subjects and probably in a considerable number of coronary-prone subjects, many of whom have silent coronary disease. Long-distance running and marathon running have limited value in the rehabilitation of cardiovascular patients for the majority of occupations, which involve predominantly upper extremity effort. Fewer than 6 in 1,000 patients with coronary heart disease have been estimated as being potentially able to achieve the high level of training and maximal $\dot{V}o_2$ sufficient to complete a marathon run of 5 hours [84].

To determine whether rehabilitation efforts enhance the "quantity" of life, it is necessary to conduct prospectively planned, controlled, randomized studies, many of which are in progress. A major advance has been the institution of several cooperative randomized studies in the United States (e.g., the National Exercise and Heart Disease Project), Canada, and Europe to evaluate the effects of prescribed, supervised exercise on the clinical course of subjects who have sustained a myocardial infarction. There is a need for a sufficient number of subjects and for variations in the design of the exercise training to determine whether long-range adherence is feasible at reasonable cost. The need also exists to improve practical and optimal types of rehabilitation facilities. Should they be simple or complex, separated or integrated into the body of medical care, or located in isolated areas? Unfortunately, the concept of the spa—usually laden with mystique, dogma, pseudoscience, and empiricism—is flourishing in Germany and many eastern European countries and is now beginning to emerge in the United States. Another movement, which is less costly and potentially more widely available, has been the development of in-hospital outpatient departments, community reconditioning centers such as the YMCA and Jewish Community Center, and other urban and suburban training programs.

PATIENT AND FAMILY EDUCATION

Many cogent needs regarding patient and family education need attention. Often, the social-psychological barriers to communication may be significant when the patient and other involved health professionals have different social and cultural backgrounds. Thus, improved communication between the patient and physician is vital. The patient should be informed about the disease, the reasons for and the results of diagnostic tests, the clinical course and prognosis tests, and the clinical course and prognosis of the disease. Precise information should be provided on specific activities such as rest, work, activities of daily living, exercise, recreational and leisure activities, sexual intercourse, travel, nutrition, and smoking. There is also a need to improve and to utilize a variety of community agencies that are valuable in rehabilitation. Society should be challenged to participate by providing support for facilities for widespread education regarding nutrition, work, effort, physiology, psychology, and other aspects of health hygiene. The individual patient also needs guidance and encouragement to develop a concept of self-responsibility for health, hygiene, and the avoidance of disease.

## Conclusions

Comprehensive rehabilitation after acute myocardial infarction aims to restore the individual to an optimal functional status. It is based on the evaluation, utilization, and enhancement of the residual cardiovascular capacity. In the majority of postinfarction patients, residual capacity can be utilized and enhanced for most occupational, recreational, and social functions. The process of rehabilitation seeks to prevent the impairment of function related to physical deconditioning by promoting appropriate activity, providing early assessment of cardiovascular function and struc-ture, quantitating the severity of the illness, identifying the significant postinfarction risk factors, and instituting measures to modify them. Comprehensive therapy to enhance rehabilitation includes not only conventional medical therapy, and measures to retard or reverse the process of atherosclerosis [87], but also psychotherapy, exercise training, and surgery.

The results of rehabilitation efforts are most rewarding when the program is individualized, is pursued in a systematic and practical fashion with realistic testing related to occupational needs, and makes provisions for continued medical care. Rehabilitation programs must include patient education, selection of appropriate therapy, and societal involvement. The recent clinical trials have provided strong evidence that lipid control reduces the incidence of coronary heart disease in asymptomatic subjects and retards and in few cases reverses the progression of atherosclerosis [87]. However, there are myriad unsolved problems. Little doubt exists that active participation in a reconditioning and comprehensive rehabilitation program can go a long way toward improving the quality of life for the patient who has sustained an acute myocardial infarction.

## References

1. Wenger, N.K., Hellerstein, H.K., Blackburn, H., and Castranova, S.J. Physician practice in management of patients with uncomplicated myocardial infarction—changes in the past decade. *Circulation* 65:421, 1982.
2. McNeer, J.F., Wagner, G.S., Ginsburg, P.B., Wallace, A.G., McCants, C.B., Conley, M.J., and Rosati, R.A. Hospital discharge one week after acute myocardial infarction. *N. Engl. J. Med.* 298:229, 1978.
3. Hellerstein, H.K. and Ford, A.B. Rehabilitation of the cardiac patient. *JAMA* 164:225, 1957.
4. Blankenhorn, D.H. Reversibility of latent atherosclerosis: Studies by femoral angiography in humans. *Mod. Concepts Cardiovasc. Dis.* 47:79, 1978.
5. Naughton, J.P. and Hellerstein, H.K. (eds.) *Exercise Testing and Exercise Training in Coronary Artery Disease.* New York: Academic, 1973.
6. Hellerstein, H.K., Hornsten, T.R., Goldbarg, A.N., Burlando, A.G., Friedman, E.H., Hirsch, E.Z., and Marik, S. The Influence of Active Conditioning upon Coronary Atherosclerosis. In Brest, A.N., and Moyer, J.H. (eds.), *Atheroscle-*

rotic Vascular Disease. A Hahnemann Symposium. New York: Appelton-Century-Crofts, 1967, p. 115.

7. Heberden, W. Commentaries on the History and Cure of Diseases. Boston: Wells and Lilly, 1918.

8. Herrick, J.B. Clinical features of sudden obstruction of the coronary arteries. JAMA 59:2015, 1912.

9. Mallory, G.K., White, P.D., and Salcedo-Salgar, J. The speed of healing of myocardial infarction. A study of the pathologic anatomy in seventy-two cases. Am. Heart J. 18:647, 1939.

10. Lewis, T. Diseases of the Heart. New York: Macmillan, 1933, p. 49.

11. Dock, W. The evaluation sequelae of complete bedrest. JAMA 125:1083, 1944.

12. Harrison, T.R. Abusive bed rest as a therapeutic measure for patients with cardiovascular disease. JAMA 125:1075, 1944.

13. Taylor, H.L., Henschel, A., Brozek, J., and Keys, A. Effect of bed rest on cardiovascular function, and work performance. J. Appl. Physiol. 2:223, 1949.

14. Saltin, B., Blomqvist, G., Mitchell, J.H., Johnson, R.L., Wildenthal, K., and Chapman, C.B. Response to exercise after bedrest and training. Circulation 38 (Suppl. 7):1, 1968.

15. Levine, S.A. and Lown, B. The chair treatment of acute coronary thrombosis. Trans. Assoc. Am. Physicians 64:316, 1951.

16. Pinner, J.I. and Altman, A.H. Selective replacement in industry. J. Rehabil. 32:2, 1966.

17. Turell, D.J. and Hellerstein, H.K. Six year average follow-up of 460 consecutive cardiac patients. Circulation 18:790, 1958.

18. Parran, T.V., Hellerstein, H.K., Cohen, D., and Goldston, E. Results of Studies at the Work Classification Clinic of the Cleveland Area Heart Society. In Rosebaum, F.F. and Belknap, E.L. (eds.), Work and the Heart. New York: Hoeber, 1959, p. 330.

19. Harvey, V.K. and Luongo, E.P. Physical capacity for work: Principles of industrial physiology and psychology related to the evaluation of working capacity of the physically impaired. Occup. Med. 1:1, 1946.

20. Ford, A.B. and Hellerstein, H.K. Work and heart disease. I. A. physiologic study in the factory. Circulation 18:823, 1958.

21. Ford, A.B., Hellerstein, H.K., and Turell, D.J. Work and heart disease. II. A physiologic study in a steel mill. Circulation 20:537, 1959.

22. Hellerstein, H.K. and Goldston, E. Rehabilitation of patients with heart disease. Postgrad. Med. 15:265, 1954.

23. Fardy, P.S. and Hellerstein, H.K. A comparison of continuous and intermittent progressive multistage exercise testing. Med. Sci. Sports 10:1, 1978.

24. Day, H.W. and Averill, K.L. Recorded arrhythmias in an acute coronary care area. Dis. Chest 49:113, 1966.

25. Cain, H.D., Frasher, W.G., Jr., and Stivelman, R. Graded activity program for safe return to self-care after myocardial infarction. JAMA 177:111, 1961.

26. Hellerstein, H.K. Techniques of exercise prescription and evaluation. National Workshop: Exercise in Prevention in the Evaluation and in the Treatment of Heart Disease. Myrtle Beach, S.C., May 6–8, 1969. J. S.C. Med. Assoc. 65 (Suppl. 1–12):46, 1969.

27. Hellerstein, H.K. Exercise Therapy and Coronary Heart Disease. Rehabilitation and Secondary Prevention. In deHaas, J.H., Hemker, H.C., and Snellen, H.A. (eds.), Ischaemic Heart Disease. Leiden: Leiden University Press, 1970, pp. 406–429.

28. DeBusk, R.F., Spivack, A.P., VanKessel, A., Graham, C., and Harrison, D.C. The coronary care unit activities program: Its role in post-infarction rehabilitation. J. Chronic Dis. 24:373, 1971.

29. Ericsson, M., Granath, A., Ohlsen, P., Sodermark, T., and Volpe, U. Arrhythmias and symptoms during treadmill testing three weeks after myocardial infarction in 100 patients. Br. Heart J. 135:787, 1973.

30. Markiewicz, W., Houston, N., and DeBusk, R.F. Exercise testing soon after myocardial infarction. Circulation 56:26, 1977.

31. Sivarajan, E.S., Lerman, J., Mansfield, L.W., and Bruce, R.A. Progressive ambulation and treadmill testing of patients with acute myocardial infarction during hospitalization: A feasibility study. Arch. Phys. Med. Rehabil. 58:241, 1977.

32. Davidson, D.M. and DeBusk, R.F. Prognostic value of a single exercise test 3 weeks after myocardial infarction. Circulation 61:236, 1980.

33. Wohl, A.J., Lewis, H.R., Campbell, W., Karlsson, E., Willerson, J.T., Mullins, C.B., and Blomqvist, C.G. Cardiovascular function during early recovery from acute myocardial infarction. Circulation 56: 931, 1977.

34. Hellerstein, H.K. Exercise therapy in coronary disease. Bull. N.Y. Acad. Med. 44: 1028, 1968.

35. Hellerstein, H.K., Hirsch, E.Z., Ader, R., Greenblott, N., and Siegel, M. Principles of Exercise Prescription. Normals and Cardiac Subjects. In Naughton, J.P. and Hellerstein, H.K. (eds.), Exercise Testing and Exercise Training in Coronary Heart Disease. New York: Academic, 1973, p. 129.

36. Lampman, R.M., Santinga, J.T., Bassett, D.R., Mercer, N., Block, W.D., Flora, J.D., Jr., Foss, M.L., and Thorland, W.G. Effectiveness of unsupervised and supervised high intensity physical training in normalizing serum lipids in men with

type IV hyperlipoproteinemia. *Circulation* 57:-172, 1978.

37. Hellerstein, H.K. and Friedman, E.H. Sexual activity and the post coronary patient. *Arch. Intern. Med.* 125:987, 1970.

38. Dolkas, C.B. and Greenleaf, J.E. Insulin and glucose responses during bedrest with isotonic and isometric exercise. *J. Appl. Physiol.* 43:1033, 1977.

39. Robson, R.H. and Fluck, D.C. Autonomic blockade and coronary catecholamines and cyclic AMP in exercising man. *J. Appl. Physiol.* 43:949, 1977.

40. Hellerstein, H.K. A Misguided Goal or Unrealized Objective. Panel V: Acceleration of Collaterals Due to Physical Activity—Dogma or Fact. In Kellerman, J.J. and Denolin, H. (eds.), *Critical Evaluation of Cardiac Rehabilitation*. Basel: Karger, 1977, p. 125.

41. Mead, W.F., Pyfer, H.R., Trombold, J.C., and Frederick, R.C. Successful resuscitation of two near simultaneous cases of cardiac arrest with a review of fifteen cases occurring during supervised exercise. *Circulation* 53:1, 187, 1976.

42. Shaw, L.W., for the National Exercise and Heart Disease Project staff. Effects of a prescribed supervised exercise program on mortality and cardiovascular morbidity in patients after a myocardial infarction. The National Exercise and Heart Disease Project. *Am. J. Cardiol.* 48:39, 1981.

43. Shephard, R.J. The value of exercise in ischemic heart disease: A cumulative analysis. *J. Cardiac Rehab.* 3:294, 1983.

44. Bruce, R.A. Progress in Exercise Cardiology. In Yu, P.D. and Goodwin, J.F. (eds.), *Progress in Cardiology*. Philadelphia: Lea & Febiger, 1974, p. 113.

45. Hellerstein, H.K. and Franklin, B.A. Exercise testing and prescription. In Wenger, N.K. and Hellerstein, H.K. (eds.), *Rehabilitation After Myocardial Infarction*. New York: Wiley, 2nd ed., 1984.

46. Kitamura, K., Jorgensen, C.R., Taylor, H.L., and Wanger, Y. Hemodynamic correlates of myocardial oxygen consumption during upright exercise. *J. Appl. Physiol.* 32:516, 1972.

47. Nelson, R.R., Gobel, F.L., Jorgensen, C.R., Wang, K., Wang, Y., and Taylor, H.L. Hemodynamic predictors of myocardial oxygen consumption during static and dynamic exercise. *Circulation* 50:1179, 1974.

48. Fardy, P.S., Webb, D., and Hellerstein, H.K. Benefits of arm exercise in cardiac rehabilitation. *The Physician and Sportsmedicine*, p. 31, Oct. 1977.

49. Radke, J.E., Hellerstein, H.K., Salzman, S.H., Maistelman, H.M., and Ricklin, R. The quantitative effects of physical conditioning on the exercise electrocardiogram of subjects with atheriosclerotic heart disease and normal subjects. In Brunner, D. and Jokl, E. (eds.), *Physical Activity and Aging*. Basel: Karger, 1970.

50. Young, S.G. and Froelicher, V.F. Exercise testing: An update. *Mod. Concepts Cardiovasc. Dis.* 52:25, 1983.

51. Simoons, M.L. and Hugenholtz, P.G. Estimation of the probability of exercise-induced ischemia by quantitative ECG analysis. *Circulation* 56:552, 1977.

52. Blessey, R., Ice, R., Camp, J., Moody, K., Scharfman, S., Stein, M., and Selvester, R. Diagnostic sensitivity of a multiple lead system in maximal exercise testing: A comparison between V5 and alternative leads. *Med. Sci. Sports* 10:36, 1978.

53. Saltin, B., Nazor, K., Costill, D.I., Stein, E., Jansson, E., Essen, B., and Gollnick, P.D. The nature of the training response: Peripheral and central adaptations to one-legged exercise. *Acta Physiol. Scand.* 96:289, 1976.

54. Magel, J.R. and Faulkner, J.A. Maximum oxygen uptakes of college swimmers. *J. Appl. Physiol.* 22:-929, 1967.

55. Clausen, J.P., Trap-Jensen, J., and Lassen, N.A. The effects of training on the heart rate during arm and leg exercise. *Scand. J. Clin. Lab. Invest.* 26:295, 1970.

56. Holloszy, J.O. Long-term Metabolic Adaptations in Muscle to Endurance Exercise. In Naughton, J.P. and Hellerstein, H.K. (eds.), *Exercise Testing and Exercise Training in Coronary Heart Disease.* New York: Academic, 1973, pp. 211–222.

57. McArdle, W.D., Magel, J.R., Delio, D.J., Toner, M., and Chase, J.M. Specificity of run training on $Vo_2$ max and heart rate changes during running and swimming. *Med. Sci. Sports* 10:1, 16, 1978.

58. VanHandel, P.J., Costill, D.L., and Getchell, L.H. Central circulatory adaptations to physical training. *Res. Q. Am. Assoc. Health Phys. Educ.* 47:-815, 1976.

59. Naughton, J. Physical activity for myocardial infarction patients. *Cardiovasc. Rev. Rep.* 3:237, 1982.

60. Wilhelmsen, L., Sanne, H., Elmfeldt, D., Grimby, G., Tibbins, G., and Wedel, H. A controlled trial of physical training after myocardial infarction: Effects on risk factors, nonfatal reinfarction, and death. *Prev. Med.* 4:491, 1975.

61. Hellerstein, H.K. Anatomic Factors Influencing Effects of Exercise Therapy of ASHD Subjects. In Roskamm, H. and Reindell, R. (eds.), *Das Chronisch Kranke Herz.* Stuttgart: F.K. Schattauer, 1973, p. 513.

62. Dowell, R.T., Stone, H.L., Sordahl, L.A., and Asimakis, G.K. Contractile function and myofibrillar ATPase activity in the exercise-trained dog heart. *J. Appl. Physiol.* 43:977, 1977.

63. Hellerstein, H.K. and Cay, E.L. Psychological Aspects. In *Myocardial Infarction, How to Prevent, How to Rehabilitate.* Council on Cardiac Rehabilitation. International Society of Cardiology 1984.

64. WHO Expert Committee. Rehabilitation of patients with cardiovascular disease. W.H.O. Tech. Rep. Ser. 270, 1964.

65. Hellerstein, H.K., Brock, L.L., Bruce, R.A., Fox, S.M., III, Haskell, W.L., Naughton, J., Parmley, L.F., Jr., Taylor, H.L., and Zohman, L.R. *Exercise Testing and Training of Apparently Healthy Individuals: A Handbook for Physicians.* The Committee on Exercise. New York: American Heart Association, 1972.

66. Hellerstein, H.K., Brock, L.L., Bruce, R.A., Fox, S.M., III, Haskell, W.L., Naughton, J., Parmley, L.F., Jr., Taylor, H.L., and Zohman, L.R. *Exercise Testing and Training of Individuals with Heart Disease or at High Risk for Its Development. A Handbook for Physicians.* (The Committee on Exercise. New York: American Heart Association, 1975.)

67. DeBusk, R.F., Valdez, R., Houston, N., and Haskell, W. Cardiovascular responses to dynamic and static effort soon after myocardial infarction: Application to occupational work assessment. *Circulation* 58:368, 1978.

68. Hellerstein, H.K. Prescription of vocational and leisure activities. Practical aspects. *Adv. Cardiol.* 24:56, 1978.

69. Poulsen, E. and Asmussen, E. Energy requirement of practical jobs from pulse increase and ergometer test. *Ergonomics* 5:33, 1962.

70. Rabkin, J.H. and Struening, E.L. Life events, stress, and illness. *Science* 194:1013, 1976.

71. Coronary Drug Project Research Group. Factors influencing long-term prognosis after recovery from myocardial infarction. *J. Chronic Dis.* 27:267, 1974.

72. Coronary Drug Project Research Group. The prognostic importance of the electrocardiogram after myocardial infarction. *Ann. Intern. Med.* 77:677, 1972.

73. Brensike, J.F., Levy, R.I., Kelsey, S.T., Passamani, E.R., Richardson, J.M., Loh, I.K., Stone, N.J., Aldrich, R.F., Battaglini, J.W., Moriarty, D.J., Fisher, M.R., Friedman, L., Friedewald, W., Detre, K.M., and Epstein, S.E. Effects of therapy with cholestyramine on progression of coronary arteriosclerosis: Results of the NHLBI Type II Coronary Intervention Study. *Circulation* 69:313, 1984.

74. Blackburn, H. Personal communication.

75. Stunkard, A.J. Presidential address 1974. From explanation to action in psychosomatic medicine: A case of obesity. *Psychosom. Med.* 37:195, 1975.

76. Farquhar, J., Maccoby, N., Wood, P.D., Alexander, J.K., Breitrose, H., Brown, B.W., Jr., Haskell, W.L., McAlister, A.L., Meyer, A.J., Nash, J.D., and Stern, M.P. Community education for cardiovascular health. *Lancet* 1:1192, 1977.

77. Ruberman, W., Weinblatt, E., Goldberg, J.D., and Chaudharg, B.S. Psychosocial influences on mortality after myocardial infarction. *N. Engl. J. Med.* 311:552, 1984.

78. Blackburn, H. The Potential for Preventing Reinfarction. In Wenger, N.K. and Hellerstein, H.K. (eds.), *Rehabilitation After Myocardial Infarction.* New York: Wiley, 1979.

79. Jenkins, C.D. Psychologic and social precursors of coronary disease. *N. Engl. J. Med.* 284:244, 1971.

80. Oberman, A., Wayne, J.B., Kouchoukos, N.T., Charles, E.D., Russell, R.O., Jr., and Rogers, W. Employment status after coronary artery bypass surgery. *Circulation* 65 (suppl II):11–115, 1982.

81. Laks, H., Kaiser, G.C., Barner, H.B., Codd, J.E., and Willman, V.I. Coronary revascularization under age 40 years. *Am. J. Cardiol.* 41:584, 1978.

82. Johnson, W.D., Kayser, K.L., Pedraza, P.M., and Shore, R.T. Employment patterns in males before and after myocardial revascularization surgery: A study of 2229 consecutive male patients followed for as long as 10 years. *Circulation* 65:1086, 1982.

83. Hellerstein, H.K. Sexual Activity After Coronary Bypass Surgery. In *Proceedings Conference, Critical Evaluation of Cardiac Rehabilitation Council.* Tel Aviv: International Society of Cardiology, 1975.

84. Hellerstein, H.K. Limitations of marathon running in the rehabilitation of coronary patients. Anatomic and physiologic determinants. *Ann. N.Y. Acad. Sci.* 301:484, 1977.

85. Hellerstein, H.K. and Moir, T.W. Distance Running in the 1980s. Cardiovascular Benefits and Risks. In Wenger, N.K., (ed.), *Exercise and the Heart.* (2nd Edition), *Cardiovascular Clinics,* 15/1, Philadelphia: Davis, 1984, pp 75–86.

86. The lipid research clinics coronary primary prevention trial results. I. Reduction in incident of coronary heart disease. Lipid Research Clinics Program. *JAMA* 241:351, 1984.

87. The lipid research clinics coronary primary prevention trial results. II. The relationship of reduction in incidence of coronary heart disease to cholesterol lowering. Lipid Research Clinics Program. *JAMA* 251:365, 1984.

# 17. PSYCHOSOCIAL ASPECTS OF CORONARY ARTERY DISEASE

Joan Kirschenbaum Cohn

Most of the published data dealing with the interplay between psychosocial factors and coronary artery disease can be grouped into five distinct areas. The first is the role of stress, personality traits, and life crises as risk factors for the development of coronary artery disease. These have been discussed previously in chapters 3 and 12. The second area is the effect of emotional upheaval—with its corresponding neurohormonal stimulation leading both to increased myocardial oxygen demand and to greater vasomotor tone—as a cause of angina. This area has been discussed in chapter 2. The third area can be simply called "living with angina" and also includes the psychosocial adjustments of asymptomatic persons with coronary artery disease and silent myocardial ischemia. The fourth area concerns the psychologic problems associated with recovery from a myocardial infarction, including those involving the coronary care unit itself, as well as the rehabilitation process after myocardial infarction. Some of the latter problems have been alluded to in chapter 16. The fifth area concerns psychological adjustment following coronary bypass surgery. This chapter will focus on the last three areas, discussing current concepts as well as controversies.

## Reacting to the Diagnosis of Coronary Artery Disease: An Overview

Since the heart is the center of physiological functioning, a diagnosis indicating that one's heart is impaired is frightening at best. The two major types of psychological reaction that patients experience can be observed both in angina and silent myocardial ischemia, as well as in myocardial infarction. These two extremes of coping with the disease range from absolute denial to assuming the role of a "cardiac cripple," with various stages in between. These reactions will be described in more detail in subsequent sections, since this pattern becomes a recurrent theme of which the physician must be aware. Furthermore, because diseases of the heart imply a loss of health and prior functioning, cardiologists may see patients go through stages similar to those of mourning, as described by Elisabeth Kubler-Ross [1]: denial, anger, bargaining, acceptance, or hope.

## Is "Living With Angina" Different From "Living With Silent Myocardial Ischemia"?

In discussing therapy of angina pectoris in chapter 12, the importance of adjusting or preserving the patient's life-style within the context of the disease was stressed. This can be facilitated through good physician-patient communication, including discussion of work and leisure habits, sexual activity, and general concerns. At this point, before a myocardial infarction has ensued, the patient is more likely to deny the disease, but the knowledge that the patient may be "headed for a coronary" obviously causes a certain amount of fear and anxiety [2].

One of the areas that is currently generating considerable interest in physicians and allied health care professionals is silent myocardial ischemia in asymptomatic patients with coronary artery disease. To learn more about the psychological reactions in patients recently diagnosed with this syndrome, we used a questionnaire in 15 patients (table 17–1). Although no direct comparisons were made with a control group of patients with angina, the data have important implications for the primary physician and consulting cardiologist caring for the patient.

In this study of patients with asymptomatic coronary artery disease, we noted several trends [3]. First, as expected, surprise was the most common initial reaction to the diagnosis. Fear then became the dominant response. How could someone who felt so well have a potentially life-threatening problem? Second, we noted the desire of the patients to do something "different" in their life-style to avoid possible complications of the disease. This desire sometimes resulted in paradoxes: those who had exercised before now stopped their exercise, and those who had led sedentary lives now began to exercise.

Importantly, physicians caring for the patient should be aware of how the patient and family are coping. The physicians should also determine whether reactions of patient and family to the diagnosis are within a normal range; if not, they should suggest individual or family counseling. In patients with asymptomatic coronary artery disease, we have found a broad spectrum of individual reactions, just like those with symptomatic disease. At one end of the spectrum is the patient who is preoccupied with death and ensures that whatever his activities, they do not adversely affect his heart (the "cardiac cripple"). At the other end is the patient who denies any cardiovascular disease, thus constantly testing himself, his family, and his physician; he will do everything in an extreme manner. The patient's family reacts in many different ways to the diagnosis. The way in which disease is handled by spouse and children often reflects how the family functions, as well as any psychopathology in the relations within the family. Their attitude greatly influences the health and functioning of the patient. The fact that the major breadwinner has a potentially life-threatening disease that is asymptomatic, i.e. "silent," is often very frightening for the patient and the family to face. Self-indulgent and self-destructive behavior may be difficult to modify for the asymptomatic patient who is smoking or overweight. Furthermore, denial of the disease is easy when among one's anxieties is the knowledge transmitted by the physician that little is known of the natural history of the disease or what is the best treatment. Not surprisingly, therefore, physicians may find that this type of patient wants and needs more time, more understanding, and more detailed description of the disease, its prognosis, and the prescribed therapeutic regimen than does the

TABLE 17–1. Patient Questionnaire

1. When was the diagnosis made?
2. How was it presented to you?
3. Could it have been done differently?
4. How did you feel when you learned about the diagnosis? Fear? Sadness? Anger? Other Emotions?
5. What was your spouse's reaction?
6. What was your children's reaction?
7. Do you regularly exercise?
8. If so, what kind?
9. Has the pattern changed?
10. Has your sex life changed?
11. What were the doctor's suggestions to you about how to live your life after he told you the diagnosis?
12. Have you in fact done anything differently because of the diagnosis?
13. Would you consider taking medication for an indefinite period of time?
14. Would you consider having surgery?
15. Do you think the public should be more aware of the problem of asymptomatic coronary artery disease?

Source: Cohn, P.F., and Cohn, J.K. *J. Am. Coll. Cardiol.* 3:956, 1983.

"conventional" patient with coronary artery disease.

It should be emphasized that the family of the asymptomatic patient also needs special time. In trying to ease the family's anxiety, the physician should explain how asymptomatic disease is different, yet at the same time does exhibit common features of the usual and symptomatic forms of coronary artery disease. Discussing why the anginal sensation is protective and why patients without symptoms should be especially careful about avoiding situations where they may be overstressed or overexerted would be helpful. A hard concept for both the patient and the family to accept is that one has to cease an activity despite the lack of symptoms. It is recognized that choice of therapy is difficult in this syndrome; the patient's own thoughts and desires must be elicited to avoid further anxiety. Psychological counseling may be helpful if the physician senses that the patient and the family are excessively anxious, just as would be the case for patients with symptomatic coronary artery disease.

In summary, persons with asymptomatic coronary artery disease routinely have fears and anxieties concerning their life-style. Both patient and family may react to the knowledge of the disease by denying it entirely, by total overprotection, or by some stance in between. Physicians must be more available to this type of patient and family to present the unique aspects of asymptomatic disease. Unfortunately, physicians may have to be very assertive in direction when, because of limited knowledge of this disease, they themselves have as many questions as the patient concerning treatment.

## Recovering From a Myocardial Infarction

Patients who have a myocardial infarction may feel a sense of "being damaged, and out of control", as Stern, et al. [4] have suggested. Patients whose infarction was not preceded by other prior cardiac symptoms are caught unaware, so that their prior method of functioning is not valid for the present. A state of crisis for the patient and family is at hand.

Let us again reiterate the major mechanisms of coping, and their pitfalls, that many patients employ. The denial of symptoms that prevents the patient from going immediately to the emergency room of the local hospital may hinder full recovery and even result in death. During the next phase of the illness, when the patient is transferred to the coronary care unit, denial becomes a healthy defensive mechanism to ward off the anxiety caused by the possibility of sudden death. Later, it can reach unhealthy extremes. Patients may deny that *anything* is wrong. They may refuse to stop smoking, to become involved in exercise and to discontinue unhealthy dietary habits. They act as though they want to prove that the doctor is wrong, that they are stronger than God, nature, or fate. We may even see patients who begin regular exercise programs when they are contraindicated because of recurrent angina.

In contrast to patients who deny their heart disease are the "cardiac cripples." Upon learning that they have heart disease, patients will take to their home or even to bed, never to return to normal preinfarct functioning. Some patients, at this stage, exaggerate the extent of their disease and expect the spouse and children to reorganize their lives around their care. In between these two extremes are the patients who may become sad or depressed because of the loss of normal healthy functioning for a limited time period. They may then be able to return to normal functioning after appropriate tests, medications, or operations have been performed. The cardiologist may have to assess whether the patient is capable of performing at the level of prior normal functioning. If the patient does not "bounce back," consultation or therapy with a mental health professional may be indicated.

PSYCHOLOGICAL PROBLEMS AND PSYCHOSOCIAL ADAPTATIONS AFTER A MYOCARDIAL INFARCTION

The most important prognosticator of how a patient will recover from a myocardial infarction relates to the emotional makeup of the individual who suffers the infarct, to how well the individual can adjust to living with the implications of the disease [5].

One often forgets that the patient who suffers the infarct does not live alone or work alone.

The patient is an individual who functions within the context of many interlocking systems, each of which influences the health and recovery (or lack of recovery) of the patient. How a person lived in his or her environment prior to the onset of the infarction cannot help but influence how that individual is able to recover postinfarction.

The systems that influence a patient's life are primarily the family system and economic system. How is the man or woman perceived within the context of his or her marriage and family? If prior to infarct, the man's role was that of leader and sole breadwinner, how will the crisis affect his ability to assume his role within the family? Since relationships within a marriage and family are reciprocal, the illness of one member of the system affects the homeostasis of the interlocking network. What role can the spouse play to help fill the gap of the patient without undermining his or her self-esteem and confidence? The functioning of the family prior to illness is an important diagnostic tool for the medical team to use for deciding appropriate further treatment.

The economic system greatly affects the functioning of the patient in the postinfarction period. Was the patient working before the infarct? Was the job satisfying? What financial benefits are available during convalescence or retirement? White-collar workers are more likely to return to their jobs more quickly than blue-collar workers, as Doehrman [6] notes in his review. However, one does not know why this may be true. Psychological factors appear to be more important than physiological factors in this regard, but one must also realize that blue-collar workers may have better long-term disability coverage through their union contracts. Furthermore, management positions are more sedentary and less physically taxing than most blue-collar jobs. Many first-generation American blue-collar workers, embarrassed by their vulnerability to illness, believe they may be interpreted as less powerful, masculine, and dynamic.

When assessing the impact of a myocardial infarction on the future life of the patient, another system, the medical or hospital system, is a powerful element to consider. The way in which a patient is handled from the very beginning of emergency room treatment may affect the outcome of the crisis. It is imperative that the patient and family be well informed about what is expected and what is not during the course of the hospital stay. Hackett [7] cited the example of cardiac resuscitation, a procedure that is not uncommon and does not necessarily alter progress toward recovery but is a frightening experience for the patient to undergo and the family to witness. Lack of information, partial disclosures, and conspiracies of silence can lead to fantasies that are detrimental to the emotional health of the patient [7].

After the emergency room, the patient is usually sent to the coronary care unit. The unit can be seen by the patient as either a frightening or safe environment. Patients may be reassured that while they are in the coronary care unit, the constant beeps and "space-age" monitors that appear so intimidating actually serve as "guardian angels" for their safety [7]. Families need reassurance, as well, through physicians or nurses taking time to explain the various functions of the machines and other personnel. If the family is unduly concerned, the patient may become more anxious than necessary.

Stern et al. [8] state that patients who have an absence of depression and anxiety during their hospital stay, including time spent in the coronary care unit, have a good psychological response in their posthospitalization period. They base this finding on a study they performed at George Washington University Medical Center. The study eventually included 68 patients and was an extension of their earlier study [4]. These 68 patients included 55 males and 13 females and had a mean age of 53 years. They were predominantly middle class. The authors found no relation between denial, depression and anxiety, and the severity of the myocardial infarction, as determined by the commonly used Peel index, in which the higher the index, the more severe the infarction (table 17–2). Table 17–3 shows the results of the in-hospital and subsequent outpatient evaluations. Anxiety and depression were reduced only slightly by 1-year postinfarction, while return to work and sexual activity increased dramatically from the 6-week measurement. Cay [5] evaluated the relation-

TABLE 17-2. Peel index scores and psychological response

| Peel index | Total patient sample | Deniers | Depressed | Anxious |
|---|---|---|---|---|
| 1–8 | 15 | 6 | 1 | 2 |
| 9–12 | 23 | 6 | 3 | 3 |
| 13–16 | 16 | 4 | 2 | 3 |
| 17+ | 7 | 0 | 2 | 1 |
| Mean score | 11.5 | 9.8 | 13.2 | 12.0 |

Source: Stern, M.J., Pascale, L., et al. *J. Chron. Dis.* 29:513, 1976.

TABLE 17-4. Return to work related to initial reaction to an infarction

| Emotional upset 5–8 days after MI | Return to full activity by 4 months | Return to full activity within 1 year |
|---|---|---|
| Absent | 52% | 88% |
| Present | 36% | 31% |

Source: Cay, E.L., *Adv. Cardiol.* 29:108, 1982.

ship between return to work and emotional upset. Patients whose emotional upset had subsided by 5 to 8 days were likely to resume full activity (table 17–4).

Stern and colleagues feel that patients' denial of the seriousness of a myocardial infarction can help them deal with the situation and can actually be beneficial. As we have noted, denial is seen as being especially helpful during the coronary care unit stay, when things are most frightening. However, it is our experience that in addition to denial, one should *expect* to have a certain degree of fear, anxiety, and depression because one's heart, and therefore general functioning, has been impaired, even if temporarily. If symptoms are denied excessively, however, patients may be tempted to retain harmful habits such as smoking and poor nutritional habits. The depression one sees in most myocardial infarction patients is a reactive depression, which usually lasts around 6 months to a year. It, therefore, is time limited and within normal expectations.

Transfer to a regular medical floor from the coronary care unit is another potentially trau-

matic experience. Even if a patient has successfully used denial previously, the reality of the loss of one's intact health now becomes apparent and is often mourned. However, it can be reassuring to the patient and family to acknowledge (with the physician's or mental health professional's assistance, if necessary) that some sadness and anxiety is also normal and appropriate at this stage.

Once the patient is well established on the medical floor, it is often helpful for patient and spouse individually or together to join a quasi-therapeutic group. These groups provide a forum for airing questions, concerns, and anxieties about the patient's and family's future. Often these groups are set up, at least initially, to be medically and educationally oriented. Just what is permissible and advisable when I leave the hospital? How does the heart work and why and how do heart attacks occur? How can I delete or decrease the stress from my life and adjust to my life now? It is essential to include the spouse and family in educational and therapeutic situations. They are very much affected by the sickness of the patient. Group psychotherapy will be discussed further in the chapter.

Often patients become very manipulative

TABLE 17-3. Posthospital follow-up (expressed in %)

| | In-Hosp. | 6-weeks | 3-months | 6-months | 1-year |
|---|---|---|---|---|---|
| Anxiety | 42.0 | 30.0 | 17.6 | 21.5 | 16.7 |
| Depression | 29.0 | 15.4 | 11.8 | 9.8 | 13.0 |
| Return to work | | 19.1 | 59.5 | 71.4 | 63.8 |
| Return to sex | | 26.5 | 58.1 | 71.4 | 68.7 |
| Mortality | | | 1.6 | 3.2 | 4.8 |
| Patients interviewed | 98.4 | 95.2 | 96.8 | 93.7 | 92.1 |

Source: Stern, M.J., Pascale, L., et al. *J. Chron. Dis.* 29:513, 1976.

upon discharge from hospital. They have had to assume a regressed, somewhat childlike posture during hospitalization, a situation they cannot tolerate for too long. Their self-esteem and self-respect are no longer intact, and they need some ego-satisfying activities. Doehrman [6] states that conflicts between patient and family members often focus upon the patient's diet, medication, and physical activity, the only areas the patient is able to "control" while convalescing. The patient may, therefore, resent the protectiveness and concern shown by the family and interpret their gestures as being demeaning. The patient wants to dominate and control as much "turf" as possible. As we shall discuss later, spouses feel both guilty and fearful about the possibility of another myocardial infarction. They become solicitous and nonconfrontational, which may anger patients even more [6].

Patients fall into three categories in their adjustment to a myocardial infarction. They can use one of the two coping strategies we have previously cited; i.e., they may assume that they are "cardiac cripples" and can no longer participate in day-to-day living or they may deny that they were ever sick and resume bad health habits. Alternatively, and preferably, they can adjust to their new life with some sadness and then resume normal life patterns. If the patient and family have not resumed a normal life within 3 to 6 months, a referral for psychotherapy with a mental health consultant is warranted.

## USE OF GROUP PSYCHOTHERAPY IN THE POST-INFARCTION PERIOD

It is important to provide a supportive network for patients who have suffered the psychological trauma that often accompanies a myocardial infarction. In addition to the help offered by the cardiologist and the family, group psychotherapy has been found to be a helpful tool in dealing with the psychosocial aspects of recovery.

Many patients have no understanding of why a myocardial infarction occurs. A lack of education and understanding often leads to denial and then inappropriate behavior on the part of the patient. A group provides a setting in which to explore the perplexing questions that arise in the patient's mind. It is particularly helpful to find

that one is not alone in the physiological and/or psychological discomfort one is having.

The aim of group psychotherapy for patients recovering from a myocardial infarction is to provide an atmosphere in which common problems and solutions can be shared [9]. Thus, patients can use the group setting to further understand their condition; receive help with specific problems such as diet, exercise, and drugs; learn how to lessen anxiety through ventilation and expression of feeling; develop awareness of behavior patterns and problems; reduce reliance upon unhealthy defense mechanisms such as hypochondriasis, depression, and excessive denial; and develop ego strengths and healthy coping mechanisms. They can also utilize the group to diminish their sense of isolation.

In contrast to strict therapy-oriented groups, cardiac patients tend to be more comfortable focusing on the reality of "here and now" problems [9, 10]. These patients have to deal with a major blow to themselves both psychologically and physiologically that may result in a crisis for both the patient and the family. Many of these patients strive to protect themselves from being viewed as anything but a "normal" person with a "minor" physical problem. Therefore, the groups are not seen as psychotherapeutic, but more of a social club or gathering. In fact, the use of "club" in the name of the group is common.

Hackett [10] has stated that "in order for a group to be successful, it should be initiated while the patient is still in the hospital. An essential is that it be introduced as a medical function, with an emphasis on teaching, answering questions and sharing experiences." Much of the educational material that is introduced soon after the myocardial infarction must be repeated because the patient may be unable to remember what has happened during that time period.

To reemphasize an important point, a myocardial infarction affects *both* the patient and family. It has been found that male patients feel more comfortable talking about the problems of recovery when their wives can receive psychological counseling in a separate group. But in actuality, the groups that have been held for wives *only* have been less than totally effective. Many wives seem reluctant to express their frustration and anger about their husband's disease. Although they may feel guilty that in some way they are responsible for the "heart attack," this information does not seem to surface. The women seem to be more comfortable with a couples group rather than a wives-only group.

The issues raised in groups vary considerably. In their study of one particular group led by a psychiatric nurse, Bilodeau and Hackett [11] listed the 15 most frequently raised issues (table 17–5). Whether or not group psychotherapy can affect prognosis was addressed in the study by Ibrahim and colleagues [9]. These investigators studied 105 patients, of which 53 were in active group psychotherapy and 52 served as controls. Patients were categorized by their severity of infarction, using the Peel index. As seen in table 17–6, there was a difference in mortality between treatment and control groups: treatment patients fared better. In addition, favorable effects were suggested by decreased length of stay in hospital and by fewer signs of social alienation. Furthermore, when patients come on a regular basis, they express more satisfaction with the helpfulness of the group and they are more apt to recommend it to other heart patients [9, 10]. Indeed, whatever reluctance exists about groups is from cardiologists who do not know how effective the group experience can be in providing a supportive network for the patient.

Most importantly, these "heart clubs" should be led by a trained mental health professional (clinical social worker, psychologist, psychiatrist) because the group dynamics seen in therapeutic groups also prevail in the more socially oriented clubs (positioning, "scapegoating," "one-upmanship," etc.). "Although one sees patients being protective of one another in the group, a reason that inward feelings are often not confronted, one needs the protection and skills of a therapist trained in group therapy" [10].

In summary, we know that patients are often burdened with the fear that they can no longer fulfill their responsibilities and enjoy their lives because they have suffered a myocardial infarction. A group network provides patients with a supportive atmosphere in which they can air their concerns about reducing stress, resuming previous lifestyles, and any other concerns related to recovery. It would be most helpful to patients in particular and the families in general if cardiologists were more active in addressing the psychosocial needs of their patients. Group "heart clubs" can serve as that vehicle; if patients are still demonstrating difficulty in coping with

TABLE 17–5. The 15 most frequently expressed issues in groups

| Issue | Percent of all issues raised | Time consumed | |
|---|---|---|---|
| | | Percent | Rank |
| Leader | 10.7 | 6.8 | 5 |
| Group cohesiveness | 7.7 | 4.2 | 10 |
| Current state of physical health | 7.3 | 5.0 | 8 |
| Medical care after discharge | 6.3 | 7.1 | 4 |
| Work | 5.7 | 8.5 | 2 |
| Medications | 5.1 | 6.0 | 6 |
| Smoking | 4.8 | 8.7 | 1 |
| Current state of emotional health | 4.5 | 2.3 | 14 |
| Death | 4.1 | 3.3 | 12 |
| Attitude of others | 3.5 | 3.5 | 11 |
| Nature of illness | 3.5 | 2.2 | 15 |
| Nutrition | 3.2 | 7.5 | 3 |
| Illness and death of others | 3.2 | 2.7 | 13 |
| Family, home, friends | 3.1 | 4.3 | 9 |
| Finances | 3.0 | 5.2 | 7 |

Source: Bilodeau, C.B. and Hackett, T.P. *Amer. J. Psychiat.* 128:1, 1971.

TABLE 17–6. 18-month cumulative survival rates by the Peel prognostic index

| | Average number of patients | Survival rate | Standard error |
|---|---|---|---|
| All patients | 94 | .882 | .033 |
| Low Peel index | 51 | .949 | .029 |
| High Peel index | 43 | .811 | .058 |
| Treatment patients | 50 | .914 | .043 |
| Low Peel index | 24 | .962 | .038 |
| High Peel index | 26 | .879 | .067 |
| Control patients | 44 | .849 | .050 |
| Low Peel index | 27 | .940 | .041 |
| High Peel index | 17 | .735 | .094 |

Adapted from Ibrahim, M.A., Feldman, J.G., et al. *Int. J. Psych. Med.* 5:253, 1974.

their situation after 6 to 9 months, however, individual, marital, or family therapy should be suggested.

EFFECTS ON THE SPOUSE AND FAMILY

Attitudes of the patient's family are very important throughout both the hospital stay and the at-home recovery period; Davidson [12] believes they are probably the most crucial influence in determining the individual's psychological adaptation and subsequent course. Similarly, others [13] also feel a spouse's understanding attitude and ability to cope may be crucial in the rehabilitation of the patient.

The medical team must realize that a patient's myocardial infarction does not occur within a vacuum. The patient has assumed a particular role prior to the illness, which may or may not be resumed. It is important for the medical team to assess family functioning so that the spouse and children can be appropriately used as allies in the recovery phase.

The nature and suddenness of a myocardial infarction put the spouse in a particularly distressful situation [13]. Often there has been no anticipatory time period, so the family is thrown into crisis. Spouses often relate a feeling of numbness, panic, sense of loss, and fear of death or permanent incapacity in the patient when the myocardial infarction occurs [13, 14]. Since they also have the same fears, lack of knowledge, and misconceptions as does the patient, the family must be kept as abreast and aware of developments as the patient [15]. This educational need

is present from the onset of the infarction. It is important to note that the fear, pain, shock, anxiety, and depression experienced by the patient and family hinder their ability to learn and incorporate the specific knowledge that is being imparted by the medical team. Thus, it is very important that verbal and even written instructions be imparted in a supportive and caring way. These instructions should be repeated over the course of the hospital and posthospital recovery period [12].

The posthospital home recovery period of convalescence is particularly difficult and stressful for the patient and family [12–15]. A stable marriage before the infarction, where communication patterns were open and helpful, usually indicates that stability will return to the family within 3 to 6 months. The home recovery period is particularly difficult because roles in the marriage and family have to be redefined. If the husband is now confined to the house and assuming household and child-care responsibilities, he may become irritable, bored, and depressed. Having been used to an active life, he may have too much time on his hands, which may cause irritation with his wife and family. The wife is often placed in a double-bind position. If she appears concerned, protective, directive, and solicitous, her husband becomes annoyed because he believes he is being dispossessed as leader and that his masculinity is being threatened. Often the wife will deny or repress her angry feelings so as not to upset her spouse, which will often result in depression. If, however, she is less protective, she may then feel guilty or be accused of not caring. Since the lines of communication during this time period are generally not good, she is also in a position of feeling alone with little or no support. It is hard for her to strike a balance between being protective and helpful versus allowing her husband to return to an appropriate level of former activity [15]. Children seem to see the patient as even more handicapped than the spouse does. They may experience guilt, denial, and anger similar to that of their mother. They may see their father as even more ill because their mother is not performing her usual role but instead is now working outside the house, managing the finances, or taking up the slack necessitated by their father's illness.

Despite medical evidence that physical recovery of the individual is usually complete within 3 months, patients and their families often consider themselves impaired for at least a year. If support groups, family therapy, or couple therapy can be implemented as soon as the patient is medically stable, a better prognosis is indicated. The more educational this experience, the more supportive it is. If the physician or mental health professional informs the patient and family that the road to recovery will not be accomplished without problems, the family will not panic and give up hope when the period is particularly stressful. The family should be made aware of particular behaviors that may be difficult for them to cope with; for example, for a while the patient will feel easily tired, depressed, anxious, and fearful. Because everyone will have to assume new and perhaps more difficult roles, the family homeostasis will change. There can never be change of this magnitude without some distress and discomfort.

## PSYCHOSEXUAL ADJUSTMENT AFTER MYOCARDIAL INFARCTIONS

When the patient recovering from a myocardial infarction returns home, a period of stress begins in the family, and especially in the marital relationship. Patients often experience a sense of loss of their healthy body, resulting in depression, anxiety, exhaustion, boredom, and feelings of hopelessness [15].

Although there are myths about hazards of

sexual activity in the cardiac patient, resumption of sexual activity helps to solidify the marital relationship during a stressful period. Most patients report either a decrease in sexual activity or total abstinence. Husbands want to assert their masculinity through sexual intercourse but are afraid of injuring themselves. Their wives, feeling guilty, also repress their sexual needs in hopes of keeping their husbands safe [12].

Patients are often uncomfortable about taking the cardiologist's time to talk about their sexual needs. At their 4-week or 6-week checkup after the infarction, the doctor should broach the subject with sensitivity. The physician should consider the patient's values and previous sex life when assessing the patient's sexual needs. As emphasized in chapter 16, very few rehabilitation programs address the patient's sexual needs, and this is detrimental to full recovery.

It is important that the physician give precise and accurate information to the couple. The goal should be to give supportive, reassuring counseling that will facilitate communication within the couple. Some drugs may tend to decrease sexual desire (particularly diuretics and beta-blockers) and this should be pointed out [12].

Two widely held sexual myths should be dispelled by the cardiologist: (1) patients recovering from cardiac illness should not be sexually active; (2) coitus promotes myocardial infarction. The reality is that intimacy can promote therapeutic recovery. Coital death is related more to intercourse performed in extramarital affairs that produce anxiety and stress than to the act itself [12].

Physiologically, sexual activity can be resumed at either 6 weeks or when a patient feels comfortable climbing stairs. Psychologically, the earlier the sexual activity can be resumed the better. In particular, the male patient will have a sense of control, masculinity, intimacy, and strength. As McLane states, "a satisfying sexual relationship can be a valuable step toward fostering self-confidence and a feeling of returning to health" [15].

## EFFECTS OF CARDIAC REHABILITATION ON PSYCHOLOGICAL FUNCTIONING

The aims of a cardiac rehabilitation program for patients recovering from a myocardial infarction are "(1) achievement of a return to the premorbid state, particularly in the physical, psychological and social sphere and/or (2) achievement of maximal functioning in the social and psychological spheres within the limits of psychosocial capacity" [16]. Cardiac rehabilitation programs have been examined in detail in chapter 16. This section will address the issue of how effective these programs are in improving psychological functioning.

Often the patient who has suffered a myocardial infarction has a lowered sense of self-esteem and an inordinate fear that his or her prior lifestyle cannot be resumed. Working with a patient in small and/or large group rehabilitation programs can often lead to restoring physical capacity, reducing fear and anxiety, and enhancing self-esteem [17]. Not only is a patient expected to participate regularly in the exercise program, but also be an ongoing member of a psychotherapeutic group. As we noted previously, within this context, patients have the opportunity of discussing a wide variety of issues that may concern them: how to reduce or eliminate stress, when and how often to have sexual relations, what physical limitations must be followed, what food restrictions are advisable, etc. If a patient and/or family is having a particularly difficult time adjusting to the aftermath of the crisis, individual or family psychotherapy may be indicated.

Participation in a cardiac rehabilitation program provides a necessary support system for the patient. It is within this context that many patients have derived the strength to give up smoking and initiate a regular physical activity program. This increased sense of control and "doing something for oneself" leads to a greater sense of self-esteem. This feeling counteracts the loss of confidence that results from a myocardial infarction. The superiority of an outpatient cardiac rehabilitation program to that of a "physician-encouraged" but nonsupervised home rehabilitation program was reported by Erdman and Duivenvoorden [17] in a study of 64 patients divided into two groups. The study compared the psychological changes in the two groups and showed the advantages of the structured outpatient program. Interestingly, no differences in work resumption were noted (table

17-7), indicating how complex the return-to-work issue is, even in presumably well-adjusted patients.

## Recovery From Coronary Bypass Surgery

Brown and Rawlinson [18] reported that surgically treated patients were significantly less depressed and more likely to report improvement in health and family function following coronary bypass surgery than were their medically treated counterparts. But recovering from surgery is not without its problems. Bruce et al. [19] describes three coping strategies that patients employ during immediate recovery from coronary bypass surgery. The first is "compartmentalization," i.e., normal behavior within the confines of the limits of the disease. "Generalization" is the second strategy: patients are totally preoccupied with their symptomatic disability and are unable to readjust to normal ordinary life activities. They are concerned about returning to work, pessimistic about the future, have inappropriate emotional reactions that then reactivate angina as if there were a self-fulfilling prophecy. The third is "vacillation," a lack of any coping strategy, which often results in severe angina and depression.

It is fascinating to find in populations of patients "rehabilitated" through bypass surgery a general lack of coping strategies and skills to improve their quality of life. Their cardiac capacities are greatly improved, but their general attitude toward life and living doesn't change. Most people who had not worked preoperatively do not return to work, while those who had worked preoperatively often return. Both physiologic

TABLE 17-7. Work resumption at the end of the study

| Work resumption | Outpatient group | Home group |
|---|---|---|
| Not at all | 11 | 12 |
| Part time | 17 | 10 |
| Full time | 4 | 10 |
| Total patients | 32 | 32 |

Source: Erdman, R.A. and Duivenvoorden, J.J. *J. Cardiac. Rehabil.* 3:696, 1983.

improvement and working status appear independent of postoperative psychosocial status [19].

We must, however, examine this issue with an open mind. Many reported studies may have study populations that are skewed toward lower-class workers who may have no motivation to return to their jobs. Their disability payments and retirement pensions may equal or exceed their salaries; their jobs may have been boring and routine. One must also look at the family dynamics and expectations of the patient. If the children have left home, and the spouse is retired or not working, a family "need" may be met by keeping the postoperative patient needy and childlike.

In a more complex stratification, Kimball[20] divided his postoperative population of 54 patients into four groups that pass through three periods of time: early, intermediate, and post-hospital. His four groups include "adjusted," "symbiotic," "anxious," and "depressed." This time course is depicted in table 17–8. The "adjusted" patients had high levels of functioning preoperatively and were able through open expression of feelings to continue to adjust to their new life-style. The "symbiotic" were content to be in a regressed stage, at which recovery took longer than necessary. They enjoyed being taken care of, just as they had when they were young. The "anxious" group functioned well both pre- and postoperatively, with attempts at controlling their anxiety through massive denial. The "depressed" group appeared clinically depressed both pre- and postoperatively. They seemed out of control, with little hope for future improvement.

In the early period following surgery, Kimball reports patients responding either "catastrophically" or "euphorically." The catastrophic response refers to an almost catatonic posture that may serve to bind anxiety in the early postoperative period. If it lasts only a short time, it can be a helpful response. The euphoria experienced by postoperative patients hastens physiological health.

It has long been appreciated that the patient in the postoperative intensive care unit experiences a sense of delirium in reaction to the massive amounts of drugs and the unfamiliarity of the

TABLE 17–8. Characteristics of groups after bypass surgery

| Postoperative period | "Adjusted," Group I (13) | "Symbiotic," Group II (15) | "Anxious," Group III (12) | "Depressed," Group IV (14) | Total (54) |
|---|---|---|---|---|---|
| EARLY | | | | | |
| Unremarkable | 6 | 5 | 0 | 4 | 15 |
| Catastrophic | 2 | 3 | 6 | 2 | 13 |
| Euphoric | 1 | 4 | 1 | 1 | 7 |
| Altered states of consciousness | 3 | 3 | 2 | 1 | 9 |
| Dead | 1 | 0 | 3 | 6 | 10 |
| INTERMEDIATE | | | | | |
| Phase I, anxiety | 0 | 0 | 4 | 2 | 6 |
| Phase II, general reaction | 12 | 15 | 9 | 8 | 44 |
| Phase III, complication | 2 | 6 | 3 | 3 | 14 |
| Dead | 0 | 0 | 0 | 2 | 2 |
| POSTHOSPITAL (3–15 month followup) | | | | | |
| Improved | 9 | 1 | 3 | 1 | 14 |
| Unchanged | 3 | 8 | 3 | 2 | 16 |
| Worse | 0 | 5 | 2 | 1 | 8 |
| Dead | 0 | 1 | 1 | 3 | 5 |
| Total dead | 1 | 1 | 4 | 11 | 17 |

Source: Kimball, C.P. *Amer. J. Psychiat.* 126:96, 1969.

environment and as a way of coping with loss and fear. When the patient leaves the intensive care unit, stress and anxiety may be the dominant response; the reality that loss of heart function may result in a need for a new life-style reawakens. Depression and withdrawal during the intermediate period may also indicate a relief that one is not dead. Importantly, staff must allow both patient and family the opportunity of expressing the fears and anxieties that are normal in this period. This is an excellent opportunity to introduce the patient and family to a reeducation of what can be expected in the future. It is a time for qualified professionals to involve the patient and/or family in group, family, or individual psychotherapy. Although not empirically proven, there is general consensus that postoperative patients and families that are involved in some kind of psychotherapeutic experience have a better prognosis than their noninvolved counterparts.

## Conclusions

In coronary artery disease, as in many disease states, the psychological ramifications of the disease are often as troublesome as are the actual medical problems. While cardiologists utilize well-defined approaches to the treatment of coronary artery disease, their understanding of the psychosocial aspects of this disease are too often limited. This chapter has addressed itself to these aspects, as well as to the need to see patients and their families as units. Hopefully, acknowledgment by physicians that psychosocial factors are important will be the first step toward dealing with them.

## References

1. Kubler-Ross, E. *On Death and Dying.* New York: MacMillan, 1969.
2. Olin, B.M. Psychosomatic link in cardiovascular disorders. *Psychosomatics* 18:9, 1977.
3. Cohn, J.K. and Cohn, P.F. Patient reactions to the diagnosis of asymptomatic coronary artery disease: Implications for the primary physician and consultant cardiologist. *J. Am. Coll. Cardiol.* 1:956, 1983.
4. Stern, M.J. Pascale, L., and McLoone, J.B. Psychosocial adaptation following an acute myo-

cardial infarction. *J. Chron. Dis.* 29:513, 1976.
5. Cay, E.L. Psychological problems in patients after a myocardial infarction. *Adv. Cardiol.* 29:108, 1982.
6. Doehrman, S.R. Psycho-social aspects of recovery from coronary heart disease: A review. *Soc. Sci. & Med.* 11:199, 1977.
7. Hackett, T.P. and Rosenbaum, J.F. Emotion, Psychiatric Disorders and the Heart. In Braunwald, E. (ed), *Heart Disease* (2nd ed.). Philadelphia: W.B. Saunders, 1984, pp. 1820–34.
8. Stern, M.J., Pascale, L. and Ackerman, A. Life adjustment postmyocardial infarction: Determining predictive variables. *Arch. Intern. Med.* 137:1680, 1977.
9. Ibrahim, M.A., Feldman, J.G., Sultz, H.A., Staiman, M.G., Young, L.J., and Dean, D. Management after myocardial infarction: A controlled trial of the effect of group psychotherapy. *Int. J. Psych. Med.* 5:253, 1974.
10. Hackett, T.P. The use of groups in the rehabilitation of the postcoronary patient. *Adv. Cardiol.* 24:127, 1978.
11. Bilodeau, C.B. and Hackett, T.P. Issues raised in a group setting by patients recovering from myocardial infarction. *Amer. J. Psychiat.* 128:1, 1971.
12. Davidson, D.M. The family and cardiac rehabilitation. *J. Fam. Pract.* 8:253, 1979.
13. Skelton, M. and Dominian, J. Psychological stress in wives of patients with myocardial infarction. *Br. Med. J.* 2:101, 1973.
14. Stern, M.J. and Pascale L. Psychosocial adaptation post-myocardial infarction: The spouse's dilemma. *J. Psychosom. Res.* 23:83, 1979.
15. McLane, M., Krop, H., and Mehta, J. Psychosexual adjustment and counseling after myocardial infarction. *Ann. Int. Med.* 92:514, 1980.
16. Croog, S.H., Levin, S., and Lurie, Z. The heart patient and the recovery process. A review of the directions of research on social and psychological factors. *Soc. Sci. Med.* 2:111, 1982.
17. Erdman R.A.M. and Duivenvoorden, H.J. Psychologic evaluation of a cardiac rehabilitation program: A randomized clinical trial in patients with myocardial infarction. *J. Cardiac. Rehabil.* 3:696, 1983.
18. Brown, J.S. and Rawlinson. Psychosocial status of patients randomly assigned to medical or surgical therapy for chronic stable angina. *Am. J. Cardiol.* 44:546, 1979.
19. Bruce, E.H., Bruce, R.A., Hossack, K.F., and Kusumi, F. Psychosocial coping strategies and cardiac capacity before and after coronary artery bypass surgery. *Int. J. Psych. Med.* 13:69, 1983.
20. Kimball, C.P. Psychological responses to the experience of open heart surgery. *Amer. J. Psychiat.* 126:96, 1969.

# 18. NONATHEROSCLEROTIC CORONARY ARTERY DISEASE

## L. David Hillis
## Peter F. Cohn

Although atherosclerosis is the predominant underlying lesion in most patients with ischemic heart disease, other pathologic processes that involve the coronary arteries may cause myocardial ischemia. When the coronary arteries are involved with one of these disorders, the clinical and electrocardiographic manifestations may simulate those of atherosclerotic coronary artery disease. As outlined in table 18–1, nonatherosclerotic coronary artery disease may be congenital, associated with several hereditary metabolic derangements, or acquired as part of a variety of systemic disease processes. If coronary artery spasm is demonstrable, the patient is said to have a form of Prinzmetal's variant angina. The clinical and laboratory features as well as the therapy and prognosis of this syndrome are discussed in chapter 12. On the other hand, if coronary artery spasm is not present, the patient is said to have chest pain with normal coronary arteriograms; this entity is discussed in chapter 4.

Points of controversy concerning nonatherosclerotic coronary artery disease include (1) the clinical significance and need for surgical correction of some of the congenital disorders, (2) the origin of coronary artery emboli, (3) the pathophysiology and treatment of the coronary artery aneurysms due to the mucocutaneous lymph node syndrome, (4) the contribution of steroid therapy and irradiation to premature atherosclerosis, and (5) the relation of blunt chest trauma to coronary artery occlusion.

## Congenital Disorders of the Coronary Arteries

### ANOMALOUS ORIGIN OF A CORONARY ARTERY FROM THE PULMONARY ARTERY

Several forms of this anomaly have been described, including anomalous origin of the right [1] or left [2–5] coronary arteries, both coronary arteries [6], or an accessory coronary artery [7]. On the one extreme, when both coronary arteries arise from the pulmonary artery, death usually occurs soon after birth. On the other extreme, the patient in whom only the right coronary artery originates from the pulmonary artery is usually asymptomatic as long as right ventricular oxygen demands are not excessive; therefore, this anomaly is an incidental postmortem finding.

Of the various forms of anomalous origin of a coronary artery from the pulmonary artery, the most common is the origin of the left coronary artery from the pulmonary artery [8]. Infants with this anomaly appear normal at birth, but within 1 to 2 months they develop myocardial ischemia and congestive heart failure, from which 80 to 85 percent die during the first year [9]. The remaining 15 to 20 percent reach adulthood because of substantial intercoronary collaterals that allow arterial blood from the right coronary artery to bypass the myocardial capillaries and to enter the left coronary artery, from which, in turn, it drains into the pulmonary artery.

The adult patient with anomalous origin of the left coronary artery from the pulmonary artery may come to medical attention because of

TABLE 18–1. Etiologies of nonatherosclerotic coronary artery disease

I. CONGENITAL DISORDERS OF THE CORONARY ARTERIES
   A. Anomalous origin of a coronary artery from the pulmonary artery
   B. Anomalous origin of a coronary artery from the aorta or other coronary artery
   C. Coronary arteriovenous fistula
   D. Coronary artery aneurysm

II. HEREDITARY METABOLIC DERANGEMENTS WITH CORONARY ARTERY INVOLVEMENT
   A. Diseases causing aortic dissection
      1. Marfan's syndrome
      2. Ehlers-Danlos syndrome
   B. Pseudoxanthoma elasticum
   C. Gargoylism (Hurler's syndrome)
   D. Homocystinuria

III. ACQUIRED DISORDERS OF THE CORONARY ARTERIES
   A. Embolization
   B. Dissection
   C. Syphilitic
   D. Infiltrative
      1. Tumors
      2. Amyloidosis
   E. Connective Tissue Diseases
      1. Periarteritis nodosa
      2. Rheumatoid arthritis
      3. Systemic lupus erythematosus
   F. Miscellaneous
      1. Irradiation
      2. Chest trauma
      3. Nitrate withdrawal

angina pectoris, myocardial infarction, a murmur of mitral regurgitation (due to dysfunction of the papillary muscle supplied by the anomalous coronary artery), left ventricular failure, or sudden death. On physical examination, the patient usually has a holosystolic murmur of mitral regurgitation. In addition, a continuous or diastolic murmur may be audible, reflecting retrograde flow through the intercoronary anastomoses that connect the right and left coronary arteries. A third heart sound due to left ventricular dysfunction may be audible. The electrocardiogram may demonstrate left atrial enlargement, left ventricular hypertrophy, and anterolateral ischemia or infarction. The chest x-ray and echocardiogram show left atrial and ventricular enlargement. At cardiac catheteriza-

tion, selective injection of contrast material into the right coronary artery usually opacifies the entire coronary arterial system. The right coronary artery is dilated and tortuous, and there are extensive collateral vessels that connect the distal right coronary artery to the left circumflex and left anterior descending coronary arteries. If opacification of the left coronary artery is optimal, one may visualize the efflux of contrast material from the left main coronary artery into the pulmonary artery. The left ventriculogram demonstrates mitral regurgitation and left ventricular dysfunction.

Once the origin of the left coronary artery is shown to be from the pulmonary artery, surgical correction is indicated. If possible, operative therapy should be delayed until the patient is at least 18 months of age, since coronary arterial surgery in the first year of life—especially in infants with severely depressed left ventricular function—carries a very high mortality [10]. If there is adequate collateral flow from the right to the left coronary artery, ligation of the anomalous left coronary artery may be sufficient [11–14]. Alternatively, the left main coronary artery may be detached from the pulmonary artery and anastomosed to the ascending aorta [15, 16]. However, such a transposition may be technically impossible, so that a segment of saphenous vein may require interposition from the ascending aorta to the ligated left main or left anterior descending coronary artery [17]. In addition to angina relief, symptoms of congestive heart failure often improve following operative repair, since such failure may be due to reversible myocardial ischemia or papillary muscle dysfunction.

ANOMALOUS ORIGIN OF A CORONARY ARTERY FROM THE AORTA OR OTHER CORONARY ARTERY.
The incidence of one or more coronary arteries arising aberrantly from the aorta is .6 to 1.2 percent [18–20]; thus, it is much more common than the anomalous origin of a coronary artery from the pulmonary artery. The most common such anomaly is the origin of the left circumflex coronary artery from the right sinus of Valsalva or proximal right coronary artery (figure 18–1). Less commonly, one may see the origin of the left main coronary artery from the right sinus of

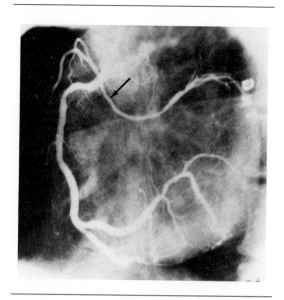

FIGURE 18–1. Anomalous origin of the left circumflex artery (arrow) from the proximal right coronary artery as demonstrated by selective right coronary angiography.

Valsalva or the origin of the right coronary artery from the left sinus of Valsalva.

The course taken by the coronary artery after its aberrant origin determines whether symptoms of ischemic heart disease develop. On the one hand, if the artery passes from its aberrant origin to its proper anatomic location by traversing anterior or posterior to the aorta and right ventricular infundibulum, no manifestations of ischemic heart disease arise, and the anomaly has no clinical significance. On the other hand, angina pectoris or sudden death with exertion has been reported in patients in whom the right or left coronary artery arises from the opposite sinus of Valsalva and passes *between* the aorta and right ventricular infundibulum [21–27]. In those individuals whose left main coronary artery arises aberrantly from the right sinus of Valsalva and passes between the aorta and right ventricular infundibulum, sudden death may occur in association with vigorous physical exertion, and it is postulated that the aortic dilatation that accompanies exercise somehow "kinks" the left main coronary artery, causing global left ventricular ischemia and ventricular fibrillation [27]. On occasion, sudden

death via a similar mechanism may occur in individuals whose right coronary artery arises from the left sinus of Valsalva and passes between the aorta and right ventricular infundibulum [28, 29].

If a patient is found at cardiac catheterization to have a left coronary artery originating from the right sinus of Valsalva and passing to its normal anatomic location between the aorta and right venticular infundibulum, coronary artery bypass grafting should probably be performed to avoid sudden death. In contrast, bypass grafting is usually not required for the patient in whom the right coronary artery arises from the left sinus of Valsalva and passes between the aorta and right ventricular infundibulum unless angina pectoris or ventricular ectopy during physical exertion are inadequately controlled on medical therapy.

## CORONARY ARTERIOVENOUS FISTULA

A coronary arteriovenous fistula is said to exist when a coronary artery communicates directly with the right atrium, coronary sinus, right ventricle, or (rarely) the pulmonary artery [3, 4, 30]. The involved coronary artery is dilated, elongated, and tortuous. The fistula's clinical significance is determined in part by the amount of blood flowing through it. If flow is large, a substantial left-to-right shunt is present and may cause symptoms of left ventricular failure (dyspnea, orthopnea, and peripheral edema) or angina (due to a diversion of blood from other coronary arteries to the low-resistance fistula) [31, 32]. An occasional patient with a coronary arteriovenous fistula develops bacterial endocarditis. On physical examination, the left ventricular impulse is hyperdynamic if the intracardiac shunt is large. A continuous murmur is audible over the anterior precordium. The electrocardiogram is usually normal, and the chest x-ray may demonstrate mild cardiomegaly.

The morbidity and mortality related to a coronary arteriovenous fistula may be due to high-output congestive heart failure, fistula-related ischemic heart disease, or bacterial endocarditis. In the past, surgical therapy was not recommended unless the intracardiac shunt was at least 2:1 in magnitude. More recently, however, elective ligation during childhood of all coronary arteriovenous fistulae—even those that are small, uncomplicated, and asymptomatic—has been recommended, since most unoperated patients eventually develop symptoms and fistula-related complications with increasing age [33]. The preferred operative procedure is ligation of the fistula as close as possible to its entrance into the right-sided cardiac chamber [34]. This can often be accomplished without cardiopulmonary bypass [35].

## CORONARY ARTERY ANEURYSM

Congenital coronary artery aneurysms are uncommon in comparison to those that result from atherosclerosis or trauma. Most are discovered incidentally at postmortem, but an occasional one comes to attention antemortem because of the patient's symptoms (angina) or signs (an unusual murmur or an abnormal chest x-ray). If such an aneurysm causes severe symptoms, surgical therapy can be used to excise it [36].

The mucocutaneous lymph node syndrome (so-called Kawasaki disease) is a febrile illness of infants and young children that closely resembles periarteritis nodosa. It always occurs in children less than 10 years of age, and most patients are under age 2. Its clinical characteristics include fever unresponsive to antibiotics; bilateral congestion of the ocular conjunctiva; indurative peripheral edema and erythema of the palms and feet; dry, erythematous, and fissured lips; injected oropharyngeal mucosa and tongue; and exanthema of the trunk. In addition, the patient often has cervical adenopathy, diarrhea, arthralgias, pyuria, proteinuria, leucocytosis, and thrombocytosis. Although the disease occurs most frequently in Japan, it has been reported in the United States and other countries [37, 38].

The major pathologic changes of the mucocutaneous lymph node syndrome are limited to the cardiovascular system and especially to the coronary arteries [39]. In infants dying of this syndrome, the postmortem examination reveals coronary arterial aneurysms with occlusion due to thromboendarteritis. Of those with the disease who do not die, such aneurysms are demonstrable angiographically or echocardiographically in 15 to 20 percent [40, 41]. During subsequent follow-up, these aneurysms spontaneously regress in about half the patients,

whereas in the remainder the persistent aneurysmal alterations may lead to premature atherosclerosis [42]. The propensity for infants or children with this syndrome to develop coronary artery aneurysms may be lessened by low-dose aspirin, which may also influence regression of the aneurysm over the weeks to months after the acute illness. Coronary artery bypass grafting has been performed in patients with severe coronary narrowings, with beneficial effects in most instances [43].

# Hereditary Metabolic Derangements with Coronary Artery Involvement

## DISEASES CAUSING AORTIC DISSECTION

Dissection of the ascending aorta may cause narrowing or obliteration of the coronary arterial ostia, with resultant myocardial ischemia or infarction. Aortic dissection is a well-recognized occurrence in patients with certain inherited disorders of connective tissue, including Marfan's syndrome (in which the pathologic alterations in the aortic media are identical to those of cystic medial necrosis) [44] and the Ehlers-Danlos syndrome. In addition, an occasional patient with Marfan's syndrome has cystic medial necrosis of the coronary arteries themselves [45]. Aneurysms of the sinuses of Valsalva, with resultant rupture or thrombosis, have been described in patients with Marfan's syndrome and the Ehlers-Danlos syndrome [46]. The patient with an aortic dissection and coronary ostial involvement should be placed on intravenous trimethaphan (to reduce systemic arterial pressure) and β-blockers (to diminish left ventricular contractility), and then should undergo emergent aortography and surgical repair [47, 48].

## PSEUDOXANTHOMA ELASTICUM

Individuals with pseudoxanthoma elasticum often have diffuse arterial degeneration and calcification at a young age. As a result, claudication, hypertension, and angina pectoris are common [49]. For the patient with limiting angina, β-adrenergic blockers, calcium antagonists, and nitrates are often efficacious. If necessary, coronary artery bypass grafting may be employed for anginal relief [50].

## GARGOYLISM (HURLER'S SYNDROME)

Inherited as an autosomal recessive trait, gargoylism is characterized clinically by dwarfism, mental retardation (often severe), grotesque facial appearance (typified by a large head, hypertelorism, thickened lips, and hypertrophied gums), corneal clouding, deafness, and joint contractures, most often involving the hips, knees, ankles, elbows, and fingers. In addition, these individuals may have several cardiac abnormalities [51]. The deposition of mucopolysaccharides may induce valvular abnormalities, most frequently left-sided regurgitation; an infiltrative cardiomyopathy; and coronary arterial stenoses or total occlusions, caused by intimal infiltration of dense, wavy, collagenous fibers and swollen, vacuolated fibroblasts (so-called Hurler cells). As a result of such encroachment, angina pectoris and myocardial infarction have been reported in a patient as young as 4 years [52, 53]. Angina pectoris due to coronary artery involvement is best treated medically (with $\beta$-adrenergic blockers, calcium antagonists, and nitrates). The aggressiveness with which coronary artery bypass grafting is undertaken depends on the clinical situation.

## HOMOCYSTINURIA

Among adult patients, homocystinuria is the most common inborn error of amino acid metabolism. It is inherited as an autosomal recessive trait. The hepatic enzyme cystathionine synthase, which converts homocystine and serine to cystathionine, is deficient or totally absent. As a result, an excessive amount of homocystine is excreted in the urine, and large amounts of homocystine and methionine are present in plasma.

The clinical characteristics of homocystinuria include ectopia lentis, mental retardation of varying severity, and skeletal abnormalities. These individuals often have arterial and venous thromboses, including renal artery thrombosis with resultant hypertension, vena caval and portal vein thrombosis, and coronary artery stenosis or occlusion with resultant myocardial ischemia or infarction [54].

The therapy of homocystinuria centers on manipulation of the dietary intake of cystine, cystathionine, and methionine. Excellent results have been obtained when these patients have been placed on a diet low in methionine and high in cystine. In addition, some patients with homocystinuria are improved by massive doses of pyridoxine (250 to 500 mg daily); for unclear reasons, others are "pyridoxine resisitant" [55, 56].

## Acquired Disorders of the Coronary Arteries

### EMBOLIZATION

Embolization of a coronary artery may cause acute myocardial infarction and its sequelae. Coronary artery embolization with subsequent fatal infarction is not uncommon, occurring in as many as 13 percent of patients with infarction who are examined at postmortem [57]. Valvular heart disease is the most frequent underlying disorder with which such embolization occurs, but it may also be seen in individuals with cardiomyopathy and idiopathic paroxysmal atrial fibrillation. Since embolization occurs abruptly, collateral coronary blood flow is not extensively developed, so that the resultant infarction is often large and therefore, fatal. Coronary arterial emboli may originate from one of several sources [58]. First, fragments of vegetations of bacterial or fungal endocarditis may occlude a large coronary artery [59]. In fact, endocarditis is responsible for 65 to 70 percent of all coronary embolic events [60]. In postmortem analyses, embolization from endocarditis most often involves the left anterior descending coronary artery.

Second, thrombi that have formed in the left atrium, left ventricle, or sinuses of Valsalva may dislodge and embolize to the coronary arteries. Alternatively, peripheral venous thrombi may embolize "paradoxically" to the systemic circulation in patients with an abnormal communication between the right and left heart chambers (most commonly a patent foramen ovale) [61, 62]. Since coronary embolism may result from thrombus formation on a prosthetic valve [63], adequate anticoagulation (with coumadin) is necessary in all patients with prosthetic valves except those with porcine heterografts [64]. Even in these individuals, however, an enlarged left atrium and continued atrial fibrillation after insertion of a mitral heterograft probably make full anticoagulation mandatory [65].

Third, embolization of calcific material or valvular debris to the coronary arteries may occur at the time of valvular surgery [66], and embolization of prosthetic material (fragments of a ball or disc) has rarely occurred in patients with prosthetic valves in place. Fourth, embolization of a coronary artery may occur with small pieces of tumor (most commonly a left atrial myxoma) or air, the latter usually introduced during selective coronary arteriography or cardiac surgery.

The therapy of coronary artery embolization centers on the elimination of its source. For example, embolization due to endocarditis is best prevented by treating the endocarditis with proper antimicrobials, and anticoagulation is often associated with hemorrhage. However, if coronary artery embolization is due to platelet thrombi from the left atrium, left ventricle, sinuses of Valsalva, a prosthetic valve, or the deep veins of the pelvis or legs, long-term systemic anticoagulation should be instituted. Coronary artery embolization from a left-sided intracardiac tumor is treated most effectively by surgical excision of the tumor. If acute coronary embolization is recognized immediately, it may be treated surgically with embolectomy and aortocoronary vein bypass grafting [67].

### DISSECTION

*Primary* spontaneous dissection of a coronary artery is an extremely rare occurrence. It usually begins near the coronary ostium and extends 2 to 4 centimeters distally. About 75 percent of the reported cases have occurred in young females, many of whom were pregnant or immediately postpartum [68]. Systemic arterial hypertension is not a predisposing factor in patients with primary coronary artery dissection. Of the 3 major coronary arteries, the left anterior descending is most frequently involved [69, 70].

*Secondary* coronary artery dissection occurs most commonly as an extension of a dissecting aortic aneurysm. Rarely, it may occur during cannulation of a coronary ostium at the time of arteriography [71–73] or cardiac surgery [74]. If coronary arterial dissection of any etiology causes myocardial ischemia, the patient should immediately undergo coronary artery bypass grafting.

### SYPHILITIC

Syphilis may involve the coronary arteries in two ways. First, about one-third of patients with syphilitic aortitis have coronary artery ostial involvement, and severe ostial narrowing is present in 20 to 25 percent of these patients [75]. Most patients with coronary ostial stenosis have concomitant aortic regurgitation. Since coronary ostial narrowing develops slowly in these individuals, coronary collaterals are extensive, and therefore, myocardial infarction is uncommon. Second, syphilitic coronary arteritis involving the proximal portions of the major epicardial coronary arteries occurs rarely [76].

The patient with syphilitic coronary artery involvement should be treated with a proper antibiotic regimen to eliminate the causative organism. However, coronary ostial stenoses are not affected by antibiotic therapy, and as a result, coronary artery bypass grafting must be employed in those patients with limiting angina despite medical therapy. Bypass grafting is often performed in conjunction with aortic valve replacement, since many of these patients have concomitant severe aortic regurgitation [77].

### INFILTRATIVE

Metastatic tumor tissue may encroach on the epicardial coronary arteries, causing coronary insufficiency or even myocardial infarction [78]. The most common tumors to involve the heart by metastatic spread are malignant melanoma and carcinoma of the bronchus [79]. In addition, malignant lymphoma often involves the heart, usually by direct extension from the mediastinal lymph nodes [80].

Although amyloidosis usually involves the heart via diffuse myocardial infiltration, an occasional patient has amyloid deposition within the lumina of the epicardial coronary arteries [81]. These individuals often complain of classic angina pectoris or may even sustain a myocardial infarction. Since their long-term prognosis is guarded, every attempt should be made to control the symptoms of their ischemic heart disease with medical therapy.

## CONNECTIVE TISSUE DISEASES

The coronary arteries are involved by an inflammatory, necrotizing, obliterative arteritis in 60 to 70 percent of adults with *periarteritis nodosa* [82]. Some of these patients develop nodular aneurysms of the epicardial coronary arteries, which may rupture (causing hemopericardium and tamponade) or thrombose (resulting in myocardial ischemia or infarction). Although corticosteroids have been administered to patients with periarteritis nodosa, their effect on coronary arterial involvement is unknown.

As many as 25 to 50 percent of patients with *rheumatoid arthritis* have some morphologic evidence of systemic arteritis [83], and the heart is the most frequently affected visceral organ. Although this arteritic process is usually confined to the arterioles, it may occasionally involve the large epicardial coronary arteries, leading to myocardial ischemia or infarction [84]. Some patients with active *systemic lupus erythematosus* develop an acute inflammatory arteritis of the large coronary arteries, with resultant myocardial infarction [85, 86]. Apart from this, severe atherosclerotic coronary artery disease occurs in many patients with systemic lupus who have received long-term, high-dose corticosteroid therapy [87, 88].

The patient with coronary arteritis and resultant myocardial ischemia or infarction should receive $\beta$-adrenergic blocking agents, calcium antagonists, and nitrates to control symptoms. Bypass surgery should be performed only as a last resort, since the arteritic process is usually diffuse.

## MISCELLANEOUS

Many patients who have previously received large amounts of mediastinal *irradiation* develop angina pectoris or myocardial infarction. High-dose irradiation of the coronary arteries produces luminal narrowing in two ways. First, irradiation induces severe thickening of the coronary arterial wall because of intimal and adventitial fibrous proliferation, thus encroaching on the coronary arterial lumen [89]. Second, large doses of irradiation greatly accelerate the atherosclerotic process; in fact, irradiation and hypercholesterolemia act synergistically to produce more atherosclerosis than that caused by

either stimulus alone [90]. Many patients with coronary artery narrowing due to previous mediastinal irradiation are excellent candidates for coronary artery bypass grafting, since they are often young and since their stenoses are frequently confined to the proximal portions of the major epicardial coronary arteries [91].

In a rare individual, *blunt trauma to the chest* may cause coronary artery occlusion with resultant infarction [92, 93]. The pathophysiologic mechanism by which this occurs is not understood. More commonly, a *penetrating injury of the chest* may lacerate a major epicardial coronary artery. Because of its location, the left anterior descending coronary artery is most frequently involved [94]. A coronary artery laceration may be repaired surgically via one of several techniques, including direct reanastomosis of the damaged vessel, patch angioplasty, or ligation of the vessel at the site of laceration followed by saphenous vein grafting to its distal portion.

*Withdrawal from chronic nitroglycerin exposure* may induce angina pectoris or even myocardial infarction in patients without atherosclerotic coronary artery disease [95]. The initial exposure to nitroglycerin causes coronary artery dilatation, in response to which compensatory vasoconstriction occurs. When nitroglycerin is withdrawn, this vasoconstrictive response is unopposed, leading to coronary arterial constriction. Typically, the individual who is chronically exposed to nitroglycerin develops symptoms of myocardial ischemia 48 to 60 hours after it is withdrawn, and these symptoms, in turn, are promptly relieved by nitroglycerin.

## References

1. Tingelstad, J.B., Lower, R.R., and Eldredge, W.J. Anomalous origin of the right coronary artery from the main pulmonary artery. *Am. J. Cardiol.* 30:670, 1972.
2. Ogden, J.A. Congenital anomalies of the coronary arteries. *Am. J. Cardiol.* 25:474, 1970.
3. Levin, D.C., Fellows, K.E., and Abrams, H.L. Hemodynamically significant primary anomalies of the coronary arteries. Angiographic aspects. *Circulation* 58:25, 1978.
4. Flamm, M.D., Stinson, E.B., Hultgren, H.N., Shumway, N.E., and Hancock E.W. Anomalous origin of the left coronary artery from the pulmo-

nary artery. Surgical treatment by ostial occlusion through pulmonary arteriotomy. *Circulation* 38:-113, 1968.

5. Donaldson, R.M., Raphael, M., Radley-Smith, R., Yacoub, M.H., and Ross, D.N. Angiographic identification of primary coronary anomalies causing impaired myocardial perfusion. *Cath. Cardiovasc. Diag.* 9:237, 1983.

6. Colmers, R.A. and Siderides, C.I. Anomalous origin of both coronary arteries from the pulmonary trunk. Myocardial infarction in otherwise normal heart. *Am. J. Cardiol.* 12:263, 1963.

7. Edwards, J.E. Anomalous coronary arteries with special reference to arteriovenous-like communications. *Circulation* 17:1001, 1958.

8. Askenazi, J. and Nadas, A.S. Anomalous left coronary artery originating from the pulmonary artery. Report of 15 cases. *Circulation* 51:976, 1975.

9. Wesselhoeft, H., Fawcett, J.S., and Johnson, A.L. Anomalous origin of the left coronary artery from the pulmonary trunk. Its clinical spectrum, pathology, and pathophysiology, based on a review of 140 cases with 7 further cases. *Circulation* 38:403, 1968.

10. Driscoll, D.J., Nihill, M.R., Mullins, C.E., Cooley, D.A., and McNamara, D.G. Management of symptomatic infants with anomalous origin of the left coronary artery from the pulmonary artery. *Am. J. Cardiol.* 47:642, 1981.

11. Harthorne, J.W., Scannell, J.G., and Dinsmore, R.E. Anomalous origin of the left coronary artery. Remediable cause of sudden death in adults. *N. Engl. J. Med.* 275:660, 1966.

12. Likar, I., Criley, J.M., and Lewis, K.B. Anomalous left coronary artery arising from the pulmonary artery in an adult. A review of the therapeutic problem. *Circulation* 33:727, 1966.

13. Roche, A.H.G. Anomalous origin of the left coronary artery from the pulmonary artery in the adult. Report of uneventful ligation in two cases. *Am. J. Cardiol.* 20:561, 1967.

14. Summer, G.L. and Hendrix, G.H. Surgical ligation of an anomalous left coronary artery arising from the pulmonary artery in an adult. Report of a case and review of the literature. *Am. Heart. J.* 76:812, 1968.

15. Cooley, D.A., Hallman, G.L., and Bloodwell, R.D. Definitive surgical treatment of anomalous origin of left coronary artery from pulmonary artery: Indications and results. *J. Thorac. Cardiovasc. Surg.* 52:798, 1966.

16. Grace, R.R., Angelini, P., and Cooley, D.A. Aortic implantation of anomalous left coronary artery rising from pulmonary artery. *Am. J. Cardiol.* 39:-608, 1977.

17. Evans, J.J. and Phillips, J.F. Origin of the left anterior descending coronary artery from the pulmonary artery: 3 year angiographic follow-up

after saphenous vein bypass graft and proximal ligation. *J. Am. Coll. Cardiol.* 3:219, 1984.

18. Liberthson, R.R., Dinsmore, R.E., Bharati, S., Rubenstein, J.J., Caulfield, J., Wheeler, E.O., Harthorne J.W., and Lev, M. Aberrant coronary artery origin from the aorta. Diagnosis and clinical significance. *Circulation* 50:774, 1974.

19. Engel, H.J., Torres, C. and Page, H.L. Major variations in anatomical origin of the coronary arteries. Angiographic observations in 4250 patients without associated congenital heart disease. *Cath. Cardiovasc. Diag.* 1:157, 1975.

20. Kimbiris, D., Iskandrian, A.S., Segal, B.L., and Bemis, C.E. Anomalous aortic origin of coronary arteries. *Circulation* 58:606, 1978.

21. Liberthson, R.R., Dinsmore, R.E., and Fallon, J.T. Aberrant coronary artery origin from the aorta. Report of 18 patients, review of literature and delineation of natural history and management. *Circulation* 59:748, 1979.

22. Thompson, S.I., Vieweg, W.V.R., Alpert, J.S., and Hagan, A.D. Anomalous origin of the right coronary artery from the left sinus of Valsalva with associated chest pain: Report of 2 cases. *Cath. Cardiovasc. Diag.* 2:397, 1976.

23. Benge, W., Martins, J.B., and Funk, D.C. Morbidity associated with anomalous origin of the right coronary artery from the left sinus of Valsalva. *Am. Heart. J.* 99:96, 1980.

24. Bloomfield, P., Ehrlich, C., Folland, E.D., Bianco, J.A., Tow, D.E., and Parisi, A.F. Anomalous right coronary artery: A surgically correctable cause of angina pectoris. *Am. J. Cardiol.* 51:-1235, 1983.

25. Benson, P.A. and Lack, A.R. Anomalous aortic origin of the left coronary artery. Report of two cases. *Arch. Pathol.* 86:214, 1968.

26. Moodie, D.S., Gill, C., Loop, F.D., and Sheldon, W.C. Anomalous left main coronary artery originating from the right sinus of Valsalva. Pathophysiology, angiographic definition, and surgical approaches. *J. Thorac. Cardiovasc. Surg.* 80:198, 1980.

27. Cheitlin, M.D., DeCastro, C.M., and McAllister, H.A. Sudden death as a complication of anomalous left coronary origin from the anterior sinus of Valsalva. A not-so-minor congenital anomaly. *Circulation* 50:780, 1974.

28. Isner, J.M., Shen, E.M., Martin, E.T., and Fortin, R.V. Sudden unexpected death as a result of anomalous origin of the right coronary artery from the left sinus of Valsalva. *Am. J. Med.* 76:-155, 1984.

29. Roberts, W.C., Siegel, R.J., and Zipes, D.P. Origin of the right coronary artery from the left sinus of Valsalva and its functional consequences: Analysis of 10 necropsy patients. *Am. J. Cardiol.* 49:863, 1982.

30. Baim, D.S., Kline, H., and Silverman, J.F. Bilat-

eral coronary artery-pulmonary artery fistulas. Report of five cases and review of the literature. *Circulation* 65:810, 1982.

31. Jaffe, R.B., Glancy, D.L., Epstein, S.E., Brown, B.G., and Morrow, A.G. Coronary arterial-right heart fistulae. Long-term observations in seven patients. *Circulation* 47:133, 1973.

32. Morgan, J.R., Forker, A.D., O'Sullivan, M.J., and Fosburg, R.G. Coronary arterial fistulas. Seven cases with unusual features. *Am. J. Cardiol.* 30:432, 1972.

33. Liberthson, R.R., Sagar, K., Berkoben, J.P., Weintraub, R.M., and Levine, F.H. Congenital coronary arteriovenous fistula. Report of 13 patients, review of the literature, and delineation of management. *Circulation* 59:849, 1979.

34. Effler, D.B., Sheldon, W.C., Turner, J.J., and Groves, L.K. Coronary arteriovenous fistulas: Diagnosis and surgical management. Report of 15 cases. *Surgery* 61:41, 1967.

35. Edis, A.J., Schattenberg, T.T., Feldt, R.H., and Danielson, G.K. Congenital coronary artery fistula. Surgical considerations and results of operation. *Mayo Clin. Proc.* 47:567, 1972.

36. Lim, C.H., Tan, N.C., Tan, L., Seah, C.S., and Tan, D. Giant congenital aneurysm of the right coronary artery. *Am. J. Cardiol.* 39:751, 1977.

37. Brown, J.S., Billmeier, G.J., Cox, F., Ibrahim, M., Stepp, W.P., Jr., and Gibson, R. Mucocutaneous lymph node syndrome in the continental United States. *J. Pediat.* 88:81, 1976.

38. Fukushige, J., Nihill, M.R., and McNamara, D.G. Spectrum of cardiovascular lesions in mucocutaneous lymph node syndrome: Analysis of eight cases. *Am. J. Cardiol.* 45:98, 1980.

39. Fujiwara, H. and Hamashima, Y. Pathology of the heart in Kawasaki disease. *Pediatrics* 61:100, 1978.

40. Kato, H., Koike, S., Tanaka, C., Yokochi, K., Yushioka, F., Takeuchi, S., Matsunaga, S., and Yokoyama, T. Coronary heart disease in children with Kawasaki disease. *Jap. Circ. J.* 43:469, 1979.

41. Maeda, T., Yoshida, H., Funabashi, T., Nakaya, S., Takabatake, S., Ohno, T., and Taniguchi, N. Subcostal 2-dimensional echocardiographic imaging of peripheral left coronary artery aneurysms in Kawasaki disease. *Am. J. Cardiol.* 52:48, 1983.

42. Kato, H., Ichinose, E., Yoshioka, F., Tukechi, T., Matsunaga, S., Suzuki, K., and Rikitake, N. Fate of coronary aneurysms in Kawasaki disease: Serial coronary angiography and long-term follow-up study. *Am. J. Cardiol.* 49:1758, 1982.

43. Kitamura, S., Kawachi, K., Harima, R., Sakakibara, T., Hirose, H., and Kawashima, Y. Surgery for coronary heart disease due to mucocutaneous lymph node syndrome (Kawasaki disease). Report of 6 patients. *Am. J. Cardiol.* 51:442, 1983.

44. Pyeritz, R.E. and McKusick, V.A. The Marfan syndrome: Diagnosis and management. *N. Engl. J. Med.* 300:772, 1979.

45. Becker, A.E. and Van Mantgem, J.P. The coronary arteries in Marfan's syndrome. A morphologic study. *Am. J. Cardiol.* 36:315, 1975.

46. Cupo, L.N., Pyeritz, R.E., Olson, J.L., McPhee, S.J., Hutchins, G.M., and McKusick, V.A. Ehlers-Danlos syndrome with abnormal collagen fibrils, sinus of Valsalva aneurysms, myocardial infarction, panacinar emphysema and cerebral heterotopias. *Am. J. Med.* 71:1051, 1981.

47. Wheat, M.W., Jr. Treatment of dissecting aneurysms of the aorta. Current status. *Prog. Cardiovasc. Dis.* 16:87, 1973.

48. Wheat, M.W., Jr. Acute dissecting aneurysms of the aorta: Diagnosis and treatment—1979. *Am. Heart J.* 99:373, 1980.

49. Przybojewski, J.Z., Maritz, F., Tiedt, F.A.C., Vander Walt, J.J. Pseudoxanthoma elasticum with cardiac involvement. *S. Afr. Med. J.* 59:268, 1981.

50. Bete, J.M., Banas, J.S., Jr., Moran, J., Pinn, V., and Levine, H.J. Coronary artery disease in an 18-year-old girl with pseudoxanthoma elasticum: Successful surgical therapy. *Am. J. Cardiol.* 36:515, 1975.

51. Lindsay, S. The cardiovascular system in gargoylism. *Br. Heart J.* 12:17, 1950.

52. Craig, W.S. Gargoylism in a twin brother and sister. *Arch. Dis. Child.* 29:293, 1954.

53. Brosius, F.C., III and Roberts, W.C. Coronary artery disease in the Hurler syndrome. Qualitative and quantitative analysis of the extent of coronary narrowing at necropsy in six children. *Am. J. Cardiol.* 47:649, 1981.

54. Schimke, R.N., McKusick, V.A., Huang, T., and Pollack, A.D. Homocystinuria. Studies of 20 families with 38 affected members. *JAMA* 193:711, 1965.

55. Perry, T.L., Dunn, H.G., Hansen, S., MacDougall, L., and Warrington, P.D. Early diagnosis and treatment of homocystinuria. *Pediatrics* 37:502, 1966.

56. Barber, G.W., and Spaeth G.L. Pyridoxine therapy in homocystinuria. *Lancet* 1:337, 1967.

57. Prizel, K.R., Hutchins, G.M., and Bulkley, B.H. Coronary artery embolism and myocardial infarction. A clinicopathologic study of 55 patients. *Ann. Intern. Med.* 88:155, 1978.

58. Roberts, W.C. Coronary embolism: A review of causes, consequences, and diagnostic considerations. *Cardiovasc. Med.* 3:699, 1978.

59. Weinstein, L. and Rubin, R.H. Infective endocarditis—1973. *Prog. Cardiovasc. Dis.* 16:239, 1973.

60. Wenger, N.K., and Bauer, S. Coronary embolism. Review of the literature and presentation of 15 cases. *Am. J. Med.* 25:549, 1958.

61. Steiger, B.W., Libanoff, A.J., and Springer, E.B. Myocardial infarction due to paradoxical embolism. *Am. J. Med.* 47:995, 1969.

62. Meister, S.G., Grossman, W., Dexter, L. and Dalen, J.E. Paradoxical embolism. Diagnosis during life. *Am. J. Med.* 53:292, 1972.

63. Friedli, B., Aerichide, N., Grondin, P., and Campeau, L. Thromboembolic complications of heart valve prostheses. *Am. Heart. J.* 81:702, 1971.

64. Kloster, F.E. Diagnosis and management of complications of prosthetic heart valves. *Am. J. Cardiol.* 35:872, 1975.

65. Edmiston, W.A., Harrison, E.C., Duick, G.F., Parnassus, W., and Lau, F.Y.K. Thromboembolism in mitral porcine valve recipients. *Am. J. Cardiol.* 41:508, 1978.

66. Steiner, I., Hlava, A., and Prochazka, J. Calcific coronary embolization associated with cardiac valve replacement. Necropsy x-ray study. *Br. Heart J.* 38:816, 1976.

67. Pifarre, R., Grieco, J., Sullivan, H.J., Scanlon, P.J., Johnson, S.A., and Gunnar, R.M. Coronary embolism: Surgical management. *Ann. Thorac. Surg.* 30:564, 1980.

68. Shaver, P.J., Carrig, T.F., and Baker, W.P. Postpartum coronary artery dissection. *Br. Heart J.* 40:83, 1978.

69. Smith, J.C. Dissecting aneurysms of coronary arteries. *Arch. Pathol.* 99:117, 1975.

70. Rabinowitz, M., Virmani, R., and McAllister, H.A., Jr. Spontaneous coronary artery dissection and eosinophilic inflammation: A cause and effect relationship? *Am. J. Med.* 72:923, 1982.

71. Meller, J., Freidman, S., Dack, S., and Herman MV. Coronary artery dissection—a complication of cardiac catheterization without sequelae: Case report and review of the literature. *Cathet. Cardiovasc. Diagn.* 2:301, 1976.

72. Silverman, J.F., Gnekow, W., and Pfeifer, J.F. Iatrogenic dissection of the right coronary artery. *Radiology* 110:712, 1974.

73. Geraci, A.R., Krishnaswami, V., and Selman, M.W. Aorto-coronary dissection complicating coronary arteriography. *J. Thorac. Cardiovasc. Surg.* 65:695, 1973.

74. Bulkley, B.H., and Roberts, W.C. Isolated coronary arterial dissection. A complication of cardiac operations. *J. Thorac. Cardiovasc. Surg.* 67:148, 1974.

75. Heggtveit, H.A. Syphilitic aortitis. A clinicopathologic autopsy study of 100 cases, 1950 to 1960. *Circulation* 29:346, 1964.

76. Moritz, A.R. Syphilitic coronary arteritis. *Arch. Pathol.* 11:44, 1931.

77. Sakashita, I., Asano, K., Aoki, Y., Yamazaki, Y., and Terashima, M. A case report of syphilitic aortic insufficiency treated by simultaneous prosthetic valve replacement, aortoplasty, and re-

versed aorto-right coronary bypass procedure. *Jap. Heart. J.* 14:554, 1973.

78. Harris, T.R., Copeland, G.D., and Brody, D.A. Progressive injury current with metastatic tumor of the heart. Case report and review of the literature. *Am. Heart. J.* 69:392, 1965.

79. Hanbury, W.J. Secondary tumors of the heart. *Br. J. Cancer.* 14:23, 1960.

80. Roberts, W.C., Glancy, D.L., DeVita, V.T., Jr. Heart in malignant lymphoma (Hodgkin's disease, lymphosarcoma, reticulum cell sarcoma, and mycosis fungoides). A study of 196 autopsy cases. *Am. J. Cardiol.* 22:85, 1968.

81. Barth, R.F., Willerson, J.T., Buja, L.M., Decker, J.L., and Roberts, W.C. Amyloid coronary artery disease, primary systemic amyloidosis, and paraproteinemia. *Arch. Intern. Med.* 126:627, 1970.

82. Holsinger, D.R., Osmundson, P.J., and Edwards, J.E. The heart in periarteritis nodosa. *Circulation* 25:610, 1962.

83. Schmid, F.R., Cooper, N.S., Ziff, M., and McEwen, C. Arteritis in rheumatoid arthritis. *Am. J. Med.* 30:56, 1961.

84. Swezey, R.L. Myocardial infarction due to rheumatoid arteritis. An antemortem diagnosis. *JAMA* 199:855, 1967.

85. Bonfiglio, T.A., Botti, R.E., and Hagstrom, J.W.C. Coronary arteritis, occlusion, and myocardial infarction due to lupus erythematosus. *Am. Heart J.* 83:153, 1972.

86. Heibel, R.H., O'Toole, J.D., Curtiss, E.I., Medsger, T.A., Jr., Reddy, S.P., and Shaver, J.A. Coronary arteritis in systemic lupus erythematosus. *Chest* 69:700, 1976.

87. Bulkley, B.H., and Roberts, W.C. The heart in systemic lupus erythematosus and the changes induced in it by corticosteroid therapy. A study of 36 necropsy patients. *Am. J. Med.* 58:243, 1975.

88. Haider, Y.S., and Roberts, W.C. Coronary arterial disease in systemic lupus erythematosus. Quantification of degrees of narrowing in 22 necropsy patients (21 women) aged 16 to 37 years. *Am. J. Med.* 70:775, 1981.

89. Stewart, J.R. and Fajardo, L.F. Radiation-induced heart disease: An update. *Prog. Cardiovasc. Dis.* 27:173, 1984.

90. Amromin, G.D., Gildenhorn, H.L., Solomon, R.D., Nadkarni, B.B., and Jacobs, M.L. The synergism of x-irradiation and cholesterol-fat feeding on the development of coronary artery lesions. *J. Atheroscl. Res.* 4:325, 1964.

91. Brosius, F.C. III, Waller, B.F., and Roberts, W.C. Radiation heart disease. Analysis of 16 young (aged 15 to 33 years) necropsy patients who received over 3500 rads to the heart. *Am. J. Med.* 70:519, 1981.

92. Oren, A., Bar-Shlomo, B., and Stern, S. Acute

coronary occlusion following blunt injury to the chest in the absence of coronary atherosclerosis. *Am. Heart. J.* 92:501, 1976.

93. Stern, T., Wolf, R.Y., Reichart, B., Harrington, O.B., and Crosby, V.G. Coronary artery occlusion resulting from blunt trauma. *JAMA* 230:-1308, 1974.

94. Rea, W.J., Sugg, W.L., Wilson, L.C., Webb, W.R., and Ecker, R.R. Coronary artery lacerations. An analysis of 22 patients. *Ann. Thorac. Surg.* 7:518, 1969.

95. Lange, R.L., Reid, M.S., Tresch, D.D., Keelan, M.H., Bernhard, V.M., and Coolidge, G. Nonathromatous ischemic heart disease following withdrawal from chronic industrial nitroglycerin exposure. *Circulation* 46:666, 1972.

# INDEX